Shimizu's Dermatology

Shimizu's Dermatology

Hiroshi Shimizu MD, PhD

Department of Dermatology
Hokkaido University Graduate School of Medicine
Sapporo, Japan

SECOND EDITION

WILEY Blackwell

This edition first published 2017 © 2017 by John Wiley & Sons, Ltd.
Previous edition: Nakayama Shoten Co., Ltd.

Registered Office
John Wiley & Sons, Ltd, The Atrium, Southern Gate, Chichester, West Sussex, PO19 8SQ, UK

Editorial Offices
9600 Garsington Road, Oxford, OX4 2DQ, UK
The Atrium, Southern Gate, Chichester, West Sussex, PO19 8SQ, UK
111 River Street, Hoboken, NJ 07030-5774, USA

For details of our global editorial offices, for customer services and for information about how
to apply for permission to reuse the copyright material in this book please see our website at
www.wiley.com/wiley-blackwell

Library of Congress Cataloging-in-Publication Data

Names: Shimizu, Hiroshi, 1954– author.
Title: Shimizu's dermatology / Hiroshi Shimizu.
Other titles: Shimizu's textbook of dermatology | Dermatology
Description: 2nd edition. | Chichester, West Sussex ; Hoboken, NJ : John Wiley and Sons, Inc., 2016. |
    Includes index. | Preceded by Shimizu's textbook of dermatology / Hiroshi Shimizu.
    Hokkaido University. 2007.
Identifiers: LCCN 2016015879 | ISBN 9781119099055 (pbk.)
Subjects: | MESH: Skin Diseases
Classification: LCC RL74 | NLM WR 140 | DDC 616.5–dc23
LC record available at https://lccn.loc.gov/2016015879

A catalogue record for this book is available from the British Library.

Wiley also publishes its books in a variety of electronic formats. Some content that appears in print may not
be available in electronic books.

Cover image: shironosov/gettyimages

Set in 10/12pt Meridien by SPi Global, Pondicherry, India

1   2017

Contents

Contents

CHAPTER 1
Structure and function of the skin

The skin is the largest organ of the human body, covering a surface area of approximately 1.6 m² and accounting for about 16% of an adult's body weight. The skin is in direct contact with the outside environment and helps maintain four key functions:

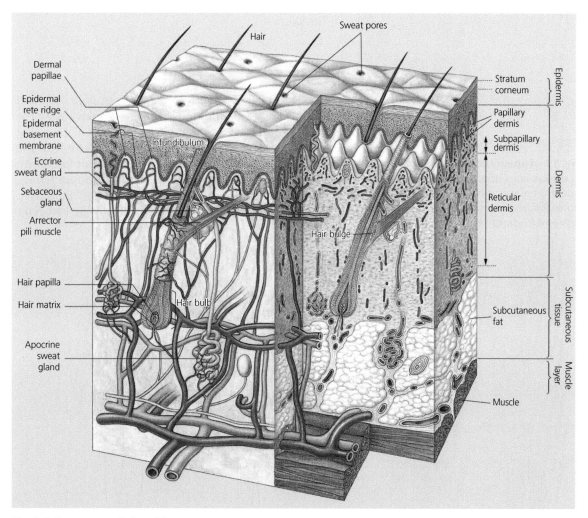

Fig. 1.1 Structure of the skin.

Shimizu's Dermatology, Second Edition. Hiroshi Shimizu.
© 2017 John Wiley & Sons, Ltd. Published 2017 by John Wiley & Sons, Ltd.

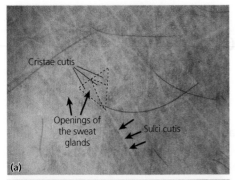

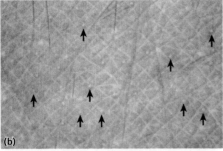

Fig. 1.2 Appearance of the skin surface.
a: Cristae cutis (triangle), sulci cutis and
openings of the sweat glands. b: Sweat
pores fed by sweat glands open to the
cristae cutis (arrows).

- retention of water and other molecules
- regulation of body temperature
- protection of the body from invading microorganisms and other harmful external factors
- sensory perception.

The horny cell layer plays a crucial role in maintaining the human body's water balance. To gain insight into cutaneous biology and skin diseases, an understanding of the structure and functions of normal human skin is essential. This chapter discusses the structure and function of normal skin and skin appendages, and the basics of immune mechanisms that mainly relate to the skin.

Overview of the skin

The skin is the largest human organ in both area and weight. It has the important function of separating the body from the external environment and maintaining homeostasis in the body. In order to achieve this, the skin has a complicated structure and various functions. Skin consists of a three-layer structure of epidermis, dermis, and subcutaneous tissue (Fig. 1.1). The cells in the epidermis are keratinocytes (~95%), melanocytes

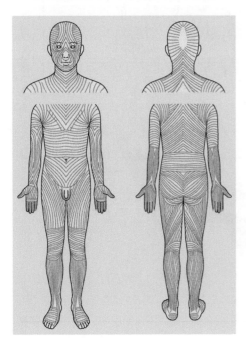

Fig. 1.3 Cleavage lines (Langer cleavage lines).

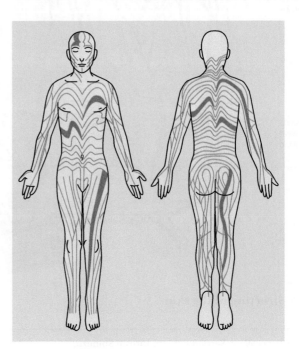

Fig. 1.4 Blaschko's lines.

(~5%), and Langerhans cells. The horny cell layer, formed by the keratinization of keratinocytes, is the outermost skin layer and is in direct contact with the external environment. It has the important functions of moisture retention and protection against the external environment, such as foreign substances and ultraviolet radiation. The major dermal components are collagen fibers, elastic fibers, blood vessels, and the components that maintain the skin, such as the extracellular matrix. The dermal appendages include the sweat glands, sebaceous glands, and hair follicles. At the boundary between the epidermis and dermis are finger-like projections, called dermal papillae, that project into the epidermis (see Fig. 1.1). The epidermis also projects into the dermis, producing the epidermal rete ridge. The main component of subcutaneous tissue is fat tissue, which stores neutral fat and provides protection from external impacts and heat/cold.

The skin surface is not smooth; it is laced with networks of fine shallow and deep grooves called sulci cutis. Sweat ducts open onto the skin surface in the center of the crista cutis, which is formed by the borders of the sulci cutis (Fig. 1.2).

The orientation of the sulci cutis is site dependent and is called the dermal ridge pattern. Fingerprints and patterns on the palms and soles, which are unique to each person, are formed by the sulci cutis. Langer's lines, also called cleavage lines, is a term used to define the direction within the human skin along which the skin has the least flexibility (Fig. 1.3). Elastic fibers are aligned in specific site-dependent orientations in the dermis. Several skin diseases, such as epidermal nevi, occur along specific lines called Blaschko's lines. These lines are distributed all over the body (Fig. 1.4) and are thought to be associated with the direction taken by the migrating differentiated cell clones during fetal skin development.

Epidermis

Structure and cells of the epidermis

The epidermis is approximately 0.2 mm thick. It consists mainly of keratinocytes (~95%), which proliferate and divide in the basal layer and move outward as they mature to form the cornified layer. This process takes 45 days in normal skin. In the epidermis, keratinocytes are therefore at different stages of maturation and are arranged in four main layers (Fig. 1.5 and

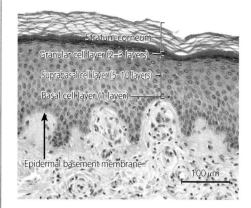

Stratum corneum
Granular cell layer (2–3 layers)
Suprabasal cell layer (5–10 layers)
Basal cell layer (1 layer)

Epidermal basement membrane

100 μm

Fig. 1.5 The four layers of the epidermis.

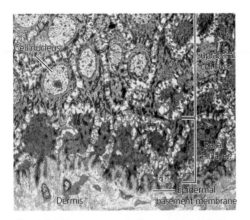

Fig. 1.6 Ultrastructural anatomy of the epidermis.

Fig. 1.6). Cytokeratins such as keratin intermediate filaments and tonofilaments are found abundantly in the cytoplasm of many epidermal keratinocytes and are distributed in bundles around the nuclei, from which they distally connect with hemidesmosomes and desmosomes to form a rigid and robust cellular cytoskeleton.

Basal cell layer

The basal cell layer, or stratum basale, consists of a single layer of cubical and/or columnar cells that replicate and migrate outward. It also comprises the epidermal stem cell subpopulation. Basal cells contain a basophilic (or darkly staining) cytoplasm and an elliptical nucleus rich in chromatin. These cells have desmosomes for cell-to-cell attachment, gap junctions for cell communication and hemidesmosomes for connection with the extracellular matrix and the underlying basal membrane (Fig. 1.7).

Prickle cell layer

The prickle cell layer, or stratum spinosum, consists of 5–10 layers that appear connected to each other by

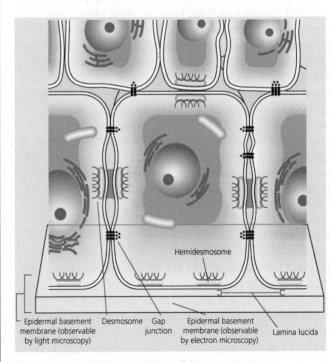

Fig. 1.7 Intercellular positions of desmosomes, gap junctions, and hemidesmosomes.

prickle-like structures that correspond to the location of desmosomes. Prickle cells in the lower layer are polygonal and those in the upper layers have a flattened morphology. They are larger than basal cells and contain small amounts of chromatin in their round nuclei.

Granular cell layer

The granular cell layer, or stratum granulosum, consists of two or three layers of cells containing basophilic keratohyalin granules. Granular cells and their nuclei are even flatter than those in the suprabasal layer. Spherical lamellar granules (also known as Odland bodies or keratosomes) have a diameter of approximately 300 nm and can be observed in the granular cell layer by electron microscopy. The main component of lamellar granules is stratum corneum lipid, which is released into the intercellular space of horny cells.

Horny cell layer

The horny cell layer, or stratum corneum, consists of about 10 sublayers. Enucleated keratinocytes become membranous and multilayered, resembling fallen leaves; they exfoliate sequentially from the outermost layer. The horny cell layer, which is very thick in the palms and soles, is underlain by the stratum lucidum (Fig. 1.8). Horny cells are flat, and their cytoplasm is filled with aggregated keratin fibers. The stratum corneum appears as an eosinophilic layer in hematoxylin and eosin staining. The horny cells gradually change into membranous structures in the upper layers. By electron microscopy, the clear contrast between electron-dense interfibrous substances and electron-sparse keratin fibers is called the keratin pattern.

The cell membrane is thickest in the horny cell layer and forms the cornified cell envelope or marginal band (Fig. 1.9 and Fig. 1.10). The protein component of the cornified cell envelope is extremely stable against physicochemical degradation.

Other cells

Keratinocytes account for 95% of all epidermal cells. The remaining 5% consists of melanocytes, Langerhans cells, and Merkel cells, which are respectively involved in melanin formation, antigen presentation, and sensation.

Adhesion of keratinocytes

The epidermal basement membrane plays a key role in dermal-epidermal adhesion.

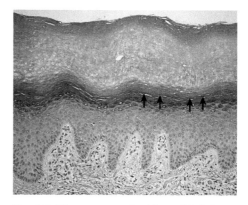

Fig. 1.8 The stratum lucida, which is found in the palms and soles (arrows).

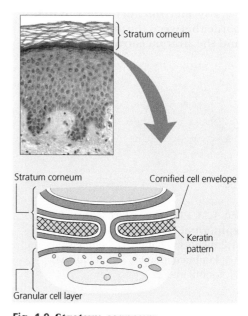

Fig. 1.9 Stratum corneum.

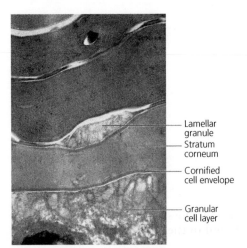

Fig. 1.10 Electron microscopy of the border between the granular cell layer and the stratum corneum.

Labels: Lamellar granule; Stratum corneum; Cornified cell envelope; Granular cell layer

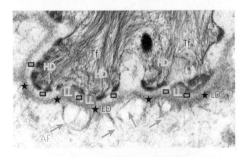

Fig. 1.11 Electron microscopy of the epidermal basement membrane.
AF, anchoring fibril; HD, hemidesmosome; LD, lamina densa; LL, lamina lucida; Tf, tonofilament.

Epidermal basement membrane

This underlies the epidermis and is revealed by periodic acid–Schiff (PAS) staining under light microscopy. The structure of the epidermal basement membrane includes the lamina densa (LD) and the lamina lucida (LL), which are observed by electron microscopy (Fig. 1.11 and Fig. 1.12).

The lamina densa is approximately 60–80 nm thick and consists mainly of fibronectins, heparan sulfate proteoglycan, type IV collagen, and laminin-332. By electron microscopy, it appears as an electron-dense lattice network. While desmosomes are important for cell-to-cell adhesion, hemidesmosomes mediate adhesion between the basal cells and the underlying lamina densa. Although a hemidesmosome resembles a bisected desmosome, its molecular composition is very different from that of a desmosome. Keratin fibers within the basal cells link hemidesmosomes, which maintain the structure of the cell (Fig. 1.13).

The lamina lucida is composed of a large glycoprotein called laminin-332, in addition to type XVII collagen (BP180; BPAG2). Type XVII collagen projects directly into the lamina lucida/lamina densa interface and connects hemidesmosomes with the lamina densa. Anchoring fibrils, which form semi-circular loop structures, link the dermis with the lamina densa by associating with type I and III collagens.

Adhesion between keratinocytes

Intercellular adhesion between keratinocytes is mediated by several cell-to-cell junctions, including desmosome junctions, adherens junctions, gap junctions, and tight junctions.

The desmosome consists of an inner and an outer plaque (attachment plaque) that are mainly composed

---

MEMO 1–1 Blister formation caused by inherited abnormalities or autoantibody deposition

Blisters can form as a result of an inherited abnormality or autoantibody deposition targeting various components of the cutaneous basement membrane which weakens the dermal-epidermal junction. For example, autoantibodies against type XVII collagen and BP230, which are components of hemidesmosomes, result in bullous pemphigoid. Inherited mutations in *KRT5*, *KRT14*, *COL17A1* encoding BP180, laminin-332, or *COL7A1* encoding type VII collagen cause epidermolysis bullosa (see Chapter 14). Blisters can also form as a result of weakened intercellular adhesion in the epidermis resulting from autoantibody deposition against desmogleins, which are structural components of desmosomes. Autoantibodies targeting desmoglein 1 cause pemphigus foliaceus whilst autoantibodies against desmoglein 3 result in pemphigus vulgaris.

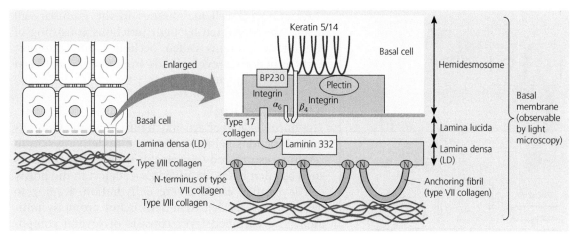

Fig. 1.12 Microstructure of the basement membrane zone.

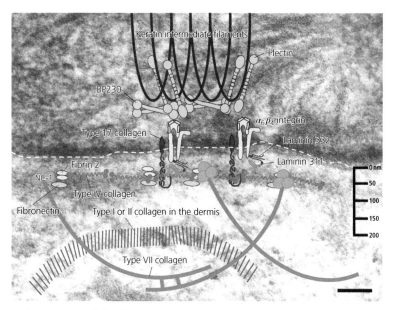

Fig. 1.13 Electron microscopy of the basement membrane zone.

of desmoplakin. Desmoplakin connects keratin fibers and strengthens the cytoskeleton. Transmembrane proteins such as desmogleins and desmocollins form homophilic connections to the same molecules by a calcium ion-dependent mechanism (Fig. 1.14).

The gap junction consists of several connexin subunits (forming a connexon) and has a structure in which cell membranes are linked with each other by a 2–3 nm gap. Gap junctions are involved not only in connecting cells but also in transporting small molecules and ions between cells (Fig. 1.15).

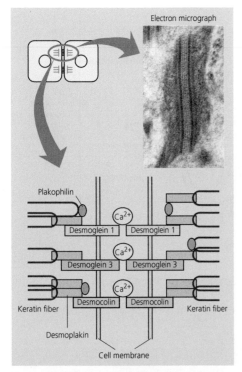

Fig. 1.14 Ultrastructural image and illustration of the desmosome.

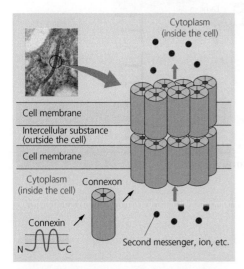

Fig. 1.15 Molecular components of the gap junction.

Keratinocyte cell membranes in the granular cell layers are connected by tight junctions consisting of membrane proteins called occludins and claudins. Tight junctions prevent fluids from leaking between cells (tight conjugation).

Keratinization

The horny cell layer acts like a film of plastic wrap, its main functions being to allow the underlying skin to retain moisture and to protect it from external factors such as microbes. Extensive loss or defect in the horny cell layer may cause severe dehydration, leading to death within 24 h if treatment is not promptly initiated. The cornified layer consists of several components, including keratins (produced by epidermal keratinocytes) and lipids. During keratinization, the epidermal keratinocytes divide in the basal layer, produce keratins, undergo differentiation, and migrate to the upper layers as they mature. Studies have demonstrated that epidermal keratinocytes secrete various cytokines.

Keratin

Keratin tonofilaments form a cytoskeletal network that is essential for maintaining the structure of the keratinocyte. Keratins are classified as type I (acidic) or type II (neutral to basic). Type I and type II keratins bind to each other in pairs to form intermediate filaments. Keratins can associate with each other to form keratin pairs, and this process is dependent on the state of differentiation of the keratinocytes. For example, K5/K14 pairs are found in basal cells whereas K1/K10 pairs are present in the suprabasal cell layers (Table 1.1, Fig. 1.16).

When keratinized, keratin fibers in the granular cell layer aggregate in association with filaggrin to form a characteristic condensed keratin pattern. Profilaggrins, abundantly present in keratohyalin granules, are cleaved into filaggrins by the action of the protease peptidylarginine deiminase during keratinization (Fig. 1.17). Released filaggrins aggregate keratin fibers in the horny cell cytoplasm, and the keratins are converted into amino acids in the upper layer of the stratum corneum. The cleaved filaggrins, which function in moisture retention and ultraviolet absorption, are called natural moisturizing factors (NMF).

Table 1.1 Expression regions of main keratin pairs, and congenital disorders from mutations of keratins.

Keratins	Main area of expression	Genetic disorder	Indirect reference
K1, K10	Suprabasal cell layer	Epidermolytic ichthyosis	Chapter 15
K2	Granular cell layer	Superficial epidermolytic ichthyosis	Chapter 15
K3, K12	Anterior epithelium of the comea	Juvenile epithelial corneal dystrophy (Meesman)	
K4, K13	Mucosa	White spong nevus (on tongue)	Chapter 22
K5, K14	Keratinocytes in the basal cell layer	Epidermolysis bullosa simplex	Chapter 14
K6, K16	Nails	Pachyonychia congenita	Chapter 19
K9	Keratinocytes in the suprabasal cell layer and granular cell layer on the palmoplantar region	Palmoplantar keratoderma (Vömer)	Chapter 15

Cornified cell envelope

The cornified cell envelope (marginal band) is an extremely large, strong and insoluble structure lining the horny cell membrane. By electron microscopy, it appears as an electron-dense structure at the periphery of the horny cells (Fig. 1.18). The main structural components of the cornified cell envelope are involucrins, produced in the lower keratinocyte prickle cells, and loricrins, produced by keratinocytes in the granular layer. The cornified cell envelope forms when these proteins are successively cross-linked by enzymes such as transglutaminases during keratinization. Transglutaminases are calcium-dependent enzymes that are activated by calcium influx into cells that undergo apoptosis during keratinization.

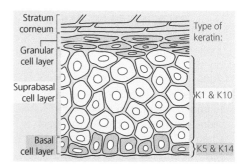

Fig. 1.16 Expression of keratin types in the epidermis.

MEMO 1–2 Ichthyosis caused by enzyme deficiency

- **Transglutaminase 1:** this is an enzyme that allows cell membrane components to link with protein molecules such as loricrin, involucrin, cystatin-α, and small proline-rich proteins. Without this activity, a normal cornified cell envelope does not form. For example, deficiency of transglutaminase 1 results in various ichthyoses, such as autosomal recessive lamellar ichthyosis and bathing suit ichthyosis (see Chapter 15).
- **ABCA12:** deficiency of the lipid transporter ABCA12 results in abnormal production of lamellar granules and incomplete formation of intercellular lipids, which is the underlying molecular basis of harlequin ichthyosis (see Chapter 15). The skin thickening seen in this condition is thought to result from a compensatory increase in the number of horny layer cells or an inhibition of the normal exfoliative process.
- **Steroid sulfatase:** deficiency of steroid sulfatase, which metabolizes sulfate cholesterol, inhibits normal exfoliation of horny cells and causes X-linked recessive ichthyosis (see Chapter 15).

MEMO 1–3 Activities of vitamin A

Vitamin A inhibits cholesterol sulfotransferases and decreases cholesterol sulfates, which is thought to stimulate exfoliation of the horny cell layers.

MEMO 1–4 Ceramide and its moisturizing function

The ceramide content of the horny cell layer is reduced in patients with atopic dermatitis. Ceramide is thought to be involved in disorders of dry skin and skin barrier function. In 2006 it was clarified that 20–50% of patients with atopic dermatitis had mutations in filaggrin genes, which reduces skin moisture retentivity (see Chapter 7).

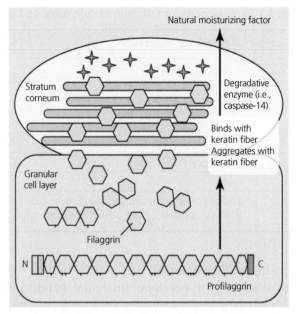

Fig. 1.17 Profilaggrin and filaggrin. Profilaggrin, which is in phosphorylated form, is stored in the keratohyalin granules of the granular cell layer. Profilaggrin is degraded into filaggrin through the process of dephosphorylation at the time of keratinization. Filaggrin aggregates and binds with keratin fibers in the stratum corneum to form the keratin pattern. Filaggrin ultimately degrades to low molecular weight substances such as urocanic acid and becomes a natural moisturizing factor that is involved in moisture retention and ultraviolet absorption.

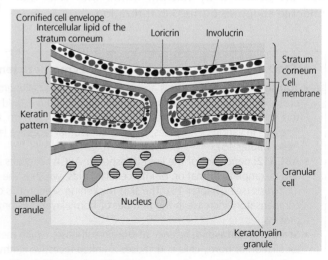

Fig. 1.18 The border between the epidermis and stratum corneum.

Horny layer (stratum corneum intracellular lipids)

The main function of intercellular lipids in the stratum corneum is to prevent excessive transepidermal water loss. These lipids consist mainly of ceramides (~50%), followed by cholesterols (~30%), free fatty acids, and cholesterol sulfates. Lamellar granules are found abundantly in the cytoplasm of the granular cell layers. These granules are released when the granular cells undergo apoptosis. The enzyme ABCA12 plays a significant role in the release of lipids from lamellar granules in granular cells. Ceramides are released by lamellar granules; free fatty acids are secreted from granular cell membranes. Cholesterol sulfates connect and stabilize the lipid structures between horny cells.

Exfoliation of horny cells

A key factor in the exfoliation of the stratum corneum is the degradation of horny cell intercellular lipids by lipases, a group of catabolic lipid enzymes and steroid sulfatases. Adhesion between keratinocytes is subsequently disrupted by proteases in the upper skin surface, resulting in the gradual exfoliation of the horny cell layer.

Melanocytes and melanin synthesis
Form and distribution of melanocytes

Melanocytes (pigment cells) are neural crest (ectoderm)-derived dendritic cells found in the basal cell layer and hair matrix (Fig. 1.19). Melanocytes (and Langerhans cells) are referred to as clear cells, since their cytoplasm contracts during dehydration and fixation in hematoxylin and eosin staining. Melanocytes display a characteristic brownish-black color in dopa oxidase staining. Approximately 1000–1500 melanocytes are seen per square millimeter of skin. An increase in melanocyte density is found in sun-exposed sites of the body, such as the face, and in physiologically pigmented sites, such as the external genitals.

The Golgi apparatus in the melanocyte is well developed and contains melanosomes in various stages of development (stages I, II, III, and IV). Melanin is produced in melanosomes from the amino acid tyrosine. Mature melanosomes are packaged and transported to the neighboring basal cells and suprabasal cells. Melanosomes transported to

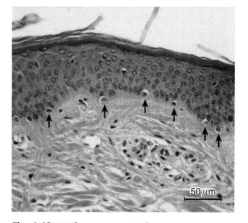

Fig. 1.19 Melanocytes. Melanocytes are seen as clear cells (arrows) under hematoxylin and eosin staining, because the cytoplasm of melanocytes shrinks during fixation.

MEMO 1–5 Causes of enhanced pigmentation

Adenocorticotropic hormones (ACTH), melanocyte-stimulating hormones (MSH), thyroid hormones, estrogens, ultraviolet rays, and X-rays are known to increase pigmentation of the skin.

MEMO 1–6 Association of tyrosinase with albinism

A child that has a congenital lack of tyrosinase is born with pale skin due to the lack of melanins (oculocutaneous albinism). In patients with Menkes' disease, there is extreme copper deficiency, which causes tyrosinase activity to decrease, resulting in reduced pigmentation

MEMO 1–7 Increase of 5-S-cysteinyl dopa (5-S-CD) in serum

In malignant melanomas, there is generally an increase in pheomelanin production, resulting in an increase of 5-S-CD in blood and urine. Therefore, an increase of 5-S-CD in the blood indicates metastasis of a malignant melanoma and its degree of spreading.

the basal epidermal keratinocytes aggregate in the upper part of the cytoplasm of the basal cells, forming a melanin cap to protect their DNA from UV radiation.

Racial differences in skin color are determined by the number and size of melanosomes. There is no difference in the distribution or density of melanocytes between races.

Biosynthesis of melanin

Melanin is a generic term for a group of substances called pigmented molecular phenolic polymers, which are indole compounds synthesized from tyrosines through polymer formation (Fig. 1.20).

Melanins in humans are broadly classified as eumelanin (black or intrinsic melanin) and pheomelanin (yellow melanin). Melanins in human skin and hair are complexes of these two types, and their ratio determines skin and hair color.

Tyrosines are supplied by blood, are subsequently oxidized by tyrosinase, which contains copper, and are finally metabolized into dopas and then into dopaquinones. Tyrosinase is the rate-limiting enzyme that catalyzes these two reactions during melanin synthesis (see Fig. 1.20).

Dopaquinones are automatically oxidized to become indole compounds that bind together to synthesize eumelanins. The presence of cysteine at this stage enables the conversion of dopaquinones, through their binding to cysteine, into 5-S-cysteinyldopa, which polymerizes to produce pheomelanins.

Melanosomes

These subcellular organelles are enclosed by a lipid double membrane in which melanins are exclusively produced. Melanin synthesis occurs when tyrosinases, which are synthesized by the Golgi apparatus, are carried to premelanosomes in the agranular endoplasmic reticulum. As melanin production increases, melanosomes enlarge. The formation of melanosomes is divided into stages I–IV by the degree of melanin deposition (Fig. 1.21). For example, a melanosome in stage IV is football shaped and measures approximately 500–700 nm along its major axis. It is transported from the dendrites to the neighboring epidermal keratinocytes.

Functions of melanin

The most important role of melanin is to confer protection to the skin from UV irradiation and thus to reduce the occurrence of malignant tumors and sunlight injury. The darker the skin, the lower the incidence of skin cancer caused by UV light.

Exposure to sunlight darkens the skin, and this process can occur rapidly due to oxidation of melanins or can happen several days after exposure, when there is an increase in melanin synthesis and mature melanosome formation.

Melanins can also absorb harmful active enzymes, metals, and drugs.

Langerhans cells

Langerhans cells are bone marrow-derived dendritic cells specific to stratified squamous epithelia such as the skin. Discrete Langerhans cells are frequently seen in the middle and upper suprabasal cell layers (Fig. 1.22). The cells are distributed at a density of 400–1000/mm². They lack tonofilaments and cell attachment structures, such as desmosomes, and they migrate. By electron microscopy, a few fibrillary components and Birbeck granules, whose cross-section is a characteristic tennis racket shape, are observed in the cytoplasm (see Fig. 1.55). Birbeck granules may be either Golgi apparatus derived or membrane derived, and are thought to be involved in receptor-mediated endocytosis.

Langerhans cells present antigens to T cells and can be easily distinguished from other cell types since they are ATPase, CD1a and S-100 protein positive.

Merkel cells

Merkel cells are found in the epidermal basal cell layer and are involved in touch sensation. They are seen at particularly high density in the finger pulps, oral mucosa, and hairy areas (the hair roots). They have angular plasma membrane projections and connect to adjacent keratinocytes by desmosomes (Fig. 1.23). Sensory (free) nerve endings are connected by synapses beneath the Merkel cells. Multiple dense-core granules (Merkel cell granules) are found in the cytoplasm. Following physical stimulation, they secrete neurotransmitters that convey tactile information to the underlying sensory nerve.

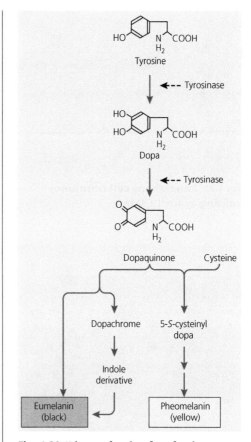

Fig. 1.20 Biosynthesis of melanin.

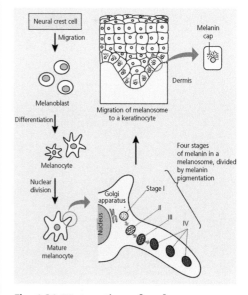

Fig. 1.21 Maturation of melanosomes.

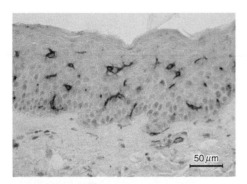

50 μm

Fig. 1.22 Langerhans cell (immuno-staining against CD1a).

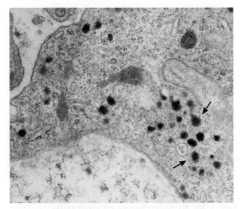

Fig. 1.23 Birbeck granules of Langerhans cell (arrows).

Dermis

Structure of the dermis

The dermis is the structure beneath the epidermis, and the two are separated by the basement membrane (see Fig. 1.1). The dermis is approximately 15–40 times thicker than the epidermis and consists of three layers.

- **Papillary layer:** this is the dermal area that projects between the epidermal ridges. It consists of thin fiber components and sensory nerve endings and is richly supplied with capillary blood vessels.
- **Subpapillary layer:** this area is subjacent to the epidermis and has the same components as the papillary layer.
- **Reticular layer:** this layer accounts for the largest part of the dermis. It has dense connective tissue consisting of fiber components. The lowermost part is in contact with the subcutaneous fat. There are also blood vessels and nerves in parts of the reticular dermis.

The dermis is composed of fibrous tissue and dermal matrix formed by cells in the interstitium (Fig. 1.24). The major dermal components are collagen fibers (mainly collagen types I and III), with smaller amounts of elastic fibers, reticular fibers, and matrix. Fibroblasts, macrophages, mast cells, plasma cells, endothelial cells, and nerve cells make up the cellular composition of the dermis.

Interstitial components
Collagen fibers

Collagen fibers account for 70% of the weight of dry dermis (Fig. 1.25) and appear white to the naked eye. The collagen fibrous component is poorly extensible; however, it is extremely tough and especially resistant to tension applied parallel to the fibers. This characteristic is important in maintaining the dynamic strength of the skin.

Collagen fibers form from aggregations of thin fibrils. The strength and thickness of the collagen fiber correlate with the number of fibrils. Thin collagen fibers are sparsely seen in the papillary and subpapillary layers; however, collagen bundles with thick, fully developed collagen fibers are densely distributed in the reticular upper dermal layers.

By light microscopy, the proteinaceous collagen fibers appear pink with hematoxylin and eosin staining, red with Elastica van Gieson staining, and blue with Azan

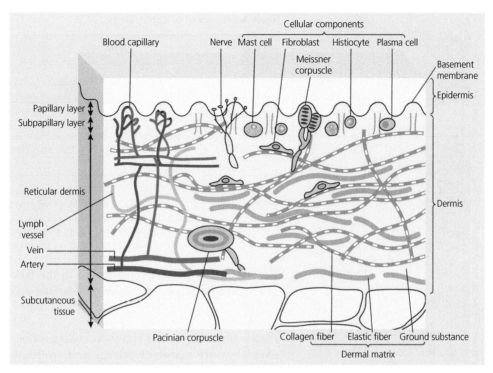

Fig. 1.24 Structure of the dermis.

or Masson trichrome staining. By electron microscopy, collagen fibrils appear as long fibers with a diameter ranging between 100 and 500 nm and display cross-striations that repeat at intervals of 60–70 nm (see Fig. 1.25). Fibrils become collagen fibers by aggregating with glycoproteins. A thick collagen bundle can reach a diameter of 2–15 µm.

Collagens are produced in the rough endoplasmic reticulum of fibroblasts. Helical procollagens with three α-chains are first secreted, and their molecular ends are cut by procollagen peptidase to become tropocollagens. The molecules then cross-link to each other with regular gaps that form the striped collagen fiber (Fig. 1.26).

Twenty subtypes of collagen molecules with α-chains of different molecular structures have been discovered (Table 1.2); however, type I collagen accounts for 80% of the collagen fibers that make up the dermis. Reticular fibers, which are distributed in the perivascular regions, are thin argyrophilic fibers that do not form thick fiber bundles. They are composed of type III collagen and account for about 15% of all fibers. The remaining 5% of collagen fibers are thought to be type V collagen. Types

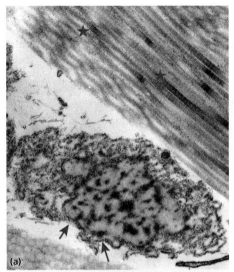

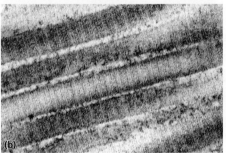

Fig. 1.25 Electron microscopy of the dermal matrix. a: Collagen fibers (stars) and elastic fibers (arrows). b: High-power magnification of collagen fibers. Stripes approximately 60–70 nm in width are seen.

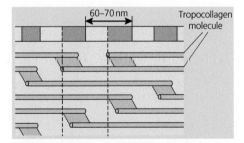

Fig. 1.26 Stripes of collagen fibers. Fine fibrils (tropocollagens) have cross-links, giving the fibers the appearance of stripes with intervals of 60–70 nm.

Table 1.2 Types of collagen fibers.

Fiber	Type
Fibrillar	I (dermis), II, III, V, XI
Basement membrane	IV
Anchoring fibril	VII (basement membrane)
Network-forming	VIII, X
FACIT*	IX, XII, XIV, XVI, XIX, XX
Microfibril	VI
Multiplexin	XV, XVIII
Other	XIII, XVII (basement membrane)

* Fibril associated collagen with interrupted triple helix.

IV, VII, and XVII are mainly found in the basal membranes in association with epidermal keratinocytes.

Elastic fibers

Elastic fibers are not as tough as collagen fibers; however, they are extremely elastic and are found abundantly in the dermis of the scalp and face, as well as in extensible structures such as arteries and tendons.

Elastic fibers found in the reticular dermis tend to be thicker than those in the papillary dermis. In the reticular layers, elastic fibers are scattered among collagen bundles and are orientated parallel to the skin surface. In the papillary layer, elastic fibers tend to be thinner and are orientated perpendicular to the skin surface. Nearer the skin surface, the elastic fibers form arches from which thin fibers project perpendicularly to reach the lamina densa. Elastic fibers are also connected to the lamina densa of sweat ducts, smooth muscle, nerves, and blood vessels.

Elastic fibers vary between 1 and 3 μm in diameter. They cannot be differentiated from collagen fibers by hematoxylin and eosin staining. Elastic fibers stain black in Elastica van Gieson or Weigert staining, and reddish-violet in aldehyde fuchsin staining. By electron microscopy, the striped pattern that characterizes collagen fibers is not observed (see Fig. 1.25).

Ground substance (extracellular matrix)

Ground substance (extracellular matrix) is a gelatinous amorphous compound of sugar and proteins that is found between fibers and cells in the dermis. The components of ground substance are principally pro-teoglycans and glycoproteins whose molecular weights range from 150,000 to 250,000 kDa and whose sugar content is between 2% and 15%.

These molecules stabilize the dermal fibers to give flexibility to the skin. Fibronectin is a glycoprotein that contains a domain connecting fibrin, heparin, and col-lagen. It also binds integrin receptors on the cell sur-face and is involved in cell proliferation, differentiation, and wound healing. In addition to proteoglycans and glycoproteins, lymph-derived tissue fluid and blood make up the remainder of ground substance and are involved in the transport of substances essential to cellular activities and metabolism.

Proteoglycans are large molecules made up of multiple glycosaminoglycans (mucopolysaccharides) connected with backbone proteins. Glycosaminoglycans are mostly produced by fibroblasts in the dermis and are rich in hyaluronic acids, which are associated with moisture retention.

Cellular components
Fibroblast
Fibroblasts originate from mesenchymal cells and pro-duce collagen and elastic fibers as well as glycosamino-glycans. They appear as thin spindle-shaped cells interspersed amongst collagen fibers (Fig. 1.27). By electron microscopy, multiple Golgi apparatuses and granular endoplasmic reticuli are seen in fibroblast. When collagen fibers are produced and the dermis matures, fibroblasts stop their activities and become fibrocytes. At this stage, their cell nuclei shrink and fewer endoplasmic reticuli are seen. Adrenal cortex hormones and thyroid hormones are involved in this process.

Histiocytes
Histiocytes are macrophages that are involved in antigen presentation to T cells. They are broadly distrib-uted in the connective tissue and intermingle with fibroblasts on the outside of endocapillary cells (Fig. 1.28). By light microscopy, histiocytes are seen to have a large spindled or star shape with a small, round nucleus. By electron microscopy, concave nuclei and pseudopodial protrusions are observed. Histiocytes con-tain Golgi apparatuses, smooth and rough endoplasmic reticuli, and lysosomes. The lysosomes contain hydro-lases and active acid phosphatases. Histiocytes release

MEMO 1–8 Abnormal-ities of elastic fibers or collagen fibers

If elastic fibers are decreased, lost or denatured, dermatolysis or senile cutis rhomboidalis nuchae may occur. Congenital abnormalities of the fibrillin protein result in Marfan syndrome (see Chapter 18). Abnormalities in dermal collagens may cause Ehlers–Danlos syndrome.

MEMO 1–9 Histiocytes, monocytes, macro-phages

Macrophages are large phagocytic cells of which there are two types.
- **Free macrophages:** e.g., monocytes in blood, and migrating macrophages in granulomas.
- **Fixed macrophages:** e.g., histiocytes in the dermis and subcutaneous tissue, and Kupffer cells.

MEMO 1–10 Histiocytes, the key to pathological diagnosis

Epithelioid cells, Touton giant cells, xanthoma cells, and foreign body giant cells in an epithelioid cell granuloma are histiocytes that are pathologically present in an atypical form (see Chapter 2).

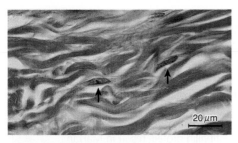

Fig. 1.27 Fibroblasts (arrows).

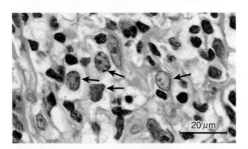

Fig. 1.28 Histiocytes (arrows).

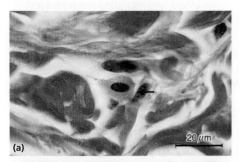

(a)

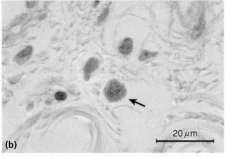

(b)

Fig. 1.29 Mast cells. a: Hematoxylin and eosin staining. b: Metachromasia is seen by toluidine blue staining.

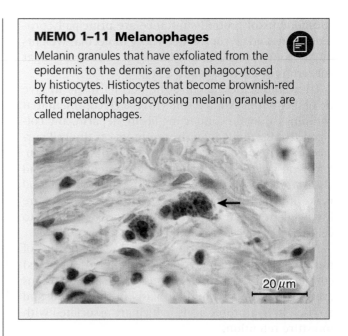

MEMO 1–11 Melanophages

Melanin granules that have exfoliated from the epidermis to the dermis are often phagocytosed by histiocytes. Histiocytes that become brownish-red after repeatedly phagocytosing melanin granules are called melanophages.

collagenase and lysosomal enzymes, such as elastase, to digest the interstitium. They are also involved in organ repair, and they degrade and phagocytose foreign bodies and present them as antigens to T cells.

Mast cells

Mast cells are found in the dermis around capillaries and in the periphery of subcutaneous tissue. The shape is round to spindled, and the diameter is 10 μm (Fig. 1.29). Mast cells produce various vasodilatory and hyperlucent chemical mediators. Mast cell granules stain reddish-violet in toluidine blue and methylene blue, and exhibit metachromasia. Cutaneous mast cells resemble basophils in form and function; however, their characteristics differ slightly from those of other organs, because they differentiate in skin during intrauterine life.

Mast cells contain intracytoplasmic granules that appear by electron microscopy as round structures, each with a diameter of 0.3–0.5 μm, evenly distributed in the cytoplasm. Chemotransmitters in the granules are released outside the cell under various stimuli, such as in type I allergic reactions (Fig. 1.30). The main components of the released substances are histamines and heparins, followed by enzymes, including neutrophil chemotactic factors (NCF), eosinophil chemotactic factors of anaphylaxis (ECF-A), tryptase, chymase, and tumor necrosis factor (TNF)-like substances. The mast cell may also produce and release inflammatory substances such as prostaglandins, leukotrienes, and platelet-activating factors.

Plasma cells

Plasma cells are differentiated B cells that have been stimulated by an antigen. They produce antibodies and are involved in humoral immunity. The shape varies from round to pear-shaped, and the diameter ranges from 8 to 14 μm, which is twice that of a leukocyte. They have a wheel-shaped nucleolus and many Golgi apparatuses (Fig. 1.31).

Dermal dendrocytes

Dermal dendrocytes are found in the dermal upper layer (in and between the papillary layer and the reticular layer). Thought to be immunocompetent cells, they are characterized by the presence of clotting factor XIIIa.

Vascular channels and nerves
Blood vessels

Arterial branches distributed in the skin (Fig. 1.32 and Fig. 1.33) are connected with each other in the deep dermal layer to form a horizontal network (subcutaneous plexus). From the subcutaneous plexuses, branches ascend to form a second vascular network in the lower papillary layer (subpapillary plexus). These

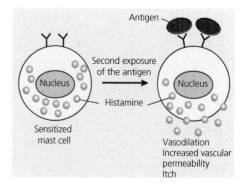

Fig. 1.30 Mast cell sensitization.

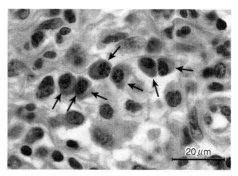

Fig. 1.31 Plasma cells (arrows).

MEMO 1–12 Discriminating between blood vessels and lymph vessels

The important points in discriminating between these are tabulated below.

Item	Blood vessel	Lymph vessel
Podplanin	Negative	Positive
Factor VIII	Positive	Basically negative
Basal layer	Extended and multi-layered	Intermittent
Intercellular connection	Developed	Weak
Lumen shape	Round	Irregular
Elastic fiber stain	Arteries: Positive in the internal elastic layer	Negative
	Veins: Negative	

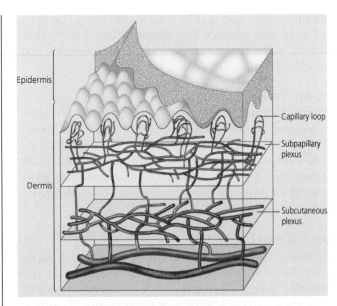

Fig. 1.32 Distribution of blood vessels in the dermis.

arteries in the dermis are arterioles. The subpapillary plexus gives rise to arterioles that ascend through the papillary layer, forming capillary loops in the upper papillary layer before anastomosing with venules that connect to each other to form two types of venous plexuses, whereby the blood flows into the cutaneous veins (see Fig. 1.32).

There are also distinctive vascular plexuses in the vicinity of the cutaneous appendages. For example, the peripheral regions of the eccrine glands are particularly rich in vascular networks, which control blood flow volume and body temperature. Moreover, hair follicles in the anagen (growth) stage are richly supplied with blood vessels in the surrounding dermal tissue.

Blood can also circulate directly from arteries to veins by means of arteriovenous anastomoses, which are supplied by sympathetic nerves. These anastomoses control peripheral blood flow and are involved in the regulation of body temperature. Glomus apparatuses, which have spherical anastomotic branches, are widely seen in the skin. They are particularly well developed in the fingers, at the apical ends of the toes and below the nails.

By electron microscopy, endothelial cells, pericytes, and the multilayered basement membrane in the peripheral interstitium may be observed in the

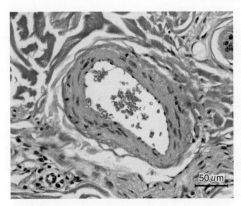

Fig. 1.33 Cross-section of a blood vessel (hematoxylin and eosin).

capillaries. In the endothelial cells, stick-shaped Weibel–Palade granules (diameter ~200 nm; length ~1 μm) containing factor VIII associated with histamines and blood coagulation may be seen. Pericytes have a vasoconstrictive effect and are observed along the walls of endothelial cells.

Lymphatic vessels

Lymphatic vessels are distributed around the subpapillary layer and are categorized as postcapillary, dermal or subcutaneous. The endothelial cells of the lymph capillaries are thin and are not associated with pericytes or the basal membrane. They are partly ruptured and are surrounded by loose collagen and elastic fibers (Fig. 1.34). The structure of lymph vessels is not as regular as that of blood vessels. Aggregated cutaneous lymphatic fluid passes through the regional lymph nodes and flows into the blood vessels. Podplanin is known to be a lymphatic endothelial cell marker.

Nervous system

The nerve fiber bundle is covered with a membrane in the lower dermal layers. The nerve fibers change from myelinated to non-myelinated in the upper dermal layers, where the nerve bundles branch into numerous fibers that then innervate the superficial dermis and peripheral appendages (Fig. 1.35). sensory nerves transmit tactile, pressure, pain, and temperature sensation. Autonomic nerves innervate blood vessels, sweat glands, and other appendages.

Sensory nerves

Sensory nerve structures include free nerve endings, which sense pain, Merkel cells (described earlier), which perceive tactile sensation in the epidermal basal layers, and nerve end bulbs, which transmit tactile, pressure, and vibration sensation.

Free nerve endings

Free nerve endings are distributed in the upper dermal and papillary layers. Some adhere to Merkel cells in the dermal papillary layer, whereas others infiltrate the dermis directly. Non-myelinated nerves transmit pain sensation.

End corpuscles

The end corpuscle is a specific sensory nerve terminal that consists of different types as described below.

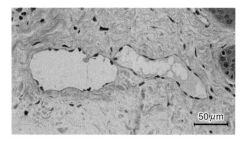

Fig. 1.34 Cross-section of lymphatic vessels (hematoxylin and eosin).

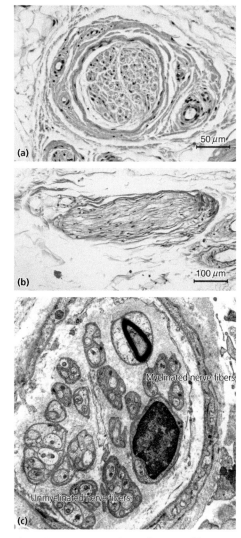

Fig. 1.35 Cross-section of nerve fibers. a: Myelinated nerve fibers. b: Unmyelinated nerve fibers. c: Electron microscopy.

MEMO 1–13 Sympathetic nerves distributed in the eccrine sweat glands

The sympathetic nerves are generally adrenergic; however, sympathetic innervation in the eccrine glands is cholinergic.

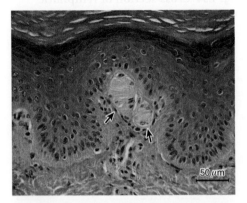

Fig. 1.36 Meissner corpuscles (arrows).

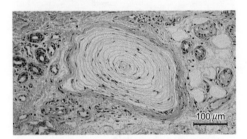

Fig. 1.37 Pacinian corpuscle (hematoxylin and eosin staining).

Meissner end corpuscles are present in the dermal papillae of the palms, soles, lips of the mouth, and external genitals. They perceive tactile and pressure sensations (Fig. 1.36). Pacinian corpuscles are seen in the deep dermal layer and subcutaneous tissue of the palms, soles, and external genitalia. They have an oval structure, measure approximately 1 mm along the major axis and can be clearly observed by light microscopy (Fig. 1.37). The central nerve fiber has a multilayered concentric structure. They are involved in vibratory perception.

Autonomic nerves

Autonomic nerves are principally distributed in the sweat glands, arrector pili muscles, blood vessels, and glomus apparatus. They control the functions of these structures. Cholinergic non-myelinated sympathetic nerves are distributed in the eccrine sweat glands. The adrenergic sympathetic nerves are distributed in the arrector pili muscles and blood vessels.

Subcutaneous fat tissue

The subcutaneous tissue is the layer between the dermis and the fascia. It cushions the skin against external physical pressure, retains moisture, and generates heat.

The subcutaneous tissue is largely composed of fat cells. Assembled fat cells are separated by a connective fibrous septum to form fat lobules. Fiber bundles called retinaculae cutis produced in the dermis firmly connect the dermis to the underlying fascia and periostea. These bundles run through the subcutaneous tissue. The main component of the fat droplet is triglyceride, composed of olein acid and palmitin acid. Since a large droplet accounts for most of the contents of the cellular cytoplasm in the fat cell, other cellular organelles are pushed to the edge. Multiple smooth muscles called tunicae dartoses are characteristically seen in the dermal deep layers and subcutaneous tissues of the scrotum, penis, labia majora, and nipples (Fig. 1.38). The boundary between the subcutaneous tissue and skeletal muscle is called the musculus cutaneous. It is not apparent at sites where muscles of expression (e.g., the face) are found.

The thickness of the subcutaneous tissue depends on several factors, including the body site and age.

The subcutis is particularly thick in the cheeks, breasts, buttocks, thighs, palms, and soles; it is thin in the eyelids, dorsal aspect of the nose, lips of the mouth, and labia minora, and absent in the foreskin. Subcutaneous tissue tends to develop and enlarge in newborns and at puberty. In embryos and newborn infants, heat is produced at a rapid rate by brown fat tissue in the dorsal region.

Appendages

Hair apparatus

The hair apparatus protects the scalp from external forces such as sunlight and controls the amount of heat produced in the head. Eyelashes protect the eyes from dust, and armpit and pubic hair absorb mechanical friction. The number of hairs on the scalp averages 100,000. The hair apparatus, which consists of hair and hair follicles, is distributed throughout the skin, except on the lips of the mouth.

Hair follicle

The structure that encloses the hair shaft is the hair follicle. It is aligned oblique to the skin surface. Part of the hair follicle is slightly enlarged to form a hair bulge to which the base of the arrector pili muscle is connected (Fig. 1.39 and Fig. 1.40). Dermal stem cells reside in the hair bulge. Sebaceous glands are seen above the bulge area and apocrine glands open farther above. The base of the hair root during the anagen (growth) stage bulges out and is called the hair bulb. It contains a group of cells that form the hair papilla. The hair follicle has a funnel-shaped appearance (hair infundibulum). The hair follicle is surrounded by two layers: an epithelial inner layer and a connective tissue outer layer. The epithelial inner layer consists of an inner and an outer root sheath. The connective tissue component is called the connective tissue sheath.

Connective tissue sheath

The connective tissue sheath (CTS) covers the external aspect of the hair follicle and is in contact with the dermis. Collagen fibers are arranged concentrically within the CTS but are oriented longitudinally outside the CTS. Elastic fibers can be found among these collagen fibers.

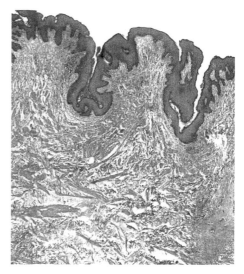

Fig. 1.38 Tunica dartos.

MEMO 1–14 Unusual keratinization of the outer root sheath

When cells in the outer root sheath denucleate and keratinize without passing through the granular layer or becoming flat, it is called trichilemmal keratinization.

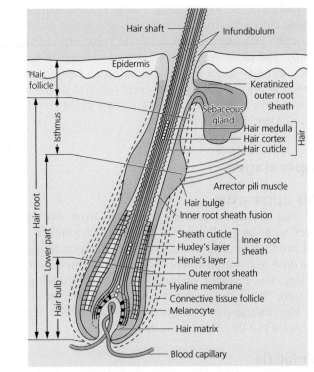

Fig. 1.39 Longitudinal section of the hair follicle.

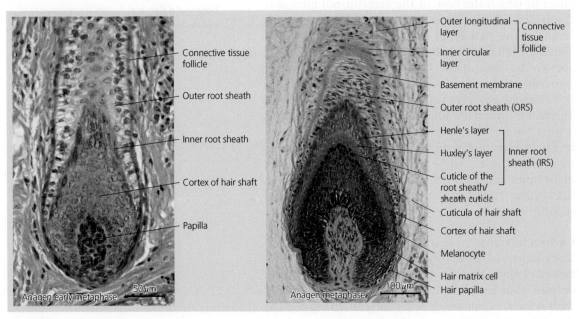

Fig. 1.40-1 Longitudinal cross-section of the structure of the hair follicle (hematoxylin and eosin staining).

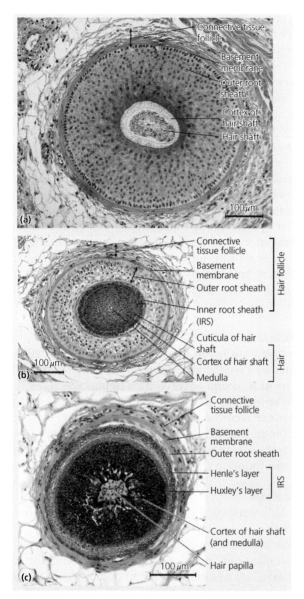

Fig. 1.40-2 Cross-section of the structure of the hair follicle (hematoxylin and eosin staining). a: Hair follicular isthmus. b: Lower part of a hair follicle. c: Hair bulb. (See Fig. 1.39 for the longitudinal positions.)

Outer root sheath

The outer root sheath (ORS) is the outermost part of the hair infundibulum (the innermost two layers). A keratinized structure, it contains keratinocytes that have light cytoplasm without keratohyalin granules. The outer aspect of the ORS is separated from the CTS by a basement membrane. The inner aspect of the ORS is connected by desmosomes with the Henle's layer, which is the outermost layer of the inner root sheath.

Inner root sheath

The inner root sheath (IRS), found within the ORS, consists of capsular layers, Huxley's layer (consisting of a double layer of cells), and Henle's layer (containing a single layer of cells). The capsular cuticles anchor and entangle with each other, and their apical tips function as hooks to stabilize the hair. Henle's layer is connected with the ORS by desmosomes.

Keratinization occurs in the IRS close to the interfollicular epidermis. By hematoxylin and eosin staining, eosinophilic trichohyalin granules are seen in the IRS, especially within the Henle's and Huxley's layers. The process of keratinization terminates at the level of the opening of the sebaceous gland and is followed by exfoliation.

Hair bulb

The hair bulb is the bulge of the hair follicle, with a dermal hair papilla at its center. The dermal hair papilla is surrounded and covered by a hemi-spherical structure known as the hair matrix layer, where hair and inner root sheath cells grow and extend upward. The outer root sheath forms the outermost layer of the hair bulb. Melanocytes that provide hairs with melanin are also found in the hair matrix.

Hair shaft

The hair shaft consists of a three-layered structure of medulla (inner layer), cortex (middle layer), and cuticle (outer layer, also called the cuticula).

Tonofilaments are aligned in the direction of the cortical axis, and a pattern similar to that observed for keratin by electron microscopy is seen at the tips of the tonofilaments. Keratinization occurs in the cortex; however, unlike in the epidermis and inner root sheath, keratohyalin and trichohyalin granules are not seen. In addition, the keratins produced in the hair cortex are rich in cysteines, glycines, and tyrosines. The hair keratins are generally known as hard keratins, and they also can be seen at other sites, such as the nails.

Within the hair shaft cuticle, the cortex is covered in a scale-like pattern of flattened cells that are attached to the capsular cuticles of the inner root sheath. This connection becomes the outermost layer of the hair shaft, protecting that shaft. Excessive physical damage to hair, for example from overbrushing and excessive use of hair dyes and other chemicals, may damage the hair cuticles, resulting in loss of the natural glow of the hair.

Hair color differs according to the size and number of melanosomes. Dark hair contains large and/or numerous melanosomes; red hair contains large amounts of pheomelanins.

Hair cycle

The hair cycle can be subdivided into the anagen (growth), catagen (transition), and telogen (rest) phases (Fig. 1.41). About 85% of scalp hairs are in the anagen phase, which generally lasts for several years after the emergence of the hair. This is followed by a slowing of the growth rate during the catagen phase, which lasts between 2 and 3 weeks. About 1–2% of scalp hairs are in the catagen phase and grow 0.3–0.5 mm in length per day. The hair then stops growing and remains in the telogen phase for several months. Approximately 15% of scalp hairs are in this phase. As new hairs are produced, hair within the same follicle in the telogen phase falls out. About 100 hairs are lost per day. As hair follicles transition from the anagen to the catagen phase, they begin to contract and cell division stops. The cells in the hair follicle also lose their ability to divide in the telogen phase, and they ascend to the elevated part of the hair. The hair root then has a stick-like appearance and is called a club hair. In the telogen phase, macrophages phagocytose melanin pigments and cell fragments in the hair papilla. During the anagen phase, cell division begins at the surface of the hair follicle.

The part of the hair below the hair bulge contains stem cells, and expands and contracts during the hair cycle. The human hair cycle differs for each hair; however, the overall number of hairs remains roughly constant.

Arrector pili muscle

The arrector pili muscle consists of a strand of smooth muscle that connects at the level of the hair bulge. It contracts in response to cold and to emotional factors such as fear and surprise, and that contraction pulls the hair upwards, causing "goose bumps." Goose bumps may accompany shivering that occurs to raise the body temperature. The arrector pili muscle is controlled by adrenergic sympathetic nerves.

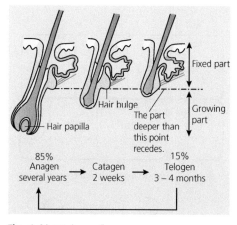

Fig. 1.41 Hair cycle.

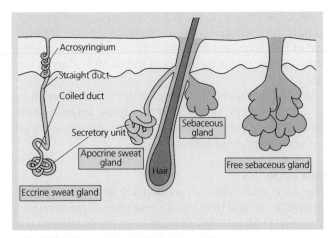

Fig. 1.42 Sebaceous and sweat glands.

Sebaceous glands

Sebum is produced by the sebaceous glands (Fig. 1.42) and is emulsified on the skin surface to form fatty acids, wax esters, and triglycerides that coat the skin surface. This coat is acidic, with a pH ranging from 4 to 6, and it has bactericidal properties (acid mantle). Sebum and sebaceous glands prevent invasion and infection by pathogens and toxic substances. Additionally, the sebaceous glands control water loss from the skin and help maintain moisture in the horny cell layers.

The sebaceous glands are widely distributed throughout the skin, except in the palms and soles and some mucous membranes. Mostly associated with hair follicles, they release sebum in the infundibular portion of the hair follicle. Sites at which there is a high density of sebaceous glands are called seborrheic zones. These are seen in the scalp, face (the T zone, which includes the forehead, regions of the glabella, and the nasolabial groove), sternal regions, armpits, navel, and external genitalia. The seborrheic zone is very densely distributed with sebaceous glands ($400–900/cm^2$). These glands are called free sebaceous glands because they are not attached to hair follicles. Meibomian glands, found in the eyelids, are a type of free sebaceous gland.

The sebaceous gland is composed of sebaceous lobules and a duct that carries sebum to the hair follicle. Sebocytes produced by cell division migrate into the lobules during maturation and acquire fat droplets. As they migrate towards the center of the gland, the cells rupture, releasing sebum in a process called holocrine secretion (Fig. 1.43).

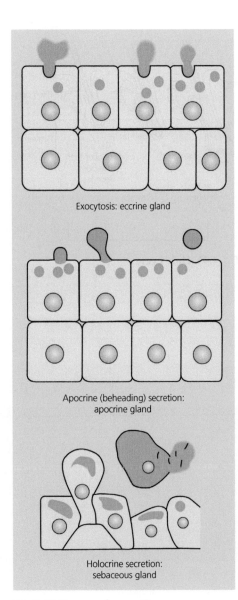

Exocytosis: eccrine gland

Apocrine (beheading) secretion:
apocrine gland

Holocrine secretion:
sebaceous gland

Fig. 1.43 Types of secretion.

The amount of sebum secretion changes with age. Large amounts of sebum are produced in newborn infants. Production begins to increase again from puberty. The secretion of sebum peaks in women in their second and third decades of life and in men in their third and fourth decades of life, decreasing thereafter. The amount of sebum secretion is controlled predominantly by sex hormones: testosterone in men and adrenal androgens in women. Hormones derived from the mother are thought to influence sebum secretion in the newborn.

Sweat glands

There are two main types of sweat glands in humans: eccrine glands, which are distributed throughout most of the body, and apocrine glands, which are found at specific sites of the body. Both are hair follicle-associated glands consisting of a secretory part and a sweat duct. The secretory parts are coiled and extend in the deep dermal layer and subcutaneous tissue (see Fig. 1.42).

Eccrine sweat glands

Eccrine sweat glands are found over the entire body, especially in the palms, soles, and armpits, at a density ranging from 130 to 600/cm². Approximately 3 million eccrine glands are found in the human body. Perspiration is enhanced by thermal stimulation, which is associated with body temperature control, and may also be stimulated by mental strain or gustatory stimulus (gustatory sweating). The total amount of perspiration in a day is controlled by acetylcholines and averages 700–900 mL in adults.

The secretory portion of the eccrine gland consists of two cell types within a single layer. These cells are surrounded by flat myoepithelial cells (Fig. 1.44a). Cells on the basal layer side contain few subcellular organelles and large amounts of glycogen. Since these cells secrete large amounts of serous sweat by eccrine secretion (see Fig. 1.43), they are also called serous cells. Cells on the luminal side secrete mucus. The myoepithelial cell is a smooth muscle cell that pushes the accumulated sweat out of the lumen into the sweat ducts by contraction.

The eccrine secretory unit consists of a proximal coiled portion found in the deep dermis and subcutaneous fat, and eccrine ducts that ascend perpendicularly in the dermis (straight ducts). In the epidermis,

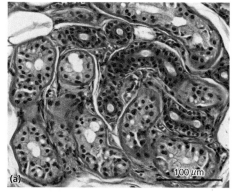
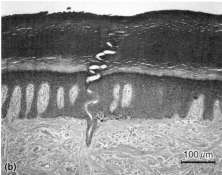
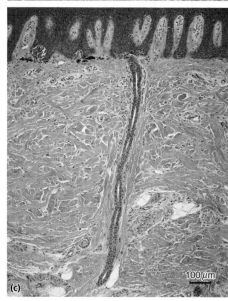

Fig. 1.44 Eccrine sweat gland. a: Cross-section. b: Longitudinal section of the duct in the epidermis. c: Longitudinal section of the duct in the dermis.

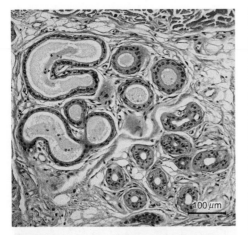

Fig. 1.45 **Apocrine sweat gland.**

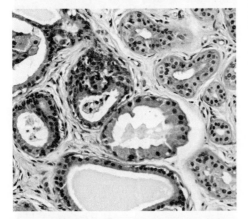

Fig. 1.46 **Apocrine (beheading) secretion of the sweat gland.**

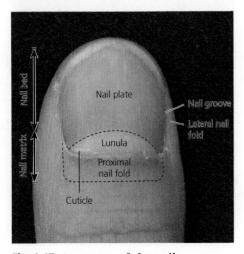

Fig. 1.47 **Anatomy of the nail.**

the duct becomes coiled again like a corkscrew and opens onto the skin surface (see Figs 1.42 and 1.44). The sweat duct contains two cell layers, consisting of intraluminal cells and peripheral cells, but it lacks myoepithelial cells. The sweat that is produced in secretory areas (known as precursor sweat) is slightly hypertonic; therefore, sodium ions and chlorine ions are reabsorbed by intraluminal cells in the coiled ducts, and hypotonic sweat is finally secreted.

Apocrine sweat glands

Apocrine sweat glands, which are fewer than eccrine glands, are degenerated pheromone-producing mammary glands found at specific sites such as the armpits, external ear canals, areola mammae, external genitals, and anus. They are always associated with hair follicles and enlarge during puberty through hormonal stimulation. Mammary glands and Moll's glands of the eyelids are modified apocrine glands. Apocrine glands produce small amounts of viscous and odorless sweat. However, the breakdown of several sweat components such as glycoproteins and fat by commensal skin bacteria produces odor.

The secretory portion of the apocrine gland is larger than that of the eccrine gland. Secretory cells are aligned as a single-layer epithelium surrounded by myoepithelial cells (Fig. 1.45). Sweat is secreted in a process called apocrine or decapitation secretion, during which the luminal surface of the cells bulges, blebs, and separates from the cell (apocrine secretion; Fig. 1.46) (see Fig. 1.43).

The sweat ducts do not open to the skin surface directly, but into the upper parts of the sebaceous glands (see Fig. 1.42).

Nails

The nail apparatus consists of the nail plate, nail matrix, nail folds, and nail bed. Each of these parts is made up of several more detailed structures (Fig. 1.47). The nail differentiates from the primitive epidermis around the third month of fetal development. Recent studies have shown that the nail has characteristics of both the dermis and the hair. The fingernail grows 0.1 mm per day, and it takes about 6 months to regrow an entire nail plate. The growth of nails is slower in the elderly, whose nails tend to be thick and brownish. Nails are important in protecting the digits and in assisting subtle sensation in the fingertips.

Nail plate

The nail plate, which can vary in size, shape, and thickness, is usually a rectangular plate of tightly organized keratinized cells (onychocytes) that rests on the dorsal tip of the digits. It is a three-layered structure of dorsal, intermediate, and ventral parts. In the proximal area, the nail plate is covered by the proximal nail fold, where the nail matrix is found. Proliferating cells within the nail matrix become keratinized to form the nail plate. Keratohyalin granules are not involved in this keratinization process. An opaque white half-moon shape (lunula) may appear at the root of the nail plate as a result of inadequate keratinization.

Nail matrix

Keratinocytes are produced in the nail matrix. The cells that differentiate and proliferate in the nail matrix extend and keratinize to form the nail plate; however, the ventral aspect of the nail plate is thought to originate from the nail bed.

Nail fold

The two edges of skin that border the nail plate and the nail bed are called the nail folds. The cuticle is the keratinized layer of skin that extends to partly cover the nail plate.

Nail bed

The nail bed is found at the base of the nail plate. It has the same components as the epidermis, except that it lacks the granular layer. It is continuously keratinized to connect with the nail plate.

Immunology of the skin

Basics of immunology
Immune system

Immunity is crucial in protecting the human body from invasion by pathogenic microorganisms. One of the main functions of the skin is to physically prevent such invasion. However, the human body can tolerate microorganisms known as commensals that are present on the skin surface, in the intestines, and in the mucous membranes. Disruption of the relationship between the human body and its commensals can result in invasion by these organisms, triggering the activation of immune mechanisms.

MEMO 1–15 Bleeding in the cuticle

Hemorrhagic puncta in the cuticle may be seen in collagen diseases (e.g., systemic lupus erythematosus, dermatomyositis, scleroderma). It is thought to result from angiitis occurring in the microvessels.

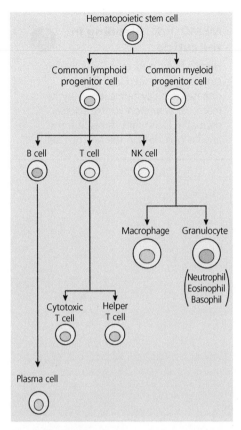

Fig. 1.48 Myelogenous cells composing the immune system.

The immune system performs the following functions.
- Distinguishing between "self" and "non-self."
- Excluding "non-self."
- Remembering what has invaded (immunological memory).

These functions are performed by immunocompetent cells such as lymphocytes and antigen-presenting cells, both of which are derived from the bone marrow (Fig. 1.48).

Reaction pattern

Foreign substances (or antigens) including bacteria, viruses, transplanted tissue, and certain proteins are distinguished as "non-self" by the immune system. The major histocompatibility complex (MHC) plays a critical role in identifying whether an antigen is self or non-self. In humans, the MHC is called HLA (human leukocyte antigen) because it was first discovered in leukocytes. HLA is categorized as class I (HLA-A, -B, -C) or class II (HLA-DP, -DQ, -DR) (Fig. 1.49). Each of us is characterized by a different HLA pattern. However, certain individuals have specific HLA patterns that increase their susceptibility to certain immunological disorders (Table 1.3).

Exogenous antigens that are recognized as non-self undergo phagocytosis by histiocytes (macrophages) or dendritic cells, such as cutaneous Langerhans cells. These cells, also known as antigen-presenting cells, process the antigen into short peptides that are then displayed on the surface nestled within a MHC class II molecule. The information of the antigen is conveyed by the combination of a T cell receptor (TCR) and MHC, resulting in immune activation and reaction (Fig. 1.50).

MEMO 1–16 Acquired and natural immunity

The antigen-specific immune system that acts through the MHC molecules confers what is called adaptive immunity, because the system reacts and adapts to various foreign objects. Innate immunity is conferred by a system that recognizes certain molecular structures of invading microorganisms and activates neutrophils, macrophages, NK cells, and complements at the initial stages of microbial invasion. The lipopolysaccharides on the surface of bacteria, for example, join with TLR4 molecules on the surface of macrophages and trigger the acquired immune system while phagocytosing and excluding the invading bacteria. Innate immunity quickly responds to bacteria whose invasion is identified for the first time by the immune system; however, the system's ability to exclude invading bacteria is low.

Serum immune reaction

Antibodies

Antibodies are immunoglobulins produced by B lymphocytes. They are able to react against infectious agents or pathogenic proteins (antigens), inhibiting infections and neutralizing protein toxicity. B lymphocytes secrete a number of specific antibodies corresponding to the antigens they have previously encountered. There are five classes of immunoglobulins, namely IgG, IgM, IgA, IgD, and IgE, in descending order of concentration (Table 1.4). IgG, produced during infection, accounts for 75% of immunoglobulins and plays a central role in the humoral immune reaction (Fig. 1.51). IgM production occurs at the very early stage of infection and precedes the production of IgG. It strongly activates the complement system (see next section). IgA is seen abundantly in exocrine secretions, such as mucus, where it prevents invasion by pathogens. IgE elicits an immune response by binding to IgE receptors (FcεR) found on mast cells, basophils, and eosinophils. It plays an important role in type I allergy. In recent years, overproduction of IgE and interleukin (IL)-4 in atopic dermatitis has been attracting attention.

Complement system

The complement system consists of a number of proteins present in serum. It forms part of the innate immune system. The components of the complement

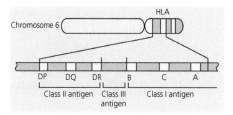

Fig. 1.49 HLA (human leukocyte antigen) genes on the short arm of chromosome 6. Genetic recombination causes the HLA pattern to differ for each individual.

Table 1.3 Association between HLA complex and skin diseases.

Disorder	Associated HLA in ethnic Japanese	Associated HLA in Caucasians	Indirect reference
Behçet's disease	B51	B51	Chapter 11
Systemic lupus erythematosus	A11, B40, DR2, DRW9	B8, DR2, DR3	Chapter 12
Neonatal lupus erythematosus	DW12		Chapter 12
Sjögren syndrome		DR3, DW3	Chapter 12
Rheumatoid arthritis	DR4	DR4	Chapter 12
Pemphigus vulgaris	A10, DR4	A10, B13	Chapter 14
Herpes gestationis		A1,B8,DR3	Chapter 14
Epidermolysis bullosa acquisita		B8	Chapter 14
Dermatitis herpetiformis (Duhring)		B8, DW3	Chapter 14
Psoriasis vulgaris	Cw6	Cw6	Chapter 15
Pustular psoriasis		B27	Chapter 15

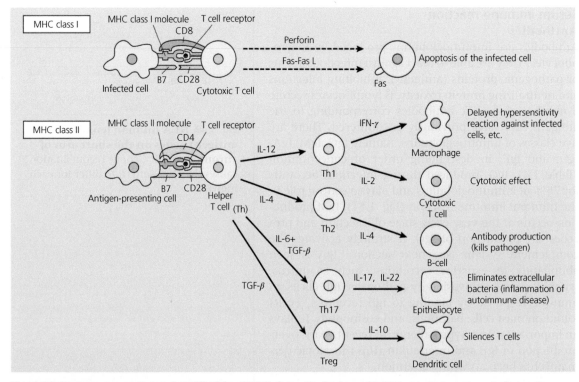

Fig. 1.50 Immune reactions classified by MHC class. Each class of MHC presents antigen information to a different type of T cell.

Table 1.4 Basic characteristics of immunoglobulins.

	IgG	IgM	IgA (secretory)	IgD	IgE
Molecular weight (kDa)	146	970	160	184	188
Serum concentration	870–1700 mg/dl	Male: 33–190 mg/dl Female: 46–260 mg/dl	110–410 mg/dl	<11.5 mg/dl	<170 IU/ml
Half-life in blood (days)	21	10	6	3	2
Antigen type of heavy chain	γ	μ	α	δ	ε
Transport across the placenta	(+)	(–)	(–)	(–)	(–)
Disorder with high value	Collagen disease	Schnitzler syndrome	Henoch-Schonlein purpura	Behçet's disease	Atopic dermatitis
Basic structure		(Monomer) (Dimer) secretory piece J chain			

system can be classified into nine types (C1–C9) and further subclassified. In the classical pathway, C1 reacts to IgG or IgM antibodies, followed by a cascade of complement activation that causes destruction of the pathogens and infected cells. In the alternative pathway, the reaction is evoked mostly by bacterial components, which directly activate C3, factor B, and factor D. A third pathway, the lectin pathway, has also been described. This pathway involves lectin, an acute-phase protein that binds to mannose residues on the microbial surface and induces the activation of the complement system by activating mannan-binding lectin-associated serine proteases 1 and 2 (MASP-1 and MASP-2).

Immunocompetent cells
Immunocompetent cells in general
T cells

T cells play a key role in cell-mediated immunity and express T cell receptors on the cell surface. These receptors allow the T cells to recognize the antigenic information associated with MHC molecules (see Fig. 1.50). T cells are produced in the bone marrow and develop in the thymus. They are classified into CD4-positive helper T cells (helper T lymphocyte; Th) and CD8-positive cytotoxic T lymphocytes (Tc).

Th expresses the cell surface marker CD4, which allows it to adhere to MHC class II molecules. Therefore, Th reacts with antigen-presenting cells and B lymphocytes, both of which contain MHC class II molecules. Th can be differentiated into the two sub-types of Th1 and Th2, depending on the surrounding cytokine environment (see Fig. 1.50). Th1 secretes cytokines such as IL-2 and IFN-γ, which are involved primarily in histiocyte (macrophage) activation as well as induction of cellular immunity by evoking various inflammatory reactions. Th2 secretes IL-4 and IL-5, activates antibody production in B cells and inactivates foreign substances (humoral immunity). Th1 is involved mostly in type IV allergy, while Th2 is involved in type I allergy (atopic diseases).

In recent years, an IL-17-producing T cell has been found; this is called Th17. Th17 activates neutrophils through epidermal cells or fibroblasts, plays a role in eliminating bacteria and fungi from cells and is thought to engage in tissue remodeling. Th17 is strongly involved in maintaining inflammation in chronic inflammatory disorders such as psoriasis and Crohn's

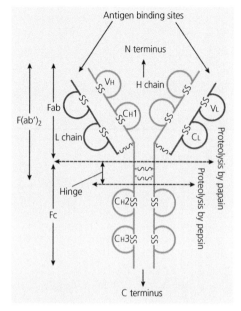

Fig. 1.51 Basic structure of human immunoglobulin (IgG). Fab, fragment antigen binding. Fc, crystallizable fragment. VL, variable light chain. CL, constant light chain. VH, variable heavy chain. CH, constant heavy chain.

disease and in autoimmune diseases including rheumatoid arthritis.

Tc expresses the CD8 molecule, which enables it to associate with MHC class I molecules and initiate cytotoxic immunity (see Fig. 1.50); in this way, non-self cells and virus-infected cells are destroyed. Tc is important in transplantation immunity, tumor immunity, and viral infections.

Recently, the presence of another T cell subtype, the regulatory T cell (Treg), has been identified. Treg is thought to be involved in immunological tolerance, including the suppression of autoimmune disease onset.

B cells

B cells are derived from hematopoietic stem cells in the bone marrow, after which they migrate to the spleen and undergo maturation. Upon activation in lymph nodes, spleen tissue and peripheral lymphoid tissue, B cells differentiate into antibody-forming cells (plasma cells). B cells express part of the ingested pathogen on the cell surface in association with MHC class II molecules. The antigen can then be detected by T lymphocytes, which in turn activate the production of antigen-specific antibodies by B cells. B cells can also be activated in a T cell-independent manner. Some B cells also differentiate into memory B cells and are able to produce specific antibodies upon reinfection.

Histiocytes (macrophages)

Histiocytes (macrophages) are bone marrow-derived cells that are induced mainly by IFN-γ. Strongly phagocytic histiocytes degrade phagocytosed antigen proteins into small peptides and present the antigenic information to T cells via MHC class II molecules (see Fig. 1.50). During inflammation, there is a proliferation of histiocytes that then migrate to the inflammatory loci. During this process, they secrete various cytokines (IL-1β, IL-6, IL-8, IFN-α) and induce phagocytosis of the pathogen, resulting in damage to the infected cells. Histiocytes may also fuse to form giant cells. They are the main cells involved in granuloma formation during chronic inflammation (see Chapter 2).

Mast cells

Mast cells play a central role in type I allergy. They contain high-affinity IgE receptors (FcεRI) and considerable amounts of histamine. When bound with IgE and further cross-linked by IgE-specific antigens, mast cells degranulate and release various cytokines (IL-3, IL-4, IL-5), which lead to dermal edema such as that seen in urticaria. Mastocytosis is caused by the malignant proliferation of mast cells.

Eosinophils

Eosinophils have both phagocytic and cytotoxic functions. They are associated with atopic diseases (type I allergy), autoimmune blistering diseases, and parasitic infections. They are morphologically characterized by multiple eosinophilic granules, and they contain cytotoxic proteins such as major basic protein (MBP) and eosinophil cationic protein (ECP) (Fig. 1.52). They are activated by IL-3, IL-5, and GMCSF. They are hardly ever found in normal skin.

Neutrophils

Neutrophils are phagocytic cells that play a crucial role in fighting bacterial infections (Fig. 1.53). They strongly phagocytose bacteria bound with IgG or C3b (opsonized bacteria) through myeloperoxidase in the granules. They are hardly ever found in normal skin. In certain skin diseases, such as psoriasis vulgaris and Sweet's disease, neutrophilic infiltration can be intense, resulting in the formation of pustules.

Basophils

Like eosinophils and neutrophils, basophils are granular leukocytes that have chemical mediators such as histamines and leukotrienes in the granules and express FcεRI on the cell surface. They are involved in type I allergy and mediate functions similar to those of mast cells.

Immunocompetent cells specific to skin
Langerhans cells

Langerhans cells are bone marrow-derived antigen-presenting cells that appear as dendritic cells. They contain the characteristic racket-shaped Birbeck granules in their cytoplasm (Fig. 1.54 and Fig. 1.55). They adhere to the epidermal keratinocytes by means of E-cadherin and guard against foreign antigens. When presenting an antigen to T cells, Langerhans cells detach from the epidermis and migrate to the regional lymph nodes via lymphatic vessels (Fig. 1.56). Human Langerhans cells express MHC class II molecules, CD1a, and S-100 proteins on their cell surface; the presence of these molecular markers is useful for the identification of Langerhans cells.

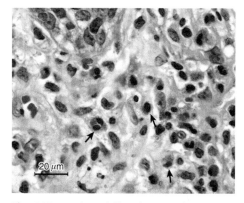

Fig. 1.52 Eosinophils. The cytoplasm is eosinophilic (red in hematoxylin-eosin staining). Note the multiple nuclei.

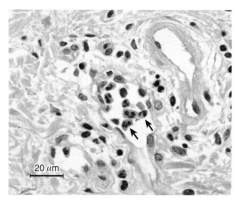

Fig. 1.53 Neutrophils. In skin, the cytoplasm of neutrophils is less eosinophilic than that of eosinophils. A neutrophil has a multi-segmented nucleus.

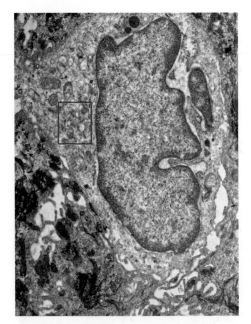

Fig. 1.54 Langerhans cell electron micrograph. A high-power magnification of the part in the red square is shown in Fig. 1.55.

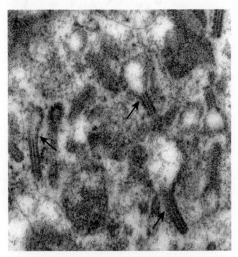

Fig. 1.55 Birbeck granules (arrows). A high-power magnification of the part in the red square in Fig. 1.54. In cross-section, Birbeck granules look like tennis rackets.

When Langerhans cells are stimulated by antigens, they express CD80 and CD86 by the functions of granulocyte macrophage-colony stimulating factor (GMCSF) and tumor necrosis factor-α (TNF-α) secreted by keratinocytes. They produce and secrete various cytokines (IL-1β, IL-6, TNF-α) to activate immune mechanisms.

Langerhans cells are not found in cutaneous lesions of graft-versus-host disease (GVHD). Ultraviolet rays, UVB in particular, suppress the numbers and functions of Langerhans cells, which is thought to be one of the mechanisms by which ultraviolet therapy works.

Keratinocytes

Keratinocytes, in addition to their role in cornification, play a crucial part in skin immunity. They produce and secrete various cytokines to stimulate immunocompetent cells (Table 1.5). IL-1α is particularly abundant in keratinocytes. When keratinocytes are destroyed by inflammation or injury, IL-1α, IL-3, IL-6, and GMCSF are released to activate lymphocytes, histiocytes, and vascular endothelial cells.

Dermal dendrocytes

Dermal dendrocytes are bone marrow-derived antigen-presenting cells found in the upper dermal layers. Since dermal dendrocytes are characterized by the cell surface expression of factor XIIIa, they are considered to be Langerhans-related cells in the dermis. They increase in number in inflammatory diseases and Kaposi's sarcoma.

Allergic reactions

The skin is a major organ where immune/allergic reactions occur. A number of skin diseases occur as a result of heightened immunological response. Such disorders, known as allergic or hypersensitivity disorders, are generally classified into the four categories established by Coombs & Gell (Table 1.6).

Type I allergy

Type I allergy is mainly mediated by mast cells. It is also called an immediate hypersensitivity reaction, since it manifests 5–15 min after an antigen (allergen) is presented. Mast cells with IgE on the surface react to a specific antigen, causing massive degranulation and the release of chemical mediators such as histamines

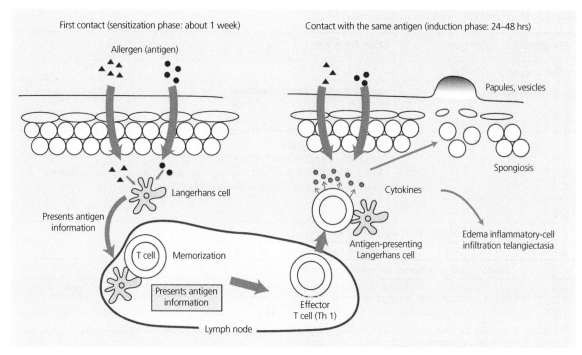

First contact (sensitization phase: about 1 week) Contact with the same antigen (induction phase: 24–48 hrs)

Allergen (antigen)

Papules, vesicles

Spongiosis

Langerhans cell

Cytokines

Presents antigen information

Edema inflammatory-cell infiltration telangiectasia

Antigen-presenting Langerhans cell

T cell   Memorization

Presents antigen information

Effector T cell (Th 1)

Lymph node

Fig. 1.56 Mechanism of allergic contact dermatitis.

and leukotrienes (see Chapter 8). These inflammatory mediators enhance vascular permeability to produce edema; in addition, they induce migration of eosinophils to evoke inflammation. The typical clinical features are nasal discharge and congestion, pruritus, conjunctivitis, and bronchial asthma. There may also be a sharp drop in systemic blood pressure due to rapid vascular dilatation. In serious cases, the patient may develop anaphylactic shock, which requires immediate treatment with epinephrine and antihistamines. In the majority of type I allergy cases, the symptoms subside within several hours.

Typical skin diseases caused by type I allergy are urticaria and certain types of drug eruptions (e.g., urticarial reaction). In atopic eczema, other factors such as filaggrin gene mutation may be involved. Additionally, allergic rhinitis (hay fever), bronchial asthma, allergic conjunctivitis, and atopic eczema are common diseases mediated by type I allergy.

Type II allergy

In type II allergy, antibodies are directed against endogenous cell surface antigens that have previously activated the complement system and cytotoxic T cells,

> **MEMO 1–17 Th1/Th2 balance**
>
> Th1 is involved in cytotoxic immunity, including apoptosis; Th2 is involved in humoral immunity, including type I allergy. Th1 and Th2 release mutually inhibitive cytokines that are thought to maintain a Th1/Th2 balance. In recent years, various allergic disorders and malignant tumors have been explained by the concept of Th1/Th2 imbalance. For example, atopic dermatitis and type I allergy are thought to be caused by a Th2-dominated immune reaction, whereas organ-specific autoimmune diseases and arterial sclerosis are thought to result from a principally Th1-mediated immune reaction.

Table 1.5 Main cytokins secreted by keratinocytes.

Classification, cytokines	Main functions
Multifunctional cytokines	
Interleukin (IL) IL-1α IL-3 IL-6 IL-7 IL-12 IL-15 IL-18 TNF-α MIF	Induction of secondary cytokines Modulation of adhesion molecules Modulation of activation and migration of T cells, B cells and macrophages Activation of endothelial cells and fibroblasts Modulation of activation and migration of Langerhans cells (IL-1α, TNF-α) Induction of fever and acute inflammatory proteins
Chemotactic factor: associated with leukocyte migration	
IL-8	Activation and migration of T cells and neutrophils
Colony stimulating factor: associated with leukocyte proliferation	
GM-CSF	Activation of granulocytes, macrophages, T cells and Langerhans cells
G-CSF	Proliferation of granulocytes
M-CSF	Proliferation of macrophages
Growth factor: associated with local cutaneous reactions	
TGF-α	Proliferation of keratinocytes
b-FGF, PDGF	Proliferation of fibroblasts and endothelial cells
Suppression factor: modulates immunity	
TGF-β	Suppression of keratinocytes and endothelial cells
IL-10	Suppression of immunity through Th1 cells

IL: interleukin, TNF: tumor necrosis factor, MIF: macrophage migration inhibitory factor, GM-CSF: granulocyte macrophage colony-stimulating factor, G-CSF: granulocyte colony-stimulating factor, M-CSF: macrophage colony-stimulating factor, TGF: tumor growth factor, b-FGF: basis fibroblast growth, PDGF: platelet derived growth factor

MEMO 1–18 Clinical symptoms resulting from abnormalities of the complement system

Several skin diseases, such as SLE, Raynaud's phenomenon, and angioneurotic edema, may be caused by congenital abnormalities and deficiencies in components of the complement system.

leading to cellular injury. Type II allergy is involved in the pathogenesis of cutaneous diseases such as autoimmune blistering diseases, e.g., bullous pemphigoid. In the case of bullous pemphigoid, autoantibodies bind to type XVII collagen, a component of hemidesmosomes in the basal cells, resulting in basal cell injury and blisters (see Chapter 14).

A drug may function as a hapten (MEMO, see Chapter 1) and bind to epidermal cells or blood cells to cause type II allergy. Drug-induced hemolytic anemia, thrombocytopenic purpura, and toxic epidermal necrosis (TEN) occur by this mechanism.

Blood group incompatibility from transfusion, autoimmune hemolytic anemia, and Goodpasture's syndrome are other type II hypersensitivity disorders.

Table 1.6 Classification of allergy.

Coombs classification	Type I	Type II	Type III	Type IV
Type of reaction	Anaphylaxis (immediate hypersensitivity)	Cytolytic reaction (cytotoxic hypersensitivity)	Immune complex reaction	Cellular immunity (delayed hypersensitivity)
Associated antibodies	IgE	IgG, IgM	IgG, IgM	-
Associated immune cells	Histiocytes, basophils, mast cells	Cytotoxic T cells, macrophages	Multinclear leukocytes, macrophages	Sensitized T cells, macrophages
Complement	Unneeded	Needed	Needed	Unneeded
Target tissues/ cells	Skin, lung, intestines	Skin, erythrocytes, leukocytes, platelets	Skin, vessel, joint, kidney, lung	Skin, lung, thyroid gland central nervous system, etc.
Disorders	Urticaria, drug eruption, asthma, pollinosis, anaphylaxis	Bullous pemphigoid, haemolytic anemia, idiopathic thrombocytopenic purpura, TEN, transfusion incompatibility	Cutaneous small-vessel vasculitis, serum sickness, glomerulonephritis	Allergic contact dermatitis, erythema induratum, GVHD
Illustration of reaction				

MEMO 1–19 Hapten

Phagocytic cells engulf antigens that contain proteins of 10,000 molecular weight or greater (complete antigen) and carry the antigenic information to the lymphocytes. Non-proteinaceous substances of low molecular weight (e.g., carbohydrates, fats, organic compounds, metallic molecules) cannot be antigens by themselves and are referred to as haptens or incomplete antigens. Haptens can elicit an immune response when they are attached to a carrier molecule such as a protein. An example of a hapten is the drug hydralazine, which can produce drug-induced SLE in certain individuals.

MEMO 1–20 Type V allergic reactions

Type V is similar to type II, in that the antigen is produced in reaction to proteins on the surface of the cells. However, in type V, a functional increase or decrease occurs in the cell when the antigen binds with the cell receptor. Graves' disease is an example of type V allergy.

Type III allergy

Type III allergy occurs when circulating antigen-antibody complexes (immune complexes) deposit in the blood vessels and other organs, such as the kidneys and joints. An infection or a drug may induce immune complex deposition in cutaneous blood vessels, resulting in fibrinoid degeneration and neutrophilic infiltration; this is called cutaneous small vessel vasculitis (see Chapter 11).

Serum sickness disease, glomerular nephritis, and lupus nephritis are other type III allergies.

Type IV allergy

Type IV allergy is an inflammation caused by a reaction between an antigen and the corresponding T cells (Th1 in particular). There are two stages in type IV allergy: a sensitization phase and an effector phase. After the initial invasion, the antigen is engulfed by antigen-presenting cells to activate T cells in the regional lymph nodes. At this time, memory T cells along with effector T cells are produced in order to enable them to respond promptly to any future exposure to the same antigen (sensitization). If future exposure occurs, memory T cells are activated by the antigen-presenting cells, inducing inflammation that peaks around 48 h after the antigenic challenge (effector phase). Since it takes a long time for the inflammation to occur, type IV allergy is also called delayed hypersensitivity (see Fig. 1.56).

Diseases caused by type IV allergy include allergic contact dermatitis and GVHD.

CHAPTER 2
Histopathology of the skin

Skin biopsy is an important procedure that is frequently used in dermatology. The skin obtained during a biopsy is processed and then examined by microscopy. In many instances, it is difficult to reach a definitive diagnosis based on history taking and examination alone. Skin biopsy can therefore help one to arrive at a final diagnosis or at a set of differential diagnoses.

Skin biopsy

Although a skin biopsy is a routine and straightforward procedure, it is essential that the biopsy site be carefully selected. For example, in dealing with inflammatory diseases, it is recommended that non-lesional skin be included in the biopsy, to allow for comparison with lesional skin. When a disease presents with multiple lesions, it may be advisable to collect several skin samples that reflect different stages of inflammation. Another important consideration is that the chosen biopsy site must be cosmetically acceptable.

The area to be biopsied is sterilized and then a local anesthetic is injected. Once the site is well anesthetized, the procedure can be performed (Fig. 2.1). The main techniques are punch biopsy (removal of a core of full-thickness skin using a circular scalpel attached to a pencil-like handle), incisional biopsy (removal of a wedge-shaped sample with a scalpel), and excisional biopsy (usually wedge-shaped removal of the entire lesion, such as a pigmented macule). Shave biopsy (superficial excision by razor blade) is another technique that is useful for lesions in the epidermis. After the specimen is taken, it is immediately placed in a 10% formaldehyde solution for fixation, to avoid secondary degeneration. Alternatively, the sample may be divided for cryofixation or 2% glutaraldehyde fixation for immunofluorescence or electron microscopy studies, respectively.

The most commonly used staining procedure is hematoxylin and eosin (HE) staining. In addition, a

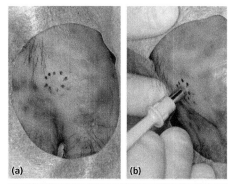
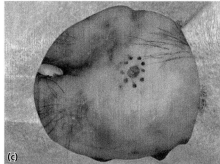
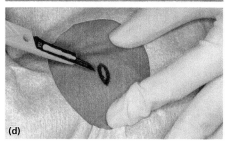

Fig. 2.1 Procedure of skin biopsy. a–c: Punch biopsy. d: Incisional biopsy with a scalpel.

Shimizu's Dermatology, Second Edition. Hiroshi Shimizu.
© 2017 John Wiley & Sons, Ltd. Published 2017 by John Wiley & Sons, Ltd.

skin specimen can be stained by other methods, collectively known as special staining procedures (Table 2.1), which are often used in combination with HE staining.

Dermatopathology

An understanding of normal skin histology is essential in dermatopathology (Fig. 2.2). This section introduces fundamental terms used to describe skin pathological changes.

Table 2.1 Specific stains used in dermatology.

Stain	Stained material	Stained color
Hematoxylin and eosin (HE)	Entire skin	Blue (nucleus), magenta (cytoplasm, etc.)
Elastica van Gieson	Collagen fibers	Red
	Elastic fibers	Black
Azan Mallory	Collagen fibers	Blue
Masson trichrome	Collagen fibers	Blue
	Smooth muscle	Red
Bodian	Nerve fibers (axons)	Black
Weigert	Elastic fibers	Black
Periodic acid-Schiff (PAS)	Basement membrane	Red
	Glycogen	Red
	Neutral mucopolysaccharides	Red
	Fungi	Red
Toluidine blue	Mast cell	Purple
	Acid mucopolysaccharides	Blue
Alcian blue	Acid mucopolysaccharides	Blue
Colloidal iron	Acid mucopolysaccharides	Blue
Fontana-Masson	Melanin granules	Black
DOPA	Melanocytes	Black
Sudan III	Fat	Reddish-orange
Congo red	Amyloid	Reddish-orange
Direct first scarlet (DFS)	Amyloid	Reddish-brown
Dylon	Anyloid	Reddish-brown
Thioflavin T fluorescence	Amyloid	Green fluorescence
Berlin blue	Hemosiderin	Blue
Von Kossa	Calcium	Brownish-black
Grocott's methenamine silver	Fungi	Black
Ziehl-Neelsen	Mycobacteria	Red
Warthin-Starry	Spirochetes, *Helicobacter pylori*	Black

Epidermis

Acanthosis

Acanthosis (epidermal hyperplasia) describes thickening of the epidermis. It is classified into flat (moderate thickening of entire lesion, e.g., in chronic eczema), psoriasiform (extension of epidermal protrusions), papillomatous (upward projection of epidermis, e.g., with viral warts or seborrheic keratosis), and pseudocarcinomatous (irregular downward epidermal projections, e.g., at the margins of chronic ulcers and in deep mycoses) (Fig. 2.3 and Fig. 2.4).

Epidermal atrophy (epidermal hypoplasia)

Epidermal atrophy is caused by a reduction of keratinocytes (Fig. 2.5) that results in thinning of the epidermis. The papillary processes are diminished or lost. It is often found in lichen planus, discoid lupus erythematosus (DLE), actinic keratosis, and photoaging.

Hyperkeratosis

Hyperkeratosis refers to an abnormal thickening of the stratum corneum and is seen in psoriasis vulgaris, ichthyosis, and callus (Fig. 2.6). In ichthyosis, hyperkeratosis is due to detachment and exfoliation of the stratum corneum, a process called retention hyperkeratosis. In psoriasis, production of the horny layer increases, a process called proliferative hyperkeratosis. Keratinization associated with hair follicles is called follicular keratosis. Hyperkeratosis that is not

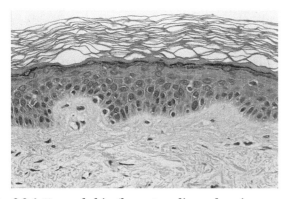

Fig. 2.2-1 Normal skin (hematoxylin and eosin staining). a: Normal skin of the forearm. The horny cell layer has a basket-weave appearance. The gaps between the stained horny cell layers are lipids that dissolved during fixation. These gaps indicate that the skin is well protected by moisturizing lipids.

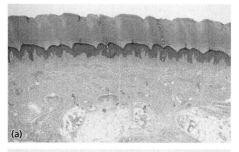
(a)
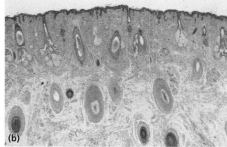
(b)
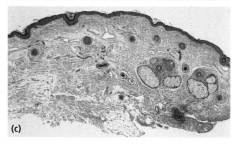
(c)

Fig. 2.2-2 Normal skin (hematoxylin and eosin staining). a: Normal skin of the sole. A thick stratum corneum is seen. b: Scalp. Many follicles can be seen. c: Face. Sebaceous glands are abundant.

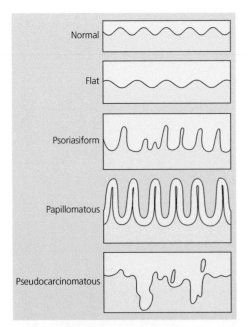

Fig. 2.3 Patterns of acanthosis.

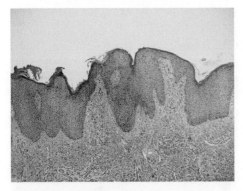

Fig. 2.4 Acanthosis (Chronic eczema)

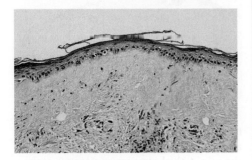

Fig. 2.5 Epidermal atrophy
(Dermatomyositis)

accompanied by parakeratosis (see next section) is called orthokeratotic hyperkeratosis.

Parakeratosis

Parakeratosis is the term used to describe incomplete keratinization of the stratum corneum. It is characterized by the presence of nuclei within the cells of the stratum corneum (Fig. 2.7). In normal skin, keratinocytes denucleate when they reach the stratum corneum; however, in inflammatory diseases such as psoriasis vulgaris, keratinocyte formation takes place so rapidly that most of the nuclei remain in the stratum corneum. Parakeratosis is frequently accompanied by hyperkeratosis and hypogranulosis. Wedge-shaped or columnar parakeratosis, called cornoid lamella, is observed in porokeratosis (see Chapter 21).

Dyskeratosis (individual cell keratinization)

Dyskeratosis occurs when keratinocytes keratinize abnormally before they reach the stratum corneum (Fig. 2.8). As the keratinocytes undergo apoptosis, their nuclei shrink. Eosinophilic cytoplasm is also seen within the dyskeratotic keratinocytes. These cells become round with the loss of intercellular bridges between the surrounding keratinocytes. Dyskeratosis is often found with inflammatory diseases and malignant tumors. The civatte bodies in lichen planus and corps ronds in Darier's disease (see Chapter 15) occur due to dyskeratosis. In erythema multiforme and graft-versus-host disease (GVHD), dyskeratotic cells accompanied by sparse lymphocytes are observed in a phenomenon called satellite cell necrosis.

Hypergranulosis

This is thickening of the granular cell layer to four or more layers, compared to the 1–3 layers of normal skin (Fig. 2.9). It is seen in lichen planus, viral warts, and congenital ichthyosis.

Granular degeneration (epidermolytic hyperkeratosis)

In granular degeneration, numerous vacuolated cells containing large keratohyalin granules appear in the granular and suprabasal cell layers (Fig. 2.10). It is characteristic of Vörner palmoplantar keratosis and epidermolytic ichthyosis (bullous congenital ichthyosiform erythroderma) (Chapter 15). It may also be found in epidermal nevus and sometimes in normal skin.

Spongiosis (intercellular edema)

Spongiosis occurs when the spaces between neighboring keratinocytes are enlarged by edema. As a result, the intercellular space becomes distended and visible (Fig. 2.11). When aggravated further, there is the formation of intradermal blisters (spongiotic bullae). Spongiosis can be found in inflammatory skin disorders such as contact dermatitis, atopic dermatitis, and acute eczema.

Intracellular edema (ballooning degeneration)

Intracellular edema results in swelling of the keratinocytes (Fig. 2.12). As the swelling increases, the cells become deformed and spherical and may develop homogeneous eosinophilic cytoplasm (ballooning degeneration). Further swelling results in cell rupture, with the remaining cell membranes becoming organized into a network pattern called reticular degeneration. Ballooning degeneration can be seen in viral eruptions such as herpes simplex infection and in hand, foot and mouth disease, and in the early stages of eczema and dermatitis.

Inclusion bodies

Inclusion bodies form by the aggregation of abnormal substances in cytoplasm (intracytoplasmic inclusion bodies) or in nuclei (intranuclear inclusion bodies). In keratinocytes, viral infection causes inclusion bodies. An example of the former is the molluscum body found in molluscum contagiosum (Fig. 23.18); the latter is found in herpes simplex and in cytomegalovirus infections as cytomegalic inclusion bodies (owl's eyes).

Acantholysis

Acantholysis refers to the separation of keratinocytes from the spinous or basal layer resulting from the dissociation of intercellular adhesion, particularly that of desmosomes. Intercellular spaces and blisters form, with acantholytic cells (spherical keratinocytes that have lost their intercellular adhesion) floating inside. Acantholytic cells have a tendency to become dyskeratotic (Fig. 2.13). This phenomenon can be observed in pemphigus, Hailey–Hailey disease, and Darier's disease.

Blisters

Blisters are subdivided into intraepidermal and subepidermal depending on the histological findings (Fig. 2.14). Intraepidermal blisters are classified by

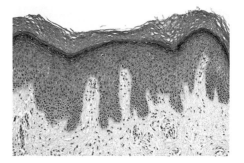

Fig. 2.6 Hyperkeratosis (Chronic eczema)

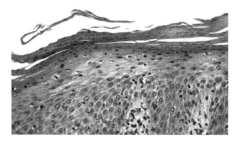

Fig. 2.7 Parakeratosis (Psoriasis vulgaris)

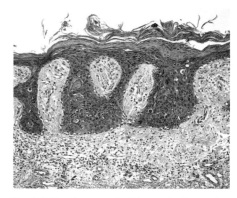

Fig. 2.8 Dyskeratosis (Bowen's disease)

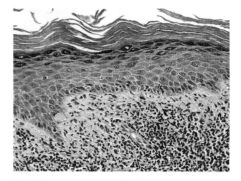

Fig. 2.9 Hypergranulosis (Parapsoriasis)

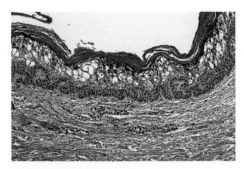

Fig. 2.10 Granular degeneration
(Epidermolytic ichthyosis)

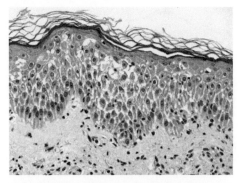

Fig. 2.11 Spongiosis (Acute eczema)

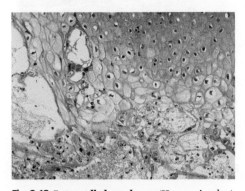

Fig. 2.12 Intracellular edema (Herpes simplex)

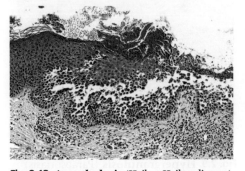

Fig. 2.13 Acantholysis (Hailey–Hailey disease)

pathomechanism into severe spongiosis (eczema/dermatitis group), prominent acantholysis (e.g., pemphigus), reticular degeneration (e.g., herpes infection), and basal cell degeneration (e.g., burns and epidermolysis bullosa simplex).

Diseases involving subepidermal blistering include burns, autoimmune bullous diseases such as bullous pemphigoid and dermatitis herpetiformis and inherited mechanobullous disorders such as epidermolysis bullosa (see Chapter 4).

Pustules

A pustule is a blister containing purulent components (mainly neutrophils). A small pustule below the stratum corneum is called a Munro's microabscess, which is a characteristic feature of psoriasis vulgaris (Fig. 2.15). A spongiform pustule is caused by damage to keratinocytes from neutrophilic infiltration and can be seen in pustular psoriasis (Kogoj's spongiform pustule) (Fig. 2.16). Pautrier's microabscess is produced by infiltration of malignant lymphocytes and is not a genuine pustule (refer to the following section).

Exocytosis (cell infiltration into the epidermis)

Exocytosis refers to the infiltration of inflammatory cells and erythrocytes into the epidermis. It is commonly seen in spongiosis. Infiltration of lymphocytes is seen in epidermal inflammatory diseases such as contact dermatitis and atopic dermatitis. Infiltration of multinucleated leukocytes is observed in impetigo contagiosa, palmoplantar pustulosis, and psoriasis.

In cutaneous T cell lymphomas such as mycosis fungoides, malignant T cells may infiltrate into the epidermis, forming a mass that does not become spongiform; this is called a Pautrier's microabscess (Fig. 2.17). In Langerhans cell histiocytosis, there is infiltration of Langerhans cells into the epidermis.

Dermal-epidermal junction
Liquefaction degeneration (vacuolar degeneration, hydropic degeneration)

Liquefaction degeneration occurs when the epidermal-dermal junction becomes vacuolated and ill-defined as a result of basal cell damage (Fig. 2.18). It is often accompanied by edema and lymphocytic infiltration and mainly occurs at the epidermal-dermal junction. When further aggravated, subepidermal blisters may form. As a result of basal cell damage, melanin granules may be released in the dermis, resulting in pigmentary incontinence (incontinentia pigmenti histologica). These granules are then phagocytosed by macrophages. Dyskeratosis caused by apoptotic keratinocytes is seen in erythema multiforme and lichen planus. An eosinophilic Civatte body with a diameter of 10 μm may be found immediately beneath the dermis (Fig. 2.18b).

Abnormalities of melanin synthesis

Production of melanin pigment in the basal epidermal layer is increased by exposure to ultraviolet radiation. Conversely, loss of melanin pigment results in leukoderma. Generally, a DOPA-oxidase or immunohistological test may be performed to diagnose abnormalities in melanin synthesis. The following are examples of disorders involving abnormalities in melanin synthesis.

- **Albinism:** a congenital abnormality of melanin synthesis (see Chapter 16).
- **Piebaldism (Waardenburg–Klein syndrome):** congenital deficiency of melanocytes in partial areas of the skin (see Chapter 16).
- **Idiopathic guttate hypomelanosis:** a functional reduction of melanocytes due to aging (see Chapter 16).
- **Nevus of Ota:** the presence of ectopic melanocytes in the dermis (see Chapter 20).
- **Chloasma:** an increase in melanin pigments in the epidermal basal cell layer caused by sex hormones (see Chapter 16).
- **Freckles:** functional increase of melanocytes (see Chapter 16).

Dermis

Inflammatory cell infiltration

Inflammatory cell infiltration occurs when inflammatory cells such as neutrophils, eosinophils, lymphocytes, plasmacytes, macrophages, and mast cells infiltrate the dermis. When the infiltrates are centered around blood vessels, it is known as perivascular infiltration. There are several infiltration patterns, including lichenoid (cells infiltrate in a band-like pattern, such as in lichen planus), vasculitic (the inflammation causes fibrinoid degeneration, blood clots or bleeding in the blood vessels; see Chapter 11) and nodular. The principal infiltrating cells and the causative diseases are shown in Table 2.2.

Granuloma

A granuloma consists of an aggregation of histiocytes (mostly macrophages) resulting in a focal chronic

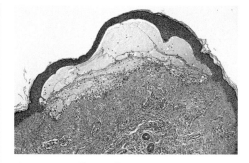

Fig. 2.14 Bulla (Bullous pemphigoid)

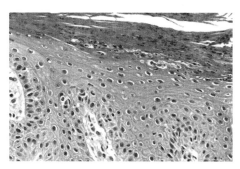

Fig. 2.15 Munro's microabscess (Psoriasis vulgaris)

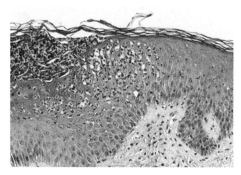

Fig. 2.16 Kogoj's spongiform pustule (Pustular psoriasis)

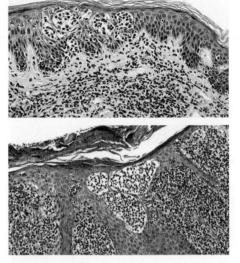

Fig. 2.17 Pautrier's microabscess (Mycosis fungoides)

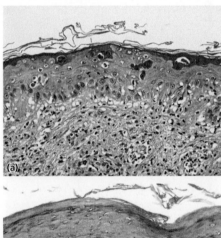

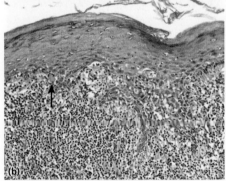

Fig. 2.18 Vacuolar degeneration. a: Graft-versus-host disease. Dyskeratosis is also seen from the apoptosis of the epidermal keratinocytes. b: Lichen planus. Civatte bodies are seen immediately below the epidermis (arrow).

inflammatory mass. The macrophages in granulomas are called epithelioid cells. In addition to macrophages, fibroblasts, degenerated connective tissue, and blood vessels may be observed in epithelioid granulomas. Granulomas are classified according to their distribution patterns and subtypes of inflammatory cells as described below.

Sarcoidal granuloma

The main components are epithelioid and giant cells. The granuloma contains few necrotic foci and slight lymphocytic infiltration. This is the typical epithelioid granuloma seen in sarcoidosis.

Tuberculoid granuloma

This is an epithelioid granuloma with caseous necrosis in the center and abundant lymphocytic infiltration at the periphery. The prototypical tuberculoid granuloma is seen in tuberculosis.

Palisading granuloma

The granuloma contains degenerated collagen fibers and mucin deposition in the center, with peripheral macrophages in a palisade or circular pattern. It is seen in granuloma annulare.

Suppurative granuloma

An abscess (neutrophilic infiltration) surrounded by macrophages and lymphocytes, it is found in deep mycoses.

Foreign body granuloma

Macrophages, neutrophils, and lymphocytes accumulate around foreign matter (e.g., glass, suture thread, animal hair, plant fibers) or an intrinsic body (e.g., elastic fibers, calcium deposits, cholesterol crystals). This inflammatory infiltrate constitutes a normal reaction to foreign bodies (Fig. 2.19). Giant cells that have phagocytosed a foreign body are often observed. The foreign body becomes buried in fibrous tissues over time.

Giant cells

Giant cell is the general term for cells that contain a characteristically large nucleus. Most giant cells are derived from macrophages and are multinucleated from the fusion of several macrophages or from repeated nuclear division (Fig. 2.20). Reed–Sternberg cells seen in Hodgkin's disease are a type of giant cell.

Table 2.2 Diseases with inflammatory infiltration into the skin.

Infiltrating cells	Disorders
Neutrophils	Early-stage inflammation: irritant contact dermatitis, erythema nodosum, etc.
	Infections: impetigo contagiosa, candidiasis, etc.
	Disorders associated with reactions of immunocomplex and complements: cutaneous small vessel vasculitis, Sweet's syndrome, Behçet's disease, dermatitis herpetiformis (Duhring)
Eosinophils	Early inflammation; incontinentia pigmenti
	Autoimmune diseases: pemphigus, bullous pemphigoid, etc.
	Type I allergy
	Malignant diseases: mycosis fungoides, Langerhans cell histiocytosis
Lymphocytes	Inflammations: allergic diseases, etc.
Plasma cells	Infections: syphilis, lymphogranuloma venereum, actinic keratosis, deep fungal infection, etc.
Histiocytes	Granulomatous diseases: sarcoidosis, granuloma annulare, etc.
Mast cells	Atopic dermatitis, chronic eczema, lichen planus, etc.
	Wounds (especially during healing), neurofibroma, etc.

Foreign body giant cells

Macrophages enlarge by phagocytosing foreign substances, and their nuclei become irregularly arranged.

Langhans giant cells

Syncytial macrophages with nuclei arranged regularly in a circular or horseshoe-shaped arrangement, they are often found in tuberculosis, sarcoidosis, and lichen nitidus.

Touton giant cells

These macrophages phagocytose fat tissue. The eosinophilic cytoplasm at the center of the cell is bordered by a ring of nuclei which are themselves surrounded by light, foamy cytoplasm. Touton giant cells are found in xanthogranuloma and xanthoma.

Changes in connective tissue

Fibrosis (irregular proliferation of fibroblasts and collagen fibers seen in scars and dermatofibroma) and sclerosis (decrease of fibroblasts, swelling or homogenization of collagen fibers seen in radiation dermatitis and systemic scleredema) are changes that affect collagen fibers. Changes that involve elastic fibers may be seen in photoaging and pseudoxanthoma elasticum.

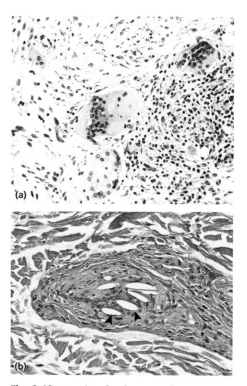

Fig. 2.19 Foreign-body granuloma.
a: Folliculitis. Giant cells are clearly seen.
b: Cholesterol crystal embolization (CCE) (blue toe syndrome). Cholesterin crystals (arrows).

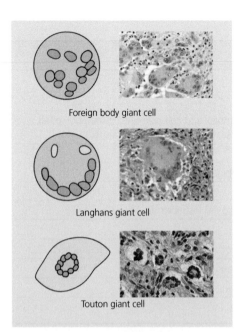

Fig. 2.20 Giant cells originating from histiocytes.

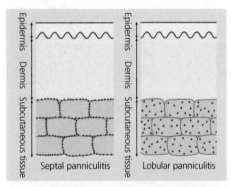

Fig. 2.21 Differences between septal panniculitis and lobular panniculitis.

Deposition of foreign substances

Deposits in the dermis include amyloids (e.g., in lichen amyloidosis), mucins (e.g., in myxedema, dermatomyositis), calcium (e.g., in pseudoxanthoma elasticum), hemosiderins (e.g., in bruising, angiitis, hemochromatosis), uric acid, and hyaline (see Chapter 17).

Subcutaneous fat tissue
Panniculitis

Panniculitis is an inflammation of the subcutaneous fat. It is classified according to the site of inflammation (Fig. 2.21). In septal panniculitis, inflammation occurs mostly in the septa of the subcutaneous fat tissue, as seen in erythema nodosum (Fig. 2.22). In lobular panniculitis, inflammation occurs in the lobules of the fat tissue such as that observed in erythema induratum (Fig. 2.23). Panniculitis can also occur in acute pancreatitis (see Chapter 18).

Other changes in fat tissue

Lipodystrophy, lipogranuloma, lipoatrophy, liponecrosis, lipolysis, lipoma, and liposarcoma are other changes that may involve fat tissue.

Immunohistochemistry

Immunohistochemical techniques are used to identify proteins in tissue by labeling them with specific antibodies. They have widespread uses in dermatology and can be employed for the identification of disease-causing autoantibodies. There are two main immunohistochemical methods: (1) immunofluorescence microscopy using fluorescent dyes, and (2) the immunoenzyme method. Antibodies frequently used in dermatology are listed in Table 2.3.

Immunofluorescence

Immunofluorescence (IF) is an immunological staining method that uses antibodies labeled with a fluorescent dye, such as fluorescein isothiocyanate (FITC), to detect a specific molecular marker. This technique is useful for detecting antigens, antibodies, and components of the complement system. IF techniques can be subdivided into the direct fluorescent antibody test, indirect fluorescent antibody test, and complement IF (Fig. 2.24).

Table 2.3 Antibodies frequently used in dermatology.

Marker	Positive skin component/ disorder
Cytokeratin (CK)	Epithelial cell
CAM5.2 (CK7+CK8)	Mesothelioma (negative in lung cancer)
Cytokeratin 20	Merkel cell
EMA (epidermal membrane antigen)	Epithelial cell
Vimentin	Mesenchymal cell
Desmin	Striated muscle, smooth muscle
α smooth muscle actin (SMA)	Striated muscle, smooth muscle
neuron-specific enolase (NSE)	Schwann cell, melanocyte cartilage
S-100 protein	Nerve fiber, paraganglionic cells, melanocyte
HMB45, MELAN A	Malignant melanoma
CEA (carcinoembryonic antigen, CD66e)	Sweat gland, gastrointestinal stromal tumor (GIST)
Ki-67 (Mib-1)	Proliferation marker of tumor cell
Factor VIII	Endothelial cell of the vessel
Factor XIIIa	Endothelial cell, dendritic cell, dermatofibroma
Gross cystic disease fluid protein (GCDFP)-15	Sweat gland
CD1a	Langerhans cells
CD3	T cell
CD4	Helper T cell
CD8	Cytotoxic T cell
CD20 (L26)	B cell
CD30 (Ki-1)	Hodgkin's disease, anaplastic large cell lymphoma
CD31	Leukemia
CD34	Endothelial cell, hemangioma, dermatofibrosarcoma protuberans
CD56	Natural killer cell
CD68	Macrophage, myeloid cell
CD79a	B cell
Cyclin D1	Mantle cell lymphoma

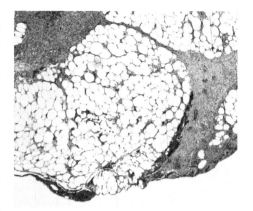

Fig. 2.22 Septal panniculitis (Erythema nodosum)

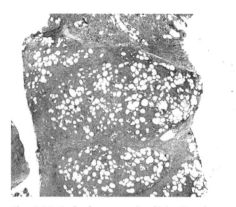

Fig. 2.23 Lobular panniculitis (Erythema induratum)

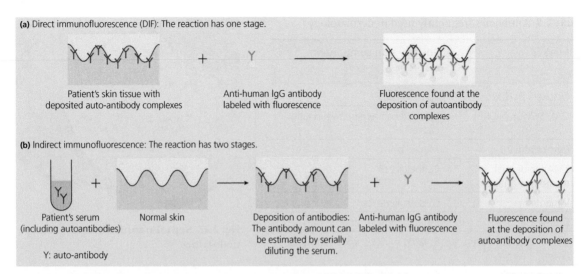

(a) Direct immunofluorescence (DIF): The reaction has one stage.

Patient's skin tissue with
deposited auto-antibody complexes

Anti-human IgG antibody
labeled with fluorescence

Fluorescence found at the
deposition of autoantibody
complexes

(b) Indirect immunofluorescence: The reaction has two stages.

Patient's serum
(including autoantibodies)   Normal skin

Deposition of antibodies:
The antibody amount can
be estimated by serially
diluting the serum.

Anti-human IgG antibody
labeled with fluorescence

Fluorescence found
at the deposition of
autoantibody complexes

Y: auto-antibody

Fig. 2.24 Mechanisms of immunofluorescence (bullous pemphigoid)

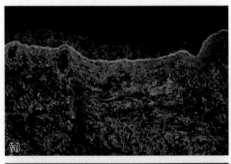

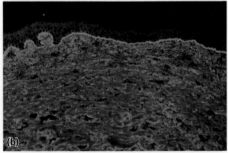

Fig. 2.25 Immunofluorescence (bullous pemphigoid). a: Direct immunofluorescence. Linear IgG deposition is seen along the basement membrane of the patient's skin. b: Indirect immunofluorescence (IIF). A 1/320 dilution of the patient's serum is used on the skin sample from a healthy person. Anti-basement membrane antibodies are seen in the blood.

Direct IF

This technique makes use of a single fluorescent-labeled antibody that detects a specific antigen. Detection of the antigen results in the release of fluorescence that can then be observed by fluorescence microscopy. This type of test is used for the in vivo detection of an autoantibody present in autoimmune diseases such as lupus erythematosus and bullous pemphigoid. Direct IF is also used for the detection of pathogenic microbes in tissues.

Indirect IF

Indirect IF is a two-phase technique in which a specific protein is bound with an unlabeled primary antibody which is then conjugated with a labeled secondary antibody (e.g., coupled with a fluorescent dye).

For example, in bullous pemphigoid, a circulating IgG autoantibody reacts directly with the cutaneous basement membrane of the patient (see Chapter 14). To diagnose bullous pemphigoid, both direct and indirect IF are used. Direct IF enables the detection of the antibody that reacts in the patient's skin in vivo. In contrast, using the indirect IF technique, normal human control skin is incubated with the patient's serum followed by labeling with a fluorescent-labeled secondary antibody (Fig. 2.25). Indirect IF is widely used not only in dermatology but also in other areas, including syphilis FTA-ABS tests (see Chapter 27), using normal skin as the substrate.

Complement IF

This technique involves a reaction between an unlabeled primary antibody and a target antigen. The antigen-antibody complex is then bound to the active serum complement. The final reaction involves the use of a labeled secondary antibody against a complement component, e.g., labeled anti-C3.

Immunoenzyme methods

In immunoenzyme methods, an enzyme rather than a fluorescent dye is conjugated with the antibody. Antigens, immunoglobulins, and complements can be detected using the enzyme reaction. Enzymes such as peroxidase are conjugated with an antibody to react against the target molecules in the tissue in the same way as in IF techniques. This enzyme catalyzes a color-producing reaction that allows the presence of the specific marker and its distribution to be detected.

Immunoenzyme methods have the following advantages over IF:

- the enzymatic reaction makes electron microscopic observation possible
- the reaction is easy to observe and has a high detection range
- the samples can be stored longer than those of IF.

Immunoenzyme methods can also be used on electron microscopic sections.

Electron microscopy and immunoelectron microscopy

The electron microscope allows the visualization of ultrastructural details in tissues by making use of electron beams instead of visible light. Electron microscopy (EM) and immuno-EM achieve magnifications of 1000 times and greater; therefore, they can be used to observe fine intracellular and intercellular structures that are not visible by light microscopy (Fig. 2.26).

The transmission electron microscope exposes an ultra-thin specimen to an electron beam. It is possible to achieve magnifications of 500,000 times. Immuno-EM makes use of a combination of immunostaining and electron microscopic observation and has greatly contributed to the advancement of dermatological science.

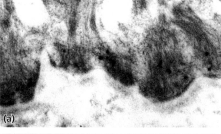

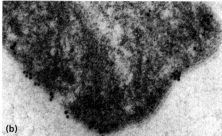

Fig. 2.26 Immunoelectron microscopy of the bullous antigen in normal human skin labeled with gold colloid. a: BP230 is immediately inside the basal cell membrane, a component of the hemidesmosome.
b: BP180 (type XVII collagen), a transmembrane protein in the basement membrane zone. NC16a, the most important domain for BP pathogenesis, is in the basal cell membrane.

In scanning EM, electron beams reflected from exposed tissue are captured. This technique is useful in revealing three-dimensional structure. However, the magnifying power is not as high as that of transmission EM.

MEMO 2–1 Skin biopsy considerations

A skin biopsy will result in scarring. The site and biopsy method must be carefully chosen in order to gain maximum information during histological examination as well as to minimize scar formation, especially when the biopsy is performed on cosmetically important sites or if the patient has a predisposition to keloid formation. It is also essential to keep good clinical records, e.g., photographing the lesion and obtaining informed consent from the patient after thoroughly explaining the necessity of the biopsy and the risks involved.

CHAPTER 3
Dermoscopy

Conventionally, megascopic inspection of the skin lesion has been the first step in diagnosing skin diseases, followed by pathological inspection using skin biopsy. In recent years, dermoscopy has become widespread as a third way of viewing skin lesions. Functionally, dermoscopy has a place between naked-eye observation and invasive skin biopsy. Dermoscopy is particularly useful for diagnosing pigmented lesions and skin tumors. The benefits of dermoscopy include the following:

- the relatively short time required for observation of the lesions
- the low cost and pocket-sized compactness of the devices
- the possibility of non-invasive examination.

To understand dermoscopic images, it is important to know the three-dimensional structure of normal skin and the pathology of diseases. This chapter discusses basic dermoscopic knowledge and representative diagnostic findings.

Dermoscope

A dermoscope is a magnifying glass with a light source. It magnifies by a factor of 10. Dermoscopy employs a simple, fundamental principle, and various types of products are commercially available (Fig. 3.1). To make records of findings, it is possible to take photos by using a camera attached to the eyepiece of the dermoscope. Specialized adaptors for cameras are also available. Commercially available models include those specially made for use with a camera (Fig. 3.1c) and digital all-in-one models.

A standard contact dermoscope (Fig. 3.1a), whose light is reflected by the stratum corneum, is used mainly for observation of the skin surface (Fig. 3.2a). Observation of skin lesions at the depth of the superficial dermis is possible by applying a transparent jelly to suppress skin surface reflectivity (Fig. 3.2b). This is the biggest difference between observation by dermoscopy and by simple magnifying glass.

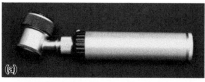
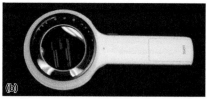
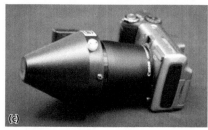
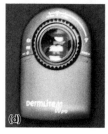
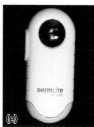

Fig. 3.1 Dermoscopes. a: Delta10 (Heine). b: Lumio (3Gen). c: Derma9500 (Derma Medical). d: DermLite II Pro (J. Hewitt). e: DermLiteDL100 (J. Hewitt).

Shimizu's Dermatology, Second Edition. Hiroshi Shimizu.
© 2017 John Wiley & Sons, Ltd. Published 2017 by John Wiley & Sons, Ltd.

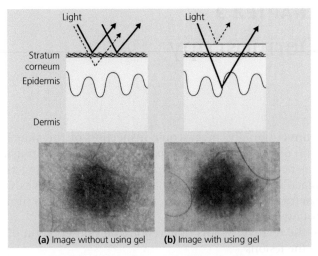

(a) Image without using gel   **(b)** Image with using gel

Fig. 3.2 Dermoscopic images (clarification by using gel)

Basically, it is the suppression of the reflection at the stratum corneum that enables dermoscopic examination. A widely used non-contact dermoscopy using cross-polarized light can show the subsurface morphology (Fig. 3.1d, e) in a simple way, which makes examination easier.

Diagnostic algorithm

Dermoscopy is particularly useful in diagnosing brown to black skin lesions. Four possibilities are considered as the first step. The four categories of features to be considered are melanocytic lesions, which show distinctive clinical features, are most commonly observed and can be benign or malignant (see Chapter 20); seborrheic keratosis (Chapter 21); basal cell carcinoma (see Chapter 22); and vascular lesions, including various types of hemangioma (see Chapter 21). When the lesion is melanocytic, for example, benignancy or malignancy is determined based on pattern analysis (the second step).

Observation should be done while keeping this two-step diagnostic procedure in mind (Fig. 3.3).

Among the benign or inflammatory lesions, which do not require the second step, there are some disorders for which clear clinical features for identification have not been established. This textbook discusses important clinical features necessary for two-step diagnosis.

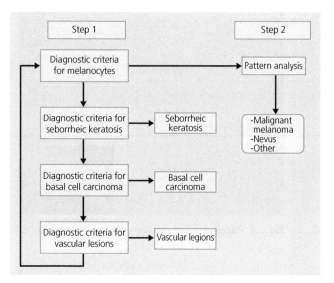

Fig. 3.3 Diagnostic algorithm (two-phase diagnosis)

Dermoscopic findings in melanocytic lesions

Parallel pattern
The sulci cutis and cristae cutis are parallel on skin of the palms and soles, and the epidermal rete ridges project into the dermis in both areas. The sweat glands open in the central zone of the crista cutis (Fig. 3.4).

Parallel furrow pattern (Fig. 3.5)
In benign nevus cell nevus, nevus cells, which have melanins, tend to aggregate in the epidermal rete ridges of the sulci cutis. The pigments are observed in the sulci cutis.

Parallel ridge pattern (Fig. 3.6)
Melanomas do not have regular patterns in the proliferation of their tumorous cells, and they show pigmentation that is irregular in shape and uneven in color. Denser pigmentation is observed in the cristae cutis, which are wider than the sulci cutis. Parallel ridge patterns are observed in the benign pigmented macules seen in patients with Peutz–Jeghers syndrome and drug eruptions. The pigmentation patterns of inherited nevus cell nevus, in which cells proliferate around the sweat ducts, often follow the parallel ridge pattern.

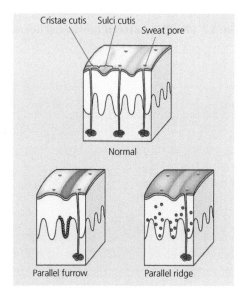

Fig. 3.4 Parallel pattern

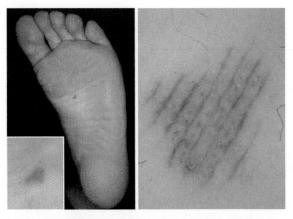

Fig. 3.5 Parallel furrow pattern (nevus cell nevus)

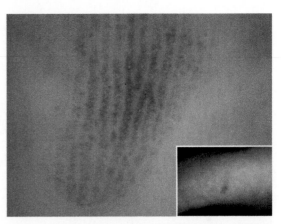

Fig. 3.6 Parallel ridge pattern (malignant melanoma)

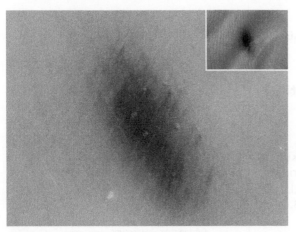

Fig. 3.7 Fibrillar pattern (nevus cell nevus)

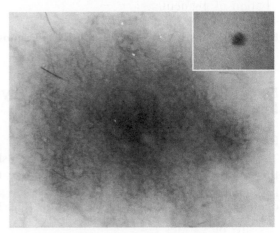

Fig. 3.8 Pigment network (nevus cell nevus)

Fibrillar pattern (Fig. 3.7)

In benign nevus cell nevus, a pigmented area that resembles a scratch mark is often observed, which is the result of external pressure that has caused diagonal migration of pigments from the original pigmentation, which was parallel to the sulci cutis.

Pigment network

Density variations in melanins are expressed in pigmentation that resembles a network (Fig. 3.8).

The typical pigment network has a symmetrical structure, whereas an atypical pigment network has an asymmetrical and inhomogeneous structure. In benign melanocytic nevi, the nevus cells tend to aggregate in the epidermal rete ridges, which results

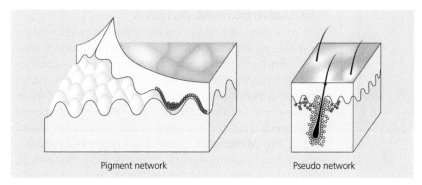

Fig. 3.9 Pigment network

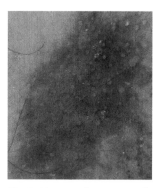

Fig. 3.10 Pseudo-network
(malignant melanoma)

in increased brownish pigmentation in those ridges and lighter pigmentation in the dermal papillae. The variation of pigmentation gives a network structure of homogeneous round or polygonal lines (Fig. 3.9). The nevus cells around the hair follicles have low melanin-producing ability, which results in lighter pigmentation around the follicles (pseudo-network; Fig. 3.10).

Dots and globules

Pigment cells that proliferate in the dermal papillae distribute as dots. The dots often aggregate densely. The larger dots are called globules (Fig. 3.11), and uniform globules make up what is called a cobblestone pattern (Fig. 3.12). These dots are often uniform in size in benign melanocytic nevi, but in melanomas the dots are of various sizes as a result of abnormal production of pigment cells and melanophages.

Streaks

Streaks are pigmentation that branches out or projects like sticks at the periphery of a lesion. In Spitz nevus, fine projections of pigmentation are observed at the entire periphery of the lesion, and this is referred to as a starburst pattern (Fig. 3.13). In melanomas, the streaks often form irregular shapes and are found at the periphery of the lesion.

Homogeneous pattern

Homogeneous pigmentation without any defined structure forms when pigment or cells that contain pigment proliferate in the epidermis or dermis. In blue nevus, the nevus cells of the dermis are seen as homogeneous blue pigmentation underlying epidermis that resembles a white veil (Fig. 3.14).

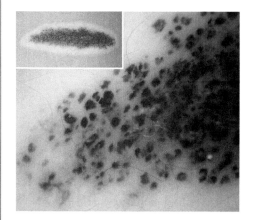

Fig. 3.11 Globules

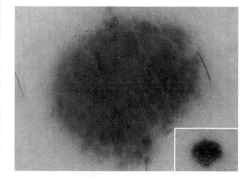

Fig. 3.12 Cobblestone pattern (nevus cell nevus)

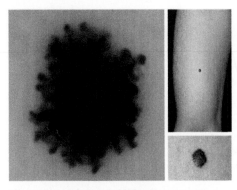

Fig. 3.13 Streaks: starburst pattern
(Spitz nevus)

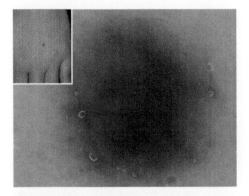

Fig. 3.14 Homogeneous pattern:
homogeneous blue pigmentation
(blue nevus)

Multicomponent pattern

The majority of benign melanocytic nevi present as dermoscopically homogeneous. Multicomponent patterns may be found in one or two types of the melanocytic lesions described above. Multicomponent pattern refers to a condition of lesion in which three or more dermoscopic features are present. Melanoma should be suspected if a multicomponent pattern is found (Fig. 3.15). Melanoma is suspected when the melanocytic lesion presents dermoscopically as asymmetrical, irregular, partly faded or without any commonly observed patterns.

Dermoscopic findings in seborrheic keratosis

Comedo-like opening

A comedo-like opening corresponds to the keratotic plug that is pathologically observed in seborrheic keratosis (see Chapter 21). Brownish to black, sharply circumscribed keratin plugs of various sizes are found (Fig. 3.16: arrows).

Multiple milia-like cysts

Multiple milia-like cysts correspond to the pseudo-horn cysts of seborrheic keratosis. White, vaguely circumscribed dots are found in a brownish lesion (Fig. 3.17: arrows). The name comes from the resemblance to the milium (see Chapter 21). This type of lesion is sometimes found in basal cell carcinoma and squamous cell carcinoma.

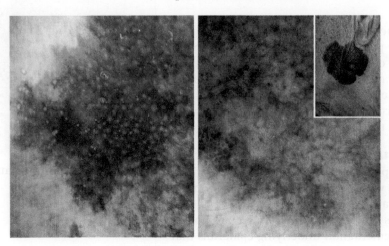

Fig. 3.15 Multicomponent pattern: malignant melanoma

Fingerprint-like structures (light brown)

Fingerprint structures are observed in early seborrheic keratosis. They have a flat appearance. Light brown macules with clear boundaries are found at the peripheries of the lesion. The macules have a fingerprint-like pattern (Fig. 3.18: arrows). It is thought that the fingerprint structures reflect senile lentigo as a precursory symptom of seborrheic keratosis (see Chapter 16).

Cerebriform pattern, brain-like appearance (fissured and ridged)

When seborrheic keratosis exhibits papillomatosis, the surface of the lesion takes on a wrinkled, brain-like appearance (Fig. 3.19).

Dermoscopic findings in basal cell carcinoma

Arborizing vessels

Branching or lightening bolt-like vessels of irregular thickness are observed, which indicate extensions of the capillary blood vessels into the dermal papillae. This feature is useful in diagnosing basal cell carcinomas in people with lightly pigmented skin (Fig. 3.20). It is necessary to place the dermoscope carefully on the lesion to view the capillary vessels. If too much pressure is applied to the lesion, the extended vessels are not visible.

Spoke wheel areas

Spoke wheel areas are observed in superficial basal cell carcinomas. Radial projections form, which reflect a tumorous lesion in the epidermis. Generally, multiple wheel-like pigmentations connect to form rings (Fig. 3.21).

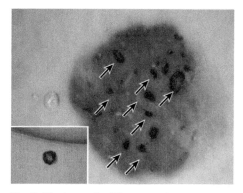

Fig. 3.16 Comedo-like opening.

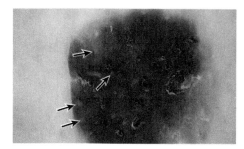

Fig. 3.17 Multiple milia-like cysts.

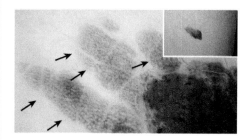

Fig. 3.18 Fingerprint-like structures: light-brown

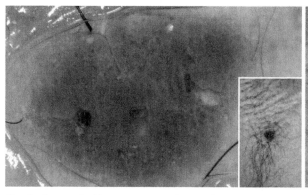
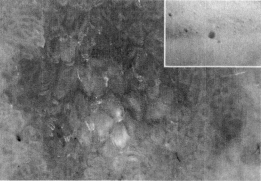

Fig. 3.19 Cerebriform pattern/brain-like appearance (with fissure and ridges).

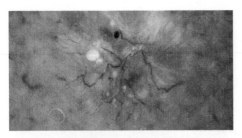

Fig. 3.20 Arborizing vessels

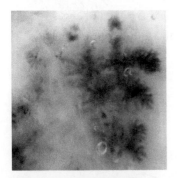

Fig. 3.21 Spoke wheel areas

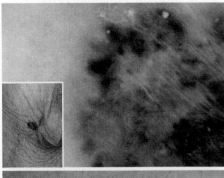

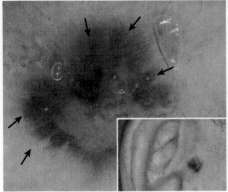

Fig. 3.22 Leaf-like structures

Leaf-like structures

When the tumorous cells in the surface area of the epidermis, which appear as spoke wheel areas, further proliferate throughout the epidermis, the pigmentation forms a structure that resembles a leaf (Fig. 3.22).

Multiple blue-gray globules/large blue-gray ovoid nests

Both of these represent essentially the same clinical condition. When light is shone on the tumorous lesion in the dermis, an aggregation of bluish pigmentation covered with a white veil is observed (Fig. 3.23). When a single nest is formed, the dermoscopic findings resemble those of blue nevus, but differentiation is possible in many cases because these lesions often have arborizing vessels.

Ulcer

Rodent ulcers tend to form in basal cell carcinomas, and it is possible to find early ulcers by dermoscopy.

Dermoscopic findings in vascular lesions, including hemorrhages

Red-blue lacunae

Angiokeratomas (see Chapter 21) appear blackish to the naked eye, which makes it necessary to differentiate them from basal cell carcinomas.

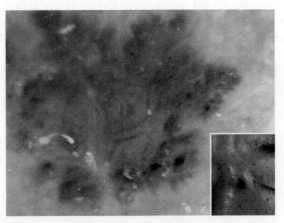

Fig. 3.23 Multiple blue-gray globules/large blue-gray ovoid nests.

In dermoscopy, however, an aggregation of round reddish-blue structures is shown, which reflects the dilated vascular cavity in the upper dermal layer (Fig. 3.24).

Reddish-blue to reddish-black homogeneous areas

Some hematomas without subjective symptoms blacken over time and require differentiation from melanocytic lesions. In dermoscopic images, a blackish hematoma has reddish parts that reflect the color of blood, based on which it is possible to determine that the blackish lesion arises from bleeding (Fig. 3.25). Black heel or subcutaneous hemorrhage on the heel caused by trauma is hard to differentiate from nevus cell nevus or melanoma by the naked eye; however, it is easily differentiated by dermoscopy.

Dotted vessels in the paronychium

Dotted vessels or extended capillaries may be observed in collagen diseases including systemic scleredema and dermatomyositis. The dotted vessels are easily observable by dermoscopy (Fig. 3.26).

Linear vessels

In spider telangiectasia (see Chapter 21), dermoscopy provides a detailed observation of radially extending vessels (Fig. 3.27).

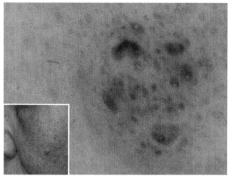

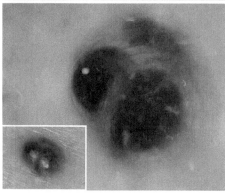

Fig. 3.24 Red-blue lacunae (angiokeratomas)

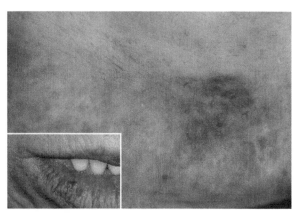

Fig. 3.25 Red-bluish to reddish-black homogeneous areas (venous lake)

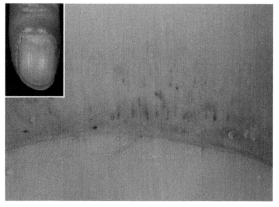

Fig. 3.26 Dotted vessels in the paronychium (dermatomyositis)

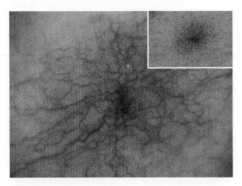

Fig. 3.27 Linear vessels (spider telangiectasia)

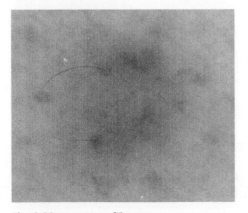

Fig. 3.28 Dermatofibroma

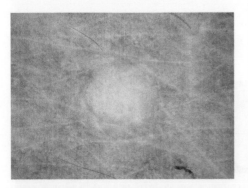

Fig. 3.29 White fibrous papulosis of the neck

Dermoscopic findings in other cutaneous diseases

Dermatofibroma
In dermatofibroma (see Chapter 21), which is not melanocytic, a delicate pigment network that reflects pigmentation in the basal cell layer forms (Fig. 3.28). The central white patch reflects the fibrosis.

Plantar wart
Diagnosis for plantar wart (see Chapter 23) often requires differentiation from clavus (see Chapter 15). Surface scraping of the plantar wart causes petechiae.

Scabies
Identification of scabies (see Chapter 28) is possible by careful observation for the presence of mite burrows and the brown, triangular mite at the leading end of the burrow.

White fibrous papulosis of the neck
Dermoscopic findings of white fibrous papulosis of the neck (see Chapter 18) are unique white homogeneous patterns with clear boundaries (Fig. 3.29).

CHAPTER 4
Description of skin lesions

Cutaneous examination involves thorough visual inspection, as well as palpation, of any skin lesions. Although developments in immunohistochemistry and histology have greatly assisted the diagnosis of skin diseases, physical examination coupled with dermoscopic examination provides important information on the nature of skin lesions, including their distribution, form, color, shape, and firmness.

Visible skin lesions are called eruptions. Eruptions are divided into primary lesions and secondary lesions. This chapter covers the terminology used for describing the various skin lesions.

Primary skin lesions

An eruption that occurs in normal skin is called a primary lesion. These include patches, where the only change is color; papules, nodules, and tumors, which are elevated; blisters, cysts, and pustules, which contain serum, keratinized substances, pus, etc.; and wheals, which are temporarily elevated.

Erythema

Erythema is a patchy redness produced by vasodilation and hyperemia in the dermal papillae and subpapillary layer (Fig. 4.1 and Fig. 4.2). Although the blood volume increases in the dermal blood vessels, there is no blood leakage in the dermis. Thus,

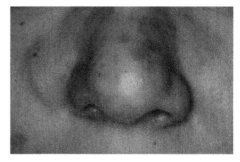

Fig. 4.1 Erythema (Annular erythema in a patient with Sjögren syndrome)

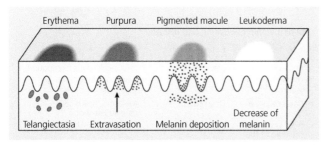

Fig. 4.2 Skin lesions. Macule colors and their respective changes.

MEMO 4–1 Unusual erythema and purpura

Bleeding may occur in the superficial epidermis, making the epidermis appear red. Unlike in the usual erythema, the redness does not fade by diascopy. Vasodilation may occur in the deep dermal layer, making that layer appear purple.

Shimizu's Dermatology, Second Edition. Hiroshi Shimizu.

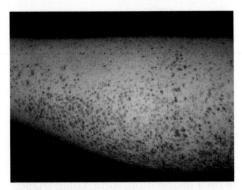

Fig. 4.3 Purpura (Henoch–Schönlein purpura)

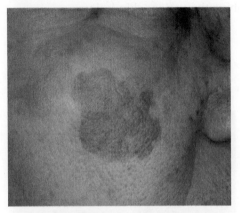

Fig. 4.4 Pigmented macule (Senile freckle)

erythema fades when a glass slide is pressed against the skin surface (diascopy).

Purpura

A purpura is a purple to bright red hemorrhagic lesion in the skin (Fig. 4.3; see also Fig. 4.2). The color of the blood does not fade during diascopy, because of blood leakage in the dermis, which distinguishes it from erythema. A purpura of 2 mm or less in diameter is called a petechia. A large purpuric lesion (10–30 mm) is called an ecchymosis, and an even larger elevated purpura is called a hematoma. A purpuric lesion is bright red (from the hemoglobin) shortly after bleeding begins but becomes brown (from hemosiderin) over time. When macrophages phagocytose and decompose the leaked blood cells, the color gradually fades.

Macule

A macule is a small flat skin lesions (less than 10 mm in diameter). Its color depends on the deposited substance (Fig. 4.4; see also Fig. 4.2). It is most commonly caused by the deposition of melanin. Other causes include hemosiderin, carotene, bile pigments, drugs, and other foreign substances (e.g., metal, charcoal).

Increased melanin deposition in the epidermal basal layer results in the formation of a brown to black macule, whereas increased deposition in the papillary

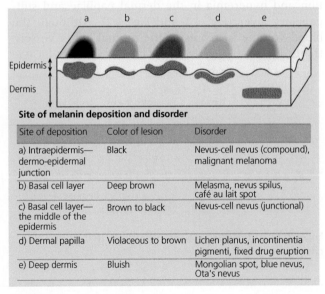

Site of melanin deposition and disorder

Site of deposition	Color of lesion	Disorder
a) Intraepidermis—dermo-epidermal junction	Black	Nevus-cell nevus (compound), malignant melanoma
b) Basal cell layer	Deep brown	Melasma, nevus spilus, café au lait spot
c) Basal cell layer—the middle of the epidermis	Brown to black	Nevus-cell nevus (junctional)
d) Dermal papilla	Violaceous to brown	Lichen planus, incontinentia pigmenti, fixed drug eruption
e) Deep dermis	Bluish	Mongolian spot, blue nevus, Ota's nevus

Fig. 4.5 Association between the site of melanin deposition and the color of the lesion.

dermis produces a gray to purplish-brown macule. Melanin deposition in the deep dermal layer results in the formation of a bluish macule. The sites of melanin pigmentation in various diseases are listed in Fig. 4.5.

Leukoderma

Leukoderma is a white patch produced by the total absence of melanin (a completely hypopigmented macule). Oculocutaneous albinism type 1A, congenital absence of melanin, piebaldism, and acquired vitiligo (Fig. 4.6) are disorders with total depigmentation (see Chapter 16). Whitish patches from decreased melanin after inflammation are called partial depigmentation. Depigmentation surrounding an eruption is called a white halo.

White patches sometimes result from ischemia (nevus anemicus: see Chapter 2).

Papule

Papules are localized elevated lesions with a diameter of 10 mm or less (Fig. 4.7 and Fig. 4.8). The surface can be smooth, eroded, ulcerated, hyperkeratotic or crusted. They may be caused by a proliferative lesion or by an inflammatory process in the epidermis, or even by dermal edema. Papules can be characterized as serous (with a vesicle on the top, e.g., eczema and dermatitis), solid (without blistering, e.g., neoplastic lesions, dermal edema), follicular (associated with hair follicles) or nonfollicular (not associated with hair follicles).

Nodule and tumor

Nodules are localized elevated lesions of 10–20 mm in diameter (Fig. 4.9). An intensely proliferative nodule with a diameter of 30 mm or more is called a tumor.

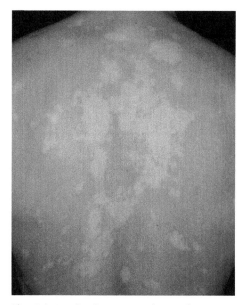

Fig. 4.6 Leukoderma (Vitiligo vulgaris)

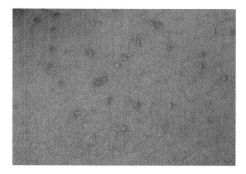

Fig. 4.8 Papule (Lichen nitidus)

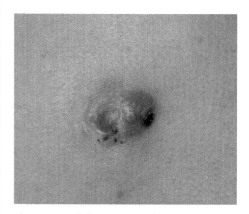

Fig. 4.9 Nodule (Dermatofibrosarcoma protuberans)

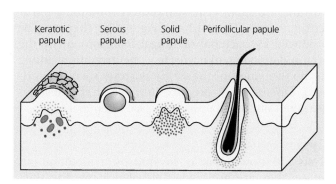

Keratotic papule   Serous papule   Solid papule   Perifollicular papule

Fig. 4.7 Various papules.

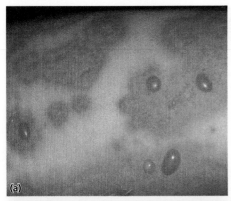

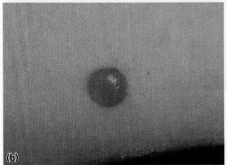

Fig. 4.11 Blisters. a: Bullous pemphigoid. b: Insect bite.

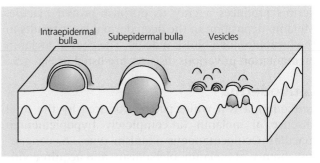

Fig. 4.10 Blisters.

Blister and vesicle

A blister is an elevated skin lesion that is enclosed by a membrane and contains transparent fluid consisting mainly of plasma and cellular material. A small blister of less than 5 mm in diameter is called a vesicle (Fig. 4.10 and Fig. 4.11).

A blister with a flaccid covering breaks easily. A flaccid blister is often produced by separation of the prickle cell layer (e.g., in pemphigus or impetigo contagiosa). A tense blister forms beneath the dermo-epidermal junction and has a thick, tight covering (e.g., in pemphigoid or dermatitis herpetiformis). It does not break as easily as a flaccid blister. During an infectious episode, a blister with a central concavity may be observed.

Blisters on the palms and soles present a droplet-like appearance, since they are surrounded by thick palmar and plantar hyperkeratosis. Such blisters are called pompholyx. Pompholyx with painful erosion and peripheral erythema in the mucous membrane is categorized as aphthae (see Fig. 4.25).

Pustule

Pustules are small yellowish blisters containing purulent materials (Fig. 4.12 and Fig. 4.13). They may be produced by bacterial or fungal infections or by the accumulation of leukocytes (e.g., neutrophils resulting in the formation of the sterile pustules seen in psoriasis). Diseases that produce multiple sterile pustules are generally called pustuloses (see Chapter 14).

Cyst

Cysts are closed lesions covered by a membranous lining; they are not always elevated above the skin. The covering consists of epithelial or connective tissue that encloses keratinized substances (e.g., in epidermal

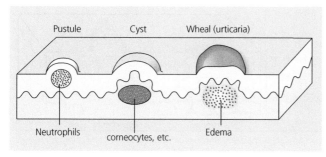

Fig. 4.12 Pustule, cyst, and wheal.

cysts) or fluid (e.g., in eccrine and apocrine hydrocystomas) (Fig. 4.14; see also Fig. 4.12).

Wheal

Wheals are localized edema that disappears after a short period of time (usually within several hours, and always within 24 h). They usually appear light pink and slightly elevated. They are accompanied by itching and heal without scarring (Fig. 4.15; see also Fig. 4.12). The terms "wheal" and "urticaria" are often use synonymously, although the former refers to a skin lesion, whereas the latter is the name of the disorder that presents with this eruption (see Chapter 8).

Secondary skin lesions

A secondary skin lesion is an eruption that occurs after a primary skin eruption.

Atrophy

Atrophy occurs when the skin becomes thin, resulting in a smooth or finely wrinkled surface (Fig. 4.16 and Fig. 4.17). The secretory function is also reduced, producing dryness of the skin surface. Processes that can lead to skin atrophy include aging, lipoatrophia, striae distensae, and atrophoderma maculatum.

Scales

Scales are produced by abnormal thickening of the skin surface that results in the formation of white lamellae from the accumulation of stratum corneum. Detachment of the stratum corneum from the skin surface is called desquamation. Under normal circumstances, desquamation of the stratum corneum cannot be observed by the naked eye, since each layer exfoliates individually. However, in diseases such as

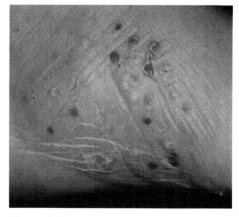

Fig. 4.13 Pustule (Palmoplantar pustulosis: localized pustular psoriasis)

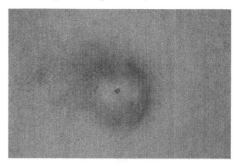

Fig. 4.14 Cyst (Epidermal cyst)

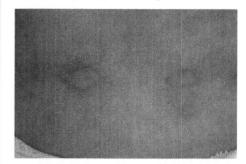

Fig. 4.15 Wheal (Acute urticaria)

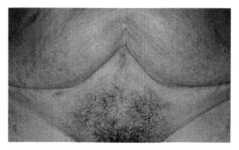

Fig. 4.16 Atrophy (Widespread striae atrophicae)

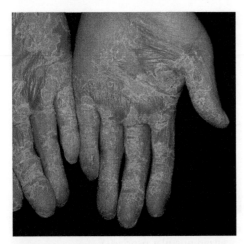

Fig. 4.18 Scaling (Psoriasis vulgaris)

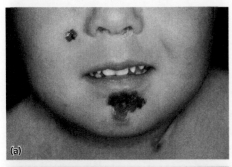

(a)

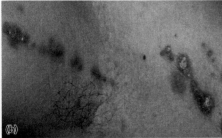

(b)

Fig. 4.19 Crusts. a: Epidermolysis bullosa simplex. b: Psoriasis vulgaris.

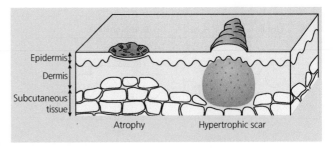

Fig. 4.17 Atrophy and hypertrophic scar.

psoriasis, scales are seen from the simultaneous exfoliation of multiple layers (Fig. 4.18).

Fine scaling is called pityriasis. Thick silver-gray scales called micaceous scales may be visible in psoriasis. Fish-like scales are called ichthyosiform scales.

There are two mechanisms of scale formation: retention hyperkeratosis and proliferation hyperkeratosis. In retention hyperkeratosis, such as in ichthyosis (see Chapter 15), the layers in the stratum corneum are too cohesive to desquamate individually and so detach as large scales after abnormal accumulation. In proliferation hyperkeratosis, such as in psoriasis (see Chapter 15), the epidermis exfoliates abnormally from overproliferation of keratinocytes.

Crust

Crusts are produced from solidified keratin and exudates; they form on eroded or ulcerated skin (Fig. 4.19). A crust consisting of dried blood is called a scab.

Callus

A callus is a localized, thickened hyperkeratotic lesion. A corn is one type of callus (see Chapter 15).

Clavus

In clavus, the stratum corneum becomes wedged into the skin by prolonged physical stimulation, such as pressure produced by wearing shoes for long periods of time. It is commonly called a corn (see Chapter 15).

Scar

Scarring is a reactive process that occurs when there is damage to the dermis. It results in the proliferation of dermal fibroblasts and the production of collagen fibers (see Fig. 4.17). A hypertrophic scar is a thickened scar that is confined to the margin of the wound.

In contrast, a keloid scar is a thickened scar that extends beyond the wound site (Fig. 4.20). The tendency of keloid scars to spread into surrounding normal skin distinguishes them from hypertrophic scars.

Excoriation

Excoriations are the result of partial damage to the epidermis by injury or scratching.

They heal without scarring since tissue damage is superficial.

Erosion

Erosions are an epidermal excoriations that extend down to the basal cell layer and heal without scarring. They often develop after the rupture of a blister or pustule (Fig. 4.21 and Fig. 4.22) and are commonly seen in the mucous membranes. They appear red and are infiltrated with serous fluid in most cases. They occur in diseases that cause intraepidermal blistering, such as impetigo contagiosa, pemphigus, epidermolysis bullosa simplex and herpes simplex infection, and in conditions that cause subepidermal blistering, such as pemphigoid, burns, and spontaneous intensely itchy eruptions (e.g., dermatitis herpetiformis, atopic dermatitis).

Ulcer

Ulcers form as a result of the complete loss of epidermis and/or a part of dermis, and they may even extend down to the subcutaneous fat (Fig. 4.23; see also Fig. 4.22). During the healing process, granulation tissue forms at the ulcer site and a scar forms. The base of an ulcer often has bleeding points, serous exudates, and crusts. Ulceration occurs as a secondary phenomenon, such as in vascular disorders (e.g., stasis dermatitis, collagen vascular diseases, vasculitis, peripheral arterial disease, and diabetes), infections, and malignancies.

Fissure

A fissure is a thin linear cleavage running through the deep epidermal layer and the dermis (Fig. 4.24; see also Fig. 4.22). It may be seen in disorders such as chronic eczema involving the hands and feet, psoriasis, and angular cheilitis. It tends to occur in the hands and feet, in intertriginous areas, near joints, and at mucocutaneous junctions.

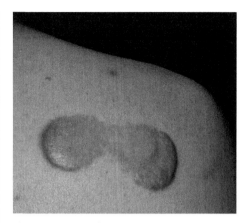

Fig. 4.20 Keloid

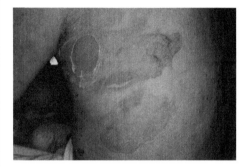

Fig. 4.21 Erosion (Bullous pemphigoid)

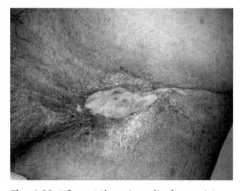

Fig. 4.22 Ulcer (Chronic radiochematic)

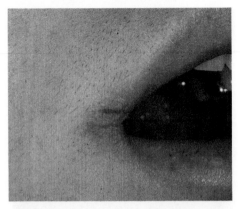

Fig. 4.24 Fissure (Angular cheilitis)

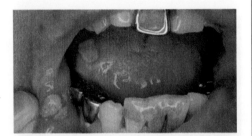

Fig. 4.25 Aphtha (Patient with Behçet's disease)

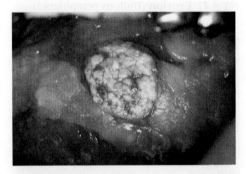

Fig. 4.26 Leukoplakia.

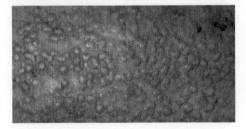

Fig. 4.27 Lichen (Lichen amyloidosis)

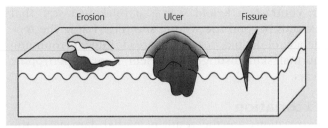

Fig. 4.23 Ulcer. Chronic radiation dermatitis. [was Fig. 4.22]

Enanthema

An enanthema is a lesion of the mucous membranes such as the oral mucosa, conjunctiva, and external genitalia. Specific types are listed below.

Aphtha

An aphtha is a painful, sharply circumscribed, round erosion of 1 cm or less in diameter in the mucous membrane (Fig. 4.25). It is accompanied by a peripheral inflammatory flush. It heals without scarring. Deep ulcers are not considered aphtha. Diseases that cause aphtha are viral infections (e.g., herpes simplex, varicella, hand-foot-and-mouth disease) and Behçet's disease (see Chapter 11). Physical irritation by poorly fitting dentures is another cause.

Leukoplakia

A leukoplakia is a white patch of abnormal keratinization of the mucosal epithelium (Fig. 4.26). It may be benign or precancerous (see Chapter 22).

Lesions with elevation of the skin

Lichen

Lichens are multiple aggregated papules of 5 mm or less in diameter that persist longer than 1 month without progressing to another type of lesion (Fig. 4.27). Lichens are classified into lichen planus, lichen nitidus, lichen spinulosus, lichen striatus (see Chapter 15), lichen amyloidosis, lichen sclerosus (see Chapter 18), lichen myxedematosus (see Chapter 17), and lichen scrofulosorum (see Chapter 26). Atypical lichen-like skin lesions are called lichenoid eruptions.

Lichenification

Lichenification refers to the thickening and hardening of skin resulting from chronic scratching or rubbing. Both the sulci cutis and cristae cutis are clearly observed (Fig. 4.28). Lichenification is often produced as a plaque (see next section) that is called a lichenified plaque. Lichenification is seen in chronic eczema, lichen simplex chronicus (lichen Vidal), and atopic dermatitis (see Chapter 7).

Plaques

A plaque is a slightly elevated skin lesion of 2–3 cm in diameter (Fig. 4.29). The surface may be flat or papillomatous, and the shape may be round, oval or atypical.

Papilloma

A papilloma is a protrusion that is covered by either epidermal or mucosal epithelium. Connective tissue containing capillaries may also be present. Since it is protrusive, a papilloma is susceptible to injury and infection. Elevated lesions arising from the glandular epithelium are usually called polyps.

Condyloma

Condylomas are aggregations of soft nodules with a papillary or granular surface (Fig. 4.30). They are mostly seen in the mucous membranes, such as those of the external genitals. Typical condylomas are condyloma acuminatum, caused by human papilloma virus (HPV) (see Chapter 23), and condyloma lata, caused by syphilis (see Chapter 27).

Lesions associated with hair follicles

Acne

Acne is an inflammatory lesion arising at a hair follicle; it is characterized by erythema or pustules (Fig. 4.31). It is usually accompanied by blackheads or whiteheads (comedones) and frequently occurs in seborrheic zones of the skin. The term "acne" usually refers to acne vulgaris (see Chapter 19); other types of acne include oil-induced acne, iodine-induced acne (the follicle is blocked by iodine secreted after chronic ingestion of iodine), steroid-induced acne (from chronic use of topical and systemic corticosteroids), and drug-induced acne (see Table 10.1).

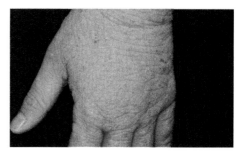

Fig. 4.28 Lichenification (Atopic dermatitis)

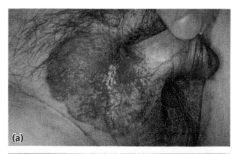

(a)

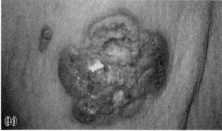

(b)

Fig. 4.29 Plaque. a: Extramammary Paget's disease. b: Mycosis fungoides.

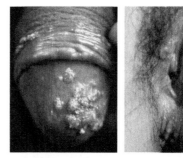

Fig. 4.30 Condyloma (Left: Condyloma acuminatum. Right: Condyloma latum)

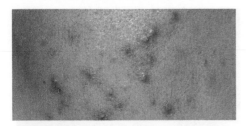

Fig. 4.31 Acne (Acne vulgaris)

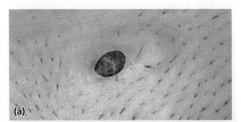

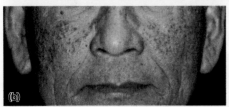

Fig. 4.32 Comedo. a: Solitary giant comedo. b: Favre–Racouchot syndrome.

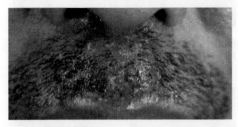

Fig. 4.33 Sycosis (Sycosis vulgaris)

Fig. 4.34 Erythroderma (Patient with Hodgkin's disease)

Comedo

Comedones are small papules that result from the blockage of a hair follicle by sebum (Fig. 4.32). They can be closed (whitehead) or open (blackhead). Comedones frequently occur on the face of elderly persons. A plaque of multiple aggregated comedones on the face of chronically sun-exposed individuals is observed in Favré–Racouchot disease.

Sycosis

Sycosis is a chronic inflammation of the hair follicles of terminal hair; it is characterized by nodules and pustules that may coalesce into a plaque (Fig. 4.33). The main types are sycosis vulgaris and sycosis trichophytica (see Chapter 25).

Lesions with color changes

Erythroderma

Erythroderma occurs when more than 90% of the skin surface develops erythema (Fig. 4.34). Often accompanied by scaling, erythroderma may also be called exfoliative dermatitis (see Chapter 9).

Melanosis

Melanosis is large and vaguely marginated pigmentation on the skin surface and includes friction melanosis and Riehl's melanosis (see Chapter 16).

Livedo (livedo reticularis)

Livedos are large networks of red to light brown lesions caused by the hypotonicity of the venous network and hypertonicity of the arterial network at the junction of the dermis and subcutaneous fat (Fig. 4.35). They occur as a physiological response or as a secondary symptom of an underlying medical condition, such as vasculitis (see Chapter 11).

Lesions accompanied by multiple blisters and pustules

Herpetiform lesion

Herpetiform lesions are characterized by aggregated vesicles and small pustules (Fig. 4.36). They resemble the lesions seen in cutaneous herpes simplex and herpes zoster infections (see Chapter 23). Herpetiform lesions may also be observed in dermatitis herpetiformis and herpes gestationis (see Chapter 14).

Impetigo

Impetigo is a combination of pustules and crusts that may be accompanied by erythema and small blisters (Fig. 4.37). Impetigo may be seen in highly infectious dermatitis, such as impetigo contagiosa (see Chapter 24).

Lesions associated with changes in the stratum corneum

Pityriasis

Pityriasis is characterized by fine scaling caused by abnormal keratinization (Fig. 4.38). It includes pityriasis rosea (see Chapter 15), pityriasis simplex faciei (see Chapter 7) and pityriasis rotunda.

Xerosis

Xerosis refers to rough, dry skin caused by diminished secretion of sebum and sweat. Pityroid scales and shallow cracks may develop, giving an ichthyosis-like appearance and mild itching. In winter, severely itchy asteatotic eczema (see Chapter 7) may occur as a complication because of the decreased skin barrier function. Aging and excess washing of sebum relate to this symptom. Hereditary xeroderma pigmentosum is a type of xerosis (see Chapter 13).

Ichthyosis

Ichthyosis is thick, dry scaling that causes the skin to resemble glued-on fish scales (Fig. 4.39). The various ichthyoses include congenital and acquired disorders (see Chapter 15).

Lesions accompanied by other changes

Poikiloderma

Poikiloderma describes the combination of skin atrophy, hypopigmentation, hyperpigmentation, and telangiectasia (Fig. 4.40). It is often observed at the terminal stages of several skin disorders. Poikiloderma

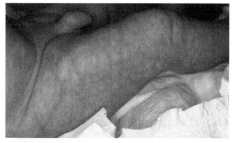

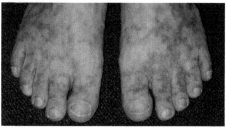

Fig. 4.35 Livedo reticularis.

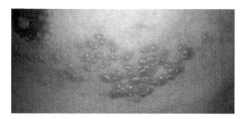

Fig. 4.36 Herpes (Herpes zoster)

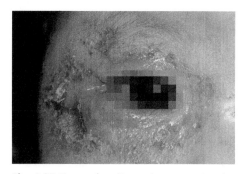

Fig. 4.37 Impetigo (Impetigo contagiosa)

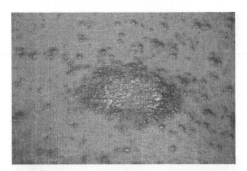

Fig. 4.38 Pityriasis (Pityriasis rosea)

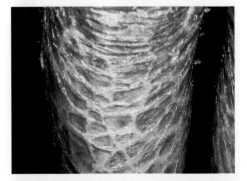

Fig. 4.39 Ichthyosis (Lamellar ichthyosis)

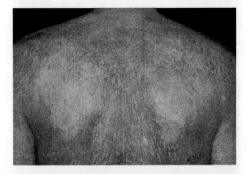

Fig. 4.40 Poikiloderma (Dermatomyositis)

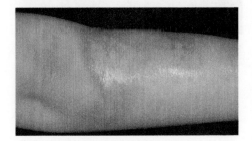

Fig. 4.41 Sclerosis (Morphea)

occurs in dermatomyositis, scleroderma, systemic lupus erythematosus (SLE) (see Chapter 12), chronic radiodermatitis and xeroderma pigmentosum (see Chapter 13), and mycosis fungoides (Chapter 22). Congenital poikiloderma is seen in Rothmund–Thomson syndrome (see Chapter 18).

Sclerosis

Sclerosis is the thickening of the skin caused by proliferation of connective tissues such as collagen and extracellular matrix (Fig. 4.41). It is seen in scleroderma, scleredema adultorum, and lichen myxedematosus (see Chapter 17). Pathologically, there is a decrease in the number of fibroblasts, and collagen fibers become swollen or uniform in size.

Seborrhea

Seborrhea occurs when there is an increase in sebum accumulation on the skin surface as a result of increased secretion. This tends to lead to bacterial infection, acne vulgaris (see Chapter 19), infantile eczema, and seborrheic dermatitis (see Chapter 7); however, seborrhea itself does not present with inflammatory symptoms. Sites that are densely distributed with sebaceous glands, such as the head, face, upper chest, middle of the back, armpits, and external genitalia, are called seborrheic zones.

The severity depends greatly on genetic factors and predisposition. Androgens are known to enhance sebum discharge. Physiologically, seborrhea is most prevalent in newborn infants and in adolescents. Seborrhea is known to have an increased incidence in patients with Parkinson's disease or AIDS.

Alopecia

Alopecia is a condition in which there is sparse or absent hair growth (Fig. 4.42). The major types of alopecia are alopecia areata, male-pattern baldness, and telogen effluvium (see Chapter 19).

Pruritus

Pruritus is itching without eruptions. It is also called pruritus cutaneous (see Chapter 8), and it may occur secondarily in various systemic disorders and local lesions, such as in urogenital diseases.

Dermatological phenomena

Nikolsky sign
When skin that appears normal is rubbed or pinched, the upper layer easily detaches and blisters occur. It is positive in the skin of patients with toxic epidermal necrolysis (see Chapter 10), staphylococcal scalded skin syndrome (see Chapter 24), pemphigus, and epidermolysis bullosa (see Chapter 14).

Köbner phenomenon
Lesions occur by stimuli such as friction or sunlight on normal skin (Fig. 4.43). It is positive in psoriasis and lichen planus (see Chapter 15), and in verruca plana (see Chapter 23).

Darier's sign
Gentle rubbing of a lesion in a patient with mastocytosis (urticaria pigmentosa; see Chapter 21) causes mast cell degranulation, and the site may become markedly elevated to form an urticarial lesion. This phenomenon is called Darier's sign (Fig. 4.44), which distinguishes mastocytosis from other pigmented lesions. Urticarial lesions are usually produced shortly after rubbing in mastocytosis.

Auspitz phenomenon
Auspitz phenomenon is the occurrence of small bleeding points after the cutaneous basement membrane zone is exposed. In psoriasis, Auspitz phenomenon may be positive after scales are lifted off (see Chapter 15). However, the test may also be positive in cases of eczema. Auspitz phenomenon is not necessarily specific to psoriasis.

Pathergy test
When the skin of a patient with Behçet's disease (see Chapter 11) is pricked with a needle, erythema, papule or pustule appears after 24–48 h. It is positive if reddening of 2 mm or longer occurs 48 h after pricking of the flexor surface of the forearm for about 5 mm in length with a 21G hypodermic needle. This test is positive for about 70% of patients with Behçet's disease, which reflects the skin irritability of patients with the condition.

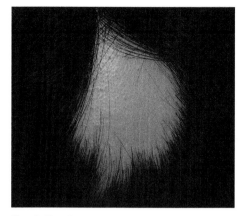

Fig. 4.42 Alopecia (Alopecia areata)

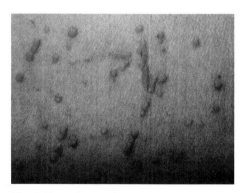

Fig. 4.43 Köbner phenomenon (Verruca plana)

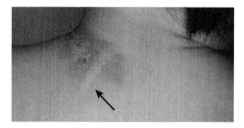

Fig. 4.44 Darier's sign (Mastocytosis.) Edema is marked.

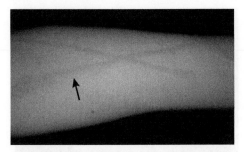

Fig. 4.45 Dermographism (Factitious urticaria)

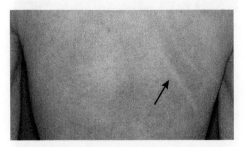

Fig. 4.46 White dermographism (Atopic dermatitis)

Dermographism

Dermographism is a reaction produced on the skin after it has been rubbed by a blunt object such as a fingernail. If the rubbed site becomes red and elevated, it is called red dermographism, which is a diagnostic finding of physical urticaria (Fig. 4.45). If the site becomes white, it is called white dermographism, which is usually seen in patients with atopic dermatitis (Fig. 4.46). Mild dermographism is found in about 74% of healthy persons.

Raynaud's phenomenon

See Chapter 11.

CHAPTER 5
Diagnosis of skin diseases

Accurate history taking and thorough skin examination (inspection and palpation) are important in reaching the correct dermatological diagnosis. Examination of the skin is aided by dermoscopy and in some cases by the odor emanating from the skin. Additional tests may be performed according to the presenting symptoms.

General diagnostic methods (Fig. 5.1)

History taking

History taking begins with a detailed inquiry into the nature of the presenting symptoms, followed by an assessment of any previous medical or dermatological diseases. It is important to look into any significant drug, family, social, recreational, and occupational history that may have triggered the onset of skin disease. The inquiries that should be included in history taking are listed below.

Chief complaint

What is the main reason for the patient's visit?

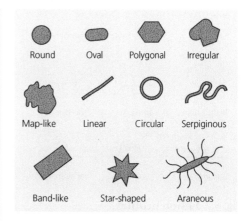

Fig. 5.1 **Lesion shapes.**

> **MEMO 5–1 Specialized terms used to describe eruptions**
>
> Some terms are more frequently used in dermatology than in other medical fields. They are described here.
> - **Shagreen patch:** a rough, elevated plaque that looks like orange peel, such as seen in tuberous sclerosis.
> - **Oystershell-like skin:** the surface is thick with rough and uneven crusts that resemble the shell of an oyster. It is seen in severe psoriasis and Norwegian scabies.
> - **Beaded skin:** multiple circular eruptions fuse to form an irregularly shaped eruption that resembles a map-like eruption.

Shimizu's Dermatology, Second Edition. Hiroshi Shimizu.
© 2017 John Wiley & Sons, Ltd. Published 2017 by John Wiley & Sons, Ltd.

Present illness
- When did the patient first notice the symptoms?
- Are there any subjective symptoms?
- Is there a presumed cause?
- Are there any systemic symptoms (e.g., high fever, fatigue, headache, aching joints, muscle pain, insomnia)?
- Were there any precursory symptoms?
- How has the lesion progressed? (Has it improved or worsened? Does it worsen at night?)
- How has the lesion spread? (Is it spreading? Does it come and go?)

Family history
Do any family members have similar symptoms? (Check the hereditary and allergic background of the patient.)

Past history
What diseases and medical treatments has the patient had? (Have topical or oral medications been used?)

In addition, the patient should be asked whether they have been in contact with people with similar symptoms at home, at school or in the workplace, to determine whether the condition is infectious or environmental.

Inspection and palpation
Physical examination should be conducted in a bright room. It is important to examine not only the site of the complaint but also the entire skin surface and mucous membranes. It should be remembered that an eruption may show its distinguishing features secondarily only after rubbing (Darier's sign). For accurate identification, it is important to examine an eruption that has not been influenced by any changes. Terms used to describe the nature and features of eruptions are listed below.
- **Eruption type:** spot, papule, nodule, blister (see Chapter 4).
- **Number of eruptions:** single or multiple.
- **Eruption shape:** round, oval, polygonal, irregular, geographical, linear, circular, serpiginous (Fig. 5.2).
- **Eruption size:** numerical values (millimeters and centimeters) are used in this textbook to describe the sizes of eruptions, thereby avoiding ambiguous expressions such as coin-sized, egg-sized, finger-sized, etc.

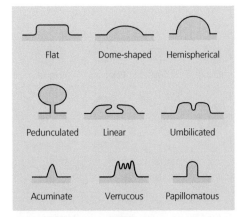

Fig. 5.2 Lesion profiles.

Flat   Dome-shaped   Hemispherical
Pedunculated   Linear   Umbilicated
Acuminate   Verrucous   Papillomatous

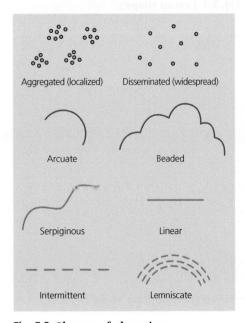

Fig. 5.3 Shapes of elevation.

Aggregated (localized)   Disseminated (widespread)
Arcuate   Beaded
Serpiginous   Linear
Intermittent   Lemniscate

- **Elevation profile:** flat, domed, hemispherical, pedunculated, linear, umbilicated (Fig. 5.3).
- **Eruption surface:** smooth, rough, warty, papillary, markedly uneven, granular, lichenoid, shagreen patch-like, oystershell-like, dry, moist, exudative, hemorrhagic (bloody, bleeding), scaly, crusty, erosive, ulcerated, cracked, atrophic, shiny, necrotic, elevated.
- **Eruption color:** erythematous, violaceous, purple, depigmented, hyperpigmented, pale.
- **Eruption texture:** soft, firm (stiff), fragile, tense, elastic, undulating, movable.
- **Eruption distribution:** localized, widespread, aggregated, plaque-like, diffuse, centrifugal, beaded, circular, serpiginous, linear, symmetrical, asymmetrical (Fig. 5.4).
- **Eruption site:** face, head, extremities, hand, sole, fingertip, toe, extensor surface, flexor surface, exposed, unexposed, groin, mucocutaneous junction, intertriginous area.
- **Subjective symptoms:** itching, pain (tenderness), numbness, crawling, hyperesthesia, hypoesthesia, burning, cold.
- **Eruption progress:** rapid versus gradual, with versus without recurrence, with versus without precedent eruption, affected versus unaffected by treatment.
- **Other:** sharply circumscribed, mildly circumscribed.

Odor assessment

Osmidrosis axillae (armpit odor) may be examined by swabbing the affected site with absorbent cotton or gauze and smelling for odor. In infectious diseases, microbial species may produce a distinctive smell. Fluid and color of pus in the eruption may also provide clues to the diagnosis.

Allergy test

The tests for allergic reactions to a specific antigen are largely divided into those for type I allergy (immediate) and those for type IV allergy (delayed). A scratch test and an intracutaneous reactivity test are conducted for a type I allergy; a patch test and an intracutaneous reactivity test are used for the investigation of a type IV allergy. For autoimmune blistering disease, ELISA and Western blot analysis are performed to detect the causative autoantibody.

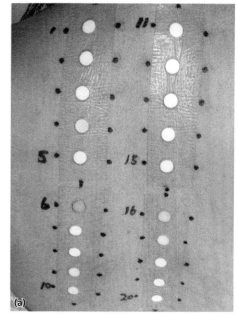

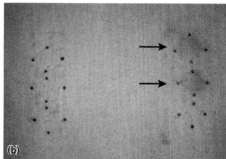

Fig. 5.4 Patch test. a: The antigens are spread on adhesive plasters that are included in the patch test unit. These are then stuck to the back of the patient. b: If the patient is allergic to the antigen, various allergic reactions (edematous erythema and papules (arrows)) are seen 48 hours later.

IgE radioallergosorbent test

This test, generally called IgE RAST, can identify a substance-specific IgE by blood test. Quantification of 200 or more substance-specific IgEs is possible. Interpretation of each IgE value depends largely on the total serum IgE (e.g., all IgE RAST results are strongly positive when the total serum IgE is high). A positive result in IgE RAST for a certain substance does not mean the inevitable onset of type I allergy against the substance. IgE RAST, which measures substance-specific IgEs for main allergens, is widely used as a screening test.

Patch test

The patch test is used for detecting the pathogenic allergen in allergic contact dermatitis. It is performed by applying the suspected allergen to normal skin in an appropriate vehicle such as white petrolatum, which is spread on an adhesive plaster or put in a Finn chamber (a plaster to which an aluminum plate is affixed). The plaster is adhered to a site of normal skin (usually the back or the upper inner arm). The patch is removed after 48 h and the test result is determined 30 min to 2 h after removal of the patch to allow the pressure caused by the patch to subside (Table 5.1). If reddening, edema, papules or erosions are present, the test is considered to be positive for allergy (Fig. 5.5). The site may be reobserved at 72 h and 96 h after patch removal for more reliable results. Diluted test substances are used in series for the test. In cases in which the result is positive only when the test substance is diluted to a certain level, that substance is regarded as the primary irritant.

Scratch test, prick test

The scratch test is a simple test to investigate type I allergy. The flexor surface of the forearm is firmly scratched with a blunt instrument, and a small amount of solution containing the allergen is applied (see Fig. 5.5). If the patient is allergic, reddening or swelling is immediately produced. The longest diameter of the reddening or swelling is measured 15–20 min after application of the allergen for identification of the allergy (Table 5.2).

A scratch test may cause anaphylactic shock in patients with a history of anaphylaxis. Therefore, the solution containing the allergen should be tested first on normal skin to determine whether urticaria is

Table 5.1 Readings and interpretation of patch test reactions.

Japanese criterion		ICDRG criterion	
−	Negative	−	Negative
±	Faint erythema	+?	Doubtful reaction; faint erythema only
+	Erythema	+	Weak positive reaction; palpable erythema, infiltration, possibly papules
‡	Edematous erythema	‡	Strong positive reaction; erythema, infiltration, papules, vesicles
‡‡	Infiltrative erythema, papules, vesicles	‡‡	Extreme positive reaction; intense erythema and infiltration and coalescing vesicles
‡‡	Coalescing vesicles	IR	Irritant reaction of different types
		NT	Not tested

ICDRG: International Contact Dermatitis Research Group

produced after 30 min (open test). If the result of the open test is positive, a scratch test or intracutaneous reactivity test is unnecessary.

Intracutaneous type I allergy test

Type I allergens can be detected by an intracutaneous test. For this test, 0.02 mL of a solution containing the suspected substance is injected intradermally. If an urticarial lesion or pseudopodia-like projection occurs within 15 min, the result is considered positive (Table 5.3). Since there is a risk of anaphylactic shock from this test, it is desirable to perform a scratch test in advance to gauge the severity of the reaction.

Intracutaneous type IV allergy test

The intracutaneous test can also be used to examine the strength of cellular immunity (type IV allergy) against an allergen. Forty-eight hours after an intradermal injection of 0.1 mL of the solution containing the suspected allergen, the major and minor axes of the reddening or swelling are measured and the average of the two values is obtained. An averaged value of 10 mm or more is usually considered a positive. Common type IV allergy tests are listed in Table 5.4.

Drug-induced lymphocyte stimulation test (DLST)

The drug-induced lymphocyte stimulation test (DLST) is useful in identifying drug-induced eruptions associated with T cells. However, the test has a low sensitivity so a negative result does not rule out the involvement of a drug. DNA synthesis accompanying a lymphocyte proliferative reaction can be determined by 3H-thymidine after peripheral blood lymphocytes are cultured with a drug. Patients with drug-induced toxic epidermal necrolysis or Stevens–Johnson syndrome tend to show positive reaction in a very short time, but those with drug-induced hypersensitivity syndrome (DIHS) often do not show a positive reaction until a few weeks after the onset of the disorder.

Drug challenge test

The drug suspected of causing allergy is administered to the patient to determine whether the eruptions will recur. One-hundredth to one-tenth of the usual dose is given orally. In serious drug eruptions, there is a high risk that a drug challenge test will induce

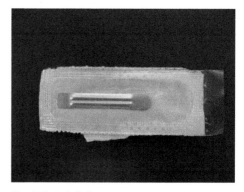

Fig. 5.5 Prick lancet.

Table 5.2 Readings of scratch test reactions.

Reading	Wheal diameter (mm)	Erythema diameter (mm)
Negative (−)	<5	<15
Positive (+)	≧5	≧15

Table 5.3 Readings of intradermal test reactions (in 15 minutes).

Reading	Wheal diameter (mm)	Erythema diameter (mm)
Negative (−)	<7	<15
Doubtful(±)	<9	<20
Positive (+)	<15	<40
Strongly positive (╫)	≧15	≧40

Table 5.4 Typical type IV allergy tests.

Tuberculin skin test (PPD skin test)
A tuberculin skin test is used to detect delayed hypersensitivity to tuberculosis, by injecting tuberculosis antigen intradermally. 0.1 ml of tuberculosis antigen (purified protein derivative; PPD, 0.05 μg/ml) is injected into the inner side of the forearm. The long diameter of the erythema 48 h after injection is used for interpretation: less than 10 mm is negative, and more than 10 mm as positive. Positive reaction is sometimes categorized into weak (only erythema), moderate (erythema and induration), and strong (erythema with vesicles and necrosis). Tuberculin skin test is specific to tuberculosis.However, patients with measles, sarcoidosis, Hodgkin's disease, severe tuberculosis, and serious malignancies may show weak reaction or false negative.
Trichophytin reaction
An antigen derived from *Trichophyton* (*Trichophyton* antigen) may be used to test intradermally for trichophytid and tinea profounda.
Sporotrichin reaction
Sporotrichin antigen is injected intradermally for diagnosis of sporotrichosis.
Ito's reaction
Haemophilus ducreyi antigen is used for diagnosis of chancroid.
Frei reaction
Frei reaction is an intradermal test for lymphogranuloma venereum.
Lepromin reaction (Mitsuda reaction)
Lepromin reaction (Mitsuda reaction). Antigen derived from leproma is intradermally injected for diagnosis and classification of leprosy.

anaphylactic shock. The drug challenge test is the most reliable allergy test.

Photosensitivity test

Photosensitivity tests are conducted by examining the reaction of the skin to irradiation. Ultraviolet radiation is divided into ultraviolet A (UVA; operative wavelength of 320–400 nm), ultraviolet B (UVB; 290–320 nm) and ultraviolet C (UVC; 100–290 nm). UVA, UVB, and visible light are the most frequently used in photosensitivity testing.

Photo test

The degree of photosensitivity and the suitable operative wavelength can be determined by the amount of radiation that causes cutaneous reactions such as pigmentation and erythema. By testing patients for the operative wavelength, it is possible to determine and therefore eliminate the radiation exposure to which the patient is sensitive.

The most widely conducted photo test is exposure to a minimum dose of UVB irradiation sufficient to cause erythema in 24 h (minimal erythema dose; MED) (Fig. 5.6). The MED varies by skin type. When the MED is low, involvement of a photosensitive disease is suspected.

Patients with drug-induced photosensitive dermatosis often show symptoms after receiving UVA radiation. The average minimal response dose (MRD) also differs by skin type. When an erythema and other reactions are observed within 24–72 h after testing a dose lower than the average MRD, the involvement of a photosensitive disease is suspected.

Chronic actinic dermatitis and some cases of porphyria cutanea tarda are diseases in which there is sensitivity to visible light. There is no standard technique for measuring MRD for photosensitive diseases; they are generally observed in the cutaneous reaction induced by 15–20 min of exposure to projector light.

A photo-provocation test of exposure to 2–3 MED of UVB irradiation for 3 consecutive days may be performed in cases of photosensitive disease, especially when the sunburn reaction is normal, such as in polymorphic light eruption.

Photo-patch test

The photo-patch test is performed to examine the influence of UV irradiation after a chemical substance is placed on the skin. Twenty-four to 48 h after a material suspected of causing photosensitivity is pasted on the skin, the site is exposed to UV irradiation (about half the MRD/MED for normal skin). If reddening or swelling occurs within 24 h, the result is considered positive (see Chapter 13).

Photo-drug test

The influence of photo irradiation in the presence of a drug can be examined by a photo-drug test. A drug that is suspected of causing a photosensitive disease is taken orally instead of topically. The photo-drug test is generally used for the diagnosis of drug-induced photosensitive diseases.

Ultrasonography

To visualize the subcutaneous structure, ultrasound is applied on the body surface and the echo is analyzed. In dermatology, ultrasound at 10–30 MHz is used. B-mode scanning for two-dimensional tomographic images is used for diagnosing and measuring the depth of neoplastic lesions. Some ultrasonography devices are equipped with a Doppler function (color and/or power Doppler) to analyze the blood flow or with an elastography function (Fig. 5.7).

Skin function test

Tests for measuring various skin functions, such as temperature control, secretion, and vascular regulation, are described below.

Measurement of skin temperature and thermography

Thermography is a technique that uses an emission pyrometer equipped with an infrared camera to express the distribution of skin temperature two-dimensionally. It is used for diagnosing diseases such as those associated with blood vessels, inflammatory disorders, and tumors (Fig. 5.8).

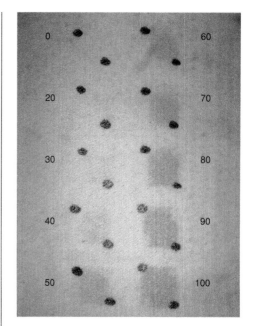

Fig. 5.6 Ultra-violet photo test for minimal erythema dose (MED). Erythema appears at the site of 30 mJ/cm^2 irradiation. The MED for this patient is 30 mJ/cm^2.

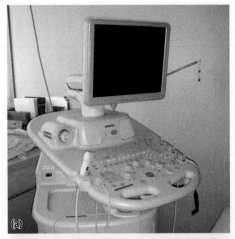

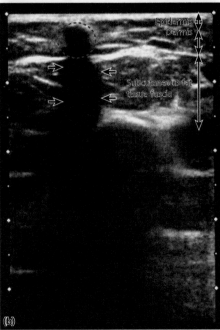

Fig. 5.7 Ultrasound test. a: Equipment. b: Pilomatricoma in the upper arm (the area encircled by the broken line; see Chapter 21). An area with acoustic shadow that reflects calcification is observed (arrows).

Sweat function test

The sweat function test is used for evaluating the severity and coverage of skin sweat function abnormality for patients with hyperhidrosis or anhidrosis (see Chapter 19). Perspiration is induced by heat stimulation (sauna, etc.) or drug stimulation (intradermal injection of pilocarpine), and the sweat is detected using starch-iodine (Fig. 5.9). Abnormality in sweat function is determined by comparing the results with those of a normal control.

Transepidermal water loss (TEWL)

Transepidermal water loss (TEWL) from the skin surface is measured by electric hygrometer (Fig. 5.10). This test is effective in determining the clinical condition of keratinization. The TEWL value is usually elevated in dyskeratoses, such as in ichthyosis.

Skin capillary resistance test

The fragility of skin capillaries can be determined by measuring ecchymosis produced in artificially pressured blood vessels. In the Rumpel–Leede test, the upper arm is compressed by a blood pressure cuff to cause congestion of the blood vessels. Pressure is applied to the patient's upper arm for 5 min to cause constriction of the blood vessels. If 10 or more hemorrhagic spots are produced within 2 min of applied pressure, the test is positive for dysfunction of vascular regulation. It may also be positive if there is abnormality in the capillaries or platelets, such as Henoch–Schönlein purpura or thrombocytopenic purpura.

Fungal examination

A potassium hydroxide (KOH) solution may be used for the detection of fungi and mites. Scales or the blister cover is swabbed (Fig. 5.11) and applied to a glass slide onto which a 20% KOH solution is dripped, and a slide cover is placed on top. The slide is placed on a hotplate at 70–80° for 5–10 min. The components of skin such as the stratum corneum are hydrolyzed, and the fungal components become easily observable. Mites may also be observed using this procedure. Dimethylsulfoxide (DMSO) added to the KOH solution reduces the dissolution time and eliminates the need to use a hotplate.

Diascopy

During diascopy, a skin lesion is pressed with a transparent glass slide to determine whether the coloration of the lesion disappears (Fig. 5.12). If the color of the erythematous lesion disappears, the diagnosis is erythema. Otherwise, the diagnosis is purpura.

Wood's lamp test

When skin of a particular patient with erythrasma, pityriasis versicolor, tinea capitis or porphyria is exposed to a Wood's lamp with a 365 nm UV light source, a characteristic fluorescence color is emitted (Fig. 5.13, Table 5.5).

Cytological diagnosis (Tzanck test)

The Tzanck test is performed by applying a glass slide to the base of a broken blister and staining the adhered cellular components using Giemsa for observation by light microscopy. Acantholytic cells called Tzanck cells are observed in pemphigus. In herpes simplex and herpes zoster, balloon cells may be observed.

Enzyme-linked immunosorbent assay

Enzyme-linked immunosorbent assay (ELISA) is a method for measuring the amount of specific proteins, using enzymes and antibodies that are associated with fluorescent substances. For the diagnosis of pemphigus, it is necessary to identify whether there are autoantibodies to desmogleins 1 and 3. For the diagnosis of bullous pemphigoid, it is necessary to identify whether there are autoantibodies to type XVII collagen.

Western blot

Western blot (immunoblotting) is a method of identifying and determining the amounts of specific proteins extracted from the skin. The protein lysates are electrophoresed and then transferred onto a membrane

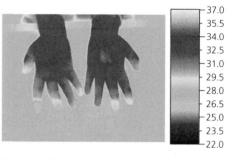

Fig. 5.8 Thermography. The hands of a patient with systemic sclerosis (see Chapter 12). The second and third fingers of the right hand show markedly low skin temperature.

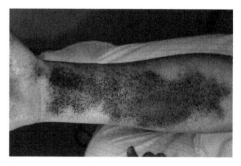

Fig. 5.9 Sweat function test. The forearm of a patient with cholinergic urticaria. Sweat is detected by using starch-iodine.

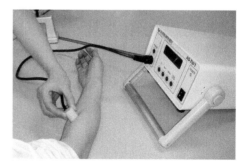

Fig. 5.10 Electric hygrometer: Measuring transepidermal water loss (TEWL).

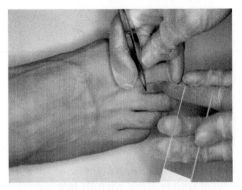

Fig. 5.11 Diagnosing tinea pedis. Scales or swabbed blister contents are sampled from the interdigital area. Microscopic examination is made with potassium hydrate.

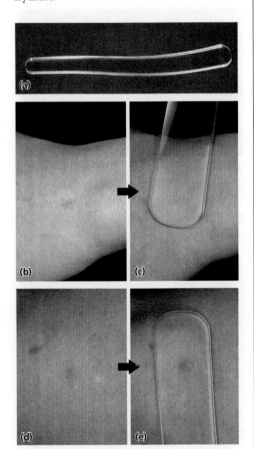

Fig. 5.12 Diascopy. a: Transparent glass plate for diascopy. b,c: Erythema disappears with pressure from the glass plate. d,e: Purpura does not disappear with such pressure.

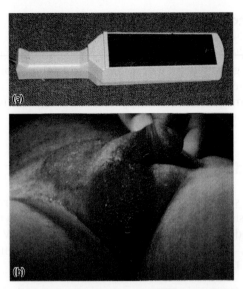

Fig. 5.13 a: Wood's lamp. b: Photodynamic diagnosis of extramammary Paget's disease. Wood's lamp reveals the area of the lesion, after δ-aminolevulinic acid ointment is applied in an occlusive dressing.

such as nitrocellulose. The membrane is then incubated with a specific antibody and developed using a chemiluminescence technique to reveal the protein bands of interest (Table 5.6, Fig. 5.14).

DNA analysis

DNA analysis is an important test for diagnosing monogenic inherited skin diseases such as epidermolysis bullosa, particularly when the causative gene is known (Fig. 5.15). The characteristic configuration of DNA in tuberculosis and non-tuberculous mycobacterial infections can also be detected by amplifying the DNA extracted from the lesion using the polymerase chain reaction (PCR).

Other general medical tests

Diagnostic imaging, such as X-ray imaging, computed tomography (CT), magnetic resonance imaging (MRI), positron emission tomography (PET), and scintigraphy, is important for the diagnosis of skin tumors and metastases, and of complications with fractures in cases of trauma with or without foreign objects. A general blood test, polymerase chain reaction (PCR) test, bacterial culture, and urinalysis may be useful in the diagnosis of skin diseases.

Table 5.5 Fluorescence under Wood's lamp.

Disorder	Fluorescence
Pityriasis versicolor	Yellow-orange
Erythrasma	Coral pink
Porphyria	Red
Tinea capitis	Yellow green-viridian

Table 5.6 Major autoantibodies detected in Western blot and their molecular weights.

Molecular weight	Antibody molecule	Target	Major disorder that produces the autoantibody
290 kDa	Type VII collagen	Epidermal anchoring fibril	Epidermolysis bullosa acquisita
250 kDa	Desmoplakin 1	Desmosome	Paraneoplastic pemphigus
230 kDa	BP230 (BPAG1)	Hemidesmosome	Bullous pemphigoid
210 kDa	Desmoplakin 2	Desmosome	Paraneoplastic pemphigus
210 kDa	Envoplakin	Marginal band	Paraneoplastic pemphigus
200 kDa	Laminin γ1	Basal membrane	Anti-laminin γ1 bullous pemphigoid
190 kDa	Periplakin	Marginal band	Paraneoplastic pemphigus
180 kDa	Type VXII collagen (BPAG2, BP180)	Hemidesmosome	Bullous pemphigoid
160 kDa	Desmoglein 1	Desmosome	Pemphigus foliaceus
130 kDa	Desmoglein 3	Desmosome	Pemphigus vulgaris

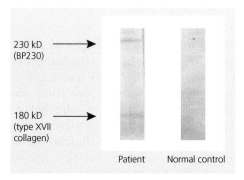

230 kD (BP230)

180 kD (type XVII collagen)

Patient   Normal control

Fig. 5.14 Western blotting. Serum from a bullous pemphigoid patient reacts against skin antigens (molecular weights of 180 kDa (type XVII collagen) and 230 kDa (BP230)).

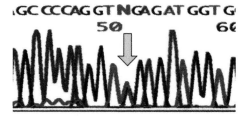

Fig. 5.15 DNA analysis of type VII collagen in a patient with dystrophic epidermolysis bullosa. A point mutation (6781 in exon 86) causes a nonsense mutation. Instead of arginine (CGA), a stop codon (TGA) occurs at 2261 amino acid.

CHAPTER 6

Treatment of skin diseases

Dermatological treatments are divided into topical, systemic (oral administration of drugs and injections), physical, laser, and surgical therapies. Of these, topical drug application is the most common treatment modality in dermatology. Physical therapies such as irradiation and warming/cooling of affected sites are also frequently used.

Table 6.1-1 Principles of adsorption and infiltration of topical medicine.

- Topical agents penetrate more easily through skin with a thin stratum corneum, such as the face and scrotum, and less readily through skin with a thick stratum corneum, such as the palms and soles (Table 6.1-2)
- Absorption of a topical agent is also dependent on the molecular weight of the agent. Generally, substances whose molecular weight is 1 kDa or more do not permeate the stratum corneum even at the site of dermatitis (see Fig. 6.1).
- The absorption of a topical agent is increased at sites where there is damage or loss of the stratum corneum, such as at sites of erosions and ulcerations. Oleaginous compounds act relatively slowly on these lesions
- The absorption of a topical agent tends to increase with the duration of contact with the skin. This characteristic is taken advantage of in occlusive therapy
- The type of vehicle and the consistency of the active ingredient are chosen depending on the state and site of the skin eruption.

Topical therapies

Topical therapies involve the external application of a drug on affected skin. Topical agents are composed of a main agent or active ingredient mixed with an appropriate vehicle or base.

The stratum corneum has water-repellent properties and prevents evaporation from the skin. It therefore represents the strongest physical barrier for the penetration of a topical agent. The water-repellent stratum corneum has a thin sebum membrane on the surface that also functions as a physical barrier. The site below the granular cell layer is hydrophilic and can readily absorb a topical agent.

The adsorption of topical agents varies by the region and condition of the skin, and the relationship between the penetrance and the molecular size of the topical agent varies by the condition of the skin (Table 6.1, Fig. 6.1).

Forms and vehicles for topical agents

Vehicles are important in helping the active ingredient to permeate the skin. They may also have a role in hydration, cooling, lubrication, protection, softening, and purification of the skin, and in itch relief. A vehicle can be applied without any active ingredient in many cases. Vehicles should be non-stimulating, colorless and odorless, stable (non-denaturing), able to retain the main agent evenly, moderately viscous, appropriately firm, and moderately absorbable.

Shimizu's Dermatology, Second Edition. Hiroshi Shimizu.
© 2017 John Wiley & Sons, Ltd. Published 2017 by John Wiley & Sons, Ltd.

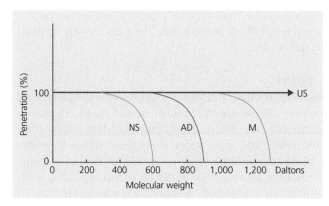

Fig. 6.1 Size of molecule versus estimated permeability in skin under various conditions. AD, atopic dermatitis skin; M, mucosa; NS, normal skin; US, ultrasound-treated human skin without stratum corneum. Source: Bos & Meinardi. *Exp Dermatol* 2000; 9(3): 168. Reproduced with permission of Wiley.

The same main agent may be combined with different vehicles to produce topical agents of various consistencies that can be used for different applications (Fig. 6.2 and Fig. 6.3, Table 6.2).

Ointments

Ointments are the most frequently used topical agents. They are generally more inert than other vehicles. There are two types of ointments.

Oleaginous ointments

These are the most commonly used ointments. Oils such as Vaseline, paraffin, olive oil, and Plastibase are the most frequently used hydrophobic bases for oleaginous ointments. These are water insoluble and do not contain or absorb water. The vehicle may protect and soften the skin. Oleaginous ointments are the most inert and may be applied on all types of eruptions. (Examples include various steroid ointments, petroleum jelly, and zinc oxide ointments.)

Water-in-oil emulsion, emulsified ointments

Emulsifiers such as polyethylene glycol are used in some oleaginous ointments. These emulsified ointments contain fine droplets of water (see Fig. 6.2) and are called water-in-oil (w/o) emulsion ointments. They induce a cooling sensation upon application and are also called cold creams. They are more protective

Table 6.1-2 Relative absorption rate of topical steroids by skin region (forearm=1).

Region	Relative absorption rate
Plantar area	0.1
Palms	0.8
Flexor side of forearm	1
Back	1.7
Scalp	3.5
Axilla	3.6
Cheek	13
Scrotum	42

Source: Feldmann RJ et al. Regional variation in percutaneous penetration of 14C cortisol in man. *J Invest Dermatol* 1967;48:181–183.

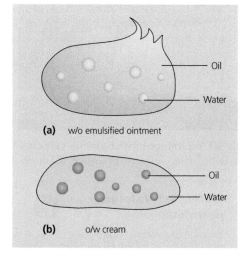

Fig. 6.2 Illustration of water-in-oil (w/o) emulsified ointment and oil-in-water (o/w) cream. a: w/o emulsified ointment. Water granules are dispersed in oil by emulsion. b: o/w emulsive cream. Oil granules are dispersed in water.

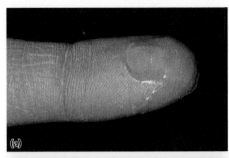

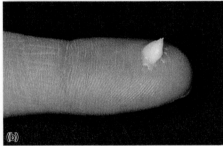

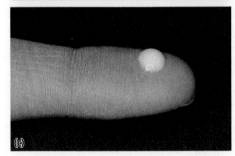

Fig. 6.3 Topical agents with various vehicles.
a: Oleaginous ointment. b: Cream. c: Lotion.

MEMO 6–1 Vaseline, petroleum jelly

Vaseline (petroleum jelly) is a semi-solid compound derived and refined from petroleum. It is often used as a vehicle for topical agents. It comes in yellow and white, and there is no essential difference between the two.

MEMO 6–2 Ointments

"Ointment" in dermatology usually refers to an oleaginous ointment. However, some water-in-oil emulsive creams (cold cream) and oil-in-water creams (vanishing cream) may also be regarded as "ointments" by patients.

and less sticky than creams (see next section), and are easily washed off with water. They are mostly applied on dry lesions.

Creams

Most creams use emulsifiers to admix fine droplets of oil in water. These are called oil-in-water (o/w) emulsified ointments (see Fig. 6.2). Creams are less sticky than ointments, and their color disappears when they are applied thinly. Since they do not stain clothes, creams are readily accepted by patients, and compliance with application is ensured. Although creams are useful for erythema and papules, they should not be used on eroded or moist sites because they may cause irritation.

Gels

The main agents are mixed in hydrogel bases, such as polyvinyl alcohol and agar. After application, the gel dries out to produce a thin adhesive film on the skin. Gels with a high solvent content may be used on mucosal lesions to protect them from friction.

Lotions

Lotions are liquids (usually water) admixed with an active ingredient. When applied topically, the liquid component evaporates, thereby inducing a cooling sensation. Lotions are astringent and can protect the skin. The active agent left on the skin acts pharmacologically. In addition to water, liquid vehicles include alcohol, propylene glycol, glycerin, and zinc oxide oil (a 1:1 mixture of zinc oxide and olive oil). Some lotions require shaking prior to application.

Emulsion lotions

These are emulsions of oil in water. They are used for non-moist lesions and are often applied on the hairy scalp. (Example: steroid lotions.)

Alcohol solution

The agent is dissolved in an alcohol solvent. The solution dries soon after application, which is convenient, although the alcohol can cause irritation. It is mainly used on the scalp and nails.

Plasters

A plaster is a medicated cloth, paper or plastic film onto which a particular active ingredient is placed. One example is 50% salicylic acid plaster, which may be used on hyperkeratotic lesions such as callus and

Table 6.2 Characteristics of vehicles.

Vehicle	Form of administration	Base	Characteristics	Drawbacks
Hydrophobic base	Ointment (oleaginous ointment)	Vaseline and Plastibase	Least irritating, superior in skin protection	Greasy feeling, not water absorbent, tends to be used in a smaller amount than prescribed
Hydrophilic base	Emulsifying base	Ointment, cold cream (water-in-oil emulsion)	Hydrophilic ointment	Induces a cooling sensation upon application, less sticky than oleaginous ointment, readily penetrates the skin	Less protective, contact dermatitis may occur due to additives
		Vanishing cream (oil-in-water emulsion)	Absorptive ointment, hydrophilic petrolatum	Less greasy than oleaginous ointment, readily penetrates the skin	More irritating than ointments, contact dermatitis may occur due to addititves, excess amounts tend to be used on the face
	Water-soluble base	Water-soluble ointment	Macrogol	Strongly water absorptive, used on wet lesions, easily removed with water	Weak adhesion to the skin, excess water adsorption may cause cracking of the skin.
	Gel base	Gel, jelly	Hydrogel	Less greasy than oleaginous ointment, readily penetrates the skin	Tends to cause irritation on the cracks, less penetrative than ointments
Other	Emulsified lotion	Lotion	Water and emulsifier	Less greasy, able to be applied to the scalp	The drug affects only the skin surface, excess amounts tend to be used
	Alcoholic solution	Solution, liquid	Volatile alcohol	Dries soon after application, which provides a favorable sensation	Strong irritation
	Plaster	Tape	Plastic film	Strongly protective, readily penetrates the skin	Unable to be used on wet legions or the scalp

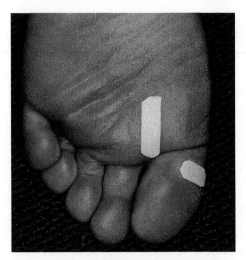

Fig. 6.4 30% Salicylic acid plaster.

MEMO 6–3 Other forms of topical agents

- **Water-soluble ointments:** water-soluble substances, including macrogol, are used for the vehicle. These ointments wash off easily.
- **Liniments:** liniments consist of a formulation of quickly evaporating solvents, such as alcohol and acetone. They have the same viscosity as lotions but, unlike lotions, they are rubbed into the skin. They dry fast on the skin and are effective in cooling the skin and relieving itching. Carbolic acid liniments are used for eruptions of, for instance, varicella.

---

clavus (Fig. 6.4). Adhesive plasters containing steroids or lidocaine are also useful. Adhesive plasters may be applied to the skin for transdermal drug delivery (e.g., nitroglycerine and fentanyl patches for the relief of angina and opiate-sensitive pain, respectively).

Frequently used topical agents
Corticosteroids

The main purpose of steroid topical application is to reduce inflammation. Mechanisms by which steroids inhibit inflammation include vasoconstriction, diminution of membrane permeability, inhibition of inflammatory chemical mediators, reduction of arachidonic acid metabolism by phospholipase A inhibition, immunosuppression, and inhibition of cell division.

Topical steroids are classified by strength: strongest, very strong, strong, mild, and weak (Table 6.3).

Topical steroid application may have side effects. Particular care should be taken when topical steroids are applied on the face and flexural areas. Systemic side effects are rare, provided that the dosage and usage of steroids are appropriate. However, when strong steroids are applied on a large area for a prolonged period or when they are used in occlusive therapy, side effects similar to those caused by systemic steroid administration may occur. Moreover, special care should be taken when topical steroids are used on infants, since systemic side effects may be produced.

Side effects of topical steroids include cutaneous atrophy, striae distensae, telangiectasia, purpura, hypertrichosis, steroid acne, rosacea-like dermatitis, and cutaneous infections (e.g., tinea incognito, candidiasis) (Table 6.4).

Immunosuppressants

Topical calcineurin inhibitors, such as tacrolimus (molecular weight: 822 Da), selectively inhibit T cell functions. They are effective for the treatment of atopic dermatitis, chronic actinic dermatitis, and lichen planus. Topical immunosuppressants must be avoided in patients with ichthyosis syndromes, such as Netherton syndrome (see Chapter 15), because absorption is enhanced in these patients.

Antifungal agents

Antifungal agents are widely used in dermatology. They may contain compounds such as imidazole, benzylamine or morpholine and act by attaching to the

Table 6.3 Topical steroids.

Brand name and form	Corticosteroid	Potency
Betnovate cream/ointment/lotion	Betamethasone valerate 0.1%	Very strong
Betnovate RD cream/ointment	Betamethasone valerate 0.025%	Strong
Bettamousse	Betamethasone valerate 0.12%	Very strong
Cutivate cream/ointment	Fluticasone propionate	Very strong
Dermacort cream	Hydrocortisone 0.1%	Mild
Dermovate cream/ointment/ scalp application	Clobetasol propionate 0.05%	Strongest
Dioderm cream	Hydrocortisone 0.1%	Mild
Diprosone cream/ointment/ lotion	Betamethasone dipropionate 0.05%	Very strong
Efcortelan cream/ointment	Hydrocortisone 0.5%, 1%, 2.5%	Mild
Elocon ointment/scalp ointment	Mometasone furoate 0.1%	Very strong
Eumovate eczema and dermatitis cream	Clobetasone butyrate 0.05%	Strong
Eumovate cream/ointment	Clobetasone butyrate 0.05%	Strong
Haelan cream/ointment/tape	Flurandrenolone (fludroxycortide)	Strong
Halciderm cream	Halcinonide 0.1%	Strongest
Locoid cream/ointment/ lipocream/scalp lotion	Hydrocortisone 17-butyrate 0.1%	Very strong
Metosyn cream/ointment	Fluocinonide 0.05%	Very strong
Mildison lipocream	Hydrocortisone 1%	Mild
Modrasone cream/ointment	Alclometasone dipropionate 0.05%	Strong
Nerisone cream/oily cream/ ointment	Diflucortolone valerate 0.1%	Very strong
Nerisone forte oily cream/ ointment	Diflucortolone valerate 0.3%	Strongest
Propaderm cream/ointment	Beclometasone dipropionate 0.025%	Very strong
Stiedex LP cream	Desoximetasone 0.05%	Strong
Synalar cream/ointment/gel	Fluocinolone acetonide 0.025%	Very strong
Synalar 1:4 cream/ointment	Fluocinolone acetonide 0.00625%	Strong
Synalar 1:10 cream/ointment	Fluocinolone acetonide 0.0025%	Mild
Ultralanum cream/ointment	Fluocortolone	Strong

(Adapted from; http://www.netdoctor.co.uk/skin_hair/eczema_corticosteroids_003762.htm).

cellular walls of fungi and inhibiting biosynthesis. These agents may be used topically (as creams, lotions or ointments) for superficial mycoses, and systemically for recalcitrant mycoses, such as tinea unguium and deep fungal infections.

MEMO 6–4 Wound dressings

The conventional wisdom was once to treat wounds and bedsores by disinfecting and drying them. However, it has become clear that, when the site is not infected, allowing them to retain their natural moisture is advantageous in promoting healing. Based on this new understanding, various types of wound dressing materials have been developed and used (See figure).

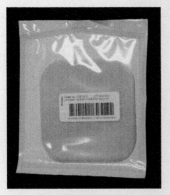

Wound dressing.

Dressing type	Example	Uses/advantages
Polyurethane film	Tegaderm®	Closely covers superficial wounds
Hydrocolloid	DuoActive®	Closely covers fresh wounds and absorbs exudates
Polyurethane foam	Hydrosite®	Absorbs exudates by its spongy structure
Alginate	Sorbsan®	Highly hemostatic
Hydrogel	Granugel®	Gel can cover concave wounds
Hydropolymer	Tielle®	For highly exudative bedsores
	DuoActive®	

MEMO 6–5 Mixing of topical agents

It was once common to mix topical agents (e.g., steroids and moisturizer). However, such mixing should be avoided. It causes the stability and behavior of the vehicle to change, which can greatly alter the skin penetration ability of the main agent. It reduces the effectiveness of the antiseptic component, which can promote bacterial infection. Dilution does not tend to reduce the side effects of topical steroids. Prescription medications are less stable when mixed. Mixing has not been shown to improve effectiveness. Topical agents are developed based on individual use.

Table 6.4 Side effects of topical steroids.

Local
Atrophy
Steroid purpura
Rosacea-like dermatitis, perioral dermatitis
Steroid acne
Hypertrichosis
Infection (bacterial, fungal, viral)
Contact dermatitis
Rebound (exacerbation of disease after sudden cessation)

Systemic
Suppression of adrenal gland function

Antibiotics

Topical agents containing antibiotics are used against superficial bacterial infections. The antibiotic should be effective against the targeted bacteria and have good transdermal sensitization capability. Macrolide and new quinolone antibiotics are effective against folliculitis and acne vulgaris. As antibiotic resistance among bacteria has been increasing in recent years, ointments containing antibiotics are not always effective in treating superficial infections.

Vitamin D analogues

Activated vitamin D3 may be used to treat hyperkeratotic and proliferative diseases such as psoriasis, ichthyosis, and palmoplantar keratosis, because of its ability to induce differentiation and inhibit the proliferation of epidermal keratinocytes. It is useful as a first-line treatment for psoriasis. It is important to note that prolonged, high doses of activated vitamin D3 may cause hypercalcemia.

Retinoids

Vitamin A acts by decreasing sulfate cholesterols, which are structural components of the stratum corneum that promote exfoliation. Topical retinoid preparations are used to treat acne vulgaris. Retinoids combine selectively with retinoic acid receptors and prevent inflammatory and non-inflammatory eruptions by inhibiting the keratinization of epithelial cells of follicles and the formation of comedones.

Imiquimods

In recent years, topical imiquimods, which act as immunostimulators, have been used in treating malignant cutaneous tumors and viral warts, including condyloma acuminatum. Imiquimods are antiviral and antitumor agents that activate immune cells through toll-like receptor 7 (TLR7) and induce the secretion of proinflammatory cytokines.

Urea

Urea is used as a moisturizer for its water retention properties. Ointments containing urea are frequently used to treat senile xerosis, ichthyosis, palmoplantar keratosis, and atopic dermatitis. Urea may, however, produce irritation on cracked or moist skin.

Zinc oxide

Zinc oxide is frequently used as a vehicle or base. It can also be used as a main agent because of its desiccation, astringency, anti-itching, cooling, and radiation-blocking properties. Zinc oxide spread on cotton lint is available commercially (Fig. 6.5). Zinc oxide adhesive plasters are used in occlusive dressing therapy as a sealing material to cover the topical agent that is directly applied to the skin.

Salicylic acid

Salicylic acid is a keratolytic compound used to treat keratoderma. A plaster containing 50% salicylic acid is often used to soften and remove callosities.

Sunscreen

For patients with photosensitive disorders or xeroderma pigmentosum, it is extremely important to protect the skin from UV rays. Suntan protection is important in reducing the risk of skin cancer and

MEMO 6–6 Tars

Tars such as coal tar, wood tar, and glyteer can be applied topically on moist eruptions as well as lichenified lesions. Because of their carcinogenicity when used for long periods, they are no longer used in Japan. Tars may also cause photosensitive diseases. As tars have antiproliferative effect, they can be used in combination with ultraviolet rays (UVB) for the treatment of psoriasis (Goeckerman therapy).

MEMO 6–7 Instructing patients on the daily dosage of topical medicine

For oral medicines, it is easy to specify the precise daily dosage in the prescription. For topical medicines, it is more complex, and dermatologists must give careful instructions not only on the daily dosage but also on the amount of the topical preparation (e.g., the number of grams and how much of the tube) to be applied on the affected skin. For proper application of topical agents, careful instructions must be given to the patient, often with demonstration of proper application.

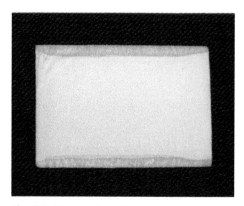

Fig. 6.5 Zinc oxide sheet.

MEMO 6–8 Fingertip unit

The amount of topical steroid that should be applied is commonly measured by fingertip units (FTUs). When prescribing topical medicines, it is important to determine the daily dosage and to give the patient proper instruction on application of the medicine. Without proper instruction, the patient may use too little or too much for proper medicinal effects.

The standard measure for topical steroid is the FTU, the amount squeezed from a standard 25 g tube with a 5 mm nozzle along an adult's fingertip. "Fingertip" means the entire length of the distal phalange of the index finger (See figure). An FTU is about 0.5 g, which is enough to spread over both palms (about 2% of the total surface area of the body). The FTU is based on a tube with a standard 5 mm nozzle. The size of the nozzle should be carefully checked when the FTU is used.

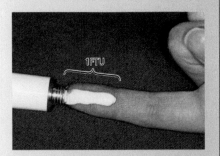

Fingertip unit.

preventing skin photoaging. Commercially available sunscreens can be classified roughly into two types by the main component: UV-reflecting/scattering agents (e.g., titanium oxide) and UV-absorbing agents (e.g., paraaminobenzoic acid: PABA). Non-chemical products made with UV-scattering agents are available. Products that contain UV-absorbing agents have high light-blocking ability but can irritate the skin.

The sun protection factor (SPF) indicates protection against UVB; the protection grade (PA) indicates protection against UVA.

Other agents

Antiviral drugs, sulfur, phenol, antihistamines, antitumor drugs, psoralen, vitamins, and non-steroidal anti-inflammatory drugs (NSAIDs) are other commonly used topical preparations.

Application

Care should be taken in the application of agents for which there are restrictions on dosage and use frequency. For agents whose dosage is not specified, it is necessary to determine the daily dosage for each patient.

Direct application

A topical agent is applied directly to a skin lesion. This is the most common application method. For proper topical treatment, careful instructions must be given to the patient, often with demonstration of the correct application. The concept of a fingertip unit (FTU) is helpful in giving instructions.

Plaster

This is applied directly to the skin lesion and is effective in removing crusts and protecting erosions and ulcers.

Occlusive dressing therapy (ODT)

A topical agent is directly applied to the skin and the site is tightly sealed with polyethylene film. Steroid adhesive plasters are sold commercially and are useful for treating thick lichenified or hyperkeratotic skin lesions. By enhancing the absorption of the main agent, ODT has increased likelihood of side effects.

Chemical and mineral bath

Chemicals and minerals are dissolved in warm water for soaking. They can also be used for disinfecting burns. A PUVA bath is useful for the treatment of psoriasis; the patient is soaked in a psoralen solution and then irradiated with UV rays.

Systemic treatments

Antihistamines
There are several types of antihistamines, which bind to histamine receptors to inhibit their function. H1 receptor-inhibiting drugs are widely used in dermatology and are extremely effective in treating inflammatory and allergic reactions. Second- and third-generation antihistamines inhibit the release of a chemical mediator from mast cells. Third-generation antihistamines such as loratadine, cetirizine, and fexofenadine have only a slight depressant action on the central nervous system (Table 6.5) and have a long serum half-life: one or two doses per day is effective in relieving itching from urticaria, dermatitis, and other pruritic conditions. Drugs with anticholinergic side effects must be avoided in patients with glaucoma and enlarged prostate.

Antibiotics
Antibiotics are used to treat superficial skin infections, such as impetigo contagiosa, and deep ones, such as cellulitis. Most skin infections tend to respond to internal systemic antibiotics; however, drug-resistant bacteria such as methicillin-resistant *Staphylococcus aureus* (MRSA) are becoming more prevalent. For this reason, it is important to perform appropriate culture tests (e.g., blood culture and skin swabs from pus or exudates) to determine the antibiotic sensitivity of the bacteria. History taking is necessary to inquire about allergic reactions. For patients with severe liver disorder or kidney dysfunction, both the dose and timing of the antibiotic administration should be taken into consideration. Types of antibiotics and their mechanisms of action are shown in Table 6.6.

Antifungal agents
Systemic antifungal agents with a narrow antifungal spectrum include griseofulvin, amphotericin B, nystatin, flucytosine, and miconazole. Recently developed antifungal agents such as itraconazole and terbinafine hydrochloride have a broad antifungal spectrum and fewer side effects. Highly keratinophilic, they concentrate in skin lesions and nails.

Table 6.5 Common antihistamines.

Non-sedating
Acrivastine (Semprex)
Cetirizine hydrocholoride (Zirtek)
Fexofenadine hydrocholoride (Telfast)
Loratadine (Clarityn)
Mizolastine (Mistamine, Mizollen)
Terfenadine
Sedating
Alimemazine tartrate/trimeprazine tartrate (Vallergan)
Azatadine maleate (Optimine)
Brompheniramine maleate (Dimotane)
Chlorphenamine maleate/ chlorpheniramine maleate (Piriton)
Cinnarizine (Stugerone)
Clemastine (Tavegil)
Cyclizine (Valoid)
Cyproheptadine hydrochloride (Periactin)
Hydroxyzine hydrochloride (Atarax, Ucerax)
Meclozine hydrochloride (Sea-legs)
Promethazine hydrochloride (Phenergan)
Promethazine teoclate (Avomine)

(http://www.bupa.co.uk/health_information/ html/medicine/antihistamine.html).

Table 6.6 Common antibiotics and their mechanisms.

Antibacterial effects	Classification by drug structure		Mechanism
Biocidal agents	β-lactams	Penicillin	Inhibition of cell wall synthesis
		Cephalosporin	
		Monobactam	
		Carbapenem	
		Penem	
	Fosfomycins		
	Aminoglycosides		Inhibition of protein synthesis
	Polypeptide antibiotics		Inhibition of cell wall synthesis
	Synthetic antibiotics	Quinolone	Inhibition of DNA synthesis
		Sulfamethoxazole/ trimethoprim	Inhibition of folic acid synthesis
Bacteriostatic agents	Tetracyclines		Inhibition of protein synthesis
	Choloramphenicols		
	Macrolides		
	Lincomycins		

They can be administered orally to patients with kerion, sycosis trichophytica or mycosis profunda. For tinea unguium, pulse therapy with itraconazole (400 mg per day, 1 week per month for 3–4 cycles) is effective.

Antiviral agents

Aciclovir, valaciclovir, and vidarabine are effective against herpes viruses, including herpes simplex and varicella zoster. Famciclovir is used for the treatment of herpes zoster.

Oral preparations of these antiviral agents, excluding vidarabine, are available and often used by outpatients. Antiviral agents are metabolized by the kidney; in patients with kidney disorder, the dose should therefore be titrated based on creatinine clearance. Ganciclovir, another antiviral agent, is effective against cytomegalovirus infection.

Corticosteroids

Corticosteroids have both anti-inflammatory and anti-immune effects. They are administered orally in collagen diseases such as systemic lupus erythematosus (SLE), in autoimmune skin diseases including pemphigus, toxic epidermal necrolysis, Stevens–Johnson syndrome and bullous pemphigoid, and in serious drug eruptions such as drug-induced hypersensitivity syndrome. Short-term oral use of corticosteroids may be prescribed for extensive drug eruptions or autosensitization dermatitis. However, systemic administration as a treatment for chronic diseases such as atopic dermatitis, chronic urticaria, and psoriasis must be carefully monitored.

Systemic use tends to cause a wider variety of side effects than topical use. Care must be taken with patients who have an underlying disease, such as diabetes mellitus or high blood pressure. The side effects of systemic steroid administration are shown in Table 6.7. The initial dose of steroids is determined according to the severity of the disease and is gradually tapered to a low maintenance dose or stopped as symptoms improve. Several oral corticosteroids (tablet or liquid) are available. One tablet is a dose equivalent to the physiological secretion for 1 day (Table 6.8). If necessary, steroid pulse therapy (1000 mg of intravenous methylprednisolone injection per day for 3 successive days) is given for severe conditions.

Immunosuppressants

Ciclosporin, azathioprine, methotrexate, and cyclophosphamide are immunosuppressants and may be used as steroid-sparing agents in the treatment of SLE, dermatomyositis, pemphigus, bullous pemphigoid, and Behçet's disease. Ciclosporin may be used alone in intractable psoriasis. Low-dose ciclosporin may be used in serious atopic dermatitis in adults during acute exacerbation; however, it tends to cause dose-dependent kidney disorders, high blood pressure, and increased risk of lymphoproliferative disorders. Therefore, blood concentration monitoring is necessary when ciclosporin is administered.

Biologics

Biologic (molecular-targeted) therapies, in which monoclonal antibodies such as rituximab, infliximab, adalimumab, secukinumab, etanercept, and alefacept are administered, have recently come into use for the treatment of severe inflammatory diseases such as Crohn's disease and psoriasis, and lymphoproliferative disorders such as B cell lymphoma (Table 6.9). These agents (except rituximab, which is not used for the treatment of psoriasis) are particularly useful in

MEMO 6–9 Dosage of oral steroids

For optimal effect, the dosage of oral steroid needs to be carefully determined for each patient depending not only on the symptoms but also, for example, on the body weight.

Table 6.7 Side effects of corticosteroids.

Severe	Relatively mild
Secondary adrenal dysfunction	Moon face, central obesity
Sideration and exacerbation of diabetes	Hyperphagia Leukocytosis
Sideration and exacerbation of hypertension	Skin streaks Subcutaneous
Hyperlipidemia	hemorrhage,
Psychiatric effects	purpura
Muscular atrophy	Steroid acne
Cataract, glaucoma	Hypertrichosis
Gastric ulcer	Alopecia
Osteoporosis	Edema
Aseptic necrosis of bone	Insomnia
Susceptibility to various infectious conditions	

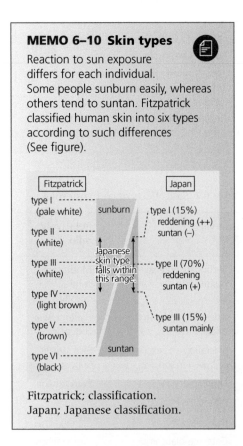

patients with severe psoriasis and psoriatic arthritis. It is expected that their use will continue to increase. However, secondary infections, such as tuberculosis, have been reported so patients must be screened for tuberculosis prior to treatment.

Retinoids

Retinoids are a class of compounds that are vitamin A derivatives. They control the proliferation and differentiation of epithelial tissues. Etretinate, acitretin, isotretinoin, and all-trans retinoic acid are used. Vitamin A acts by decreasing sulfate cholesterols, which are structural components of the stratum corneum that promote exfoliation. Retinoids are therefore useful against disorders of keratinization, such as ichthyosis, palmoplantar keratosis, Darier's disease, and severe psoriasis. Prior to starting an oral retinoid, patients must be carefully advised about the side effect profile of this class of medication. Teratogenesis and bone defects are serious side effects, and patients of reproductive age are advised to consider appropriate contraception before (1 month), during, and after stopping (2 years for women and 6 months for men) an oral retinoid. In Europe and the US, etretinate has been withdrawn from the market because of its undesirable pharmacokinetics; it has been superseded by acitretin. Care should also be taken in deciding whether to administer retinoids to children, because of the risk of premature closure of the epiphyseal line. Other side effects include epidermal exfoliation, cheilitis, nail fragility, liver disorders, and abnormal lipid metabolism.

Table 6.8 Various corticosteroids: comparison of the duration and dose for the same effects.

Duration of action	Drug	Dose needed for the same effect as 5 mg prednisolone	Dose per tablet
Short (within 8 h)	Hydrocortisone	20 mg	10 mg
Moderate (1 day)	Prednisolone	5 mg	5 mg
	Methylprednisolone	4 mg	4 mg
Long (2 days)	Dexamethasone	0.75 mg	0.5 mg
	Bethamethasone	0.5~0.6 mg	0.5 mg

(Adapted from Wallace J, et al., editors. *Dubois' lupus erythematosus*. 5th ed. Williams & Wilkins. 1997)

Table 6.9 Biologic (molecular-targeted) agents.

Drug name	Target molecule	Indication
Infliximab	TNF-α	Psoriasis, rheumatoid arthritis, ulcerative colitis, Crohn's disease, Behcet's disease
Adalimumab	TNF-α	Psoriasis, rheumatoid arthritis, ulcerative colitis, Crohn's disease, Behcet's disease
Etanercept	TNF-α	Psoriasis, rheumatoid arthritis, Crohn's disease
Ustekinumab	IL-12/23 (p40)	Psoriasis
Ixekizumab	IL-17A	Psoriasis
Brodalumab	IL-17 receptor	Psoriasis
Seculinumab	IL-17A	Psoriasis
Omalizumab	IgE	Chronic spontaneous urticaria, allergic asthma, atopic dermatitis
Canakinumab	IL-1β	Cryopyrin-associated periodic syndrome
Tocilizumab	IL-6	Castleman's disease, rheumatoid arthritis, juvenile idiopathic arthritis
Rituximab	CD20	B cell lymphoma, pemphigus vulgaris
Mogamulizumab	CCR4	Adult T cell lymphoma/leukemia, T cell lymphoma
Nivolumab	PD-1	Malignant melanoma
Brentuximab vedotin	CD30	Hodgkin's lymphoma, systemic anaplastic large cell lymphoma

DDS (4,4'-diamino-diphenyl-sulfone, dapsone)

Diaphenylsulfone, or dapsone, is a sulfa drug that inhibits folic acid synthesis and was originally used to treat leprosy (Hansen's disease). It may also be used to treat several inflammatory skin diseases characterized by neutrophilic infiltration, such as dermatitis herpetiformis (Duhring), erythema elevatum diutinum, subcorneal pustular dermatosis, vasculitis, granuloma faciale, and prurigo pigmentosa. The side effects are hemolytic anemia, methemoglobinemia, leukopenia, and liver and kidney disorders. Regular monitoring blood tests are necessary. A hypersensitivity syndrome caused by DDS, comprising skin eruptions, fever and liver dysfunction, may develop in rare cases (see Chapter 10).

Anticancer agents

Anticancer agents may be administered for skin diseases such as malignant melanoma, squamous cell carcinoma, Paget's disease, and cutaneous lymphoma,

MEMO 6–11 Skin rejuvenation

In cosmetic dermatology, various techniques and machines have been developed to respond to the needs for rejuvenating appearances, including the demand for healthy-looking skin. Skin rejuvenation achieves improvements in the skin. Hyaluronic acid filler or botulinus toxin is injected to erase wrinkles, intense pulsed light (IPL) treatment or diode laser therapy is used to improve the appearance of pigmented or photoaged skin, and chemical peeling is used to resurface the skin.

depending on the stage of the disease. Currently, many types of anticancer agents (Table 6.10) are used alone or in combination chemotherapies, with combined use of the drugs aiming to reduce side effects and drug resistance.

Table 6.10 Main side effects of anticancer agents.

Agent	Drug	Side effects			
		Myelosuppression	Nausea/vomiting	Alopecia	Other
Alkylating reagent	Cyclophosphamide	+++	++	+++	Hemorrhagic cystitis, SIADH
	Dacarbazine	+	+++	++	Flu-like syndrome, hepatic vein dysfunction
	Nimustine	++	++	++	Interstitial pneumonia, renal disorders
	Temozolomide	+	+++	++	Hematotoxicity
	Cisplatin	++	+++	+	Renal dysfunction, hypacusis, neuropathy
Antimetabolite	Methotrexate	++	+	+	Hepatic dysfunction, renal dysfunction, neuropathy
	Fluorouracil	++	+	+	Diarrhea, aphtha, cerebellar ataxia, myocardial infarction
Antimicrotubule agent	Vincristine	+	+	++	Neuropathy, constipation, SIADH
	Docetaxel	+++	+	++	Edema, eruption, allergic reaction
	Paclitaxel	+++	+	++	Allergic reaction, peripheral neuropathy
Anticancer antibiotic	Doxorubicin	+++	+++	+++	Cardiac dysfunction
	Bleomycin	+	+	++	Interstitial pneumonia, allergic reaction, fever, chills
	Mitomycin C	+++	++	++	Pneumonopathy, renal disorders
	Epirubicin	+++	+++	++	Cardiac dysfunction
	Pirarubicin	+++	++	++	Cardiac dysfunction (cummulative)
Topoisomerase inhibitor	Etoposide	+++	++	+++	Allergic reaction, hepatic dysfunction, central nervous system disorder

SIADH, syndrome of inappropriate secretion of antidiuretic hormone.
Source: Residents of the National Cancer Center Internal Medicine, *Resident's Manual for Cancer Treatment, Ver. 4*, Igaku-Shoin, 2007.

Vitamins

Skin diseases caused by specific vitamin deficiencies include angular cheilitis (ariboflavinosis, vitamin B deficiency), pellagra (niacin deficiency), and biotin deficiency (vitamin H deficiency). Vitamin C supplements are given in scurvy and may also be useful in cases of melasma, purpura, and postinflammatory pigmentation.

Chinese herbal medicine

Many types of herbal medicines may be used in treating acne vulgaris, pruritus cutaneus, urticaria, and viral warts.

Other agents

Interferons, NSAIDs, potassium iodides, zinc preparations, and prostaglandins are also used in treating various skin disorders (Table 6.11).

Laser therapies

Basics and theory of laser therapy

"Laser" is an acronym for "<u>l</u>ight <u>a</u>mplification by <u>s</u>timulated <u>e</u>mission of <u>r</u>adiation." Molecules in the laser medium, including ruby, alexandrite, and other

Table 6.11 Other dermatological drugs.

Type of drug	Main disorder
Interferon	Melanoma, mycosis fungoides
NSAID	Sweet syndrome, erythema induratum, eosinophilic pustular folliculitis
Tranexamic acid	Purpura, melasma
Ivermectin	Scabies
Potassium iodide	Sweet syndrome, Behçet's disease, sporotrichosis
Zinc preparation	Zinc deficiency disorder
Nicotinic acid amide	Pellagra, bullous pemphigoid
Finasteride	Male-pattern baldness
Liver-supporting drug	Eczema, dermatitis, urticaria, alopecia areata
Immunoglobulin	Pemphigus vulgaris, bullous pemphigoid, TEN
GCSF drug	Hematopenia after chemotherapy
Prostaglandin	Livedo vasculopathy, arteriosclerosis obliterans
Antianxiety drug, antidepressant	Postherpetic neuralgia
Antituberculosis drug	Cutaneous tuberculosis, non-tuberculous mycobacterial infections

GCSF, granulocyte colony stimulating factor; NSAID, non-steroidal antiinflammatory drug; TEN, toxic epidermal necrolysis.

Table 6.12 Common lasers.

Laser	Wavelength	Absorbed by... (chromophore)
Carbon dioxide	10600 nm	Water
Dye	577–585 nm	Hemoglobin
Ruby	694 nm	Melanin, tattooing pigments
Alexandrite	755 nm	Melanin, tattooing pigments
Nd: YAG	1064/532 nm	Melanin, hemoglobin, tattooing pigments

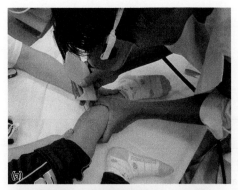

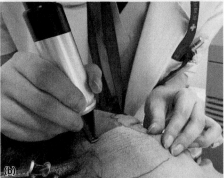

Fig. 6.6 Laser therapy. a: Dye laser. b: Alexandrite laser. Skin whitening is seen immediately after laser irradiation.

crystals, are excited in a xenon flash tube or by electric discharge. When they return to their base state, the molecules emit light that is amplified in a resonator. The emitted wavelength varies depending on the laser medium (Table 6.12). Laser energy is absorbed in tissues by heat transfer, resulting in the destruction of cells and tissues. The part of a visibly colored molecule that absorbs light in the visible range is called a chromophore. It is found in melanins and hemoglobins of normal skin. The application of a laser with a wavelength that affects melanin- or hemoglobin-containing cells causes the temperature to increase and thermal diffusion to be produced, which in turn causes the cells to burn. In this way, blood capillaries are destroyed and the unwanted color tone of the cells fades. Heat damage to the epidermis may result in adverse reactions such as blistering, scarring, and depigmentation. To reduce the risk, some lasers have cryogen spray cooling equipment (a dynamic cooling device).

Examples of laser therapy are shown in Fig. 6.6, and the laser apparatuses that are frequently used are listed in Fig. 6.7. The wavelength that is most effectively absorbed by a particular lesion is selected for irradiation (Fig. 6.8). For melanins, the proper wavelength and pulse width depend on the depth of the pigmented site from the skin surface. The degree of tissue destruction and the time necessary for the patient to recover (downtime) vary greatly depending on the laser pulse width and power. A pulse width between 100 and 500 µs (10^{-6} sec) is generally used. A Q-switched laser effectively treats deep lesions by using high energy at short pulses between 10 and 100 ns (10^{-9} sec). Long-pulse lasers are used to reduce side effects on the skin surface by using a low power output at pulses of 10 ms (10^{-3} sec) or longer.

Laser therapy on pigmented skin lesions

Alexandrite lasers (755 nm) and ruby lasers (694 nm) are used to treat pigmented skin lesions. Light at these wavelengths is not absorbed by hemoglobin. Q-switched lasers can effectively target melanosomes in the dermis and epidermis. Reduction of pigmented cells is observed in at least 80% of cases of nevus of Ota. Laser therapy is also effective for the treatment of nevocellular nevus and blue nevus. The color tone of the nevus fades in proportion to the number of irradiations. However, the therapy does not work on elevated pigmented skin lesions and is not performed in such cases; malignancy should be ruled out. Laser therapy may also be performed on ectopic Mongolian spots, senile lentigo and café au lait spots.

It can be used to remove tattoos, with the effectiveness depending on the pigment depth and color. For multicolored tattoos, a different laser should be used for each color.

Laser therapy on vascular lesions

Dye lasers (585–595 nm) are used to treat hemangiomas. These lasers target hemoglobins and damage erythrocytes. The subsequent emission of heat leads to destruction of the vascular endothelium. The lasers are effective in treating capillary malformation, infantile hemangioma, and telangiectasia. Q-switched Nd:YAG lasers (1064 and 532 nm) and diode lasers (532 nm) can be used in treating vascular lesions.

Other uses of lasers

Long-pulse 800 nm diode lasers and 1064 nm Nd:YAG lasers, which can target melanins at the hair root, are used in hair removal. The carbon dioxide laser (10,600 nm) vaporizes the skin surface and is used for excising tumors and treating scars. In photodynamic therapy (PDT), excimer dye lasers are used (see Chapter 5).

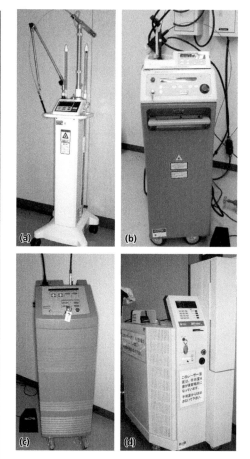

Fig. 6.7 Lasers. a: Carbon dioxide laser. b: Dye laser. c: Alexandrite laser. d: Ruby laser.

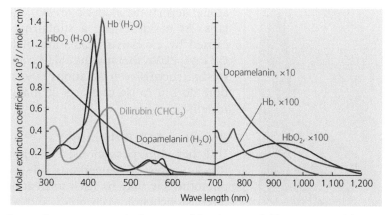

Fig. 6.8 Optical absorption spectrum in human skin. Source: Anderson & Parrish. *J Invest Dermatol* 1981; 77(1): 13–19. Reproduced with permission of *Nature*.

Physical therapies

Phototherapy

Phototherapy can be performed using ultraviolet (UV) light and infrared (IR) rays.

Ultraviolet (UV) light

Ultraviolet (UV) light is divided into three ranges of wavelength: UVA (315–400 nm), UVB (280–315 nm), and UVC (100–280 nm). The shorter the wavelength, the lower the penetration and the greater the energy. UVC light is mainly used in sterilization lamps because of its high cytotoxicity. The UV phototoxic reaction of UVA and UVB irradiation is used in dermatological laser therapies. UVA and UVB can both cause damage to DNA by exciting UV-absorbing molecules or by producing free radicals that cause cellular injury. The mechanism of UV light therapy includes local suppression of skin immunity achieved by reducing the number of Langerhans cells.

Psoralen-ultraviolet-A (PUVA) therapy

Psoralen-ultraviolet-A (PUVA) therapy (Fig. 6.9) is a routinely used treatment involving UVA in combination with psoralen in the form of 8-MOP (8-methoxypsoralen) or TMP (4,5′,8-trimethylpsoralen). UVA has a long wavelength and therefore penetrates deeply into the skin but has little energy. After oral ingestion or topical application of psoralen, a phototoxic substance, the site is irradiated with UVA. PUVA is used for the treatment of psoriasis vulgaris, vitiligo, mycosis fungoides, palmoplantar pustulosis, atopic dermatitis, alopecia areata, and prurigo nodularis. As a side effect, a sunburn reaction may be caused by excessive irradiation of long-wavelength UV rays. PUVA therapy should be carefully performed, so that successive irradiations over a long period of time do not cause cataracts or malignant cutaneous tumors.

Broadband UVB therapy

UVB has immunosuppressive properties and inhibits the functions of Langerhans cells. Broadband UVB phototherapy may be used to treat atopic dermatitis, pityriasis lichenoides chronica, and pruritus in dialysis patients. Patients with psoriasis vulgaris may also benefit from broadband UVB as well as UVB from sunlight (heliotherapy).

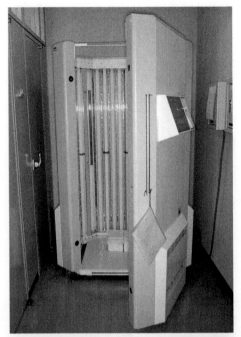
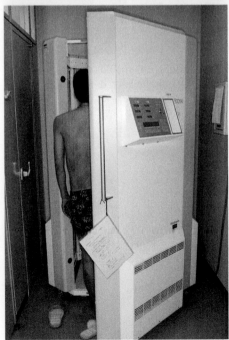

Fig. 6.9 UV irradiation instrument (narrow-band UVB/UVA).

Narrow-band UVB therapy

Narrow-band UVB has a wavelength of 311 nm ± 2 nm. It is thought to be more effective than broadband UVB as a treatment for skin diseases. It is effective against psoriasis, atopic dermatitis, early-stage mycosis fungoides, and vitiligo vulgaris.

UVA1 therapy

UVA with a long wavelength of 340–400 nm is called UVA1. Used mainly in treating patients with acute exacerbation of atopic dermatitis, it is also effective against scleroderma.

Infrared light

The patient is subjected to IR radiation at a wavelength of 760 nm or longer. This raises the skin temperature, improves blood circulation and produces an antiinflammatory effect. Transmission of IR through the skin is high, reaching a depth of several centimeters from the skin surface. This property allows IR therapy to act directly on blood vessels, nerves, lymphatic vessels, and other tissues. This treatment is effective against frostbite, chilblains, and ulcers of the lower legs.

Radiotherapy

Electron beam therapy using β rays generated by a betatron is used in treating melanoma, mycosis fungoides, and keloids. Low-tension X-rays (soft C-rays, dermopan) were once commonly used in treating various skin disorders.

Cryotherapy, cryosurgery

Cryotherapy is a method of freezing tissue using a cryogenic agent such as liquid nitrogen. It is mainly used in treating viral warts, granuloma telangiectaticum, and small soft fibromas. Nevi and hemangiomas can be treated by cryotherapy. There are two main cryotherapy methods: swabbing (a cotton swab dipped in liquid nitrogen at −196.8° is brought into contact with the lesion (Fig. 6.10)), and spraying (liquid nitrogen is sprayed on the lesion at a pressure of 0.1–0.5 kg/cm² (Fig. 6.11)).

Thermotherapy, hyperthermia

In thermotherapy, a lesion is warmed to between 42° and 47° with warm water, a body warmer or a medical exothermic sheet. This is effective in treating sporotrichosis, chromomycosis, and non-tuberculous

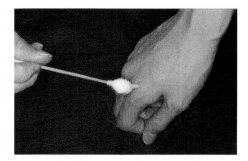

Fig. 6.10 Cryotherapy (using stype).

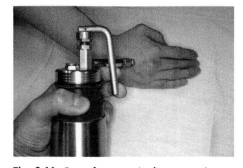

Fig. 6.11 Cryotherapy (using spray).

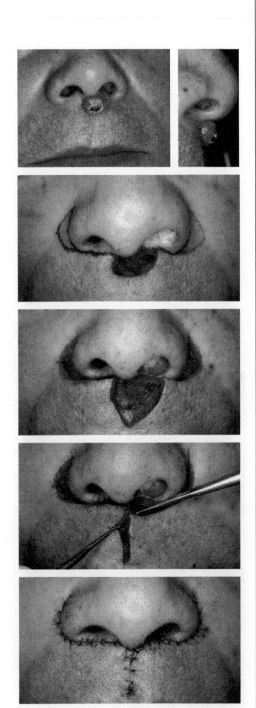

Fig. 6.13 Excision of keratoacanthoma:
Skin defect was closed by V-T flap.

mycobacterial infections. It may be used as a treatment for malignant skin tumors in conjunction with chemotherapy or irradiation therapy.

Hyperbaric oxygen (HBO) therapy

The aim of hyperbaric oxygen therapy (HBO) is to increase the amount of oxygen dissolved in the blood and thereby elevate the partial pressure of oxygen in the tissues. It may be used for peripheral circulatory disorders such as ischemic anaerobic infections (e.g., gas gangrene) or postoperatively on skin grafts.

Skin surgery

Skin surgery may be performed to treat various types of nevi, benign and malignant tumors, burn scars, intractable ulcers, chronic pyoderma, and tattoos. Preoperatively, it is important to evaluate the indication for surgery and determine whether the patient will be able to tolerate the procedure. In addition, enquiries should be made of any significant medical history, drug history, and drug allergies. The procedure and any potential complications must be thoroughly explained to the patient. It is essential to obtain written consent prior to the procedure.

Practical techniques of suturing, skin grafting, and dermabrasion are introduced briefly below. Refer to textbooks on dermatological surgery and plastic surgery for more detail.

Excision and suture

Comparatively small lesions are excised and the periphery is sutured (Fig. 6.12 and Fig. 6.13). The basic method is spindle-shaped excision and suturing. If the

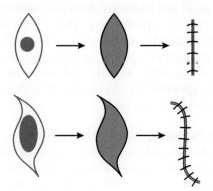

Fig. 6.12 Excision and suture.

longitudinal axis of the excision is not long enough, the ends may become elevated, producing "dog-ears" that pose a cosmetic problem. For this reason, the long axis needs to be at least three times the width. In the event that a lesion cannot be sutured in a single operation, it may be excised in two or more operations (serial excision). The skin may be extended using silicon prior to surgery (skin expansion), or skin graft may be performed. Excision is generally performed along wrinkle lines (Langer's lines: see Fig. 1.3). Excision lines must be carefully considered, especially when the excision is large or when the surgery is performed on cosmetically important sites such as the face.

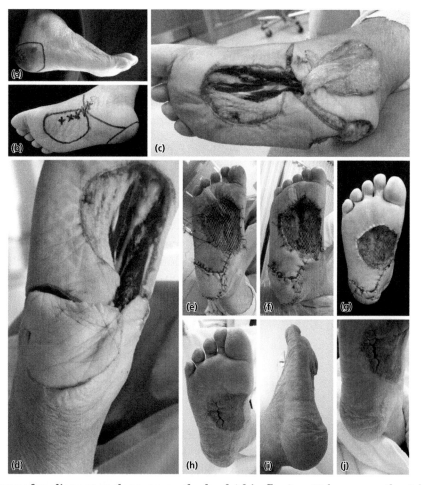

Fig. 6.14 Surgery of malignant melanoma on the heel (skin flap). a: Melanoma on the right heel. b: Presurgical design. The inner plantar artery is located by Doppler blood flow sensor (shown by the x's). c: The prepared skin flap. d: The flap is moved to the site where the melanoma was removed. e: Mesh grafting is done on the sole. f–j: Follow-up photos.

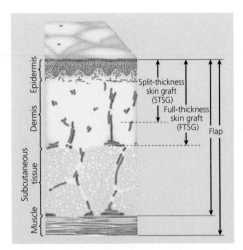

Fig. 6.15 Skin thicknesses and various graft procedures.

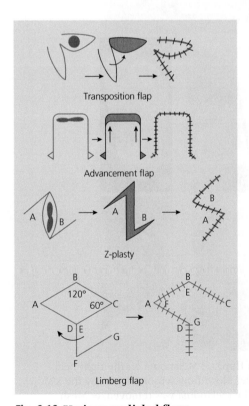

Fig. 6.16 Various pedicled flaps.

Skin grafting, skin flap

When a lesion is too large for excision and suturing, a skin graft may be performed. Skin grafting and pedicle flap reconstruction are the two main methods (Figs 6.14–6.16).

Skin grafts

Skin is removed from the donor site (Fig. 6.17) and placed in the acceptor site (tie-over method, Fig. 6.18). The removed skin remains ischemic for approximately 4 or 5 days, until blood flow is restored. Skin grafts can be full thickness (the epidermis and all the dermal layers) or split thickness (the epidermis and some dermal layers), depending on the thickness of the dermal area removed (see Fig. 6.15). In a split-thickness graft, removed skin is processed into a mesh to increase the graft survival rate (mesh skin graft). Since skin is among the organs most likely to produce immunological rejection, the patient's own normal skin is usually used as a permanent graft. Allogeneic graft, dermatoheteroplasty, and biological dressing of freeze-dried pigskin are sometimes performed to temporarily cover the body.

Pedicle flaps

Skin and subcutaneous tissues are not completely separated from the living body for the graft. The flap is supplied by blood vessels passing through the pedicle (see Fig. 6.16).

Dermabrasion, skin abrasion

Dermabrasion is a method of scraping the skin surface with a high-speed grinder, dermatome or dermal curette. Depending on the depth, dermabrasion may produce scars such as keloids, recurrent lesions or pigmentation so skillful performance is required. Instead of a high-speed grinder or dermatome, a carbon dioxide gas laser is often used to treat verrucous epidermal nevus, seborrheic keratosis, tattoos, lichen amyloidosis, porokeratosis, Darier's disease, and Hailey–Hailey disease.

Chemical peeling

The application of certain chemicals (e.g., salicylic acid, glycolic acid, trichloroacetic acid) to the skin may result in exfoliation. Chemical peeling can produce a desirable effect on lesions such as acne and senile lentigo. The depth of peeling can be varied to achieve the desired cosmetic effect.

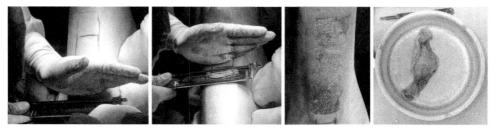

Fig. 6.17 Split-thickness skin graft was obtained using silver knife.

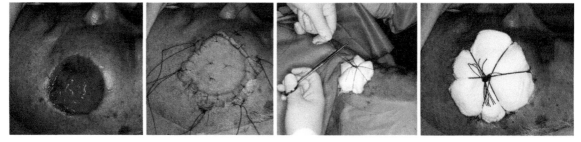

Fig. 6.18 Skin grafting and tie-over.

Electrosurgery, iontophoresis

The main types of electrosurgery are electrocoagulation, in which heat generated by an electric scalpel coagulates tissues (Fig. 6.19), and electrolysis, in which blood and tissue fluids are degenerated by the application of direct-current electricity to the skin. Iontophoresis involves the introduction of a solution of salt ions transdermally and is effective in treating palmoplantar and axillary hyperhidrosis. Several iontophoresis devices are commercially available.

Laser knife

Laser knives cauterize tissue using heat produced by a laser. Carbon dioxide gas lasers are the principal lasers used for surgery. The advantages of surgical lasers are that there is no direct contact and that they can be used without electricity, thus making them applicable for patients with pacemakers. A surgical laser is useful for treating seborrheic keratosis and verrucous epidermal nevus; moreover, the depth is easily controlled, and injury to normal tissues is minimal.

Surgitron, radiosurgery

A Surgitron uses radio waves of about 4 MHz to perform surgical treatments. Unlike an electric scalpel, it results in denaturation by heat that leaves scarring.

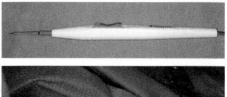
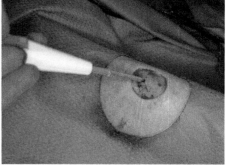

Fig. 6.19 Electrocoagulation.

CHAPTER 7

Eczema and dermatitis

Eczema and dermatitis are synonymous terms for a disease commonly seen in dermatological practice. The main clinical features are itching, erythema, scaling, and edematous papules. Histopathologically, eczema is characterized by intercellular edema (spongiosis), which can be caused by extrinsic factors such as irritants or allergens, or by intrinsic factors such as atopic diathesis. These factors interact in complex ways, and both extrinsic and intrinsic factors can often coexist. There is no international agreement on the subcategories of eczema. Eczema may be classified as acute, subacute or chronic, depending on the clinical and pathological features.

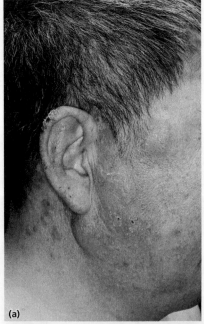

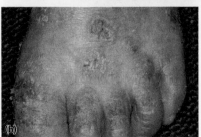

Fig. 7.1 Eczema. a: Eczema with reddening. b: Eczema with crusts and partial infiltration.

Eczema (synoym: dermatitis)

- The terms eczema and dermatitis are used interchangeably.
- The main clinical features of eczema/dermatitis are itching, erythema, scaling, and edematous papules.
- Histopathologically, it is characterized by intercellular edema (spongiosis).
- It accounts for one-third of all dermatology cases.
- Extrinsic and intrinsic factors are simultaneously involved in the onset.
- The first-line treatment is topical steroids.

Clinical features

The clinical features consist of itching and erythema on which papules, vesicles, pustules, erosions, crusts, and scales may form (Fig. 7.1). Eczema is a progressive condition, and the stages are illustrated in Fig. 7.2. In the acute stage, the symptoms may be present singly or together. In the chronic stage, in addition to the acute symptoms, there may be the lichenification, hyperpigmentation, and hypopigmentation.

Shimizu's Dermatology, Second Edition. Hiroshi Shimizu.
© 2017 John Wiley & Sons, Ltd. Published 2017 by John Wiley & Sons, Ltd.

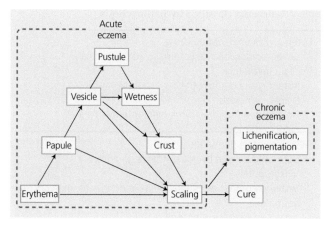

Fig. 7.2 Course and symptoms of eczema.

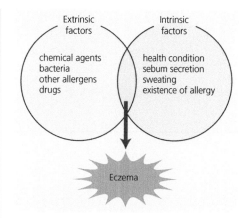

Fig. 7.3 Various factors causing eczema: Extrinsic and intrinsic factors interact, resulting in eczema formation.

Pathogenesis

Both extrinsic and intrinsic factors are involved in the pathogenesis of eczema (Fig. 7.3). When an extrinsic agent such as a drug, pollen, house dust or microorganism invades the skin, an inflammatory reaction is induced. However, the severity and type of the reaction depend on intrinsic factors such as seborrhea, dyshidrosis, atopic diathesis, and the general health of the patient.

Pathology

Eczema is characterized by intercellular edema (spongiosis) (Fig. 7.4). In the acute stage, it is accompanied by exocytosis of lymphocytes and spongiotic bullae. In the chronic stage, hyperkeratosis, parakeratosis, irregular acanthosis, and elongation of rete ridges are observed. Spongiosis and bullae are less severe in chronic eczema.

Classification

Eczema can also be classified on the basis of its etiological factors (Table 7.1). These often interact in complex ways and are not always clearly identifiable. The names used for these skin conditions vary by country.

Eczema with unidentified cause

When the cause is not identified, eczema may be classified into the subtypes of acute, subacute or chronic, according to the clinical findings, the course of the

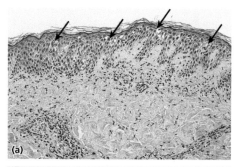

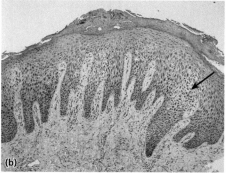

Fig. 7.4 Histopathology of eczema.
a: Acute eczema. Spongiosis (arrows) has formed from intercellular edema. Lymphocytic infiltration is also seen.
b: Chronic eczema. Hyperkeratosis, regular acanthosis and elongation of epidermal rete ridge are noted. Spongiosus is not severe.

Table 7.1 Eczema classified by pathogenesis.

Eczema with unidentified cause
Acute eczema, subacute eczema, chronic eczema
Contact dermatitis
   Irritant contact dermatitis
   Diaper dermatitis
   Housewife's (hand) eczema (keratodermia tylodes-
   palmaris progressiva)
Allergic contact dermatitis
   Dermatitis caused by vegetation (e.g., primrose,
   ginkgo nuts)
   Systemic contact dermatitis (shiitake dermatitis, mercury
   dermatitis)
   Contact dermatitis syndrome
Photocontact dermatitis (irritant, allergic)
   Contact urticaria
Atopic dermatitis
Seborrheic dermatitis
Nummular eczema
Lichen simplex chronicus (lichen Vidal)
Autosensitization dermatitis
Stasis dermatitis
Asteatotic eczema
Dyshidrotic eczema
Other
   Pityriasis simplex faciei
   Lip licker's dermatitis

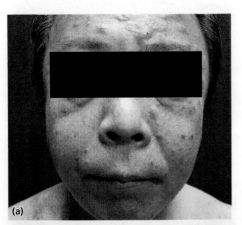
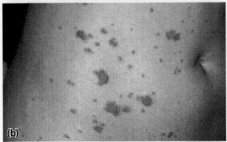

Fig. 7.5 Acute eczema. a: Multiple edematous erythema on the face. b: Pruritic erythema with scattered papules. Some vesicles are seen.

eruption, and the pathological findings. Lesions in various stages often coexist in the same individual.

Topical steroids, emollients, and oral antihistamines are the first-line treatments.

Acute eczema

Such eczema is accompanied by exudative erythema, edema, and sometimes vesicle formation (Fig. 7.5). These features develop several days after the onset of the disease. Spongiosis, intense dermal edema, and inflammation are present histologically, but acanthosis is not a feature.

Chronic eczema

Chronic eczema is characterized clinically by lichenification. When acute eczema persists for more than 1 week, the appearance of the skin may be lichenified. The main histological features are acanthosis and parakeratosis (Fig. 7.6). There are fewer inflammatory cells in the epidermis than there are in acute or subacute eczema.

Contact dermatitis

- Contact dermatitis can be divided into two main subtypes: primary irritant contact dermatitis and allergic contact dermatitis. It is localized to the site of extrinsic stimulation by a foreign substance or allergen.
- Erythema and blistering occur at the site of contact.
- It is classified roughly into irritant contact dermatitis, which is caused by toxicity of the causative substance and can affect anyone, and allergic contact dermatitis, which affects individuals who have been sensitized by contact allergy.
- There are specific types of contact dermatitis, such as diaper dermatitis and housewife's hand eczema.
- The causative substances include certain plants, chemical agents and metals, such as nickel and mercury.
- Patch testing is useful for diagnosis. The treatment consists of eliminating the causative agent and providing symptomatic relief with topical steroid ointment, antihistamines, and emollients. In severe cases, oral steroids may be used.

Clinical features

Erythema, papules, vesicles, erosions, and crusts are seen at the site of contact of the causative agent (Fig. 7.7). The eczematous lesions are relatively sharply circumscribed and are intensely itchy. The lesions may become widespread when the causative agent is spread by rubbing and scratching. If the inflammation spreads over the entire body, systemic symptoms such as fever may arise and in rare cases skin necrosis and ulceration may develop.

Atypical cases of contact dermatitis

- **Systemic contact dermatitis:** when an individual is sensitized by contact allergy and subsequently becomes exposed to the same allergen such as by inhalation, ingestion or injection, a systemic allergic reaction may be produced. Eczema or edematous erythema develops. Such contact dermatitis may be elicited by shiitake mushrooms (see Fig. 7.7-1c), mercury, and other substances. Systemic allergy caused by dental casting alloys is classified as this type of dermatitis.

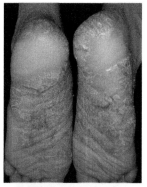
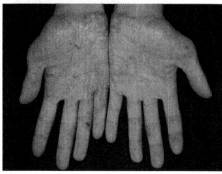

Fig. 7.6 Chronic eczema. Hyperkeratosis is severe, as in tylosis. Erythema and fissures are seen.

MEMO 7–1 Types of contact dermatitis

Contact dermatitis may be diagnosed as ginkgo nut dermatitis, rhus dermatitis, mercury dermatitis or shiitake dermatitis. The diagnosis depends on the allergen.

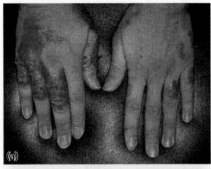

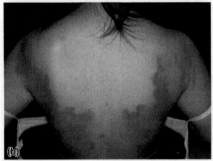

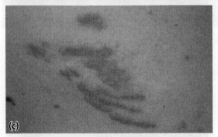

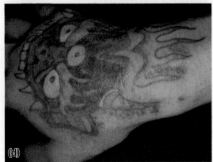

Fig. 7.7-1 Contact dermatitis. a: From an unknown cause, probably a surfactant such as soap or detergent. b: From a clothing. c: Systemic contact dermatitis called "Shiitake dermatitis", which occurs after raw shiitake mushrooms are eaten. The erythema is strongly itchy and infiltrative. d: Contact dermatitis from tattooing. Erythema with itchiness and infiltration occur as an allergic reaction to red pigments.

- **Contact dermatitis syndrome:** repeated transdermal exposure to a causative substance causes spreading of the substance by way of lymph and blood flow, and systemic skin lesions develop. Autosensitization dermatitis can be this type of dermatitis. It may appear as a symptom of erythema multiforme or erythroderma.
- **Photocontact dermatitis:** MEMO, see Chapter 13.
- **Riehl's melanosis:** see Chapter 16.
- **Gold dermatitis caused by earrings:** readily ionized metals such as nickel often cause dermatitis. In recent years, the number of dermatitis cases caused by gold earrings has increased significantly. There is intractable induration where the ear is pierced, and a lymphoid follicle-like structure may form (Fig. 7.8).

Pathogenesis

Primary irritant contact dermatitis results from an inflammatory reaction caused by lysosomes or various cytokines released from damaged keratinocytes when the skin is exposed to an external substance. If the level of irritation is high enough, contact dermatitis can occur from the very first contact. Highly toxic substances may cause chemical burns (e.g., kerosene dermatitis; see Chapter 13). In recent years, about 80% of patients with occupational skin diseases have had irritant contact dermatitis, which has been increasing because of frequent exposure to substances with low toxicity (soap, shampoo, other occupational chemicals) that reduce the skin barrier function.

Allergic contact dermatitis occurs as a type IV allergic reaction (see Fig. 1.56). The causative agent is absorbed through the skin and then captured by Langerhans cells, which are epidermal antigen-presenting cells. The Langerhans cells subsequently migrate to the regional lymph nodes and transmit information about the antigen to the thymus-derived T cells, which then proliferate in the lymph nodes (sensitization). Subsequent exposure to the same causative agent (even in minute amounts) causes the sensitized T cells to be reactivated and various cytokines to be released, which leads to a prompt inflammatory reaction and dermatitis. Table 7.2 shows examples of substances that can cause allergic contact dermatitis.

Table 7.2 Main allergens in allergic contact dermatitis.

Heavy metals	Cobalt, nickel, chrome, mercury
Plants	Sumac (urushiol), primrose (primin), ginkgo nut (ginkgolic acid), chrysanthemums, lilies
Foods	Mango (urushiol), ginkgo nut, lettuce, onion
Daily miscellaneous goods	Antimicrobial products such as desk mats, rubber products (MBT), clothing, detergents
Cosmetic items	Hair dyes (paraphenylene diamine), aromatic preparations, preservatives
Medicinal agents	Topical non-steroidal antiinflammatory drugs, medicated plasters, disinfectants, eye lotions, topical steroids
Occupationally used substances	Various metals, resins, rubber products, machine oil

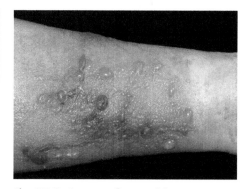

Fig. 7.7-2 Contact dermatitis. From an NSAID plaster.

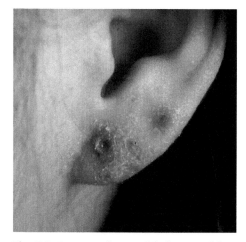

Fig. 7.8 Contact dermatitis from gold earrings.

Laboratory findings, diagnosis

Each causative agent produces a particular distribution of eruptions. Clues to the nature of the irritant or allergen can be gleaned from the history as well as by the distribution of eczema. Substances that cause contact dermatitis and are frequently used for patch testing are listed in Table 7.3 according to the body site.

Treatment

The irritant or allergen should be avoided. Topical steroids and oral antihistamines are first-line treatments. Although desensitization therapy is performed at some institutions, the efficacy varies from case to case.

Specific types of eczema

Atopic dermatitis

- Atopic dermatitis is chronic eczema/dermatitis associated with an atopic diathesis (allergic asthma, rhinitis, conjunctivitis, dermatitis).
- Eczema/dermatitis chronically recurs (for 2 months or longer in infants, and 6 months or longer in other age groups).
- Exudative eczema may develop on the face and ear pinna associated with dry pityriatic scales.
- Filaggrin plays an important role in the onset.

MEMO 7–2 Allergic contact dermatitis syndrome (ACDS)

The International Contact Dermatitis Research Group (ICDRG) uses the term "allergic contact dermatitis syndrome" to describe systemic contact dermatitis and contact dermatitis, because the ICDRG considers the two to be similar, in that the allergen has systemic effects.

There are specific names for contact dermatitis, according to patient type and the particular location on the body (See Figures).

- **Diaper dermatitis:** this occurs where the diaper comes into contact with the skin. It is irritant contact dermatitis caused by urine. Differentiation from the *Candida intertrigo* fungus (erythema mycoticum infantile; see Chapter 25) is required.
- **Housewife's hand eczema:** this affects the hands of those who frequently work with water. It is thought to be irritant contact dermatitis that involves detergents and water.
- **Lip licker's dermatitis:** frequently seen in infants and young children, this is irritant contact dermatitis around the mouth caused by saliva and food. It involves factors similar to those for factitial dermatitis (see Chapter 13).

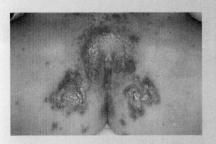
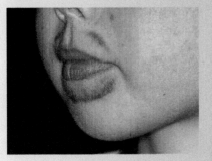

Diaper dermatitis and lip licker's dermatitis.

Table 7.3 Contact dermatitis: Locations and main causes.

Location	Cause
Scalp	Shampoos, hair dyes, hair restorers, hats, hairpins
Face	Cosmetics, medicinal agents, perfumes, eyeglasses, plants, sunscreen
Neck	Necklaces, cosmetics, perfumes, medicinal agents, clothes
Body, extremities	Clothes, cleansers, metals, medicinal agents
Hands and feet	Rubber, leather, plants, medical agents, cleansers, cosmetics, metals
Genital region	Clothes, cleansers, condoms, contraceptive devices

- White dermographism may be present, and the IgE value is high.
- The following complications can occur: Kaposi's varicelliform eruption (eczema herpetiform), cataract, and retinal detachment.
- Topical steroids, topical immunosuppressants such as tacrolimus and pimecrolimus, oral antihistamines, and emollients are the first-line treatments.

General information

The chronic lesions of atopic dermatitis develop as a result of a combination of acquired stimulatory factors and endogenous factors such as impaired skin barrier function caused by mutations in filaggrin genes and susceptibility to the production of high IgE levels. Atopic dermatitis can be defined as a disease in which the main lesions are itchy and erythematous, with recurrent remissions and exacerbations. Most patients have an atopic tendency. Atopic diatheses include a familial or personal history of one or more disorders such as bronchial asthma, allergic rhinitis, conjunctivitis or atopic dermatitis; and susceptibility to the production of high IgE levels. Type I allergy (atopic diathesis) and type IV allergy (contact dermatitis) are both involved in most cases.

Clinical features

Atopic dermatitis may be classified by age into three main groups: infantile (age 2 months to 4 years), childhood (early childhood to puberty), and adolescent/ adult. Different eruptions characterize each group (Fig. 7.9). Atopic dermatitis is accompanied by intense itching in all cases and tends to worsen when the skin is dry or sweaty. Although it most frequently occurs in infancy, the incidence in older children as well as in adults has been increasing in recent years.

Infantile atopic dermatitis

In the early stage of infantile atopic dermatitis, erythema, scales, and serous papules develop on the head

> **MEMO 7–4 Atopy**
>
> The term "atopy" was first proposed by Coca et al. in 1923. Atopy literally means abnormal hypersensitivity, and patients with atopic diatheses tend to suffer from bronchial asthma and hay fever. Atopic dermatitis is often hereditary.

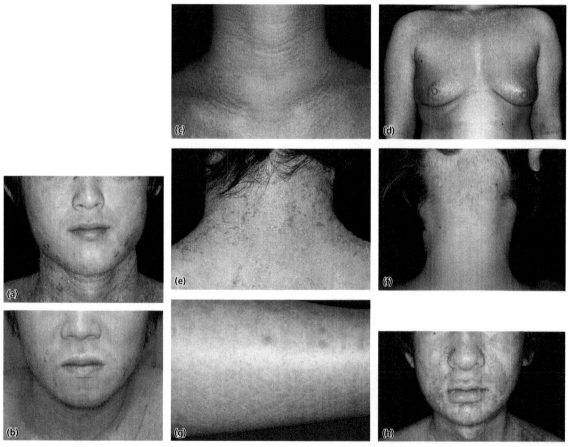

Fig. 7.9-1 Atopic dermatitis. a: Adult male. Erythema is seen on the face and neck. Erosion and infiltration from scratching are seen. Thinning of the outer edges of the eyebrows (Hertoghe's sign) is observed. b: A line in the skin below the lower eyelid (Dennie–Morgan fold) is observed. c: "Dirty neck". Poikilodermatous pigmentation is seen on the neck and upper chest. d: Poikilodermatous pigmentation is widespread on the upper body. e: Adult male. Scattered eruptions from scratching are seen. f: Scars from scratching and hair loss are seen in the occipital region of the head, a complication of trichotillomania (Chapter 19, p. 350) from mental stress. g: Complicated with ichthyosis vulgaris (Chapter 15, p. 251). h: Rapidly aggravated infiltrative erythema, consistent with non-bullous impetigo (Chapter 24, p. 489).

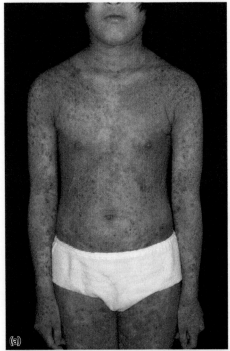

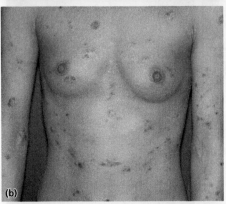

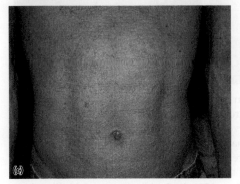

Fig. 7.9-2 Atopic dermatitis. a: Child.
b: Multiple pruritus from scratching.
c: Erythrodermic atopic dermatitis.

and face, and gradually spread to the trunk. The condition can become exudative, with crusts and scales. At this stage, it can resemble seborrheic dermatitis. Thick crusts on the head and lesions around the mouth and lower jaw (produced by causative agents in baby food) may also be observed. The trunk and extremities become dry. Follicular papules may also aggregate, giving the appearance of goose bumps. Scaly erythematous plaques may form on these lesions, and the condition may then progress to childhood atopic dermatitis.

Childhood atopic dermatitis
In childhood atopic dermatitis, the skin becomes dry. Lichenified plaques occur in the flexural areas, such as the cubital, popliteal, and axillary fossae. Fissures are often present in the auricular area. Childhood atopic dermatitis is accompanied by intense itching, and progresses rapidly to eczematous crusty lesions.

Adolescent and adult atopic dermatitis
The symptoms are similar to those seen in childhood dermatitis but tend to be more severe and widespread. Rough, dry, dark brown areas may develop all over the body. Thinning of the lateral eyebrow may be present (Hertoghe's sign, see Fig. 7.9-1a). A line in the skin below the lower eyelid (Dennie–Morgan fold) may be observed (see Fig. 7.9-1b). In severe cases, diffuse erythema occurs on the face and a mottled appearance is seen on the neck and upper chest (poikiloderma lesion, "dirty neck," see Fig. 7.9-1c, d). Prurigo nodularis may occur repeatedly on the extremities.

Pathogenesis
The pathogenesis of atopic dermatitis remains unclear but the three factors below are regarded as key. The contribution of each factor varies by case and by the growth stage of the patient. For proper treatment, it is important to consider all three factors.

Skin physiological abnormality
Skin barrier defect plays an important role in the pathogenesis of atopic dermatitis. In 2006, filaggrin gene mutations were identified as being extremely important in the development of atopic dermatitis. Filaggrin is necessary for keratinization, and it eventually metabolizes into amino acids that act as natural moisturizing factor (NMF) (see Chapter 1). Filaggrin gene mutation, which causes ichthyosis vulgaris, is

identified in 20–50% of patients with atopic dermatitis. Filaggrin works as a factor in skin barrier function,
and it is thought that decreased filaggrin production
leads to dry skin and, eventually, atopic dermatitis.
Abnormality in vascular response can be tested by
scratching the skin firmly with a blunt object, resulting
in the development of white dermographism (in atopic
dermatitis the skin may become white when scratched,
whereas normal skin becomes red; Fig. 7.10). The
atopic skin is also vulnerable to external irritation,
such as by perspiration or contact with animal fur,
wool or chemicals.

Immunological factors

Based on the intrinsic factors and the decrease in skin
barrier function, a Th2-dominated immune reaction
plays a role in the development of atopic dermatitis.
Type IV allergic reaction to external irritation is
observed. The patient is prone to overproduction of
IgE (atopic diathesis), and the IgE receptor (FceR) in
mast cells and in eosinophils is readily activated.
Positive intracutaneous reactions to various allergens
are seen in many cases, which provides evidence that
congenital immune abnormality may be involved in
atopic dermatitis.

External factors

Mites, house dust, microbes resident on the skin (e.g.,
fungi of the genus *Malassezia* and other genera),
psychological stress, and humidity are external stimuli
that can aggravate the condition.

Complications

Eye diseases such as cataracts (in 10% of severe adult
cases), keratoconus, and retinal detachment are potential complications of atopic dermatitis. These are
thought to result from prolonged eye rubbing from the
itch and oral steroid use, although this has not been
confirmed. Infectious diseases, including Kaposi's
varicelliform eruptions, molluscum contagiosum, and
impetigo contagiosa, are other important complications. Patients with atopic dermatitis may be hypersensitive to drugs and insect bites.

Laboratory findings

The serum IgE value is high, with IgE RAST for house
dust or mites being positive in most cases. An increase
in peripheral blood eosinophils may be observed.
Although the test of white dermographism is highly

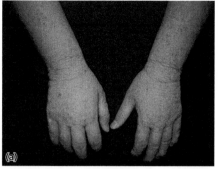

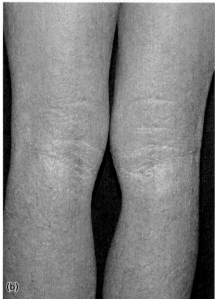

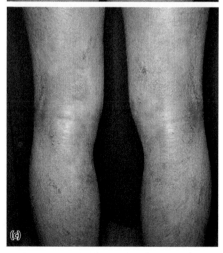

Fig. 7.9-3 Atopic dermatitis. a: Atopic
dermatitis of the hands with contact
dermatitis. b, c: Erythema, scales and
exfoliation on the flexor of the lower leg.

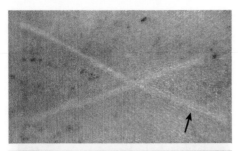

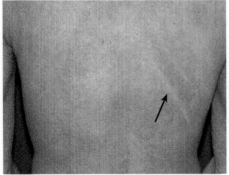

Fig. 7.10 White dermographism in a patient with atopic dermatitis.

sensitive for atopic dermatitis, it has low specificity. Serum thymus and activation-regulated chemokine (TARC) levels are closely related to disease activity.

Diagnosis

Clinically, characteristic eruptions are easy to diagnose. It is important to consider any family history of the condition. It is also important to recognize that there is an increasing incidence of adolescent and adult atopic dermatitis that did not develop in early childhood or was not recognized then. Infantile seborrheic dermatitis closely resembles infantile atopic dermatitis. Severity scoring of atopic dermatitis (SCORAD) is used for evaluating severity. Skindex-16 is used for evaluating the quality of life (QOL) of patients with atopic dermatitis.

Treatment

Topical steroid application is the primary treatment for atopic dermatitis. The strength and dosage must be chosen carefully based on the severity and course of the disease. Providing proper control and avoiding side effects and rebound phenomenon are responsibilities of the dermatologist.

Ointments containing immunosuppressants such as tacrolimus and pimecrolimus are also widely used (see Chapter 6). They are beneficial, particularly for facial lesions, and are frequently used as first-line treatments in many countries. Emollients are helpful in treating mild symptoms and dry skin in atopic dermatitis.

Oral antihistamines are effective at preventing the eruptions from becoming aggravated by rubbing and scratching. Oral steroids are used in severe cases. Ciclosporin, an immunosuppressant drug, may be administered for severe adult cases.

Improvement of the living environment (e.g., removing carpeting, keeping the temperature and humidity low to reduce perspiration) and of skin care (avoiding contact with causative agents, keeping the skin clean) is important for the management of eczema.

Prognosis

Atopic dermatitis tends to be chronic and recurrent. It mostly resolves spontaneously by the time the patient reaches the age of 10 but in some patients, the symptoms persist into adolescence or adulthood.

Seborrheic dermatitis (synonym: Seborrheic eczema)

- Seborrheic dermatitis occurs in areas where sebum is actively secreted. It is characterized by erythematous lesions accompanied by yellowish scales.
- It is one of the most common skin diseases, occurring in infants, adolescents, and adults.
- Fungi of the genus *Malassezia* resident in the skin are an etiological factor.
- Skin care and application of topical steroids and antifungal agents are the main treatments.

Clinical features

There is controversy as to whether seborrheic dermatitis in infants, adolescents, and adults is the same disease, since the clinical manifestations tend to vary with age (Fig. 7.11). Dermatitis commonly appears as eczema on seborrheic sites or intertriginous areas of the head, face, and axillary fossae. The main features are oleaginous scales and erythematous plaques that may be itchy.

In infants, yellowish crusts may develop on the scalp, eyebrows, and forehead. In addition, scaly erythematous plaques may form 2–4 weeks after birth. In most cases, the lesions resolve 8–12 months after birth. In adolescents and adults, the symptoms are chronic and recurrent, and there may be an increase in the amount of pityroid scales (also known as dandruff) and the development of scaly erythematous lesions on the eyebrows and nasolabial groove. Oystershell-like hard crusts may form on the scalp.

Pathogenesis

Triglycerides in sebum are decomposed by microbes resident on the skin to produce free fatty acids that may be associated with an abnormal immune response. Overproliferation of *Malassezia* fungi such as *Malassezia restricta* aggravates seborrheic dermatitis. Environmentally affected changes in the secretion and components of the sebum and sweat, and in vitamin metabolites, are considered to be among the causative factors.

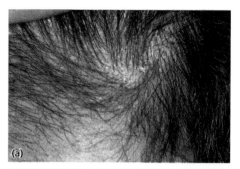
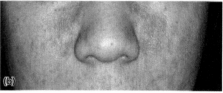

Fig. 7.11 Seborrheic dermatitis. a: Scalp. Erythema with scales. b: Face.

MEMO 7–7 *Malassezia furfur* or *Pityrosporum*

In the past, yeast detected in patients with seborrheic dermatitis and pityriasis versicolor was classified as *Malassezia furfur*; however, recent genetic analyses have clarified that these yeasts actually belong to several different species. The *Malassezia restricta* fungus predominates in seborrheic dermatitis and the *Malassezia globosa* fungus in pityriasis versicolor. Both of these species are frequently detected in atopic dermatitis. Currently, the yeast classified as *Malassezia furfur* is detected in a portion of patients with atopic dermatitis. It has been clarified that the *Pityrosporum* fungus, identified in 1904, is actually the same organism as *Malassezia furfur*, identified in 1889; both are now classified in the genus *Malassezia*.

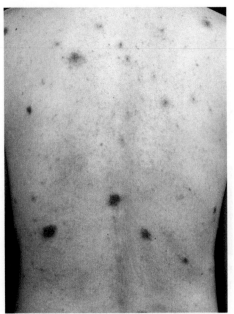

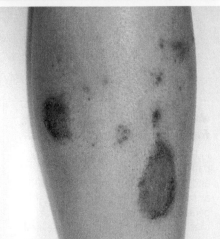

Fig. 7.12 Nummular eczema. Multiple round eczema of 1 to 5 cm in diameter.

Differential diagnosis

Dry seborrheic dermatitis closely resembles psoriasis vulgaris. It is also important to differentiate seborrheic dermatitis from pityriasis rosea and parapsoriasis en plaque. In infants, distinction from atopic dermatitis is essential.

Treatment

Proper facial cleansing with soap and hair washing with shampoo are important in keeping the seborrheic areas clean. Mild- to moderate-potency topical steroids are useful. Topical antifungal creams and shampoos are particularly effective when seborrheic dermatitis is accompanied by dandruff, especially in adolescents and older patients, because overproliferation of *Malassezia* fungi is often the cause.

Nummular eczema (eczema nummulare)

- Round, relatively large eczematous plaques are present.
- Nummular eczema may occur at any site on the body and tends to progress to autosensitization dermatitis (see later in this chapter).
- Topical steroids are the first-line treatment.

Clinical features and epidemiology

Nummular eczema is frequently seen in the winter and is characterized by multiple round lesions 1–5 cm in diameter, mostly on the extremities (particularly on the extensor surface of the lower legs), trunk, hips, and buttocks (Fig. 7.12). At the periphery of the lesions, there may be aggregations of serous papules. These may be accompanied by exudative erythema and scale formation, as well as by intense itching and multiple scars from rubbing and scratching. As the lesions progress, they may develop into autosensitization dermatitis.

Pathogenesis

Scratched insect bites may develop urticarial lesions (see Chapter 8) that progress to nummular eczema. Nummular eczema may also result from contact dermatitis or asteatotic eczema, particularly in the elderly, or it may appear as a symptom of atopic dermatitis.

Treatment

Topical steroids are effective. In cases in which infiltration and exudation are intense, the application of topical zinc ointment sheets, in addition to topical steroids, is also effective. Oral antihistamines are helpful in relieving the itch.

Lichen simplex chronicus (synonym: Lichen Vidal)

Lichen simplex chronicus is chronic eczema in which intensely itchy lichenified plaques form on the nuchal region and extensor aspect of the forearms and lower legs. Pigmentation or depigmentation may be present. A warty appearance may also develop from severe lichenification (Fig. 7.13). Repeated stimulation of the skin by friction, metal allergens and prolonged rubbing and scratching leads to chronic eczematous lesions. Topical steroids and oral antihistamines are first-line treatments for the itching.

Autosensitization dermatitis

- Multiple small papules and erythematous lesions accompanied by itching occur systemically and may result from a sudden aggravation of a localized lesion, e.g., by an infectious agent.
- This condition is thought to be mediated by an endogenous allergic reaction (id reaction).

Clinical features

Prior to the development of autosensitization reaction, there may be aggravation of a primary lesion by various stimuli, such as infectious agents (e.g., fungi and bacteria). Reddening, swelling, and exudation occur in the lower extremities in 50–60% of cases. Several weeks

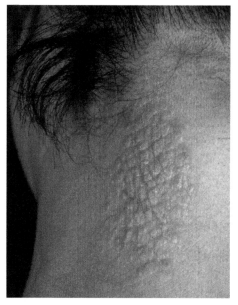

Fig. 7.13 Lichen simplex chronicus (lichen Vidal). Long-time friction from clothes is the cause. It is a chronic eczema.

MEMO 7–8 Infantile eczema

Eczema tends to occur in infants 2–3 weeks after birth, and sometimes up to several months after birth (See Figure). The differential diagnoses of infantile eczema are listed below. Differentiation among these diseases is difficult, especially in newborns.

- **Seborrheic dermatitis in infancy:** see text.
- **Atopic dermatitis:** intractable cases of infantile eczema may be atopic dermatitis.
- **Contact dermatitis:** lip licker's dermatitis and diaper dermatitis.
- **Food allergy:** eruptions caused by baby food or by changes in breast milk that may arise as a result of health problems, including nutritional imbalance in the mother.
- **Other disorders:** tinea and candidiasis. Also, Wiskott–Aldrich syndrome, hyper immunoglobulin E syndrome, Netherton syndrome (see Chapter 15) and Langerhans cell histiocytosis (see Chapter 22), which are rare.

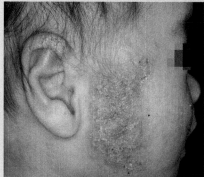

Infantile eczema.

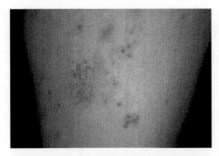

Fig. 7.14-1 Autosensitization dermatitis.
Disseminated eczematous eruptions are seen.

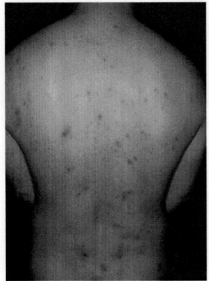

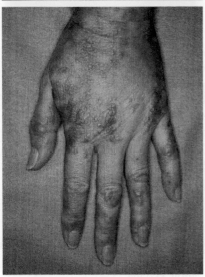

Fig. 7.14-2 Autosensitization dermatitis.

later, widespread eruptions develop on the extremities, trunk, and face. In most cases, the eruptions (id dermatitis) consist of erythema, papules, and pustules, often accompanied by intense itching (Fig. 7.14). Systemic symptoms such as fever and fatigue may occur.

Pathogenesis
Autosensitization dermatitis arises from an endogenous allergic reaction (id reaction) and is caused by sensitization against antigens thought to be decayed proteins, bacteria, fungal components, and toxins produced by injured tissues in the primary lesion. These antigens may circulate through the body by hematogenous spread from the primary lesion, or they may spread by rubbing or by an accidental intake of the causative substance (orally or intravenously). The primary lesions can be nummular eczema, stasis dermatitis, contact dermatitis, atopic dermatitis or tinea pedis.

Treatment
Topical steroids and oral antihistamines are useful for the symptomatic relief of autosensitization dermatitis. The underlying cause must also be treated. In severe cases, oral steroids may be administered.

Stasis dermatitis
- Edematous erythema or eczematous plaques form on the lower legs as a result of varicose veins or venous congestion.
- This disease tends to affect the elderly, obese individuals, and people who stand for prolonged periods.
- Stasis dermatitis may progress to autosensitization dermatitis.
- In addition to treatments similar to those for eczema, elastic bandages and varicose vein phlebectomy are effective in reducing congestion.

Clinical features
Edematous erythema occurs on the lower third of the leg, particularly near the upper ankle. The affected area gradually develops a dark red, scaly, eczematous plaque and pigmentation, and when it becomes chronic, atrophie blanche or sclerosing panniculitis may occur (Fig. 7.15). Minor trauma may induce ulceration. Treatments for stasis dermatitis may induce a secondary complication in the form of allergic contact

dermatitis from the application of an antiseptic or a topical agent (an antibiotic, or its additives or base). Aggregated serous papules often progress to autosensitization dermatitis.

Epidemiology

Stasis dermatitis is frequently found in individuals who stand for prolonged periods. Pregnancy may trigger stasis dermatitis as a complication of varicose veins.

Pathogenesis

Congestion in the cutaneous blood vessels is caused by chronic venous insufficiency (see Chapter 11), which leads to bleeding from the capillary vessel loop in the dermal upper layer. Hemosiderin deposits in the skin and gradually gives a brown appearance. The keratinocytes are injured by further impairment of blood flow. Atrophy and scaling occur in the epidermis with an increased tendency to ulceration. The skin loses its barrier function and becomes more reactive to extrinsic irritation, resulting in eczematous lesions in many cases.

Laboratory findings and diagnosis

Varicose veins in the lower extremities and the distribution of eruptions point to the diagnosis of stasis dermatitis. A Doppler test and an angiography are performed to assess the suitability of the patient for surgical treatment. A patch test is performed if allergic contact dermatitis is suspected.

Treatment

Topical steroids are effective in treating eczematous lesions. If ulceration is present, the lesion should be cleansed and dressed appropriately. The treated area should be monitored carefully for the development of allergic contact dermatitis, particularly if the lesions do not heal. In addition, compression bandaging is applied to reduce venostasis. Prior to compression bandaging, an arterial Doppler test and/or angiography must be performed to rule out peripheral arterial vascular disease, which may complicate this treatment. Pressure greater than that of elastic bandages and socks should not be applied. Bed rest and leg elevation are also advocated. Surgery such as sclerotherapy, ligation, and removal of varicose blood may be necessary for cases with severe varicosities.

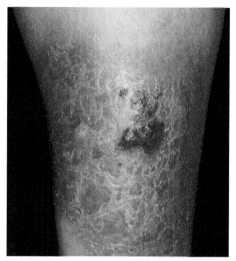
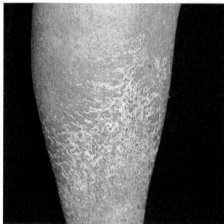

Fig. 7.15 Stasis dermatitis. Edematous, dark-red erythema with scales.

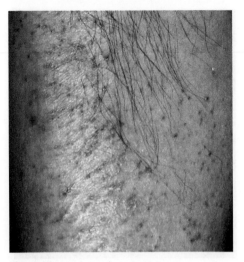

Fig. 7.16 Asteatotic eczema.

Asteatotic eczema

Skin dryness (asteatosis, xerosis; see Chapter 4) occurs when sebum decreases as a result of aging or excess washing. When the horny cell layer is destroyed, the skin becomes vulnerable to extrinsic irritation. When asteatosis becomes inflamed and eczematous, the condition is called asteatotic eczema (Fig. 7.16). This mostly affects the lower extremities of elderly people in dry seasons, especially winter (winter itch). Individuals who have a habit of excessively washing or rubbing the body with a towel may benefit from avoiding such practices. The first-line treatments are topical steroids and emollients.

MEMO 7–9 Wiskott–Aldrich syndrome

This X-linked recessive disease is characterized by increased susceptibility to infection, thrombocytopenia, and eczema (See Figure). Mutations in the WASP gene cause the disease. Lesions with eczema, petechiae, and subcutaneous bleeding appear within 1 month after birth. The symptoms are similar to those of atopic dermatitis, except that Wiskott–Aldrich syndrome is accompanied by purpura (see Fig. 7.18). The purpura is caused by the thrombocytopenia. There is a predisposition to immune deficiency-derived infections. The dermatitis is treated symptomatically with topical steroids and emollients. Hematopoietic stem cell transplantation is a drastic treatment.

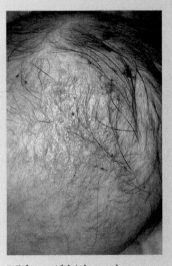

Wiskott–Aldrich syndrome.

Pompholyx and dyshidrotic eczema

Small vesicles of 2–5 mm in diameter appear suddenly on the palms and soles (pompholyx; Fig. 7.17). As a complication, irritant contact dermatitis causes the vesicles to spread to the sides of the fingers or the back of hand, and the lesions are often itchy (dyshidrotic eczema; Fig. 7.18). Scales appear during healing, which usually is completed with a few weeks. Hyperhidrosis may occur as a complication of pompholyx but the vesicles are non-follicular. Seasonal changes may induce recurrence of pompholyx. The causes have not been identified, but some cases are the result of allergic reactions to metals.

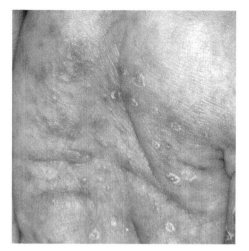

Fig. 7.17 Pompholyx. Multiple vesicles on the palm.

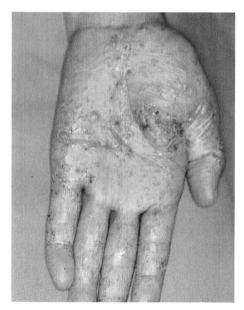

Fig. 7.18 Dyshidrotic eczema.

CHAPTER 8
Urticaria, prurigo, and pruritus

This chapter discusses three important dermatological conditions characterized by severe itching: urticaria, prurigo, and pruritus cutaneous. Each is typified by its own pathomechanism, clinical features, and histopathological findings.

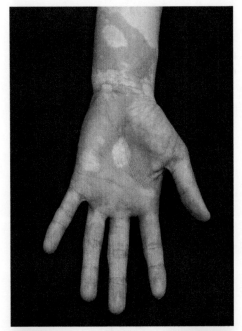

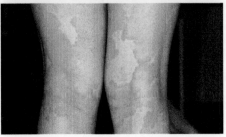

Fig. 8.1 Eruption of urticaria. It is characteristically itchy, with slightly elevated erythema and wheals.

Urticaria and angioedema

Urticaria
- Urticaria is defined as transitory localized erythema or wheals accompanied by itching. The cause is often unidentified.
- Acute urticaria occurs in episodes shorter than 6 weeks; chronic urticaria occurs in episodes of 6 weeks or longer.
- There is an increase in vascular permeability. Edema forms in the upper dermal layer. In factitious urticaria, dermographism is positive.
- Oral antihistamines are the first-line treatment.

Clinical features
There is the rapid appearance of slightly elevated, sharply circumscribed wheals or erythema with a circular, oval or map-like patterns accompanied by intense itching (Fig. 8.1 and Fig. 8.2).

Edema is the primary event. It occurs in the upper dermis and may develop at any site on the body, especially at sites subjected to rubbing or pressure. Wheals may occur not only on the skin but also in the mucosa. When wheals appear in the pharyngeal region, the urticaria causes hoarseness and sometimes breathing difficulty. The urticaria begins to subside within several hours and usually disappears within 24 h. In some cases, erythema and slightly exudative papules remain for several days.

Shimizu's Dermatology, Second Edition. Hiroshi Shimizu.
© 2017 John Wiley & Sons, Ltd. Published 2017 by John Wiley & Sons, Ltd.

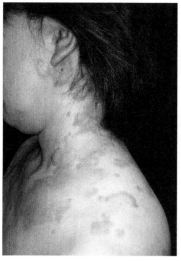
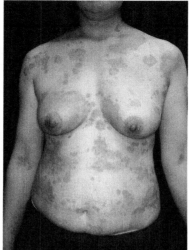
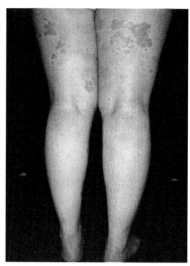

Fig. 8.2 Chronic urticaria.

Pathogenesis and classification

Chemical mediators such as histamines released from mast cells enhance vascular permeability, which causes edema to form in the upper dermal layer (Fig. 8.3). The causes are not identifiable in many cases. Some cases are antigen specific (type I allergy), and autoimmune IgE may be involved in other cases. For this reason, urticaria is often classified into the subtypes of acute (shorter than 6 weeks) and chronic (6 weeks or longer). Various factors may be involved in the activation of mast cells, including bacterial infection, systemic disease, physical irritation, foods, perspiration from exercise, circadian rhythm, mental stress, and drugs. Identifying the cause is difficult, because there may be more than one causal factor, and there may be a direct cause with indirect factors aggravating the condition. When the causal factor is identified, the disorder is called by the name of the identified factor.

Diagnosis and examinations

Urticaria is diagnosed based on the clinical findings. History taking can point to the suspected cause, such as mechanical stimuli, cold temperature, foods, and drugs. Since urticaria sometimes accompanies systemic diseases, including collagen vascular diseases, it is necessary to rule out these conditions. Dermographism is positive (i.e., when the skin is rubbed, the site turns red and becomes slightly elevated; Fig. 8.4). Tests such as those determining the serum IgE levels, IgE RAST

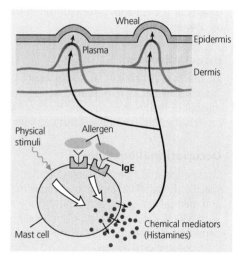

Fig. 8.3 Mechanism of urticaria.
Chemical mediators such as histamines from mast cells induce vascular hyperpermeability, which causes intradermal edema.

MEMO 8–1 Common allergic reactions

The diseases listed below can cause urticarial eruptions. The tests and treatments for these conditions are the same as for urticaria. For cases with severe respiratory symptoms or anaphylactic shock, epinephrine administration and systemic management are necessary.

Food allergies

Food allergies are hypersensitivity reactions (mainly type I allergy) to certain foods, such as eggs, milk, wheat, buckwheat, fish, poultry, shrimp, peanuts, soybeans, kiwi fruit, and papayas, or to antigens contained in food additives. An IgE RAST 5 months after birth is helpful in identifying food allergies. In addition to skin symptoms including urticaria, digestive symptoms (nausea, vomiting, abdominal pain, diarrhea), respiratory symptoms (bronchial asthma, nasal discharge, glottic edema), and anaphylaxis are found.

Latex allergy

Hev b proteins in natural rubber products cause allergic contact urticaria by inducing the production of IgE. Cross-reactions with certain kinds of foods, such as bananas, chestnuts, and avocados, are found in 30–50% of patients with latex allergy. This is called latex fruit syndrome. Erythema or wheals accompanied by itching appear immediately after contact with the allergens, and the symptoms quickly disappear immediately after removal of the allergens. Anaphylaxis may occur if the allergens are inhaled as powder.

Insect allergies

IgE reacts to histamines and other insect-derived substances in the venom of bees or the toxins in moths, inducing allergic or non-allergic immediate hypersensitivity reaction. The causes include bee stings, mosquito, flea or ant bites, and moth scale or cockroach feces inhalation. The symptoms are mainly bronchial asthma or urticaria but bee stings may cause fatal anaphylaxis.

Occupational allergies

Occupational allergies are seen in workers with certain occupations following long-term exposure to specific antigens. For example, workers in agricultural, forestry, construction, manufacturing, lumbering and medical industries, and beauticians and buckwheat noodle makers are prone to occupational allergies. Such allergies include symptoms of type I allergy, such as urticaria and bronchial asthma, irritant contact dermatitis, and allergic contact dermatitis. Photosensitive diseases are also likely to develop. Latex allergy is an occupational allergy.

Note: type I allergy is seen predominantly in food allergies. Recent studies have identified another type of food allergy in which a specific antibody can be sensitized by food intake through non-oral routes; the cross-reaction occurs with a wider range of foods (class II food allergy).

Latex fruit syndrome and oral allergy syndrome are major class II food allergies.

(radioallergosorbent test – see Chapter 5), intra-dermal allergic test, and drug induction test are helpful.

Treatment

Oral antihistamines are the primary treatment. Topical drugs are not generally used. The patient should be instructed on how to remove the aggravating factors. Oral and intravenous steroids may be necessary for severe cases. Care should be taken to avoid anaphylactic shock.

Acute and chronic urticaria

Urticaria is subdivided by duration into acute (less than 6 weeks) and chronic (6 weeks or longer). In acute urticaria, detailed history taking often reveals a history of colds or upper respiratory infection, which are important triggers for onset. Most acute urticaria episodes end within a few days to a few weeks; however, some persist longer and become chronic. Patients with chronic urticaria that follows a protracted course of 10 years or longer are not rare. Symptomatic treatment should be provided, while attention is paid to the underlying medical conditions.

Contact urticaria

Such urticaria occurs at sites where a foreign substance comes into contact with and permeates the skin or mucosa. The symptoms present a few minutes to 1 h after contact. It is classified into allergic contact urticaria and non-allergic contact urticaria. An example of the former is latex allergy and of the latter is insect allergy (MEMO, see Chapter 8).

Physical urticaria

This is urticaria caused by physical stimulation (e.g., rubbing, cold, sunlight or heat). Table 8.1 shows the subtypes and characteristics of physical urticaria. In mechanical urticaria (factitious urticaria), dermographism is positive (see Fig. 8.4).

Cholinergic urticaria

Wheals of 3–5 mm in diameter appear as a result of increased sweating following a rise in body temperature from exercise, bathing or mental stress (Fig. 8.5). Dyshidrosis or acquired anhidrosis may follow. Possible etiological factors include acetylcholines that control perspiration and type I allergy against components in sweat.

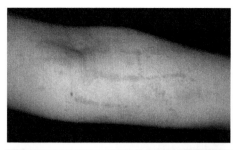

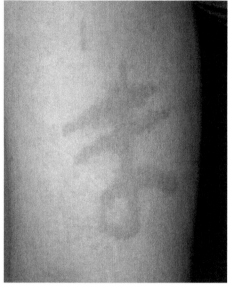

Fig. 8.4 Dermographism. Mechanical stimuli such as rubbing cause wheals (urticaria).

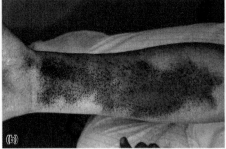

Fig. 8.5 Cholinergic urticaria. a: Small, multiple wheals are seen. b: Sweating test reveals that wheals appear at locations of sweat glands.

Table 8.1 Types and characteristics of physical urticaria.

Name	Clinical characteristics	Duration
Mechanical urticaria (factitious urticaria)	Wheals appear at sites of slight abrasion. Marked dermographic reaction is seen.	Up to 2 h
Cold urticaria	Urticaria eruptions appear at sites exposed to the cold. In systemic cold urticaria, small wheals appear on the whole body after the body is chilled.	Up to 2 h
Heat urticaria	Wheals appear at sites exposed to heat, generally within a few minutes after exposure.	Up to 2 h
Solar urticaria	Wheals appear at sites exposed to sunlight (see Chapter 13).	Up to 2 h
Delayed-pressure urticaria	Wheals appear at sites where pressure was applied, such as by underwear, at 1–2 h after pressure application. Some cases are accompanied by pain.	A few hours to a few days
Aquagenic urticaria	Small, localized follicular wheals appear at sites exposed to water (often seawater).	Up to 2 h

---

MEMO 8–2 Subtypes of hereditary angioedema

Hereditary angioedema is divided into three subtypes. In type I (85%), the production of C1-INH is decreased; in type II (15%), C1-INH is overproduced; and in type III (rare), the gene for antihemophilic factor XII is abnormal. The level of C1-INH is normal in type III.

Angioedema (synonyms: Quincke's edema, angioneurotic edema)

Edema forms by an increase in vascular permeability. Urticaria forms in the lower dermal layer and subcutaneous fat tissues. Itching tends not to present. It can be inherited or acquired. The eyelids and lips are the most frequently affected sites. The treatment for non-hereditary angioedema is the same as for urticaria.

Clinical features

Localized edema rapidly appears and can persist for 2–5 days. The size of the angioedema varies, with the diameter ranging from 1 to 10 cm. It is vaguely circumscribed, and itching does not usually present. Burning is often the chief complaint. Although it may occur at any site on the body, the most frequently affected areas are the eyelids, lips, tongue, hands, and feet (Fig. 8.6). Ordinary urticaria may accompany the condition. Angioedema may also involve the pharynx, nasal cavity, bronchial mucosa, and gut mucosa. It may cause anaphylactic shock.

Pathogenesis and classification

Angioedema is produced by increased vascular permeability in the subcutaneous tissue resulting from the release of chemical mediators by mast cells in the deep dermis or in the subcutaneous tissue or from some hereditary factor. The clinical condition is urticaria in the deep subcutaneous tissue.

Hereditary angioedema (HAE) recurs after first being triggered in the teenage years by events including trauma and mental stress. Hereditary angioedema is inherited as an autosomal dominant condition in most cases. It is caused by a congenital absence of C1 esterase inhibitor (C1-INH). The decreased activation of C1-INH leads to the production of bradykinin, which results in increases in vascular permeability and edema.

In most cases, non-hereditary angioedema is idiopathic urticaria in the deep subcutaneous tissue. In patients for whom this condition recurs in and after midlife, there are some cases with decreased C1-INH, which may be caused by underlying B cell lymphoma. ACE inhibitors may cause drug-induced angioedema.

Diagnosis

Angioedema is relatively easy to diagnose from the medical history and clinical features. When HAE is suspected, lowered levels of C1-INH and decreased complement values (especially of C4 and CH50) are helpful in diagnosing the condition.

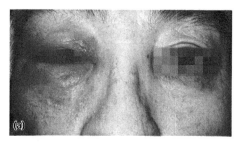

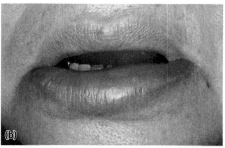

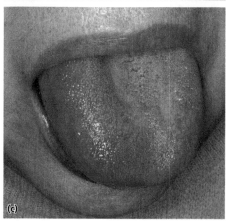

Fig. 8.6 Angioedema. a: Severe swelling on the right palpebra. b: Severe edema on the lower lip. c: Angioedema on the right side of the tongue.

MEMO 8–3 Angioedema that accompanies an increase in eosinophils

In recent years, there have been reports of episodic angioedema associated with eosinophilia in which an increase in peripheral blood eosinophils is observed and angioedema in the lower extremities recurs.

MEMO 8–4 Aspirin intolerance

This is also called NSAID (non-steroidal anti-inflammatory drug) intolerance. The mechanism of occurrence has not been identified. The symptoms are bronchial asthma or urticaria that develops after the intake of various NSAIDS or substances similar in molecular structure. In about 20% of patients with chronic urticaria, NSAIDs aggravate the condition. This phenomenon should be considered when an aspirin sensitivity test is planned after suspicion of FDEIA.

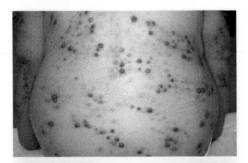

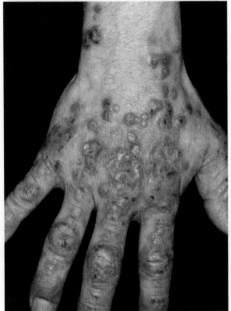

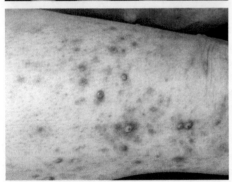

Fig. 8.7 Prurigo nodularis. Small, severely itchy nodules of 5–20 mm diameter are noted. Excoriation is also seen.

Treatment

The treatment for idiopathic angioedema is the same as that for urticaria. Antihistamines are not used for HAE or drug-induced angioedema in which C1-INH levels are low. Male hormones or tranilast are used to prevent attacks. Flash-frozen plasma or human-derived C1-INH medicines are used against acute attacks.

Food-dependent exercise-induced anaphylaxis (FDEIA)

Physical stress such as exercise 1–4 h after ingestion of certain foods may simultaneously cause anaphylaxis and urticaria. Oral aspirin aggravates the symptoms. Many cases caused by ω-5 gliadin in wheat have been reported in Japan. Shrimp, crabs, squid, oysters, and celery may produce the condition. Since exercise or ingestion of specific foods alone does not cause FDEIA, an induction test is necessary to confirm a diagnosis of FDEIA.

Urticarial vasculitis

See Chapter 11.

Prurigo

Prurigo is characterized by intensely itchy papules or small urticarial nodules. Insect bites or allergic or atopic dermatitis legions may cause prurigo, and scratching may aggravate the lesions and cause intractable nodules to form.

Clinical features and classification

An urticarial papule occurs, and nodules form in chronic cases. Prurigo is accompanied by intense itching and multiple scars from rubbing and scratching. These are called pruritic papules or nodules (Fig. 8.7). These papules or nodules do not coalesce, nor do they develop into other forms of eruptions. Intense acanthosis and inflammatory cell infiltration in the upper dermal layer are generally seen (Fig. 8.8). Prurigo is classified as acute or chronic, according to the clinical manifestations. The two types of prurigo and related disorders are outlined in this section.

Pathogenesis

Prurigo is accompanied by exudative inflammation in the upper dermal layer. Lymphocytic infiltrates may be present. The etiology is unknown in many cases. Insect bites, mechanical or electrical stimulation, certain kinds of foods and chemical stimulation, such as by histamines, are potential causative factors. Atopic dermatitis can also cause prurigo. Prurigo may also accompany malignancies, including leukemia or Hodgkin's disease.

Acute prurigo (synonyms: strophulus infantum, papular urticaria)
Clinical features
Urticarial erythema or wheals appear and become exudative papules, usually in children. Secondary infection may be caused by rubbing or scratching secondary to intense itching. Although acute prurigo lasts only several weeks, it tends to recur. Differentiation from insect bites is often difficult, but recurrence is a distinctive feature of acute prurigo.

Pathogenesis
Atopy and hypersensitivity reaction to insect bite are associated with prurigo. Children under the age of 5 are commonly affected in the summer, when insect bites are common.

Treatment and prognosis
Topical steroids and antihistamines are used. Care should be taken to prevent secondary infection.

Chronic prurigo
Classification
Chronic prurigo is subdivided into prurigo chronica multiformis, which is characterized by aggregations of individual papules coalescing into lichenoid plaques, and prurigo nodularis, which consists of sparsely distributed, itchy nodules of 5 mm to 2 cm in diameter.

Clinical features
Prurigo chronica multiformis occurs most frequently on the trunk and legs of elderly people (Fig. 8.9). Solid reddish-brown pruritic papules aggregate to form large lichenified plaques. The lesions are intensely itchy, are exacerbated by scratching and develop secondary changes, including exudates and crusts. The condition is chronic.

Prurigo nodularis most commonly affects adolescents and elderly women (see Fig. 8.7). Itchy papules resembling insect bites appear on the extremities.

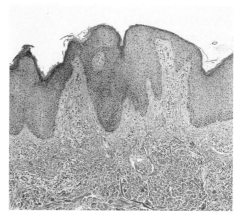

Fig. 8.8 Histopathological findings of prurigo nodularis. Acanthosis and inflammatory cell infiltration in the upper dermis are noted. Excoriation induces even more severe acanthosis.

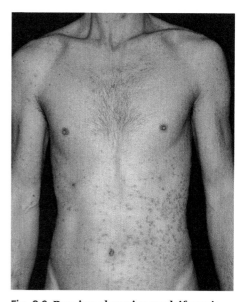

Fig. 8.9 Prurigo chronica multiformis.

MEMO 8–5 Skin disorders associated with pregnancy

MEMO 8–5 Skin disorders associated with pregnancy

- **Polymorphic eruption of pregnancy** (see Chapter 8): women in their first pregnancy often have this condition in the later stages of pregnancy. Small, itchy papules and erythematous lesions appear on the extremities and trunk.
- **Prurigo gestationis** (see Chapter 8): this is prurigo nodularis that appears on the extremities of mothers in their second or later pregnancy.
- **Pemphigoid gestationis** (see Chapter 14): this is bullous pemphigoid that affects pregnant women.
- **Impetigo herpetiformis:** this is pustular psoriasis (see Chapter 15) in pregnant women.
- **Intrahepatic cholestasis of pregnancy:** sudden itching occurs on the palms and soles and spreads to the rest of the body. Jaundice may occur.

When scratched, erosions and crusts may develop, resulting in the formation of dark brown solid nodules. These do not coalesce to form plaques, and they persist for several years.

Treatment

Direct application or occlusive dressing therapy of topical steroids is used. Application of zinc ointment sheets over the area treated with topical steroids is effective. Oral antihistamines are helpful in relieving the itch. Phototherapy may also be used for systemic lesions. Oral steroids or ciclosporin may be given for a short time in severe cases. Local injection of steroids and cryotherapy may also be used for the treatment of intractable prurigo nodularis.

Prurigo gestationis

Prurigo gestationis appears on the extremities or trunk of women in the third or fourth month of pregnancy and subsides after delivery. The likelihood increases with each successive pregnancy. Differentiation between prurigo gestationis and polymorphic eruption of pregnancy (PEP) can be difficult. The former tends to occur in the early stages of pregnancy, whereas the latter occurs in the later stages.

Polymorphic eruption of pregnancy (PEP) (synonyms: Pruritic urticarial papules and plaques of pregnancy (PUPPP))

Women who are in their first pregnancy or are pregnant with twins often have this condition. Intensely itchy small papules and erythematous lesions appear along the striae gravidarum in late pregnancy. The lesions gradually spread to the extremities and trunk, excluding the navel. They generally subside within several days after delivery. The condition may be classified as late-onset prurigo gestationis (see earlier).

Prurigo pigmentosa (synonyms: Nagashima's disease)

Prurigo pigmentosa is urticarial erythema accompanied by intense itching. Pruritic erythematous papules recur and heal with reticular pigmentation (Fig. 8.10). It most frequently occurs on the back, neck, and upper chest of adolescent females. The pathogenesis is unknown. Minocycline and DDS (dapsone) are effective treatments.

Pruritus cutaneous

- Pruritus cutaneous is characterized by intense itching without eruptions.
- It is often accompanied by dry skin.
- Eruptions, lichenification, and pigmentation may be produced secondary to rubbing or scratching.
- Oral antihistamines and psychological counseling are helpful.

Clinical features and classification

The disease is classified into pruritus universalis and pruritus localis.

Pathogenesis

Pruritus cutaneous may occur secondary to underlying systemic diseases, including liver dysfunction and renal failure (Table 8.2). Eruptions, lichenification, and pigmentation may be produced secondary to rubbing or scratching. It is often accompanied by dry skin and aggravates in winter and at bedtime.

Differential diagnosis

A systemic workup with the relevant tests is necessary to investigate pruritus cutaneous. When the genitals are affected, pruritus cutaneous should be differentiated from scabies and candidiasis.

Treatment

In addition to treatments for the primary disease, antihistamines, emollients, and UV irradiation are administered as needed. Counseling and antianxiety medication may be used for treating mental factors, if needed. Topical steroid application is effective against secondary eruptions but is ineffective against pruritus cutaneous itself. It is also important to eliminate pruritus-inducing factors such as alcohol, coffee, and spices. Maintaining proper body hygiene, wearing cotton clothes, and avoiding skin dryness are helpful. In recent years, it has been clarified that opioids play a role in the onset mechanism of itching. Nalfurafine hydrochloride, a κ receptor agonist, is used to treat itching in hemodialysis patients.

Pruritus universalis

Itching is present on the whole body surface, and this is a feature of many systemic diseases (see Table 8.2). Pruritus universalis is present in 80% of hemodialysis

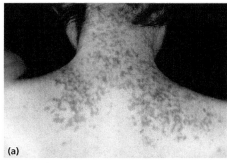

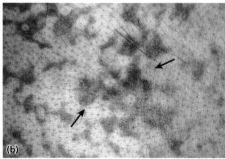

Fig. 8.10 Prurigo pigmentosa. a: Prurigo pigmentosa in a female patient in her 20s. Fresh red erythema is mixed with old lesions, which are seen as reticular hyperpigmented macules. b: Erythematous macules (arrows) are seen at the center of reticular hyperpigmentation. This is a recurrence of prurigo pigmentosa.

Table 8.2 Causes of cutaneous pruritus.

Diffuse pruritus cutaneous	
Visceral disorder	
Endocrinological dysfunction	Diabetes mellitus, diabetes insipidus, thyroid disorder, parathyroid disorder, carcinoid syndrome
Hepatic dysfunction	Hepatitis, hepatic cirrhosis, biliary atresia
Renal dysfunction	Chronic renal failure, uremia, hemodialysis
Hematological disorder	Polycythemia vera, iron deficiency anemia
Malignancy	Various carcinomas, multiple myelomas, malignant lymphoma (in particular, Hodgkin's disease and mycosis fungoides), chronic leukemia
Parasitosis	Ascariasis, ancylostomiasis
Neurological disorder	Multiple sclerosis, myelophthisis
Environmental factor	Mechanical stimuli, dry conditions, spicy foods
Drug	Cocaine, morphine, bleomycin and drugs to which the patient is hypersensitive
Food	Seafood (mackerel, tuna, squid, shrimp, clams, etc.), vegetables (aroids, bamboo shoots, eggplant, etc.), pork, wine, beer, chocolate
Pregnancy	In the third trimester
Psychogenic factor	Excessive stress, neurological symptoms, hallucinations
Skin dryness	Senile xerosis
Localized pruritus cutaneous	
Pruritus on the genital region	Urethral stricture, vaginal trichomoniasis, etc.
Pruritus on the perianal region	Constipation, diarrhea, anal prolapse, hemorrhoid, etc.

Adapted from Miyachi Y. *Minimum Dermatology*. Bunkodo, 2000.

patients. Opioids such as morphine tend to be a trigger. The elderly often have itching without any underlying medical conditions but with dry skin and/or mental stress (senile skin atrophy).

Pruritus localis

Most cases present as perianal itching. It frequently affects young and middle-aged men. It may be caused by dysuria, constipation, diarrhea, hemorrhoids or anal prolapse. In women, the labia majora and minora are predominantly affected.

CHAPTER 9
Erythema and erythroderma

Erythema is caused by hyperemia in the papillary and reticular dermis. Erythema is described as patchy redness produced by vasodilation and hyperemia in the dermal papillae and subpapillary layer. The erythema fades with the pressure of a glass slide applied to the skin surface. Erythema is seen in urticaria, psoriasis, infections, malignant lymphoma, etc. This chapter focuses on disorders whose main presenting symptom is erythema or erythroderma.

Erythema

Disorders in which erythema is the predominant symptom
Erythema multiforme (EM) (synonyms: erythema exsudativum multiforme (EEM))

- Multiple slightly elevated, round, edematous and erythematous lesions develop symmetrically on the dorsa of the hands and the extensor surfaces of the joints. It frequently occurs in the young and middle-aged.
- Infection by the herpes simplex virus or *Mycoplasma pneumoniae* is the dominant etiological factor, but drug sensitivity is also important.
- Some cases develop Stevens–Johnson syndrome or toxic epidermal necrolysis.
- Topical or oral corticosteroids are effective in the treatment of EM. Recurrence may occur.

Classification

Erythema multiforme (EM) is largely classified into localized cutaneous lesions (EM minor) and mucosal lesions with systemic involvement (EM major). EM major is considered to be synonymous with Stevens–Johnson syndrome or to be the early stage of that syndrome.

Clinical features

The eruptions occur symmetrically on the extensor aspects of the joints (e.g., the dorsal hands and feet, elbows, knees) as erythematous papules or edematous

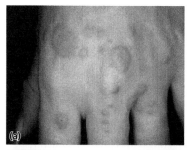

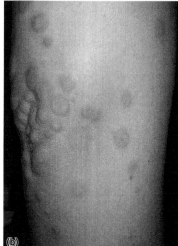

Fig. 9.1-1 Erythema multiforme.
Well-demarcated edematous exudative erythema disseminates on the dorsal hand (a) and elbow (b). The size is up to 2 cm. Note the central concavities.

Shimizu's Dermatology, Second Edition. Hiroshi Shimizu.
© 2017 John Wiley & Sons, Ltd. Published 2017 by John Wiley & Sons, Ltd.

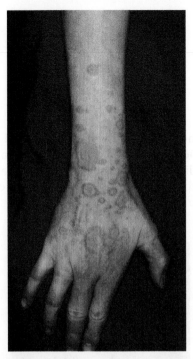

Fig. 9.1-2 Erythema multiforme. The central concavities give a characteristic iris-like appearance.

Table 9.1 Conditions associated with erythema multiforme.

Cause	Details
Infection	Virus (e.g., human herpes simplex virus), bacteria (*Streptococcus*, *Mycoplasma*, non-tuberculous mycobacteria), tinea, chlamydia, rickettsia
Drug reaction	Antibiotics, non-steroidal antiinflammatory drugs, anticonvulsants, antineoplastic agents, etc. See Chapter 10.
Collagen disease, allergic disorder	Insect bite, disease (especially systemic lupus erythematosus), sarcoidosis, Crohn's disease
Other	Physical stimulation (e.g., cold), hematopoietic malignant disorders, pregnancy, etc.

erythema, and they spread centrifugally to form sharply circumscribed, round or irregularly shaped erythema with a diameter of 6–20 mm (Fig. 9.1). The center of the eruption typically has concave or severe erythema, presenting as a bull's-eye or iris-like lesion. The affected area simultaneously shows new and old lesions that may fuse into a geographic pattern. It is accompanied by bullae when inflammation is severe. The degree of itchiness varies with the symptoms.

It frequently occurs in young and middle-aged women and tends to appear during the spring and summer. Infectious symptoms, including high fever and pharyngodynia, may precede the onset. In cases caused by herpes simplex infection, EM tends to occur 1–3 weeks after the onset of the viral symptoms (postherpetic EM).

Pathogenesis

As shown in Table 9.1, EM is caused by various factors, such as viral or bacterial infections, drugs, and malignancies. Type III allergy to the herpes simplex antigen is suspected as an etiology of erythema, because immune complexes are found in the blood or tissues of patients with erythema. The involvement of type IV allergy is also suspected, for two reasons:

- the infiltration of lymphocytes, and the expression of HLA-DR antigen and ICAM-1 in the keratinocytes are histopathologically observed
- EM is also observed in cases with contact dermatitis syndrome (see Chapter 7).

Pathology

Lymphocytic infiltration at the dermal-epidermal junction and vacuolar degeneration of the basal cells occur in the early stage. When the symptoms progress, lymphocytic infiltration reaches the epidermis, and dyskeratosis and subepidermal blisters occur. The dyskeratotic cells are accompanied by sparse lymphocytes in a phenomenon called satellite cell necrosis.

Laboratory findings

Elevated C-reactive protein (CRP) and erythrocyte sedimentation rate (ESR) are present secondary to the inflammatory process in EM. The herpes simplex virus antibody titer, *Mycoplasma* antibody titer, and anti-streptolysin O (ASO) titer may be elevated in some cases. In cases involving bacterial infection, there is an increase in neutrophils.

Diagnosis and differential diagnosis

Erythema multiforme is relatively easy to diagnose by its characteristic clinical features and by the distribution of the eruptions. A history of previous diseases such as a recent infection supports the diagnosis. When the involvement of a drug is suspected as a cause, a drug-induced lymphocyte stimulation test (DLST) or patch test may be necessary (see Chapter 5). Refer to Table 9.2 for differential diagnosis.

Treatment and prognosis

The identification of the causative factor is important not only for treatment but also for the prevention of recurrences. When infection is identified as the cause, treatment for infection will be carried out. For treating the eruptions, topical steroids or oral antihistamines are used. When an enanthema is observed, systematic steroids may be required, given that it might progress to Stevens–Johnson syndrome. EM regresses spontaneously within 2–4 weeks. When caused by herpes simplex infection, it may repeatedly recur. Preventive oral therapy for herpes simplex may be necessary.

Stevens–Johnson syndrome (synonyms: mucocutaneous ocular syndrome, EM major)

- Stevens–Johnson syndrome (SJS) is a severe acute mucocutaneous reaction with systemic symptoms such as fever and arthralgia.
- It may develop into toxic epidermal necrolysis (TEN).
- When the symptoms are severe, systemic corticosteroids or pulsed steroid therapy may be required.

Definition

Stevens–Johnson syndrome is characterized by extensive EM, including ocular and mucosal lesions, and is accompanied by systemic symptoms. Drugs are the principal cause of SJS. The disease affects 1–10 people per million per year. It may develop into TEN (see Chapter 10).

Clinical features

There is the rapid development of EM lesions associated with systemic symptoms such as high fever, general fatigue, arthralgia, myalgia, chest pain, and gastrointestinal distress (Fig. 9.2). EM is often accompanied by blistering and bleeding. The appearance differs from that of the typical target lesions seen in EM. Erosions may partially occur. The extensor surface of

Table 9.2 Erythema multiforme: differential diagnosis.

Disorder	Difference from erythema multiforme
Urticarial vasculitis	Itching. Purpura and pigmentation are left.
Systemic irritant contact dermatitis	Erythema multiforme or wet lesions that resemble erythema multiforme appear on the whole body.
Urticaria	The itching is more severe. Each lesion usually disappears within 24 h. Dermographism rubrum occurs.
Systemic lupus erythrematosus (SLE)	Systemic symptoms occur (renal, arthritic, etc.). Laboratory findings of antinuclear antibodies, etc. Erythema multiforme sometimes occurs in association with SLE.
Bullous pemphigoid	Eruptions resembling those of erythema multiforme may appear during the early stage. Laboratory findings of antinuclear antibodies by ELISA and immunofluorescence.

ELISA, enzyme-linked immunosorbent assay.

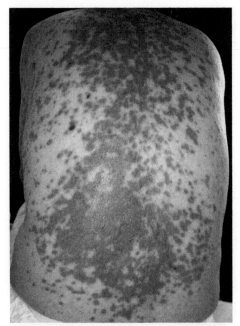

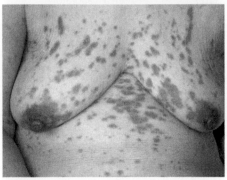

Fig. 9.2-1 Stevens–Johnson syndrome. Erythema multiforme rapidly spreads over the entire body. Some lesions overlap to form large plaques on the back. A bull's-eye pattern, characteristic of erythema multiforme, is seen at the border of a plaque.

the extremities and the entire body surface including the face and trunk may be affected. Lesions on mucosa and at mucocutaneous junctions are often severe, with edema and erosions in the eyelids, oral cavity, around the mouth, and in the external genitalia. Erosions are accompanied by pus and crusts. Patients sometimes cannot eat or excrete because of the severe pain. It may be accompanied by liver or kidney dysfunction. Eye complications include conjunctival inflammation, corneal epithelial loss, pseudomembranous conjunctivitis, and corneal opacity. These may result in visual loss. Ocular involvement in SJS requires early consultation with an ophthalmologist.

Pathology
See also the preceding section for EM. Necrosis of keratinocytes or individual cell keratinization (satellite cell necrosis) is observed, and vacuolar degeneration of the basement membrane and dermal edema is also present.

Diagnosis and differential diagnosis
Stevens–Johnson syndrome is characterized by severe lesions in the mucocutaneous junction, erythema over the entire body surface, blisters, erosions, and systemic symptoms. Histopathologically, there is epidermal necrotic degeneration. The diagnostic criteria for SJS are shown in Table 9.3. A detailed medical history is needed to identify the cause. Antibody titers of herpes simplex virus and *Mycoplasma pneumoniae* are measured, and pharyngeal culture and chest X-ray are performed. When the lesions rapidly spread, development into TEN should be considered (see Chapter 10).

Treatment
Early diagnosis and treatment are important for improving the prognosis. Systemic steroid administration (orally, intravenously or by pulse therapy) is especially important in the early stages. It is also essential to consult an ophthalmologist. When involvement of a drug is suspected as a cause, the suspected drug should be discontinued immediately, and a drug-induced lymphocyte stimulation test (DLST) should be considered (see Chapter 5). The treatment for the skin erosions is the same as that for burns. Application of topical medicine and systemic management including intravenous therapy are necessary.

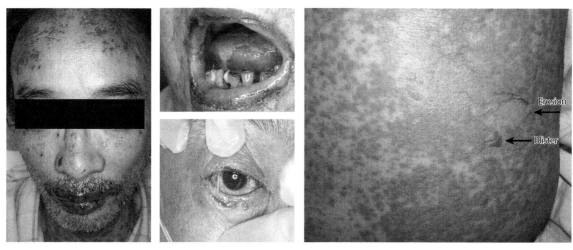

Fig. 9.2-2 Stevens–Johnson syndrome. Erosions and blistering are seen in some parts (arrows).

Table 9.3 Diagnostic criteria for Stevens–Johnson syndrome.

Major items
1 Main symptoms
(a) Erosions or blisters appear on less than 10% of the body surface. (b) Severe lesions appear on the mucosa in the mucocutaneous junction (bleeding or hyperemia is found). (c) Fever of 38°C or higher. (d) The eruptions are atypical bull's eye-shaped erythema multiforme.
2 Pathological findings
Necrotic lesions in the epidermis.
3 Ocular findings
Acute conjunctivitis in both eyes that accompanies either corneal epithelial loss (the planar lesion stains with fluorescein), pseudomembranous conjunctivitis, or both.
Other helpful items
SJS may develop into TEN. When assessment is done at the early stage, reassessment should be carried out at the peak stage.
Diagnostic criteria
When the main symptoms from (a) to (c) are all present. When the main symptoms (a), (b), and (d) are present and the condition is as described in the pathological findings. When ocular findings show abnormality and at least one of the main symptoms (a), (b) or (d) is present.

Source: Japan Intractable Diseases Information Center: www.nanbyou.or.jp/

Prognosis

Unless the patient is treated appropriately and promptly, SJS may develop into TEN and the patient may succumb to multiorgan failure. In severe cases, ocular complications such as loss of vision may result from corneal opacity and conjunctival adhesion.

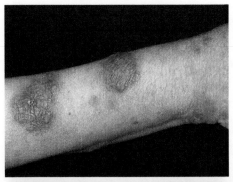

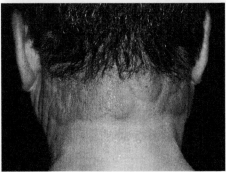

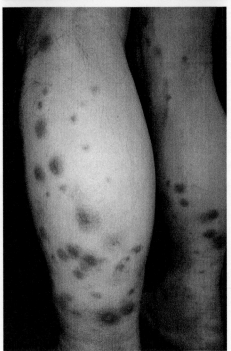

Fig. 9.3 Sweet syndrome.

Sweet syndrome (synonyms: acute febrile neutrophilic dermatosis, Sweet's disease)

- In Sweet syndrome, painful erythema with elevated borders occurs on the face and joints.
- Fever, neutrophilia, and arthralgia appear simultaneously.
- Histopathologically, there is dense neutrophilic infiltration in the dermis. Angiitis is not present.
- It is often associated with hematological malignancies (commonly acute myelogenous leukemia and myelodysplastic syndrome (MDS)).
- Oral administration of corticosteroids, potassium iodide, NSAIDs, and colchicine is the main treatment.

Clinical features

Sweet syndrome occurs most frequently on the face, neck, forearms, and dorsal aspects of the hands of persons of middle age. Several days to 4 weeks after a common cold or an upper respiratory tract infection, multiple painful, sharply circumscribed bright red to dark red edematous nodules 10–25 mm in diameter appear, accompanied by high fever (Fig. 9.3). The surface of the eruption is rough and granular, and the lesions may be surrounded by vesicles and pustules. Central clearing may lead to annular or arcuate patterns. When it occurs on the lower legs, it resembles erythema nodosum. Differentiation from Behçet's disease (see Chapter 11) is important if eruptions appear on the lower legs and oral aphtha is found.

Pathogenesis

A hypersensitivity against *Streptococcus* bacteria and other pathogens may be a possible cause of Sweet syndrome. Neutrophils that are abnormally activated as the result of involvement by granulocyte colony-stimulating factor (GCSF) or interleukin (IL)-6 possibly lead to the symptoms; however, details of the pathomechanism are unknown.

Complications

It is known that Sweet syndrome may occur secondary to underlying systemic diseases. Hematological malignancies (e.g., MDS or acute myelocytic leukemia) account for 80% of cases of complications with malignant tumors. Complications with malignant internal organ tumor or collagen vascular diseases have been reported (Table 9.4). GCSF drugs may trigger Sweet syndrome.

Table 9.4 Disorders associated with Sweet syndrome.

Classification	Details
Hematological	Myelodysplastic syndrome, acute myelocytic leukemia, myelofibrosis, etc.
Autoimmune	Sjögren syndrome, rheumatoid arthritis, systemic lupus erythematosus, ulcerative colitis, etc.
Other	Other malignancy, pyoderma gangrenosum, etc.

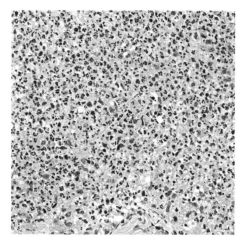

Fig. 9.4 Histopathology of Sweet's disease. Dense neutrophilic infiltration on the entire dermis without apparent vasculitis.

Pathology
Histopathologically, there is dermal edema associated with the prominent infiltration of neutrophils (Fig. 9.4). Changes in the epidermis and vasculitis (fibrinoid necrosis) are not observed. In the chronic stage, lymphocytic perivascular infiltration occurs instead of neutrophilic infiltration.

Laboratory findings and diagnosis
Peripheral leukocytosis with neutrophilia is the characteristic laboratory finding. An elevated ESR and high CRP levels are also present. High ASO values may be observed when *Streptococcus* bacteria are involved. Sweet syndrome is often associated with an underlying disease. It is necessary to determine whether the primary disease is a hematological malignancy, malignant internal organ tumor or autoimmune disease.

Treatment
Oral administration of NSAIDs, potassium iodide, and colchicine is the main treatment. Antibacterial drugs are ineffective.

Palmar erythema
Palmar erythema is observed in several conditions. It is a vascular syndrome with multiple etiologies. It is seen in pregnancy, liver disease, and collagen vascular diseases (e.g., systemic lupus erythematosus, dermatomyositis, rheumatoid arthritis). Palmar erythema may also be related to elevated serum estrogens and related 17-cetosteroid hormones. In rare cases it is observed in otherwise healthy people.

Refer to Chapter 18 for erythema nodosum and for erythema induratum.

MEMO 9–1 Paper money skin

Paper money skin is telangiectasia in which fine thread-like capillaries are visible, often on the extensor surface of the upper arm. The term comes from the resemblance of the lesion to the fine silk fibers that used to be in US paper currency (See Figure). Hyperestrogenemia is thought to cause this skin condition. As with palmar erythema, paper money skin may be caused by underlying disorders, including cirrhosis hepatitis and hyperthyroidism.

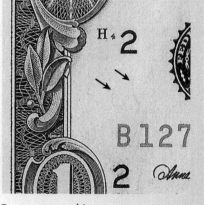

Paper money skin.

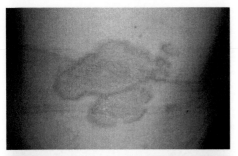

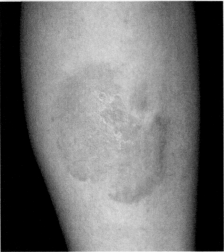

Fig. 9.5-1 Erythema annulare centrifugum.

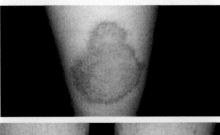

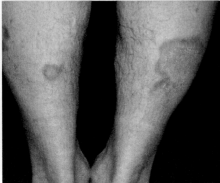

Fig. 9.5-2 Erythema annulare centrifugum.

Table 9.5 Classification of annular erythema.

Erythema annulare centrifugum
Annular erythema associated with infection
• Erythema chronicum migrans
• Erythema annulare rheumaticum
Annular erythema associated with collagen disease
• Annular erythema associated with Sjögren syndrome
• Neonatal lupus erythematosus
• Subacute cutaneous lupus erythematosus, annular/
 polycyclic
Annular erythema associated with neoplasms
• Erythema gyratum repens
• Necrolytic migratory erythema

Annular erythema

Annular erythema is a general term for diseases in which small areas of erythema appear and then spread centrifugally, resulting in an annular shape. Psoriasis, urticaria, and tinea corporis may present with annular lesions, but they should be differentiated from annular erythema. An underlying disease, such as infection, malignant internal organ tumor, drug eruption or collagen vascular disease, may be implicated. Annular erythema is classified according to the underlying disease and the clinical features (Table 9.5). Refer to Chapter 12 for collagen vascular disease associated with annular erythema.

Erythema annulare centrifugum (EAC) (synonyms: Darier's erythema annulare centrifugum)
Clinical features

Erythema annulare centrifugum (EAC) most commonly affects young and middle-aged adults. Infiltrated papules of about 2 cm diameter slowly enlarge to form an irregularly shaped ring as the central area flattens and fades (Fig. 9.5). The periphery of the lesions may be accompanied by slight scale formation. It heals in several weeks to several months, leaving light pigmentation. Ordinarily, subjective symptoms such as itching do not occur. Recurrences over several years are not uncommon.

Pathogenesis

Causes are often unidentified. It may involve interaction among inflammatory cells, their mediators and ground substance, induced by the diffusion of foreign antigens through the skin.

Pathology

The vessels of the upper and mid-dermis show dense perivascular lymphocytic sleeving.

Treatment

Topical steroids or oral antihistamines are used. A search for the underlying cause is the primary goal of treatment.

Erythema marginatum rheumaticum (synonyms: erythema marginatum (rheumatica))

Clinical features and pathogenesis

Erythema marginatum rheumaticum occurs in 5–30% of patients with active rheumatic fever, which is a streptococcal infection. It begins as an erythematous macule or papule that extends outward while the skin in the center returns to normal. The eruptions disappear in several days to several weeks at the area they first appear, but new eruptions appear in the surrounding areas. It resembles urticaria, but without the itchiness.

Treatment and prognosis

The treatment involves the systemic administration of antibiotics to treat the underlying rheumatic fever. The eruptions disappear spontaneously. The prognosis of rheumatic fever depends on the extent of coronary arterial damage.

Erythema gyratum repens

Cutaneous eruptions consisting of concentric raised erythematous bands move in waves in a "wood grain" pattern. They are accompanied by intense itching and quickly enlarge (Fig. 9.6). Over 80% of cases are associated with internal malignancy (lung, breast or bladder cancer). Some are associated with SLE, psoriasis and other disorders, or with no underlying diseases. The symptoms quickly disappear after successful treatment of the internal malignancy.

Necrolytic migratory erythema

Necrolytic migratory erythema is a cutaneous marker for glucagonoma (a glucagon-producing tumor of the pancreas). Vesicles, erosions, crusts, and pustules appear at the periphery. The lesions enlarge in annular or geographic patterns, leaving pigmentation in the central area. Recurrent remissions and exacerbations are observed over the course of several weeks. It is commonly observed in the buttocks, lower extremities and face; the symptoms may resemble those of zinc deficiency syndrome (see Chapter 17). Refer to Chapter 28 for erythema chronicum migrans (ECM).

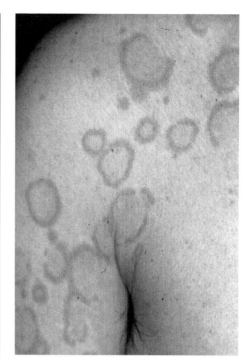

Fig. 9.6 Erythema gyratum repens.

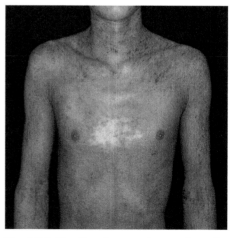

Fig. 9.7-1 Erythroderma. A case of atopic dermatitis that became erythroderma.

Table 9.6 Causative conditions of erythroderma.

Non-neoplastic
Eczema, atopic dermatitis
Drug eruption (drug-induced hypersensitivity syndrome, etc.)
Psoriasis
Erythema multiforme
Viral eruption (measles, rubella)
Pityriasis rubra pilaris
Lichen planus
Reactive arthritis
Congenital ichthyosis
Congenital ichthyosis syndrome
Bullous pemphigoid
Pemphigus
Dermatitis herpetiformis (Duhring)
Hailey-Hailey disease
Systemic lupus erythematosus
Dermatomyositis
Sarcoidosis
Fungal infections
Scabies
Staphylococcal scalded skin syndrome
Ofuji papuloerythroderma
Graft-versus-host disease
HIV infection

Neoplasm
Mycosis fungoides
Sézary syndrome
Adult T cell leukemia/lymphoma
Leukemia (chronic lymphocytic leukemia, etc.)
Malignant lymphoma, especially Hodgkin's disease
Multiple myeloma
Other malignant disorder

Erythroderma (synonyms: exfoliative dermatitis)

Erythroderma is the descriptive term used to describe erythema and scaling that affects more than 90% of the body surface as a result of an inflammatory skin disease. Erythema is caused by hyperemia in the papillary and reticular dermis. There are various etiologies.

Clinical features and pathogenesis

In erythroderma, erythema appears over 90% of the body surface and scaling occurs. The term is for describing the symptoms, and not for a specific disorder. Patchy erythemas that rapidly become generalized may be accompanied by desquamation (Table 9.6, Fig. 9.7). It may be possible to identify the underlying disorders through detailed visual inspection and history taking, but the underlying disorder is often difficult to identify. When the palms and soles are affected, erythroderma may cause acanthosis, hyperkeratosis, and fissures. There may be shedding of the scalp hair and ridging of the nails. Skin pigmentation and glossiness become noticeable as the eruptions become chronic. These may be accompanied by fever, shivering, and malaise.

Pathology

There are no characteristic pathological findings for erythroderma. Multiple skin biopsies may provide pathologies for the underlying disorder.

Laboratory findings

Various examinations may lead to identifying the underlying disorder (Table 9.7).

Treatment

Identification of the underlying disorder based on thorough examination is important. Oral antihistamines and topical steroids are useful. Side effects from topical agents may occur as a result of defective skin barrier function, which accelerates percutaneous absorption. Systemic corticosteroids are needed in severe cases. Inpatient hospital admission is advisable for cases with systemic symptoms. If identified, the underlying disorder should be treated immediately.

Eczematous erythroderma

In this condition, eczema spreads over most of the body. Eczematous erythroderma accounts for about 50% of all erythroderma cases. It can occur in patients of all ages with atopic dermatitis. Atopic dermatitis and various types of eczema become generalized as a result of intrinsic or extrinsic factors, resulting in erythroderma. Intrinsic factors include immune abnormality and liver, kidney, and adrenal dysfunction. Extrinsic factors include inappropriate topical treatment, home remedies, and environmental changes. Skin edema, erythema, and scaling are present over the entire body skin, often accompanied by intense itching and lymphadenopathy of the superficial lymph nodes. Systemic symptoms such as fever, dehydration, protein loss, body temperature instability, and opportunistic infection may occur. Skin atrophy, pigmentation, pityroid scaling, and skin glossiness become noticeable as the eruptions become chronic. Eczematous erythroderma is often caused by atopic dermatitis, contact atopic dermatitis, seborrheic dermatitis, and autosensitization dermatitis. Topical steroids are used for treatment. Oral administration of steroids should be avoided as much as possible.

Drug-induced erythroderma

Drug-induced erythroderma accounts for about 10% of all erythrodermas. It is most frequently caused by antiepileptic drugs such as carbamazepine and penicillin antibiotics. The disease often starts as erythematous papules that rapidly spread until bright red erythema involves the entire skin surface. Lichenification caused by antihypertensive drugs gradually expands and results in erythroderma that may persist for several years. When SJS or TEN is suspected, pulsed steroid therapy may be considered. Although most cases resolve relatively soon after the causative drug is discontinued, DIHS (see Chapter 10) may persist.

Psoriatic erythroderma

Refer to Chapter 15. This is a type of psoriasis. Psoriasis vulgaris or pustular psoriasis can develop into psoriasis erythroderma by inappropriate treatment, sudden cessation of oral steroids, alcohol intake or stress. Typical psoriatic lesions are often seen, and they give clues to the underlying etiology. Nail deformity frequently occurs. Oral ciclosporin or retinoid is effective.

Paraneoplastic erythroderma

T cell lymphoma (e.g., mycosis fungoides, Sézary syndrome), adult T cell leukemia, Hodgkin's disease, and chronic lymphocytic leukemia are causes of paraneoplastic erythroderma. Systemic examination

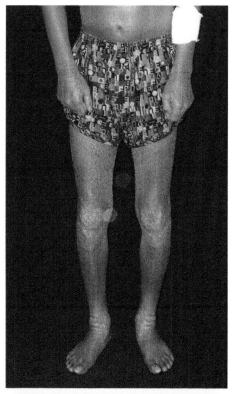

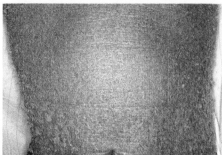

Fig. 9.7-2 Erythroderma associated with Hodgkin's disease. Flushing and marked scaling are seen on the entire body. The severity of the skin lesions mirrors that of Hodgkin's disease.

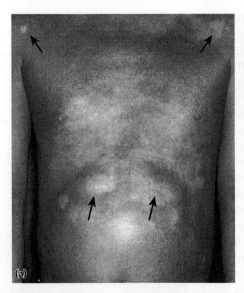 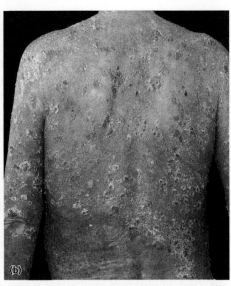

Fig. 9.7-3 Erythroderma. a: A case that accompanied Hodgkin's disease. Normal skin appears on the abdomen and shoulders, where the conditions of Hodgkin's disease are improving (arrows). b: A case that accompanied mycosis fungoides.

Table 9.7 Examinations useful for diagnosis and treatment of erythroderma.

Examination	Points
History taking	The primary disease may be estimated from the medical history and the course of progression.
Inspection and palpation	Eruptions that suggest the primary disease may be found. The diagnosis may be confirmed by conducting biopsy of the eruptions.
Biopsy	Findings characteristic of the primary disease may be found through repeated biopsy.
Microbiological examination	Culture and KOH test are done using scales and pustules. The possibility of Norwegian scabies should be considered.
Complete peripheral blood count	Indispensable for diagnosing infections, DIHS, leukemia, and Sézary syndrome. Flow cytometry is also done, if necessary.
Biochemical tests	LDH, erythrocyte sedimentation rate, and elevated CRP are non-specific. Liver dysfunction (DIHS, etc.), elevated serum CPK (dermatomyositis), etc.
Immunological tests	IgE (atopic dermatitis), Dsg/BP180ELISA, immunofluorescence (bullous dermatosis), HHV-6 (DIHS), HIV, HTLV-1, etc.
Tumor marker	The value of SCC non specifically increases as the result of extensive cutaneous lesions. sIL-2R (mycosis fungoides, Sézary syndrome) and other tumor markers.
Bone marrow examination	When hematopoietic tumors are suspected.
Serum protein fractions, kidney function, electrolytes	The systemic condition is constantly monitored for disorders, including for hypoalbuminemia.
Other	CT, MRI, and PET should be performed if necessary.

CPK, creatine phosphokinase; CRP, C-reactive protein; CT, computed tomography; DIHS, drug-induced hypersensitivity syndrome; ELISA, enzyme-linked immunosorbent assay; HHV, human herpes virus; HIV, human immunodeficiency virus; HTLV, human T cell leukemia virus type 1; KOH, potassium hydroxide; LDH, lactate dehydrogenase; MRI, magnetic resonance imaging; PET, positron emission tomography; SCC, squamous cell carcinoma.

is necessary to detect internal involvement. The primary disease should be identified and treated.

Other causes of erythroderma
Bullous dermatosis
Lupus erythematosus, bullous pemphigoid, and dermatitis herpetiformis (Duhring) may progress to erythroderma (see Chapter 14). Direct immunofluorescence antibody testing and ELISA are useful for diagnosis.

Hereditary keratosis
In non-bullous congenital ichthyosiform erythroderma, diffuse erythema, scaling, and hyperkeratosis occur at the time of birth or within several weeks after birth. Keratotic follicular papules are present on the extensor surface of the joints in pityriasis rubra pilaris and may diffuse and progress to erythroderma (see Chapter 15).

Infectious disease
Erythroderma tends to occur in immunocompromised patients, such as AIDS sufferers. Scabies (Norwegian scabies, particularly), tinea, candidiasis, and viral infections such as measles and rubella may also produce erythroderma. In children, staphylococcal scalded skin syndrome (see Chapter 24) sometimes progresses to erythroderma.

Graft-versus-host disease
Refer to Chapter 10. Erythroderma may occur as a manifestation of graft-versus-host disease (GVHD) after blood transfusion. About 10 days after transfusion, skin edema and erythema occur. The prognosis is very poor.

Papuloerythroderma of Ofuji
This is an uncommon entity of unknown etiology characterized by pruritic eruptions of flat, widespread, reddish-brown papules that spare the skinfolds (deck-chair sign) (Fig. 9.8). It may be associated with internal malignancy or malignant lymphoma.

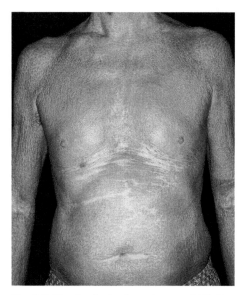

Fig. 9.8 Deck-chair sign. A case of Ofuji papuloerythroderma.

CHAPTER 10

Drug-induced skin reactions and graft-versus-host disease

Some cutaneous drug reactions present with a specific morphological pattern. However, most drug-induced skin reactions (DISRs) can present with the appearance of any cutaneous lesion (Fig. 10.1). A detailed medical and drug history is essential. It is clinically important to differentiate DISRs from viral rashes and graft-versus-host disease (GVHD).

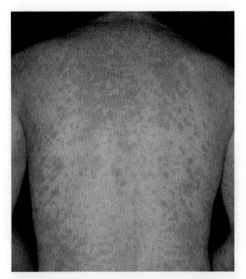

Fig. 10.1-1 Drug-induced skin reaction. Diffuse edematous erythema on the back. Each eruption was an erythema multiforme-like erythema of 1–2 cm in diameter that gradually enlarged and tended to coalesce.

Drug-induced skin reactions (DISRs)

- Drug-induced skin reaction and drug eruption are general terms for eruptions in the skin and mucosa induced by a drug or its metabolites.
- DISRs show various morphological patterns.
- Toxic epidermal necrolysis (TEN), a severe DISR with positive Nikolsky sign, has a poor prognosis.

Definition

Skin and mucocutaneous lesions induced by a drug or its metabolites are called drug-induced skin reactions. Maculopapular or morbilliform eruptions are the most common manifestations of cutaneous drug reactions. DISRs may present with the specific morphological patterns listed in Table 10.1. In diagnosing skin diseases, it is essential to consider drugs as a possible etiological factor, since DISRs can mimic any skin disorder. DISRs may be accompanied by general clinical features including fatigue, fever, lymph node enlargement, and shock, as well as internal organ dysfunction involving the liver or kidneys.

Classification and pathogenesis

Drug-induced skin reactions can be subdivided into two main types: immunological and non-immunological drug reactions. In some cases, the pathogenesis is unclear. DISRs can also be classified on the basis of their clinical features (Table 10.2; see also Table 10.1).

Shimizu's Dermatology, Second Edition. Hiroshi Shimizu.
© 2017 John Wiley & Sons, Ltd. Published 2017 by John Wiley & Sons, Ltd.

Treatment

It is essential to discontinue the causative drug. In serious cases, such as TEN or anaphylactic shock, systemic management using oral or intravenous steroids, including pulse therapy, and epinephrine may be required. Topical corticosteroids are applied for the eruptions, and the treatment for skin erosions is the same as that for burns.

Classification of DISRs by pathogenesis
DISRs with allergic pathogenesis

A drug or a drug-serum protein complex becomes antigenic resulting in a drug reaction in certain susceptible individuals in whom antibodies and lymphocytes react against specific antigens. In addition to type I–IV allergy, there are drug reactions in which Treg cells are thought to be involved (see Table 10.2).

DISRs with non-allergic pathogenesis

Drug-induced skin reactions that have no immunological basis may affect any patient irrespective of prior sensitization. The pathogenesis of non-immunological DISRs can, in some cases, be explained by the pharmacology of the drug.

- **Pharmacological effects:** DISRs may occur as a result of the direct pharmacological action of the drug. Examples include hair loss caused by anticancer agents and exfoliation on the palms and soles caused by retinoids.
- **Inappropriate use:** DISRs may occur when use instructions are not properly followed. "Red neck syndrome" or "red man syndrome" occurs when vancomycin is administered too suddenly.
- **Accumulation:** a drug may accumulate in the skin or mucous membranes from prolonged use. Argyria is an example of an accumulation disorder.
- **Drug interaction:** a drug may inhibit the metabolism or excretion of another drug or influence its protein binding. The action of a drug may be increased by alcohol intake, and fixed drug eruptions are caused by combinations of drugs.
- **Specific condition of the patient:** inherited enzyme deficiency may cause certain drug reactions. In some cases, an excessive reaction is produced even when the drug is ingested in minute amounts (intolerance).

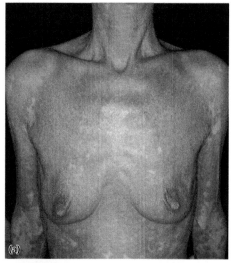

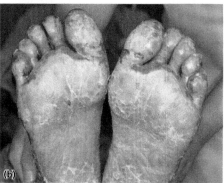

Fig. 10.1-2 Drug-induced skin reaction.
a: Drug-induced erythema enlarge and coalesce to form erythroderma.
b: Hand-foot syndrome caused by the chemotherapy drug tegafur.

Table 10.1 Drug-induced skin reactions and their typical causative drugs.

Type of eruption in the drug-induced reaction	Typical causative drug
Maculopapular	Carbamazepine, iohexol, amoxicillin hydrate, ampicillin hydrate, tiopronin, mexiletine hydrochloride
Eczematous	Ticlopidine hydrochloride, carbamazepine, tiopronin, gold sodium thiosulfate, penicillin, chlorpromazine hydrochloride
Fixed drug eruption	Acetaminophen, mefenamic acid, tetracycline, allylisopropylacetyl urea
Stevens–Johnson syndrome	Carbamazepine, allopurinol, serrapeptase, phenytoin, acetaminophen, sulindac, nevirapine
Toxic epidermal necrolysis	Phenobarbital, acetaminophen, carbamazepine, allopurinol, sulindac, diclofenac sodium
Purpuric	Interferon, digoxin, carbamazepine, gold sodium thiosulfate, prednisolone, dacarbazine, dipyridamole
Cystic	Diltiazem hydrochloride, amoxicillin hydrate, hydroxyzine pamoate, mexiletine hydrochloride, ampicillin hydrate
Acne	Prednisolone, cyanamide, gefitinib, cetuximab, imatinib mesylate, sodium bromide
Psoriasiform	Nifedipin, verapamil hydrochloride, indomethacin, terbinafine hydrochloride, interferon, isoniazid, infliximab, etanercept
DIHS	Carbamazepine, allopurinol, dapsone, salazosulfapyridine, mexiletine hydrochloride
HFS	Capecitabine, sunitinib, fluorouracil, tegafur, cytarabine, doxorubicin hydrochloride, methotrexate, docetaxel hydrate, etoposide

DIHS, drug-induced hypersensitivity syndrome; HFS, hand-foot syndrome.

Table 10.2 Drug-induced skin reactions classified by mechanism.

Mechanism	Example
Allergic	
Type I hypersensitivity	Drug-induced urticaria: penicillin, etc.
Type II hypersensitivity	Drug-induced purpura (thrombocytopenia): digoxin, etc.
Type III hypersensitivity	Drug-induced purpura (vasculitis): carbamazepine, etc.
Type VI hypersensitivity	Many types of disorders including drug-induced erythema (eczematous drug eruptions)
Other immunological mechanism	DIHS, etc.
Non-allergic	
Side effects (effect of a drug that does not fall within the purpose of administration)	Hair loss caused by anticancer agents
Excess, inappropriate administration	Red neck syndrome by vancomycin, etc.
Accumulation	Argyria, etc.
Drug interaction	Increased action by alcohol intake
Intolerance, idiosyncrasy	Aspirin intolerance
Secondary side effect	Jarisch–Herxheimer reaction, etc.

Classification of DISRs by eruption type

Although maculopapular eruption is the most commonly seen morphological pattern, DISRs can present with various skin lesions (see Table 10.1; Fig. 10.2). When assessing patients with skin eruptions, dermatologists should always consider the possibility of cutaneous drug reactions.

Identification of the causative drug

The causative drug is narrowed down based on the eruption morphology and on history taking of when the symptoms started, what drugs the patient is taking, when the patient started and stopped taking the drugs, and whether the patient has a history of similar symptoms. Examine the drug use instructions and reports on similar DISRs. Changes in symptoms from discontinuation or changes of drugs are also helpful. Relatively safe tests for identifying causative drugs include the drug-induced lymphocyte stimulation test (DLST) and patch tests. Skin tests (scratch test, prick test, intradermal test) and rechallenge tests are other options (see Chapter 5).

Specific types of DISRs
Fixed drug eruptions

Definition

Fixed drug eruptions (FDEs) are eruptions that recur at the same site whenever a certain drug is administered.

Clinical features

The lesions occur several minutes to several hours after the administration of the causative drug. FDEs frequently occur at mucocutaneous junctions such as in the perioral area, lips, and genitals, as well as in the extremities. They are characterized by itchiness and irritation, and occur as single or a few sharply demarcated red or purple patches with a diameter of 1–10 cm (Fig. 10.3). They may be accompanied by blistering or erosions. They leave pigmentation after healing. If the same drug is administered repeatedly, the pigmentation increases in darkness. The eruptions are sometimes multiple but more often single (MEMO, see Chapter 10).

Pathogenesis

Fixed drug eruptions are caused by the activation of CD8$^+$ T cells in the basal layer by drugs. Common causative agents are NSAIDs, tetracycline, and food additives. In recent years there have been many cases

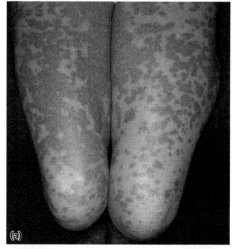
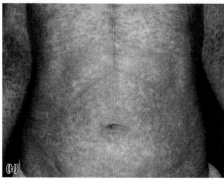

Fig. 10.2-1 Various types of drug-induced skin reaction. a,b: Erythema multiforme-like. Although uniformly colored erythematous plaques are mainly seen, newly formed erythema is seen at the periphery, some parts of which show the target-like appearance that characterizes erythema multiforme. c: Purpuric. Dark red macules up to 1 cm in diameter are observed. These do not disappear by diascopy pressure, which indicates that the eruption is purpura.

MEMO 10–1 Generalized bullous fixed drug eruption

Blistering may be present in some fixed drug eruptions and may spread over the whole body surface. Generalized bullous fixed drug eruption may be regarded as a specific type of TEN.

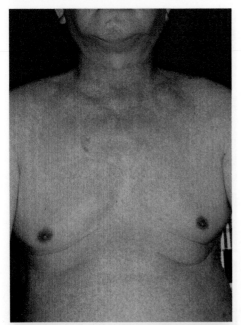

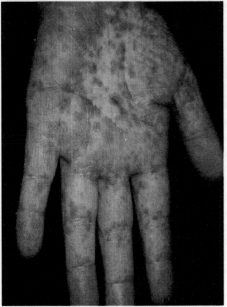

Fig. 10.2-2 Various types of drug-induced skin reactions. Urticarial drug eruptions. Edematous erythema resembling urticaria is seen on the trunk and palms.

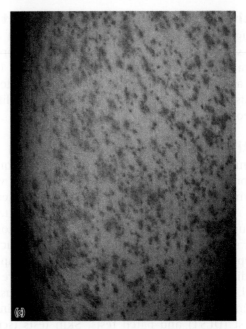

Fig. 10.2-1 (*Continued*)

caused by sedative-hypnotics in all-in-one cold and flu capsules.

Diagnosis
Fixed drug eruptions are diagnosed by a detailed drug history with particular attention to the course of the eruptions. A patch test performed on the site of the drug eruption is diagnostically useful.

Differential diagnosis
Eruptions on the extremities require differentiation from erythema multiforme.

Treatment
The causative drug should be discontinued.

Toxic epidermal necrolysis (synonym: drug-induced Lyell syndrome)
Clinical features and classification
Toxic epidermal necrolysis (TEN) is one of the most severe DISRs. It is accompanied by fever, erythema, and blistering on the whole body surface. It leads to marked epidermal necrosis and exfoliation (Fig. 10.4). TEN is classified into several types according to the clinical course (Fig. 10.5).

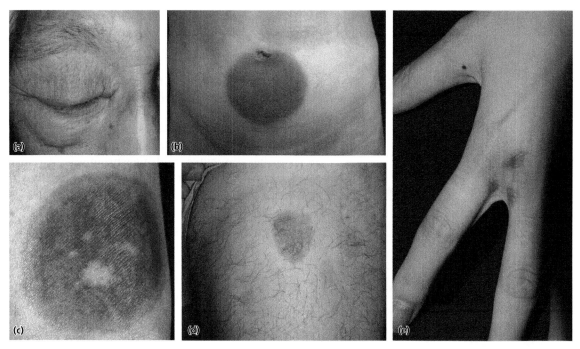

Fig. 10.3 Fixed drug eruption (FDE). a: Early FDE on the right eyelid. Early lesions are edematous erythema without pigmentation. b: FDE on the abdomen. Repeated intake of causative drug results in a severely pigmented FDE lesion. c,d: FDE on the thigh. The center of the lesion shows characteristic pigmentation caused by chronic inflammation. The periphery is erythematous, which suggests recent intake of the causative drug. e: FDE on the interdigital area. Erythema and bullous lesions are seen.

- **Toxic epidermal necrolysis developing from Stevens–Johnson syndrome (SJS):** most cases of TEN develop from SJS (see Chapter 9). Small, poorly circumscribed red edematous macular lesions gradually spread over the whole body surface. They subsequently enlarge to form blisters and erosions. Typical primary lesions are characterized by target lesions. Severe erosions develop in the oral mucosa, and systemic symptoms such as fever and fatigue may be seen. The erythema transforms into blisters and erosions with positive Nikolsky sign. SJS is characterized by dark red patches at the periphery (TEN with spots).
- **Rapid extensive type:** this is the type that Lyell first reported. Two to 3 days after intake of the causative drug, erythroderma and extensive erosions occur on the whole body and these are associated with rapid exfoliation of the skin (TEN without spots) (Fig. 10.6).
- **Specific type:** this includes generalized bullous fixed drug eruptions (MEMO, see Chapter 10).

MEMO 10–2 The threshold between SJS and TEN

Stevens–Johnson Syndrome and TEN developing from SJS are disorders with a similar spectrum of conditions, because the primary event of these two is necrosis in the skin or mucosa (see Fig. 10.5). These two are classified based on the extent of epidermal excoriation: When the area of excoriation is less than 10% of the body surface, it is defined as SJS; when it exceeds 30%, it is defined as TEN; and when it is between 10% and 30%, it is defined as SJS-TEN overlap. However, in Japanese diagnostic standards, TEN is diagnosed when the excoriation exceeds 10% (see Table 10.3).

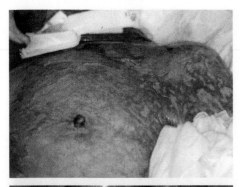

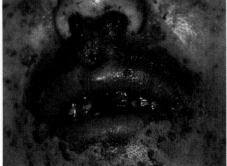

Fig. 10.4-1 Toxic epidermal necrolysis (TEN).

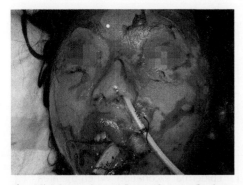

Fig. 10.4-2 Toxic epidermal necrolysis.

Pathogenesis

Many cases of TEN caused by anticonvulsants (e.g., phenobarbital, carbamazepine), acetaminophen, and allopurinol have been reported. It is widely accepted that the cellular functions of cytotoxic T cells are abnormally enhanced by certain drugs, resulting in extensive and rapid epidermal necrolysis of keratinocytes. Fas–Fas ligands and granulysin are thought to be the factors that induce apoptosis in keratinocytes, and measurements of these two proteins have been applied for early diagnosis of TEN.

Treatment and prognosis

The causative drug should be immediately discontinued. Systemic corticosteroids, including in pulse therapy, may be useful in early-stage, but not late-stage, TEN. Intensive care with topical treatment and body fluid management similar to that for patients with burns is essential. The causative drug must never be readministered. Plasma exchange and intravenous immunoglobulins may be used.

Drug-induced hypersensitivity syndrome (DIHS) (synonyms: drug rash with eosinophilia and systemic symptoms (DRESS), drug-induced delayed multiorgan hypersensitivity syndrome (DIDMOS))

There is still controversy on the terminology for this drug reaction. Drug-induced hypersensitivity syndrome (DIHS) is the term proposed by a group of Japanese dermatologists who postulate that the skin lesions result from a combination of drug allergy and reactivated latent viral infection, specifically that of human herpes virus 6 (HHV 6). Two to 6 weeks after the administration of a specific drug (see Table 10.1),

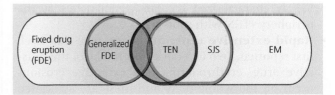

Fig. 10.5 The pathogenic association of fixed drug eruption (FDE), **toxic epidermal necrolysis** (TEN), **Stevens–Johnson syndrome** (SJS), **and erythema multiforme** (EM).

fever and generalized maculopapular erythema occur (Fig. 10.7). Liver dysfunction and hematological abnormalities (eosinophilia and the appearance of atypical lymphocytes) occur. The diagnostic criteria for DIHS are shown in Table 10.3.

Acute generalized exanthematous pustulosis (AGEP)

This is a DISR in which small aseptic pustules occur within several days after the administration of the causative drug (Fig. 10.8). It is most frequently caused by antimicrobials such as macrolide and penicillin, and by antifungal drugs and NSAIDs. The clinical features are similar to those of generalized pustular psoriasis (see Chapter 15).

Discontinuation of the causative drug and administration of topical or oral corticosteroids are effective treatments.

Hand-foot syndrome (synonyms: palmoplantar erythrodysesthesia syndrome, chemotherapy-induced acral erythema)

Painful swelling, erythema, and scaling occur on the palms and soles of a patient who is taking anticancer agents (see Table 10.1). This symptom is called hand-foot syndrome (HFS) (Fig. 10.9). In serious cases, erosions and nail loss are observed. Onset may be related to disorders in the basal cells or secretion of drugs from sweat glands. Depending on the symptoms, temporary termination or reduction of the causative drug, administration of oral NSAIDs or cooling of the lesions are the treatments.

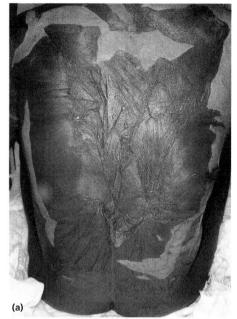
(a)

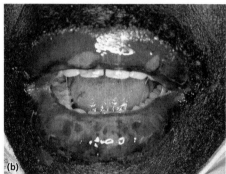
(b)

Fig. 10.6 Toxic epidermal necrolsis (Lyell's syndrome); Occurred in a black man.

Graft-versus-host disease (GVHD)

- After transplantation of hematopoietic stem cells, transplantation of organs or blood transfusion, donor lymphocytes are stimulated by major and/or minor histocompatibility locus antigens and subsequently target host tissues for cytotoxic damage.
- The three main characteristics of this disorder are eruptions (skin), jaundice (liver), and diarrhea (gastrointestinal tract).
- In acute GVHD, the main symptoms are edematous erythema and papules. In chronic GVHD, poikiloderma and lichen planus-like eruptions are found.

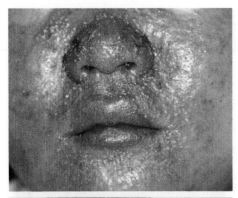

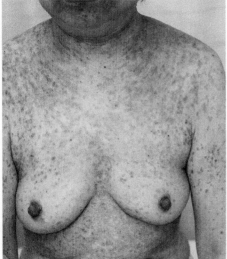

Fig. 10.7 Drug-induced hypersensitivity syndrome (DIHS).

MEMO 10–3 Drug-induced acne and tyrosine kinase inhibitor

In recent years, cases with acne-like eruptions induced by tyrosine kinase inhibitors, including gefitinib (Iressa®), cetuximab (Erbitax®), and imatinib (Glivec®), have been reported. Topical corticosteroids are more effective than antibiotics in treating these eruptions.

Table 10.3 Diagnostic criteria for drug-induced hypersensitivity syndrome (DIHS).

Concept
Drug-induced eruptions that accompany high fever and organ dysfunction. The symptoms persist after use is discontinued. Reactivation of HHV-6 occurs 2–3 weeks after the onset of the disorder in many cases.

Major findings
1 Delayed onset of erythema occurs after a certain drug is administered. The lesion rapidly enlarges. The disorder develops into erythroderma in many cases. 2 The symptoms persist 2 weeks or longer after discontinuation of use. 3 Fever of 38°C or higher. 4 Liver dysfunction. 5 Hematological abnormalities: one or more of the following: 　a. Leukocytosis (11,000/mm³ or higher) 　b. Atypical lymphocytes are found (5% or higher). 　c. Increase of eosinophils (1500/mm³ or higher). 6 Swelling of the lymph nodes. 7 Reactivation of HHV-6. Typical DIHS: all 1 to 7. Atypical DIHS: 1 to 5.

Other findings for reference
1 The causative drugs are often antiepilepsy drugs, diaphenylsulfone, salazosulfapyridine, allopurinol, minocycline, mexiletine. The period of drug intake before the onset of disorder is often 2–6 weeks. 2 The eruptions are erythematous papules and erythema multiforme in the early stage, which may develop into erythroderma later. Edema of the face, red papules around the mouth, pustules, vesicles, and scales are the characteristic symptoms. Reddening, purple spots, and slight erosion may be found on the mucosa. 3 Repeated recurrences of the clinical symptoms are often observed. 4 Reactivation of HHV-6 is determined when (1) a 4-fold or higher rise of HHV-6 IgG antibody titer is detected in pair serum test, (2) HHV-6 DNA is detected in the serum (plasma), or (3) there is an apparent increase of HHV-6 DNA in the mononuclear cells of peripheral blood or whole blood. For accurate diagnosis, the pair serum test should be done within 14 days after onset and after 28 days after onset. (The pair serum test is possible from the 21st day after onset in many cases.) 5 In addition to HHV-6, the reactivation of cytomegalovirus, HHV-7, and EB virus is found. 6 As there is multiple organ failure, some combination of renal dysfunction, diabetes, encephalitis, pneumonia, thyroiditis, and myocarditis may occur.

Source: Report on A Study on Innovative Treatments for Intractable Cutaneous Disorders (including Severe Cases of Erythema Exsudativum Multiforme (Acute Stage)), Research on Measures for Intractable Diseases, Health Labour Sciences Research Grant Project, 2005.

Pathogenesis

When donor-derived blood cells circulate in the patient's skin after transplantation of hematopoietic stem cells, the immunocompetent donor T cells may recognize the "foreign" host's histocompatibility locus antigen (HLA), triggering an immune reaction against the host's organs. It may also be caused by blood transfusions (see Chapter 9). Similar reactions may be caused by lymphocytes in the new organ in a small intestine transplant. This chapter discusses GVHD in hematopoietic stem cell transplantation.

Classification

As shown in Table 10.4, GVHD is classified on the basis of the onset and the clinical symptoms of the eruptions. Chronic GVHD was once defined as that starting at more than 100 days after transplantation, but the definition has changed as shown in Table 10.4. The skin, gastrointestinal tract, and liver are the main affected organs.

Clinical features

The severity of GVHD depends on the extent of the skin lesions and other organ involvement (Table 10.5). The grades and stages of acute GVHD are classified as shown in Table 10.6.

Acute GVHD

Edematous erythema or small light-pink papules appear on the palms and soles, extremities, and chest region. It may be accompanied by slight itching. In severe cases, the eruptions coalesce and may develop into erythroderma, blistering or erosions that may resemble the symptoms of TEN (Fig. 10.10).

Chronic GVHD

Various irreversible skin lesions are found, including poikiloderma, lichen planus-like eruptions (purplish-red plaques and oral lesions), scleroderma, hair loss, and nail deformity (Fig. 10.11). When the symptoms appear on the whole body, the result is a low quality of life in terms of cosmetic appearance.

Pathology

Dyskeratosis and intradermal lymphocyte infiltration (satellite cell necrosis) characterize the condition. Vacuolar degeneration and a decrease in the number of Langerhans cells may be seen. In chronic GVHD, there is the swelling or homogenization of collagen fibers, in addition to lichenoid reaction.

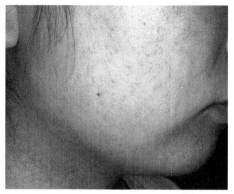
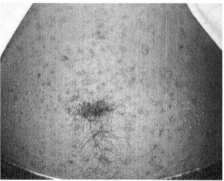

Fig. 10.8 Acute generalized exanthematous pustulosis.

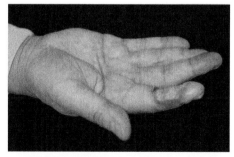
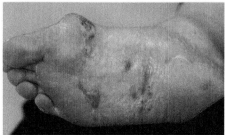

Fig. 10.9 Hand-foot syndrome.

Table 10.4 Classification of graft-versus-host disease (GVHD).

Type of GVHD		Duration after transplantation/ transfusion	Symptoms
Acute	Classic	Within 100 days	Skin eruptions, jaundice, and diarrhea are three main symptoms. Edematous erythema and papules occur on the palms and soles and other parts of the extremities. In severe cases, erythroderma occurs.
	Non-classic	100 days and later	When the above symptoms continue for 100 days or more, and cases that occur 100 or more days after transplantation
Chronic	Classic	No set duration	Various cutaneous symptoms, including poikiloderma, lichen planus-like symptoms, and scleroderma-like symptoms, are observed. Ocular symptoms, liver dysfunction, and lung symptoms
	Overlap	No set duration	When acute and chronic GVHD are present at the same time, it is called overlapping chronic GVHD.
Transfusion associated		About 10 days	Erythroderma rapidly appears. The prognosis is extremely poor.

Table 10.5 Clinical staging of organ dysfunction.

Stage	Skin: eruptions (%)	Liver: total bilirubin (mg/dL)	Digestive tract: diarrhea
1	<25	<3.0	Adult 500–1000 mL Child 280–555 mL/m² Or prolonged nausea
2	25–50	3.0–6.0	Adult 1001–1500 mL Child 556–833 mL/m²
3	>50	6.1–15.0	Adult >1500 mL Child >833 mL/m²
4	Systemic erythroderma, formation of blisters	>15.0	Severe abdominal pain (+/– obstruction of the intestines)

Source: Japan Society for Hematopoietic Cell Transplantation: Hematopoietic Cell Transplantation Guideline, GVHD, August, 2008.

Differential diagnosis

It is necessary to differentiate GVHD from DISRs, transitory eruptions associated with engraftment (engraftment syndrome), skin disorders caused by transplantation preparation such as irradiation (regimen-related toxicity), and viral infections.

Table 10.6 Grading of acute graft-versus-host disease (GVHD).

Grade	Skin stage		Liver stage		Gut stage
I	1–2		0		0
II	3	or	1	or	1
III	–		2–3	or	2–4
IV	4	or	4		–

Source: Japan Society for Hematopoietic Cell Transplantation: Hematopoietic Cell Transplantation Guideline, GVHD, August, 2008.

Treatment

Administration of systemic corticosteroids is the primary treatment; however, mild acute GVHD must be carefully monitored, because this can be the result of a graft-versus-leukemia effect. Immunosuppressants

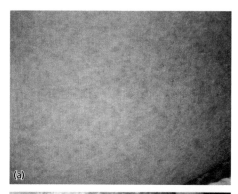

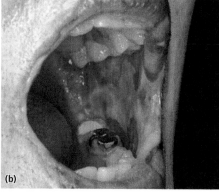

Fig. 10.10-2 Acute graft-versus-host disease. a: Small, diffuse, multiple erythema appear, and partly coalescing eruptions are seen. The eruptions coalesce and form plaques on the lower leg. b: Erosions on the lips and mucosa.

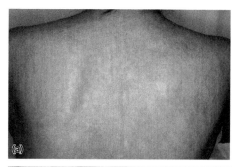

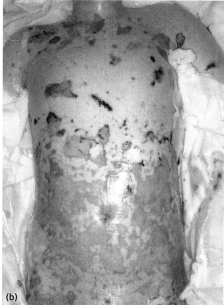

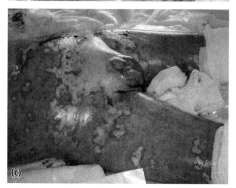

Fig. 10.10-1 Acute graft-versus-host disease. a: Diffuse erythema on the back after bone marrow transplantation. Clinically, differential diagnosis from drug eruption is almost impossible. b,c: Severe acute GVHD. Severe exfoliation similar to toxic epidermal necrolysis is seen.

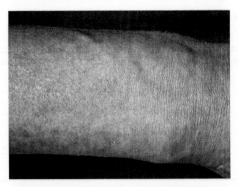

Fig. 10.11 Chronic graft-versus-host disease. Multiple purplish red plaques are seen on the forearm. The lesions are clinically similar to those of lichen planus.

(ciclosporin, tacrolimus) or antithymocyte globulin (ATG) may be administered. Topical corticosteroids are used for skin lesions but are ineffective for fixed eruptions of chronic GVHD.

CHAPTER 11
Vasculitis, purpura, and other vascular diseases

Vasculitis is an inflammatory process involving the blood vessels. It is classified according to the diameter of the artery or vein involved (Fig. 11.1). In cutaneous vasculitis, purpura or ulceration frequently develops. Purpura may be an early sign of severe systemic vasculitis.

Purpura is a descriptive term for a reddish-purple skin lesion produced by bleeding in the dermis or subcutaneous tissues. It is classified by the extent of the bleeding as petechia (up to 2 mm in diameter) or ecchymosis (2 mm or more in diameter). The major causative factors are vascular abnormality (from vasculitis or mechanical injury), blood flow abnormality (e.g., hypergammaglobulinemia, which often accompanies a systemic disease), decrease or functional abnormality of platelets, and coagulopathy. However, the etiology is unknown in many cases.

Vasculitis

Vasculitis in small vessels

Cutaneous small vessel vasculitis (synonyms: cutaneous leukocytoclastic angiitis, cutaneous leukocytoclastic vasculitis, necrotizing vasculitis, cutaneous allergic vasculitis, hypersensitivity vasculitis)

- This is a group of diseases characterized by neutrophilic infiltration into the small peripheral dermal blood vessels. Clinical features are localized in the skin.
- The clinical features of the erythema, purpura, papules, blistering, and ulceration are related to the depth and severity of the vasculitis (Fig. 11.2).

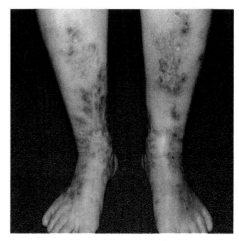

Fig. 11.1 Cutaneous small vessel vasculitis. The skin lesion presents a mix of purpura, papules, nodules, pustules, blisters, erosions, and ulcers. It is accompanied by sharp pain.

> **MEMO 11–1 Allergic vasculitis, vasculitis allergica cutis (Ruiter)**
>
> Cutaneous small vessel vasculitis that occurs mainly in the upper and middle dermal layers and is rarely accompanied by systemic symptoms is called allergic vasculitis.

Shimizu's Dermatology, Second Edition. Hiroshi Shimizu.
© 2017 John Wiley & Sons, Ltd. Published 2017 by John Wiley & Sons, Ltd.

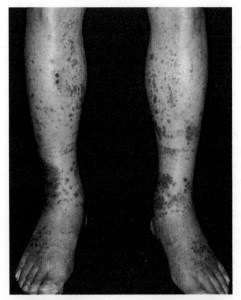

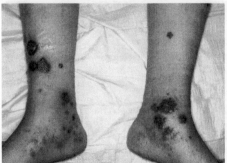

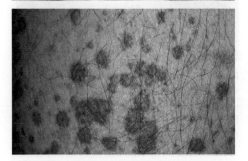

Fig. 11.3-1 Cutaneous small-vessel vasculitis (CSVV). The disease presents various cutaneous clinical features including purpura, erythema, bloody blisters, and ecchymosis.

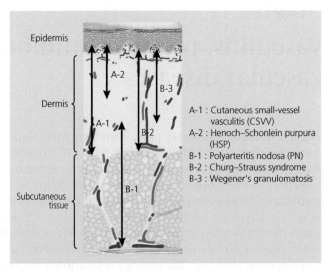

Fig. 11.2 Cutaneous vasculitis and the depth of the affected vessels.

A-1 : Cutaneous small-vessel vasculitis (CSVV)
A-2 : Henoch–Schonlein purpura (HSP)
B-1 : Polyarteritis nodosa (PN)
B-2 : Churg–Strauss syndrome
B-3 : Wegener's granulomatosis

Definition
Cutaneous small vessel vasculitis (CSVV) occurs mainly in the small vessels in the dermis (i.e., capillary and arteriovenous blood vessels) and is rarely accompanied by systemic symptoms. Urticarial vasculitis, which is described later in this chapter, is not included.

Clinical features
Purpura, urticaria, erythema multiforme-like erythema, papules, nodules, pustules, blistering, erosion, and ulceration occur mainly in the lower extremities (Fig. 11.3). It is often accompanied by itching and pain, but it may be without subjective symptoms other than the skin lesions. When it is accompanied by systemic symptoms including fever, abdominal pain or joint pain, the possibility of systemic vasculitis should be considered.

Pathogenesis
Antibody-antigen immune complexes deposit within the arteriolovenular walls and activate the immune system, resulting in vasculitis (type III allergic reaction). The antigens include antibiotics such as penicillin, chemical substances, hemolytic streptococcus, and viruses. Collagen vascular diseases and antibodies against malignant tumors are also part of the etiology.

Pathology
Vasculitis is seen mainly in the upper and middle depths of the dermis. Perivascular neutrophilic infiltration, often with fragments of leukocyte-derived nuclear

debris, is seen. Eosinophilic material deposits in the vessels or on the walls of the vessels, which is called fibrinoid degeneration. Leakage of erythrocytes and swelling of vascular endothelium are seen (Fig. 11.4).

Laboratory findings

Elevated erythrocyte sedimentation rate, increased leukocytes, and hypergammaglobulinemia are the typical findings.

Diagnosis

Cutaneous small vessel vasculitis is diagnosed by skin biopsy. It is important to differentiate CSVV from other underlying diseases, because there are many diseases that show histopathological conditions similar to those of CSVV.

Treatment and prognosis

It is essential to identify and treat the cause of the vasculitis. Causative drugs should be immediately discontinued and infections should be appropriately treated. In addition, leg elevation and bed rest may be helpful. Topical steroids, oral NSAIDs or dapsone are useful for treating skin lesions. When the symptoms are severe, oral steroids may be administered.

MEMO 11–2 Palpable purpura, non-palpable purpura

When diagnosing purpura, it is important to distinguish between purpura caused by vasculitis and purpura caused by other factors (e.g., thrombocytopenia, capillary fragility). Purpura caused by vasculitis tends to be accompanied by palpable infiltration (palpable purpura), whereas in purpura caused by other factors, infiltration is not usually present. However, infiltration is not palpable in mild vasculitis.

IgA vasculitis (synonyms: Henoch–Schönlein purpura)

- Henoch–Schönlein purpura results from IgA immune complex deposition within the vascular walls in the upper depth of the dermis (type III hypersensitivity reaction).
- Multiple palpable purpuric lesions develop on the legs.
- Joint pain, abdominal pain, and nephritis occur.
- Bed rest is the main option for treatment. The possibility of renal failure in adults should be borne in mind.

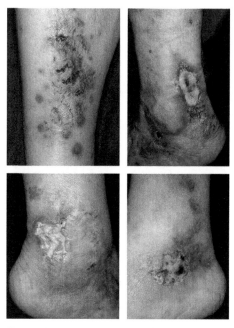

Fig. 11.3-2 Cutaneous small-vessel vasculitis (CSVV).

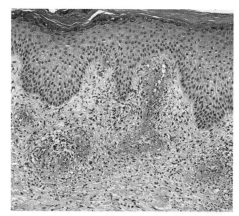

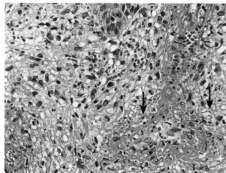

Fig. 11.4 Histopathology: Fibrinoid degeneration of the vessel walls in the upper dermis.

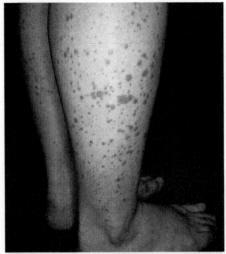

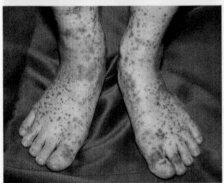

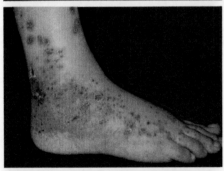

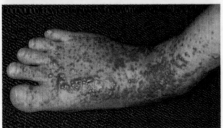

Fig. 11.5-1 Henoch–Schönlein purpura.
Palpable purpura may be accompanied by
bloody blisters in some cases.

Definition

Multiple palpable purpuric lesions develop on the lower legs, accompanied by arthralgia, gastrointestinal symptoms, and nephritis. HSP is classified as a leukocytoclastic vasculitis (see the previous section); however, the vasculitis is localized to the upper dermal layer, with IgA deposition within the vascular walls.

Clinical features

Although children are most commonly affected, HSP may also occur in adults. It may be preceded by headaches, pharyngeal pain, and flu-like symptoms. Disseminated palpable purpura ranging from several millimeters to 10 mm in diameter develops, mainly on the lower legs and dorsum of the foot, but sometimes on the thighs, upper extremities, and abdomen (Fig. 11.5). Blisters, ulcers, and a combination of old and new eruptions may be present. Sometimes there is slight pressure pain. Joint pain such as in the knees, hands, and elbows, gastrointestinal symptoms (acute or diffuse abdominal pain, and melena), and glomerular nephritis may develop.

Pathogenesis

In children, the onset occurs mostly after an acute upper respiratory tract infection. An association with hemolytic streptococcus has also been described. Drugs (e.g., penicillin, aspirin) and certain foods (e.g., milk, eggs) are also associated with HSP. These act as antigens and combine with circulating antibodies (mainly IgA), resulting in the deposition of immune complexes within the vascular walls. The subsequent induction of immunoreaction causes vasculitis and purpura.

Pathology

Leukocytoclastic vasculitis accompanied by fibrinoid degeneration is seen in the vascular walls of the upper dermis. IgA deposition is observed by direct immunofluorescence (Fig. 11.6).

Laboratory findings

When HSP is caused by a hemolytic streptococcal infection, increases in antistreptolysin O and antistreptokinase titers are seen. Decreases in blood coagulation factor XIII may be seen. The renal symptoms are closely related to the prognosis. When hematuria and proteinuria are present, special care should be taken.

Differential diagnosis

The development of palpable purpura as described above should raise the suspicion of HSP. The differential diagnoses include thrombocytopenic purpura, polyarteritis nodosa, Goodpasture syndrome, viral infection (e.g., papular purpuric "gloves and socks" syndrome), and systemic lupus erythematosus (SLE). In adults, differentiation from microscopic polyangiitis (MPA) is important.

Treatment

Bed rest is the mainstay of treatment, and agents to reinforce the blood vessels may be used. NSAIDs are useful for mild abdominal pain. When the symptoms are severe, oral steroids may be administered. Blood clotting factor XIII drugs may be useful.

Prognosis

Henoch–Schönlein purpura generally has a good prognosis and resolves within several weeks. It may, however, recur. Serious extracutaneous complications may develop in other organs, such as the kidneys (e.g., purpura nephritis), and there may be intussusception, intestinal perforation, and cerebral hemorrhage. The risk of renal failure is high in adults.

Urticarial vasculitis

When an urticarial eruption persists for more than 24 h and is associated with purpura, urticarial vasculitis should be suspected. There is the presence of urticarial or erythema multiforme-like eruptions that recur and heal with purpura or pigmentation. Histopathologically, leukocytoclastic vasculitis is seen in the upper layer of the dermis. It occurs as idiopathic urticarial vasculitis and as urticarial vasculitis with underlying disorders (e.g., SLE). It may be accompanied by hypocomplementemia and by symptoms in other organs.

Erythema elevatum diutinum

Erythema elevatum diutinum (EED) frequently occurs in middle-aged and older patients. It occurs symmetrically on the extensor surface of the elbows and knees. The original lesion appears as a slightly elevated purplish-red papule. It gradually becomes fibrotic. An atypical type of EED has been described in association with blistering or ulceration (Fig. 11.7). It may be accompanied by arthritis. Histopathologically, leukocytoclastic vasculitis is seen. It is largely asymptomatic but tends to recur. It may be accompanied by hematological malignancies. Dapsone (DDS) is an effective treatment.

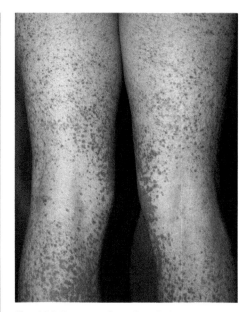

Fig. 11.5-2 Henoch–Schönlein purpura.

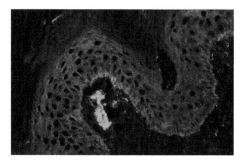

Fig. 11.6 Direct immunofluorescence of Henoch-Schönlein purpura. IgA deposition on the vascular wall in the upper dermis is observed.

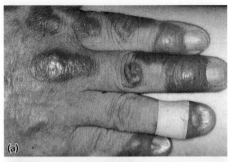

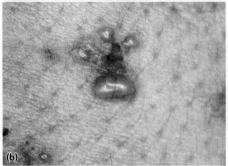

Fig. 11.7 Erythema elevatum diutinum.
a: Elevated reddish-purple plaques and fibrotic tissues are seen. b: Blisters may form.

Granuloma faciale

Granuloma faciale is described as sharply demarcated reddish-brown plaques or small nodules that develop on the face. It is associated with sun exposure, but the pathogenesis is unknown. Histopathologically, leukocytoclastic vasculitis is seen but granulomas are not. Dye laser treatment, local injection of steroids, and DDS have been used; however, granuloma faciale is a refractory disorder.

Vasculitis in small and medium-sized arteries

Polyarteritis nodosa (PN, PAN)

- Polyarteritis nodosa is a systemic vasculitis with fever, joint symptoms, kidney dysfunction, and peripheral nerve disorder.
- Histopathologically, it is characterized by leukocytoclastic vasculitis in small and medium-sized arteries.
- Cutaneous findings include subcutaneous nodules, livedo, purpura, and ulceration.

Classification

This was defined as a disorder that affects the distributing arteries and was called periarteritis nodosa. However, it has now been subclassified into the three disorders below. Before it was classified into these three, it was called classical PN.

- **Polyarteritis nodosa (PN):** this is a systemic vasculitis that affects small and medium-sized arteries in any organ.
- **Cutaneous polyarteritis nodosa (cutaneous PN):** the symptoms are localized to the skin.
- **Microscopic polyangiitis (MPA):** this is a systemic vasculitis that affects the arteriolae, venulae, and small arteries.

Clinical features and epidemiology

Polyarteritis nodosa occurs in men and women in their third to sixth decades. Cutaneous symptoms are seen in about 30–60% of patients. Livedo is often seen, mainly on the lower extremities. Subcutaneous nodules of 1–2 cm in diameter, purpura, and ulceration occur with the same orientation as the superficial arteries (Fig. 11.8). The condition is chronic. The obstruction of arteries may cause gangrene.

The symptoms of systemic vasculitis include fever, fatigue, weight loss, joint pain, renal symptoms (e.g., hypertension), polyneuropathy, cerebrovascular disorders, gastrointestinal symptoms, cardiac infarction, and lung fibrosis.

Pathology

As a skin lesion, angiitis occurs in the arteries from the deep dermal layer down to the subcutaneous tissues (see Fig. 11.1). PN is accompanied by swelling in the tunica media of small and medium-sized arteries, destruction of the elastic layer, fibrinoid degeneration, and neutrophilic cellular infiltration (Fig. 11.9). Fibrosis after granulation occurs in the late stage. Granulomas do not form.

Diagnosis and differential diagnosis

Skin disorders that must be differentiated from PN include erythema nodosum, erythema induratum, livedo vasculopathy, cryoglobulinemia, and SLE. For cases with gangrene, it is necessary to differentiate PN from pyoderma gangrenosum.

Treatment and prognosis

Administration of large doses of steroids or administration of cyclophosphamide are the first-line treatments. Inflammation causes dysfunction of the internal organs in the early stage, and the occlusion of blood vessels causes various ischemic disorders in the internal organs (e.g., renal failure, cerebral infarction, lung fibrosis, and cardiac failure) in the late stage.

Cutaneous polyarteritis nodosa

Cutaneous polyarteritis nodosa presents skin symptoms similar to those of PN; however, it lacks symptoms that involve the internal organs. The eruptions, which are triggered by hemolytic streptococcal infection, recur and follow a protracted course. Careful clinical follow-up is necessary, because cutaneous PN can worsen into systemic PN. Bed rest and elevation of the lower extremities are useful, as is the administration of vasodilators, NSAIDs or DDS.

Microscopic polyangiitis (MPA) (synonym: microscopic polyarteritis)

- A systemic vasculitis that affects the arteriolae, venulae, and small arteries, it is associated with ANCA (P-ANCA positive).
- It may quickly develop into glomerulonephritis or interstitial pneumonia. The prognosis is poor.
- Palpable purpura or livedo is seen.

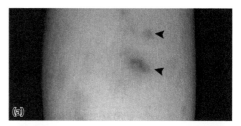

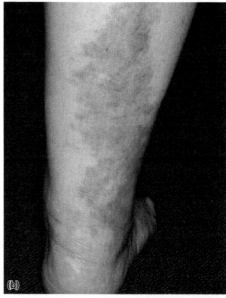

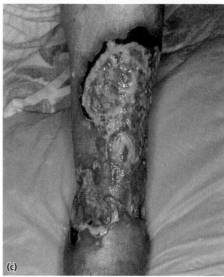

Fig. 11.8 Polyarteritis nodosa. a: Nodules with palpable, severe infiltration. b: Coalesced purpura. c: Advanced polyarteritis nodosa accompanied by ulceration.

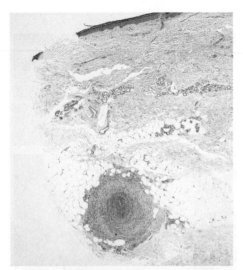

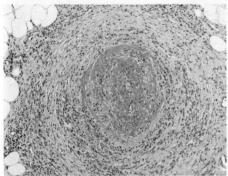

Fig. 11.9 Histopathology of PN.
Thickened vessel walls of medium-sized arteries, fibrinoid degeneration, and leukocytoclastic vasculitis are accompanied by neutrophilic infiltration.

Definition
Microscopic polyangiitis is defined as a systemic vasculitis that affects the arteriolae, venulae, and small arteries but is differentiated from classic polyarteritis nodosa. It is called ANCA-associated vasculitis, as are Churg–Strauss syndrome and Wegener's granulomatosis, because P-ANCA (MPO-ANCA), a type of anti-neutrophil cytoplasmic antibody (ANCA), is generally positive.

Clinical features
The skin lesions, which reflect the vasculitis in the arteriolae and venulae, appear as palpable purpura, mainly in the lower extremities. The palpable purpura, which is seen in 20–60% of MPA patients, appears after the systemic symptoms. Erythema, papules, livedo, nodules, and blisters may also occur.

Characteristic symptoms in other organs are acute progressive glomerular nephritis and interstitial pneumonia (pulmonary hemorrhage).

Pathology, diagnosis, and treatment
Leukocytoclastic vasculitis is seen mainly in the dermis. Granulomas do not form. Tests for MPO-ANCA, which are positive in about 60% of cases, are useful for diagnosis. The first-line treatment is the administration of high doses of steroids or immunosuppressive drugs. There have been many cases that rapidly progressed and resulted in death within a year.

Churg–Strauss syndrome (synonym: allergic granulomatous angiitis)
- This is a type of systemic vasculitis. It may be preceded by bronchial asthma, allergic rhinitis, and increased eosinophils. Called ANCA-associated vasculitis, it is generally P-ANCA positive.
- Interstitial pneumonia and lung granuloma occur.
- Multiple forms of skin lesions such as purpuras, urticaria, edematous erythema, and blood blisters occur.
- High-dose oral steroids are the main treatment.

Differential diagnosis
Churg–Strauss syndrome is a systemic vasculitis that occurs after several years of preceding disorders, including bronchial asthma and allergic rhinitis

(Fig. 11.10). Cutaneous symptoms are found in approximately half of all cases of Churg–Strauss syndrome. The skin lesions (e.g., purpura, urticaria, edematous erythema or blood blister) vary by depth. Polyneuropathy, arthritis, and lung and gastrointestinal symptoms may occur (Table 11.1).

Pathology

In Churg–Strauss syndrome, which is leukocytoclastic vasculitis mainly of the arteriolae, venulae, and small arteries, granulomas are seen outside the blood vessels, and significant eosinophilic infiltration in the tissues is seen. In many cases, granulomas are not clearly observed in the cutaneous lesions.

Laboratory findings

Leukocytosis, eosinophilia, and increased IgE levels are present. Approximately 50% of patients test positive for P-ANCA (MPO-ANCA), and they tend to develop complications such as nephritis and alveolar hemorrhage.

Treatment

Steroid pulse therapy is used. Immunosuppressants may be used in refractory cases.

Wegener's granulomatosis

- This is a type of systemic vasculitis. In many cases, upper respiratory symptoms often occur first, lung symptoms occur next, and renal symptoms follow.
- It features vasculitis accompanied by granuloma. It is a vasculitis associated with ANCA (C-ANCA positive).
- Multiple forms of skin lesions such as purpura, ecchymosis, papular erythema, and subcutaneous nodules occur.
- Multiple cavernous lung lesions are observed on the chest X-ray.
- The prognosis is improved by the combined use of steroids and cyclophosphamide.

Definition and symptoms

Wegener's granulomatosis is a systemic vasculitis that features vasculitis accompanied by granulomas in the nose, eyes, ears, upper respiratory tract, and lungs, necrotic glomerulonephritis, and vasculitis of the small

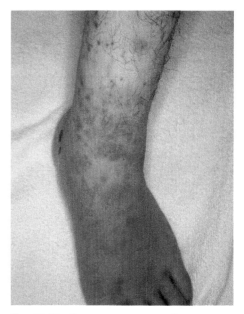

Fig. 11.10 Churg–Strauss syndrome. Infiltrative subcutaneous nodules, purpura, and erythema are seen.

Table 11.1 Main clinical symptoms and findings of Churg–Strauss syndrome (based on classification criteria proposed by the American College of Rheumatology).

Symptoms and findings	Details
Bronchial asthma	Expiratory wheezing or high-pitched rales
Eosinophilia	Eosinophils accounting for 10% or more of the fraction of peripheral leukocytes
Neuropathy, mono or poly	Numbness accompanied by pain, with glove-stocking distribution
Pulmonary infiltrates, non-fixed	Migrating or transient pulmonary infiltration (X-ray)
Paranasal sinus abnormality	Sharp pain or tenderness in paranasal sinus, or abnormal findings in X-ray
Extravascular eosinophils	Extravascular eosinophils in the skin and lung, observed pathologically

(Adapted from http://www.rheumatology.org/ publications/ classification/churg. asp?aud=mem)

and medium-sized arteries. The symptoms start as ear and upper respiratory symptoms, including nosebleeds or purulent rhinorrhea, then lung symptoms follow and kidney symptoms occur. Vasculitis symptoms such as arthralgia and polyneuropathy may also occur. Wegener's granulomatosis is classified into two types: generalized, involving all of the above organs, and localized, involving one or two organs.

Cutaneous symptoms, including palpable purpura, ecchymosis, papular erythema, and subcutaneous nodules, are found in approximately half of all cases of Wegener's granulomatosis. In the early stages, a skin lesion resembling pyoderma gangrenosum may be found, which is a clue to the diagnosis (Fig. 11.11).

Pathology
Leukocytoclastic vasculitis in the dermis is seen as a cutaneous lesion. Granulomas with giant cells may be seen in the walls of small arteries or outside the blood vessels in the subcutaneous fat tissues. Granulomas may be seen in lesions in the upper respiratory tract and lungs.

Laboratory findings
Chest X-ray shows distinctive round cavitating opacities in approximately 50% of cases. Tests for antineutrophil cytoplasmic antibody C-ANCA (PR3ANCA) are positive in 90% or more of patients in the acute phase, which is useful for diagnosis.

Treatment and prognosis
Steroids and immunosuppressants are used. Wegener's granulomatosis was once regarded as having a poor prognosis, and the majority of patients died from renal failure within a year. It can, however, be controlled with aggressive therapy initiated in the early stages.

Temporal arteritis (synonym: giant cell arteritis)
- Temporal arteritis (TA) is a vasculitis syndrome. The superficial temporal and ophthalmic arteries are affected.
- It occurs predominantly in elderly women. The typical symptoms are unexplained fever, throbbing headache, and visual impairment.

- Cord-like induration develops in the temporal region and is associated with proximal muscular pain (polymyalgia rheumatica).
- Oral steroid therapy is the mainstay of treatment.

Clinical features

Many of the patients are women in their 50s or older. TA occurs most commonly in the superficial temporal arteries. Cord-like thickening of the temporal arteries, reddening, and pressure pain are present in the temporal area. When the ischemia is marked, blisters, scalp necrosis, and hair loss occur.

Temporal arteritis is suspected when an elderly person complains of throbbing headache. When the maxillary artery is affected, pain in the masseter muscle on biting or talking (jaw claudication) occurs. When the ophthalmic artery and its branches are affected, sudden visual impairment may occur, which may lead to blindness. Symptoms of polymyalgia rheumatica are seen in about 30% of the patients. Stiffness and pain occur in the shoulders and lower back.

Laboratory findings

Elevated erythrocyte sedimentation rate and C-reactive protein (CRP) are observed. Histopathologically, infiltration of mononuclear cells and macrophages in the wall and peripheries of the blood vessels is observed, as is granulomatous angiitis with giant thrombi. Blood vessels in the other parts should be checked by MRI and FDG-PET examinations.

Treatment

Systemic steroids are used in the early stages of TA to prevent visual impairment. As the symptoms subside, the medication is gradually tapered off and is eventually discontinued.

Other diseases related to vasculitis in small and medium-sized blood vessels

Behçet's disease

- Behçet's disease is an intractable disease of recurrent acute inflammations, such as recurrent oral aphtha, and of cutaneous symptoms, genital ulceration, and ocular symptoms.

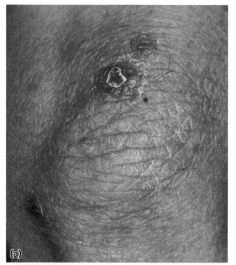

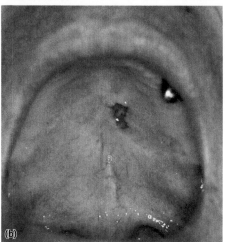

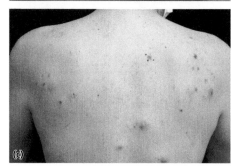

Fig. 11.11 Wegener's granulomatosis
a: Gangrenous papules. b: Ulceration in the oral cavity. c: Multiple subcutaneous nodules on the back.

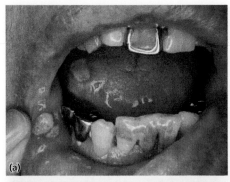

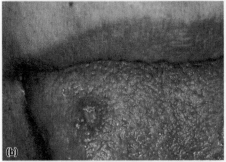

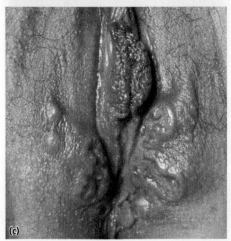

Fig. 11.12-1 Behçet's disease. a,b: Recurrent aphtha in the oral cavity accompanied by sharp pain. c: Deep ulceration in the genitalia.

- It occurs most frequently in persons in their 20s to 40s and is strongly correlated with the HLA-B51 allele. Many cases are found in the Middle East, South Asia, and the Far East.
- The typical cutaneous symptoms are erythema nodosum-like eruptions, thrombophlebitis, and folliculitis and acne-like eruptions. Needle reaction test is positive.
- There are specific severe types that severely affect the digestive tract, large arteries, and nerves.
- Colchicine and immunosuppressive therapy are the main treatment options.

Definition and symptoms

Behçet's disease manifests in individuals in their 20s, 30s, and 40s, and progresses over a long period of time with recurrent remissions and acute exacerbations (Fig. 11.12). Many cases are found in the Middle East, South Asia, and the Far East. The number of patients has been decreasing in recent years. Cutaneous and mucosal symptoms include the following.

- **Erythema nodosum-like eruptions:** erythema of 1–2 cm in diameter occurs on the lower extremities or forearms. The erythema is accompanied by pressure pain. The eruptions subside after about a week but tend to recur.
- **Thrombophlebitis:** the lesion is a palpable and painful subcutaneous linear cord in the extremities and is often migratory in nature.
- **Folliculitis and acne-like eruptions:** multiple follicular sterile pustules occur on various parts of the body. The symptoms presumably result from increased skin irritability and are similar to those observed in the needle reaction test (see Chapter 4).
- **Oral aphtha:** more than half of all patients with Behçet's disease experience oral aphtha, often as an early symptom. Single or multiple coated ulcers of 3–5 mm in diameter with red haloes form. The ulcers are painful; they heal without scarring in approximately 10 days but can recur.
- **Genital ulceration:** ulcers develop in the scrotum in men and in the labia in women. Deep and sharply demarcated ulcers form and heal, often with scarring.

Ocular symptoms such as uveitis and hypopyon are often seen in men. In acute attacks, the symptoms may lead to blindness. Arthritis or epididymitis may also occur. Symptoms with poor prognosis, which occur independently of the attacks of the above-mentioned symptoms, include disorders of the gastro-intestinal tract (e.g., ulcers in the ileocecal region), in the blood vessels (e.g., aortitis and thrombi formation in the deep veins), and nerves (e.g., meningitis and psychotic manifestations).

Pathogenesis

The pathogenesis of Behçet's disease is unknown. It has been presumed that a functional increase of neu-trophils, autoimmune reactions and angiitis occur, resulting from genetic factors (Behçet's disease has a strong correlation with HLA-B51) and environmental factors (e.g., hemolytic streptococcal infection).

Pathology

In erythema nodosum-like eruptions, septal pannicu-litis is present in which neutrophils and lymphocytes are mainly seen; however, vasculitis or thrombophle-bitis is also seen, depending on the timing of biopsy.

Diagnosis

The diagnostic criteria for Behçet's disease are out-lined in Table 11.2. When the first four typical symp-toms are present during the course of the disease, the disease is called complete Behçet's disease. In recent years, complete Behçet's disease has rarely been seen. In the international diagnostic criteria, oral aphtha is a necessary criterion and needle reac-tion is included.

Treatment

Topical steroids, oral NSAIDs, and colchicine are used for cutaneous lesions. Immunosuppressants and anti-TNF-α antibody biologics are useful for ocular symp-toms. For treating the severe specific types, high-dose steroids or oral anticoagulants are administered; how-ever, the ocular symptoms may be aggravated when the steroids are tapered off.

Kawasaki's disease (synonyms: acute febrile mucocutaneous lymph node syndrome)

- This is a disease with unknown etiology and six characteristics: (1) fever continuing for at least 5 days, (2) conjunctival reddening, particularly

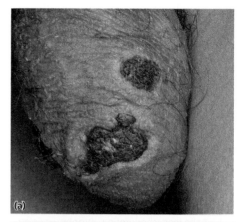
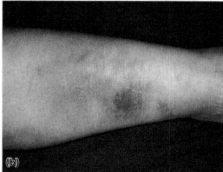
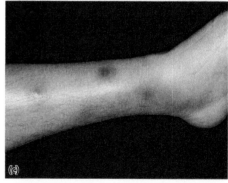
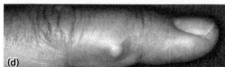
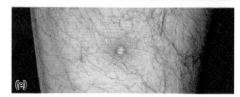

Fig. 11.12-2 Behçet's disease. a: Deep ulceration in the genitalia. b,c: Nodular erythema-like eruptions. d,e: Folliculitis-like eruptions.

Table 11.2 Diagnostic criteria of Behçet's disease.

1 Major symptoms

1 Recurrent aphthous ulceration in the oral mucosa
2 Cutaneous symptoms
  (a) Erythema nodosum-like skin lesions
  (b) Subcutaneous thrombophlebitis
  (c) Folliculitis-like eruptions, acne-like eruptions; helpful finding: enhanced sensitivity of skin
3 Ocular symptoms
  (a) Iridocyclitis
  (b) Retinouveitis (chorioretinitis)
  (c) Symptoms that suggest past occurrence of (a) and (b), such as posterior synechia of the iris, pigmentation on the lens, chorioretinal atrophy, optic atrophy, complicated cataract, secondary glaucoma or phthisis of the eyeballs
4 Genital ulceration

2 Minor symptoms
1 Arthritis that is not accompanied by articular deformity or rigidity, 2 Epididymitis, 3 Gastrointestinal lesions such as ileocecal ulcer, 4 Vascular lesions, 5 Moderate or severe central nervous symptoms
3 Diagnostic criteria for types of Behçet's disease

1 Complete Behçet's disease
  4 major symptoms during the course of the disease
2 Incomplete Behçet's disease
  (a) 3 major symptoms, or 2 major symptoms in combination with 2 minor symptoms
  (b) A typical ocular symptom in combination with another major symptom, or a typical ocular symptom in combination with 2 minor symptoms
3 Possible Behçet's disease
  1 or more major symptoms that do not meet the criteria for incomplete Behçet's disease, and recurrence or aggravation of typical minor symptoms
4 Rare symptoms of Behçet's disease
  (a) Gastrointestinal Behçet's disease: abdominal pain should be investigated, and occult blood test should be conducted.
  (b) Vascular Behçet's disease: impairment in large arteries, small arteries, or both large and small veins is noted.
  (c) Neuro Behçet's disease: headache, paralysis, and encephalomyelopathy. Investigation should be made for neurological symptoms.

Source: Japan Intractable Diseases Information Center (www.nanbyou.or.jp/top.html)

involving the bulbar conjunctivae, (3) erythema of the lips and oral cavity, flushing, and strawberry tongue edema, (4) eruptions of various shapes and erythema, (5) lesions in the distal fingers and toes starting with edema and erythema, and healing with scaling and (6) non-purulent lymph node enlargement in the neck.

- It is most common in children under the age of 4, and cases have been increasing in recent years. It may be accompanied by coronary disorders.
- The first-line treatment is high-dose intravenous immunoglobulin in the early stages.

Clinical features

Kawasaki's disease is slightly more common in males than in females (3:2). Prodromes are not present, and the onset begins with a fever of about 39°C. The symptoms are the following.

- **Erythema:** sharply marginated erythema develops on the fingers and toes. Palmoplantar hard edema, which restricts movement, is seen 3–5 days after onset. The condition lasts about 1–2 weeks, and heals with scaling starting at the tips of the fingers and toes (Fig. 11.13).
- **Eruptions of various shapes:** these are seen on the entire body at around 3–5 days after onset. They are often erythema but may manifest as various types of eruptions, including measles-like eruptions, diffuse erythema, and urticarial eruptions. Blisters are not seen. The eruptions often heal with scales in several days.
- **Lesions of the lips and oral cavity:** diffuse inflammation and cracking of the lips, and red "strawberry" tongue are seen at 2–3 days after onset.
- **Conjunctival reddening:** occurs 2–3 days after onset and lasts 1–3 weeks. Exudate is not seen.
- **Non-purulent lymph node enlargement in the neck:** often occurs unilaterally in the acute stage. The frequency of occurrence is approximately 65%.
- **Other cutaneous lesions:** erythema, vesicles, and pustules may appear at the site of BCG immunization. Transverse grooves on the nail (see Chapter 19) may be seen a few months after onset.

Joint pain and convulsions may occur. Cardiac complications are the most important. Coronary artery aneurysm or coronary stenosis may result in cardiac infarction and sudden death.

Pathogenesis

The etiology is unknown. It can be understood as an acute systemic vasculitis.

Diagnosis and treatment

The diagnostic criteria are those of the Kawasaki Disease Research Group of the Health and Welfare Ministry of Japan. The first-line treatment is high-dose intravenous immunoglobulins in the early stages (within 7 days after onset), which greatly reduces the fatality rate and the frequency of coronary arterial complications.

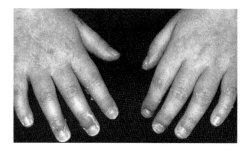

Fig. 11.13 Kawasaki's disease. Firm edema and scaling in characteristic pattern.

Pyoderma gangrenosum

- Small pustules and papules rapidly appear, forming ulcers with purplish-blue undermined edges, mainly in the lower body.
- Pyoderma gangrenosum often occurs as a complication of a primary disease such as inflammatory enteric disease, aortitis syndrome, and leukemia.
- Topical and oral steroids and oral ciclosporin are used for treatment.

Clinical features

Pyoderma gangrenosum occurs most commonly in the extremities, as well as in the lumbar and abdominal areas, particularly in females from ages 10 to 60. It may occur in the face. The symptoms start as blisters, pustules, and small hemorrhagic papules. Many eruptions gradually coalesce into ulcers and enlarge centrifugally. The edge of the eruption is dark reddish-purple and linearly elevated. Undermined edges form, and these can be palpable and visually inspected. The base of the ulcer contains brownish-yellow necrotic debris. The ulcer is painful and secretes pus when pressure is applied (Fig. 11.14). The center of the ulcer begins to heal with formation of papillary or reticular granulation tissue. The ulcer heals with scarring. Pyoderma gangrenosum can recur often in periods of several months.

Pathogenesis

The pathogenesis is unknown. Autoimmune and bacterial allergic reactions have been suspected. However, no definite cause has been identified. Skin trauma such as from biopsy may also induce pyoderma gangrenosum.

Pathology

Non-specific neutrophilic infiltration in the dermis is seen. Vasculitis is not seen. Infiltration of various inflammatory cells, including histiocytes and plasma cells, and fibrosis are found in the late stage.

Complications

Complications include inflammatory enteric diseases (e.g., ulcerative colitis and Crohn's disease), aortitis syndrome, hematological malignancies (e.g., leukemia and monoclonal IgA), and rheumatoid arthritis. Systemic examination is essential because primary diseases are found in 50–70% of patients with pyoderma gangrenosum.

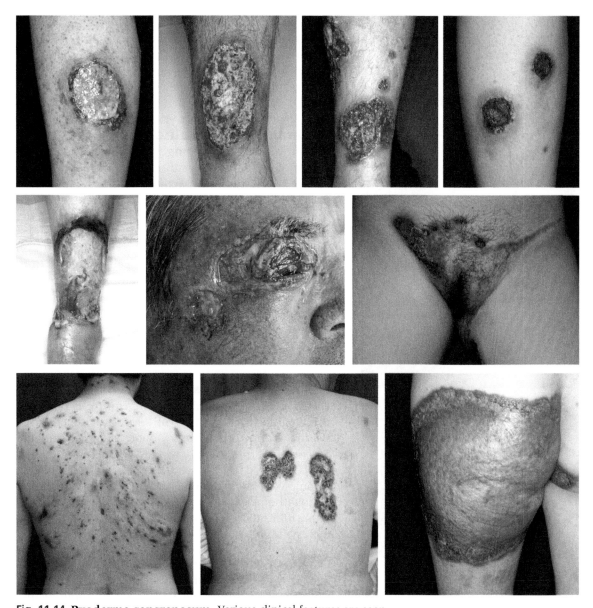

Fig. 11.14 Pyoderma gangrenosum. Various clinical features are seen.

Diagnosis

No specific examination findings have been reported but inflammation tends to produce inflammation, positive CRP, and neutrophilia. Pyoderma gangrenosum is a sterile pyoderma; nevertheless, the lesions may become secondarily infected. Differential diagnoses include deep fungal and mycobacterial infections.

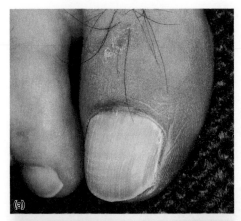

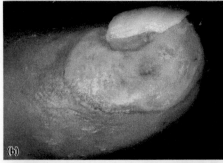

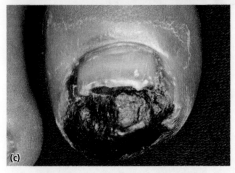

Fig. 11.15 Buerger's disease. a: Bluish discoloration (cyanosis) of the first toe. b: Progressive ulceration of the first toe. c: Necrosis of the first toe caused by impaired blood circulation.

Treatment

Topical steroids and tacrolimus are useful for local treatment. The first-line treatment is oral steroids, and oral ciclosporin and DDS should be considered when the first option is ineffective.

Buerger's disease (synonym: thromboangiitis obliterans (TAO))

Definition and symptoms

The etiology of Buerger's disease is unknown. Small arteries undergo contraction, and ischemia and occlusion of arteries and veins occur in the extremities. More than 90% of the patients are male smokers in their 20s–40s. It first occurs as Raynaud's phenomenon (see later section), a cool sensation in the fingers, intermittent claudication (pain that occurs when a person walks but subsides with rest). Over time, a minor injury may trigger ulceration with strong pain in the fingers, toes, and peripheral nails (Fig. 11.15). Deformation in the nails, which reflects ischemia, and migrating phlebitis may occur.

Laboratory findings and pathology

Observation of lowered skin temperature is done by thermography. Evaluation of superficial blood flow volume is done using a laser Doppler blood flowmeter. To check morphological changes, multiple segmental and narrowed blockages are observed by magnetic resonance (MR), 3D-CT, and other angiographies. Histopathologically, thrombus formation with neutrophilic infiltration is seen in the acute stage, and granulomas and fibrosis occur over time.

Diagnosis and differential diagnosis

Among the diagnostic criteria are those of the Research Committee of Intractable Vasculitis Syndrome of the Ministry of Health, Labor and Welfare of Japan. Differentiation from arteriosclerosis obliterans is necessary (Table 11.3).

Treatment

Smoking cessation, maintenance of warmth, and exercise therapy are the first options. Care should be taken to avoid external injury. Vasodilators and anticoagulants may be administered. Revascularization and sympathectomy are surgical treatment options.

Table 11.3 Differentiation between Buerger's disease and arteriosclerosis obliterans.

	Buerger's disease	Arteriosclerosis obliterans
Age of onset	Under 50 years of age	Aged 50 or older
Frequently affected part of the body	Small peripheral arteries	Large or medium-sized arteries
Habits, complications	Smoking	Diabetes, hypertension, hyperlipidemia
Arterial sclerosis?	(−)	+
Mobile phlebitis?	+	(−)

Mondor's disease
Clinical features and epidemiology
Many patients with Mondor's disease are females from 30 to 70 years old. Subcutaneous linear cord with a diameter of 3–10 mm appears on the chest, upper abdomen, and upper limbs (Fig. 11.16). It may also develop in men on the dorsum of the penis. It may be accompanied by spontaneous pain, and traction can also cause pain. The primary disease is thrombophlebitis or lymphangitis in the subcutaneous fat tissues. It may be induced by breast surgery (mastectomy in particular), pressure on the chest or shaving.

Pathology
The wall of the affected vein is fibrous and thick, and the lumen is narrowed or blocked. Infiltration of inflammatory cells is not seen (Fig. 11.17).

Treatment
The disease usually resolves spontaneously within several weeks. Clinical follow-up is essential.

Malignant atrophic papulosis (synonym: Degos' disease)
Multiple pink papules appear on the trunk and upper extremities followed several days to weeks later by the development of lesions about 1 cm in diameter, which form characteristic eruptions with whitish, atrophic centers surrounded by haloes or telangiectasia. The reddish color fades over time, and the papules heal with whitish atrophy. Histopathologically, mucin

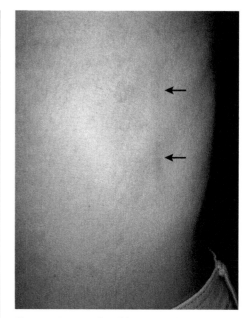

Fig. 11.16 Mondor disease. Subcutaneous, cordlike indurations (arrow) are observed.

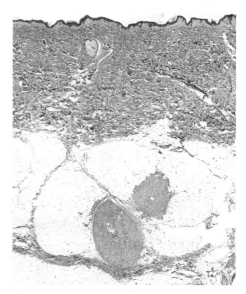

Fig. 11.17 Histopathology of Mondor's disease.

deposition and lymphocytic cell infiltrations are observed at the periphery of blood vessels. Malignant atrophic papulosis has a poor prognosis and is associated with cerebral infarction and perforative peritonitis several years after onset. A similar eruption may be seen in SLE, antiphospholipid antibody syndrome (APS), systemic scleredema, and rheumatoid arthritis. It is important to differentiate it from these primary diseases.

Thrombophlebitis (synonym: venous thrombosis)

Thrombophlebitis is a disease in which thrombi form in the superficial and deep veins. When the condition occurs in the deep veins it is called deep vein thrombosis (DVT) and may lead to serious conditions such as pulmonary embolism (PE). Superficial thrombophlebitis, which is the type most commonly treated by dermatologists, is discussed here.

Pathogenesis

Most cases of superficial thrombophlebitis result from damage to the veins by IV line placement or from the administration of vasodilators, antibiotics or anticancer agents. Varicose veins of the lower extremities, infections such as tuberculosis, and Behçet's and Buerger's disease may cause thrombophlebitis. In cases of recurring thrombophlebitis without identifiable inducing factors, the risk of DVT is high.

Clinical features

Cord-like induration parallel to the veins occurs, accompanied by tenderness and itching. Erythema is often present. Thrombophlebitis may progress and recur. In DVT of the lower extremities, rapid swelling, pain or burning sensation may occur.

Diagnosis and differential diagnosis

Thrombophlebitis is diagnosed by the distinctive clinical features. Enquiry about drug administration and investigations for Behçet's disease and tuberculosis may be necessary. Creeping eruption (see Chapter 28), in which cord-like induration is seen, can be a condition that requires differentiation from thrombophlebitis. Some cases of lower extremity DVT require differentiation from cellulitis.

Treatment
Bed rest and cooling of the affected site are the main treatments. Oral NSAIDs or steroids may be administered.

Purpura

Thrombocytopenic purpura

Clinical features and classification
Thrombocytopenic purpura is the general term for purpura that accompanies a decrease in platelet density (less than 100,000/mm³). When the platelet density is less than 100,000 per microliter, subcutaneous bleeding readily occurs. When the platelet count is less than 50,000 per microliter, the bleeding becomes marked, and petechiae and ecchymosis are produced. The purpura is non-palpable and without infiltration. Thrombocytopenic purpura is classified as either idiopathic thrombocytopenic purpura (ITP), which is caused by auto-antiplatelet antibodies, or secondary thrombocytopenic purpura, which accompanies other underlying disorders.

Idiopathic thrombocytopenic purpura
Clinical features
Based on the clinical course, ITP is classified as acute ITP, which resolves within 6 months, or chronic ITP. The former often occurs in children and is triggered by viral infections, including measles and rubella. The latter occurs in adults and is seen as the prolonged form of acute ITP. The main cutaneous symptoms are petechiae and ecchymosis, and there are no subjective symptoms. Other symptoms include bleeding in the oral and nasal mucosa and gingiva. Melena and menorrhagia may also develop. Bleeding in the joints and splenomegaly are not present. In severe cases, fatal cerebral hemorrhage may occur.

Laboratory findings
Decreased platelet density (100,000 per microliter or less) is generally the only blood cell abnormality. Platelet-associated IgG (PAIgG) is found in 80–90% of cases, with low specificity. Bone marrow biopsy shows an increase in megakaryocyte count resulting from

consumption of platelets. The coagulation system is normal. The Rumpel–Leede test (see Chapter 5) is positive.

Diagnosis and differential diagnosis

Idiopathic thrombocytopenic purpura is diagnosed by excluding other diseases such as pseudo-thrombocytopenia and secondary thrombocytopenic purpura. Henoch–Schönlein purpura and hemophilia are included in the differential diagnosis. Henoch–Schönlein purpura is distinguished from ITP by the development of relatively localized palpable purpura in the lower extremities associated with systemic symptoms such as arthralgia and abdominal pain. In contrast, in hemophilia, bleeding occurs in the joints and muscles.

Treatment

Oral steroid is the treatment of choice. Steroid pulse therapy or administration of large doses of immunoglobulin is used for severe cases. *Helicobacter pylori* eradication therapy may be done. When these drug therapies are ineffective, splenectomy may be performed.

Secondary thrombocytopenic purpura

A decrease in platelets caused by underlying disorders and other factors (Table 11.4) results in purpura.

Cryoglobulinemia

Classification

Cryoglobulinemia is a disorder with symptoms of vasculitis in which cryoglobulins (MEMO, see Chapter 11) are produced by various factors. Cryoglobulinemia is classified into types I, II, and III, depending on the cryoglobulin produced. Type I (30%), with minor symptoms of vasculitis, has symptoms that are mainly caused by blood clots. Types II (20%) and III (50%) have severe symptoms of vasculitis and are called mixed cryoglobulinemia. Cryoglobulinemia is also classified into an essential type, with unknown cause, and a secondary type, which has underlying disorders, including myeloma. In recent years, however, involvement of the type C hepatitis virus in the former has been

Table 11.4 Major causes of secondary thrombocytopenic purpura.

Abnormal production of platelets	
Production decrease	Aplastic anemia Leukemia, malignant lymphoma, bone marrow cancer Viral infection Irradiation Anticancer agents
Ineffective erythropoiesis	Myelodysplastic syndrome, paroxysmal nocturnal hemoglobinuria, vitamin B12 deficiency
Decreased platelet lifespan	
Immunological	Collagen diseases, including systemic lupus erythematosus Drugs
Enhanced consumption	Disseminated intravascular coagulation Thrombotic thrombocytopenic purpura Hemolytic-uremic syndrome Pregnancy-induced hypertension (HELLP syndrome)
Mechanical destruction	Artificial valve, artificial vessel

pointed out, and the classification is thought to be questionable.

Clinical features

Cryoglobulinemia most frequently occurs in middle-aged women. Exposure to cold results in petechiae, ecchymosis, livedo, and Raynaud's phenomenon in the lower extremities. Type I is generally mild but the blood clots may cause gangrene in the fingertips. In types II and III, the skin lesions and vasculitis are more severe, and palpable purpura, subcutaneous nodules or ulcers form. Systemic symptoms are often seen, including glomerular nephritis, joint pain, and polyneuritis.

Complications

Multiple myeloma and macroglobulinemia are often associated with type I; malignant lymphoma, rheumatoid arthritis, Sjögren syndrome and hepatitis B and C with type II; and collagen diseases (e.g., rheumatoid arthritis and dermatomyositis), infections (e.g., infectious mononucleosis and viral hepatitis) and nephritis with type III.

Pathology

Blood clots caused by cryoglobulins are seen in the cutaneous lesions in all three types, and leukocytoclastic vasculitis is seen in types II and III. Cryoglobulinemia is characterized by membranoproliferative glomerulonephritis.

Laboratory findings

Cryoglobulin is detected by the processing of sampled blood at 37°C to isolate the serum. It may be difficult to detect cryoglobulin in standard outsourced examinations. It is also necessary to test for various autoantibodies, including rheumatoid factor and hepatitis virus infections, and to conduct electrophoresis for humoral immune response.

Treatment

Exposure to cold should be avoided. If an underlying disorder is present, that disorder should be treated. Steroids are administered for the vasculitis symptoms.

MEMO 11–3 Cryoglobulin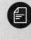

Cryoglobulin is an abnormal immunoglobulin in serum. It is a thermolabile substance, and the phase easily changes depending on the temperature. It gelates or precipitates when cooled to 4°C for 2–7 days and dissolves when warmed to 37°C. It contains a rheumatoid factor, usually IgM. There are three types.

- **Type I:** the main components are monoclonal IgM and IgG, which are seen in multiple myeloma and macroglobulinemia.
- **Type II:** the main components are monoclonal Ig, which is seen in RF, and polyclonal Ig, which is seen in malignant lymphoma, rheumatoid arthritis, and Sjögren syndrome.
- **Type III:** the main component is polyclonal Ig. It occurs with collagen disease or various infections as underlying disorders.

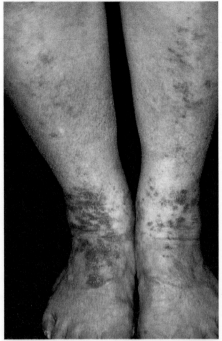

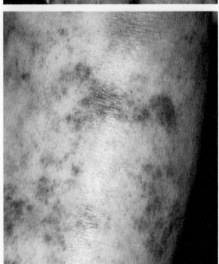

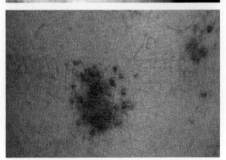

Fig. 11.18 Pigmented purpuric dermatosis.

Pigmented purpuric dermatosis (synonyms: idiopathic pigmentary purpura, purpura pigmentosa chronica)

Clinical features and classification

Pigmented purpuric dermatosis, which occurs most frequently in the lower extremities of the middle-aged, has an unknown etiology and is accompanied by petechiae and telangiectasia. It leaves pigmentation after healing (Fig. 11.18). Systemic symptoms are not present. It is a chronic condition with recurrent remissions and acute exacerbations. It is classified by the distribution of eruptions into several types: Schamberg's disease, Majocchi's disease, Gougerot–Blum syndrome, lichen aureus, and itching purpura (Table 11.5). The symptoms of these types are often mixed. Most cases of pigmented purpuric dermatosis are Schamberg's disease, and varicose veins of the lower extremities may be present.

Pathology

Lymphocytic infiltration and leakage of erythrocytes are found in the perivascular area in the upper dermal layer. Pigmented purpuric dermatosis is characterized by chronic hemorrhagic inflammation. Hemosiderin deposits are seen in old lesions (Fig. 11.19). Cells infiltrate in a band-like pattern in some cases, which makes it difficult to clinically distinguish from early mycosis fungoides.

Treatment

Topical steroids are used for relieving the symptoms. Oral vitamin C and hemostatic drugs may be useful. Bed rest with elevation of the lower extremities is helpful. When varicose veins of the lower extremities are present, the use of elastic stockings is also considered.

Senile purpura

The vascular supporting tissues weaken with age, and purpura is easily produced with minor trauma. Senile purpura occurs mostly on the dorsa of the hands and the extensor surfaces of the forearms, producing sharply marginated subcutaneous hemorrhagic spots.

Table 11.5 Major types of pigmented purpuric dermatosis.

	Schamberg's disease	Majocchi's purpura	Pigmented purpuric lichenoid dermatosis	Lichen aureus
Age of onset	40s	30s	40s	20–30s
Sex	Male > female	Female > male	Male > female	Male > female
Type of onset	Slow	Slow	Acute	Acute
Most common site	Lower extremities	Lower extremities	Lower extremities > upper extremities	One of the lower extremities
Clinical features	Petechia irregularly coalesces.	Annular purpura accompanying telangiectasia	Brownish papules. The lesion may lichenify.	Yellowish to brown plaque
Itching	±	±	+	– to ++
Course	Chronic	Chronic	Chronic	May gradually enlarge

Purpura simplex

Purpura simplex occurs frequently in the lower extremities of women. Multiple petechiae with vague margins develop. A few purpura of larger size may be seen. The lesions are not palpable and do not have subjective symptoms. Abnormality is not found by blood test. The lesions fade after bed rest. It is necessary to differentiate it from thrombocytopenic purpura and early Henoch–Schönlein purpura.

Steroid purpura

When the vascular supporting tissues are weakened by extended use of topical or oral steroids, the capillary blood vessels are readily broken by trauma, leading to purpura (Fig. 11.20). Steroid purpura most frequently occurs in the elderly. Trauma should be avoided, and steroids should be used appropriately.

For purpura in scurvy, see Chapter 17.

Other vascular diseases

Arteriosclerosis obliterans (ASO)

As a result of arteriosclerosis in medium-sized and large arteries of the lower extremities, chronic arteriosclerotic constriction or occlusion occurs. ASO in the lower extremities is discussed in this section. Ischemia in the lower extremities causes skin pallor, sensory

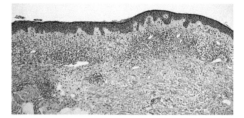
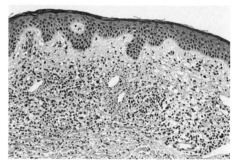

Fig. 11.19 Histopathology of pigmented purpuric dermatosis. Perivascular lymphocytic infiltration in the upper dermis, hemorrhage, and deposition of hemosiderin.

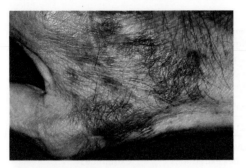

Fig. 11.20 Steroid purpura.

abnormality, pain, and ulceration. Patients often have concurrent diabetes, dyslipidemia, and obesity.

Clinical features

Arteriosclerosis obliterans most frequently occurs in men in their 60s or older. Various symptoms caused by ischemia in the arteries of the lower extremities appear.

- **Fontaine level 1:** transient cool sensation in the fingers and toes, numbness, cyanosis or whiteness of the skin, and Raynaud's phenomenon are present.
- **Fontaine level 2:** claudication is seen.
- **Fontaine level 3:** pain is present during stillness. Sharp pain and ulcers occur in the toes.
- **Fontaine level 4:** ulcers form and necrosis occurs. Amputation of the lower extremities may be necessary.

Diagnosis and differential diagnosis

The simplest, quickest, and most useful examination for ASO is the Ankle Brachial Pressure Index (ABPI). ASO is suspected when the ABPI is below 0.9. Differential diagnoses include Buerger's disease (see Table 11.3) and lumbar spinal canal stenosis, which can also cause intermittent claudication.

Treatment

For mild cases (Fontaine levels 1 and 2), antiplatelet agents, vasodilators, and exercise therapy are the first options. For severe cases with ischemia in the lower extremities, endovascular treatments including stenting and reconstructive surgery are options.

Diabetic gangrene

Diabetic gangrene results from ulcers in the toes, soles, and fingers caused by microvascular damage and sclerosis. It is accompanied by sharp pain (see Chapter 17).

Raynaud's phenomenon, Raynaud's disease

Definition

The fingers and toes become whitish. After several minutes, they progress to a purplish dark blue from cyanosis and then return to normal color through a diffuse flushing phase. The whole process takes several minutes to less than an hour. The condition may occur without any underlying disorders but it frequently occurs with underlying disorders, including collagen diseases. The former is called primary Raynaud's phenomenon/disease, and the latter is called secondary Raynaud's phenomenon/syndrome.

Clinical features

Primary Raynaud's phenomenon is frequently seen in young women, and the symptoms are generally mild. It tends to occur in cool or cold environments (in winter or in an air-conditioned workplace) or under mental strain. The fingers and toes become white, and a cool sensation, sharp pain, numbness, and edema occur (Fig. 11.21). The digits then become blue, followed by diffuse flushing and a burning sensation. In some cases, there are just one or two skin color changes instead of three, i.e., there is no cyanosis (blueness) or rubra (redness). The symptoms of secondary Raynaud's phenomenon are frequently severe, and ulcers may form in the distal fingers.

Pathogenesis

Table 11.6 shows the disorders that may cause secondary Raynaud's phenomenon. Raynaud's phenomenon is a circulatory disorder caused by various factors, with the changes occurring as a reaction to the circulatory disorder. The pallor (whiteness) reflects the ischemic condition that arises from constriction of arteries, and the cyanosis (blueness) reflects hemostasis. The diffuse flushing (redness) reflects the reactive hyperemia.

Diagnosis

It is important to make an examination for underlying disorders. Observations are done by thermography of the skin temperature during normal times to determine if the patient's skin temperature tends to become low or if there is a delay in recovery from cold stimulation. The condition may be induced by cold provocation test (soaking fingers and toes in 4°C water for 10 sec). For a young woman who has the above-described condition for 2 years without underlying disorders, the condition can be diagnosed as primary Raynaud's phenomenon.

Treatment

Causative factors should be eliminated, and the body must be kept warm. Prostaglandins may be administered. Smoking cessation is effective.

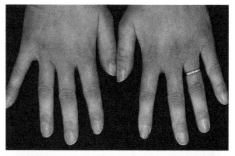
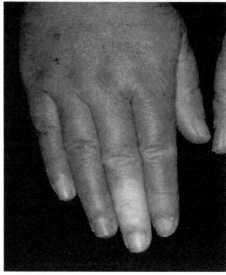

Fig. 11.21 Raynaud's phenomenon.

MEMO 11–4 Erythema ab igne, thermal burn

This is livedo caused by repeated heat exposure at the same site for a long period of time (See Figures). It is clinically livedo, but vasculitis is not found pathologically.

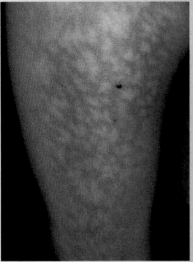

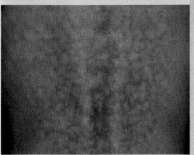

Erythema ab igne.

Table 11.6 Causes of Raynaud's phenomenon.

Disease	Causes
Primary Raynaud's phenomenon	Raynaud's disease
Secondary Raynaud's phenomenon	Physical stimulation in people who work with vibrating machinery (vibration syndrome or vibration white finger), pianists, typists, and food industry workers (meat industry, fresh fish industry)
	Drugs: ergotamine, tryptamine, β-blockers, oral contraceptives
	Collagen diseases: seen often in persons with systemic sclerosis and mixed connective tissue disease
	Blood disease: cryoglobulinemia, cold agglutinin disease
	Angiopathy: arteriosclerosis obliterans, Buerger's disease, systemic vasculitis
	Neurological disorders: carpal tunnel syndrome, multiple sclerosis
	Other diseases: malignant tumor, hypothyroidism

Chronic venous insufficiency (synonyms: venous insufficiency, venous stasis syndrome)

Definition and symptoms

Chronic venous insufficiency (CVI) is a group of symptoms with varicose veins (Fig. 11.22) as the underlying disorder. It frequently occurs in middle-aged women or elderly men, and in people who are obese or who stand for prolonged periods. Superficial veins dilate and wind in hose-like or nodular shapes. Collateral circulation may develop, and network-like venous elongations may be seen. As CVI progresses, tiredness, edema, pain, pigmentation, and stasis dermatitis occur in the lower extremities (see Chapter 7), and sclerosing panniculitis occurs, followed by the formation of non-healing ulcers (Fig. 11.23).

Pathogenesis

Varicose veins are classified as primary, occurring as valvular incompetence in the superficial and/or perforating veins from prolonged standing; secondary, occurring as a result of heightened blood pressure caused by blood clots in deep veins, broken valves after thrombophlebitis and increase in circulation during pregnancy; and congenital, occurring from Klippel–Trenaunay–Weber syndrome (see Chapter 20). Increases in the inner pressure of the great and small saphenous veins and circulatory disturbances occur from the above-described causes.

Treatment

Prolonged walking or standing should be avoided. Elevating the legs and wearing elastic stockings may be helpful. For the cutaneous symptoms of venous insufficiency, topical histamines and steroids are used. Endovascular treatments using laser or radiofrequency waves, sclerotherapy, venous stripping, and high ligation may be considered.

Livedo

Livedo is a generic term for reddish or purplish reticular spots on the skin that are caused by decreased tension in the venous network and increased tension in the arterial network at the border between the dermis and subcutaneous fat tissues. Livedo can be found as various skin conditions (Fig. 11.24) with various causes. There are three types.

- **Cutis marmorata:** this occurs as pink reticular erythema in the lower extremities of infants or young women without underlying disorders. The symptoms are transient, and there are no subjective symptoms. The erythema intensifies with cold and disappears with warming. The sympathetic nerves are thought to be involved.
- **Livedo racemosa:** this occurs on the extremities as a persistent peach-colored dendritic erythema in the shape of a horseshoe. The causes can be blockage of vascular cavities, circulatory disorders or vascular disorders (Table 11.7).

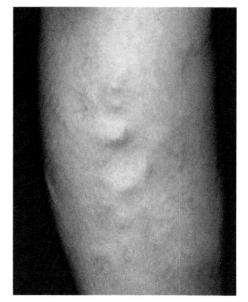

Fig. 11.22 Varicose veins. Superficial veins of lower legs enlarge in serpentine, nodular or cystiform patterns.

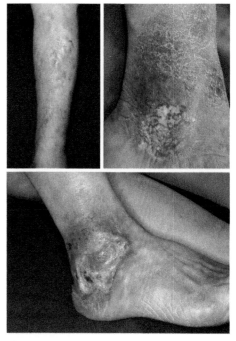

Fig. 11.23 Chronic venous insufficiency (livedo).

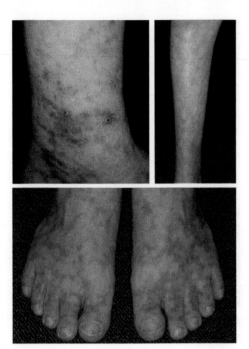

Fig. 11.24 Livedo.

Table 11.7 Conditions with livedo (reticularis).

Cause	Symptoms and diseases
Congenital	Cutis marmorata telangiectatica congenita
Physiological	Cutis marmorata (without an underlying disease)
Secondary	Livedo vasculopathy
	Collagen diseases (antiphospholipid (antibody) syndrome, systemic lupus erythematosus)
	Vasculitis (polyarteritis nodosa, in particular)
	Cryoglobulinemia
	Blue toe syndrome
	Calciphylaxis, hyperparathyroidism
	Sneddon syndrome
	Hematopoietic tumor (polycythemia vera, essential thrombocytopenia, malignant lymphoma)
	Erythema ab igne
	Infection (syphilis, tuberculosis)

- **Cutis marmorata telangiectatica congenita:** see Chapter 20.

Livedo vasculopathy (synonyms: livedo vasculitis, livedo reticularis with summer/winter ulcerations, livedoid vasculopathy)

Livedo vasculopathy is a disorder with ulcerations of unknown etiology, in which painful livedo and purpura occur mainly on the lower extremities (Fig. 11.25). Whitish atrophic scars (atrophie blanche) appear after the ulcers heal. Systemic symptoms are not present. Seasonal remissions and exacerbations may be observed. Histopathologically, vasculitis is not present but thrombi formation is observed in blood vessels in the dermis. Differentiation from antiphospholipid antibody syndrome (APS) and cryoglobulinemia is necessary. Vasodilators for peripheral vascular diseases, and oral and topical steroids are used; however, livedo vasculopathy is a refractory disorder.

Erythromelalgia (synonyms: erythralgia, acromelalgia)

Erythromelalgia occurs in the extremities, particularly in the soles. It is characterized by three main symptoms: paroxysmal burning sensation, flushing, and increase in skin temperature. The pathogenesis is unknown. Attacks often occur from exercise or bathing. Constant cooling may cause ulcers as a secondary symptom. It may occur secondarily from underlying disorders, including polycythemia vera, essential thrombocytosis, and collagen diseases. Effective treatment methods have not been established. Aspirin may be useful for cases in which thrombocytosis is the underlying condition.

Lymphangitis

Lymphangitis is inflammation of the lymphatic vessels. The cause is often hemolytic streptococcal infection. The spread of various infections, including cellulitis, trichophytic infection of the feet and parasitic infestation (e.g., filariasis), is known to cause lymphangitis, as is malignancy (e.g., breast cancer). Painful, linear, soft, palpable, cord-like erythema is accompanied by tenderness along the affected lymphatic system. Swelling of the regional lymph nodes is seen. Systemic symptoms include high fever, shivering, and loss of appetite. It is necessary to administer systemic antibiotics immediately.

Lymphedema

Lymph fluid volume increases locally from lymphatic vessel dysfunction. The causes are largely divided into congenital (e.g., hypoplasia of lymphatic vessels) and acquired (e.g., metastasis of a tumor into a lymph node, lymph node dissection, filariasis). Soft edema often develops, mainly in the lower extremities. Color changes and subjective symptoms are not present. There may be fibrosis of soft tissues as it becomes chronic. Papillary thickening of the epidermis (elephantiasis nostras verrucosa) may be seen (Fig. 11.26). Angiosarcoma may occur (Stewart–Treves syndrome; see Chapter 22).

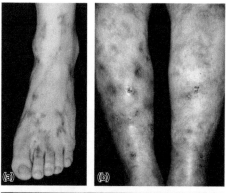
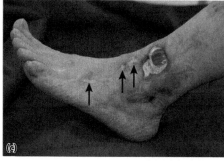

Fig. 11.25 Livedo vasculopathy. a: Livedo on the dorsa of foot. b: Ulcerations with livedo are seen on the lower legs. c: Ulceration on the lower leg, accompanied by atrophie blanche (arrows).

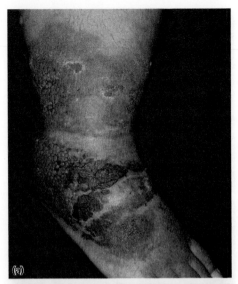

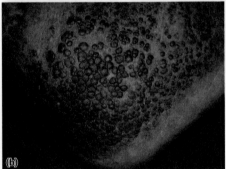

Fig. 11.26 Lymphedema. a: Marked swelling occurs secondarily in the lower leg. b: A skin lesion with extremely hypertrophic changes resembles elephant skin.

Ataxia telangiectasia (synonym: Louis–Bar syndrome)

- Ataxia telangiectasia (AT) is an autosomal recessive disease resulting from functional abnormality of the DNA repair mechanism.
- The three main symptoms are cerebellar ataxia, telangiectasia, and opportunistic infection.
- It is a type of congenital immunodeficiency syndrome.

Clinical features
Telangiectasia in the bulbar conjunctiva is seen when the patient is between 3 and 6 years old, and it appears later in the skin. The skin lesions appear first in the auricular region and cheeks, and gradually spread to the limbs. In adolescents and adults, poikiloderma and hardening of the skin occur and the patient shows a progeria-like appearance. Ataxia becomes apparent when the patient starts to walk. The patient suffers repeated respiratory and sinus infections from immunodeficiency. As the patient ages, various malignancies occur, including those in the skin.

Pathogenesis
It is an autosomal recessive disease. Mutation of the *AT* (ataxia-telangiectasia) gene on chromosome 11 causes the disease. Functional abnormalities of the DNA repair mechanism and of cell cycle control are involved. Gene rearrangement of T or B cells is inhibited by the mutation, which results in immunodeficiency and leads to increased susceptibility to cancer.

Laboratory findings
Peripheral blood T cells are reduced in number and function, and serum IgA and IgE (sometimes IgG2 and IgG4) are absent or markedly reduced. The serum α-fetoprotein value is elevated. Brain CT and MRI show atrophy in the cerebellar vermis.

Diagnosis and treatment
Ataxia telangiectasia is diagnosed on the basis of the pathological symptoms and laboratory findings. Diagnosis can also be made by *AT* gene analysis. Symptomatic therapy is the main treatment.

CHAPTER 12
Collagen diseases

Collagen diseases (connective tissue diseases) share similarities with autoimmune disorders. Multiple organs may be affected, and the site of the main lesion often differs from case to case. Diagnosis of collagen diseases is mainly based on the criteria established by the American College of Rheumatology.

Lupus erythematosus

Definition and classification

Lupus erythematosus (LE) is a diagnostic term for diseases that can cause various systemic changes, including those involving the skin. LE can also cause localized cutaneous lesions, as seen in discoid lupus erythematosus (DLE), lupus erythematosus profundus, and subacute cutaneous lupus erythematosus. Cutaneous LE is subcategorized as acute, subacute or chronic, with each subtype having characteristic features (Table 12.1). Cutaneous lesions may occur in SLE; however, the same lesions can be seen as a symptom of an intermediate LE type that does not satisfy the diagnostic criteria of SLE. In some cases, only the cutaneous symptoms occur (MEMO, see Chapter 12). Acute cutaneous LE generally occurs as a symptom of SLE and is discussed in the section on SLE. The subacute and chronic types often have only the cutaneous symptoms, and these are discussed in independent sections.

Systemic lupus erythematosus (SLE)

- Multiple organ failure occurs. The kidneys, heart, joints, and central nervous system are affected. SLE is an autoimmune disease of unknown etiology. Young women are most commonly affected.
- The typical mucocutaneous manifestations are erythema on the cheeks (butterfly rash), DLE, oral ulcerations, photosensitivity, and alopecia.
- The laboratory findings are the presence of antinuclear, anti-dsDNA, and anti-Sm antibodies, biological false-positive serological reaction for syphilis,

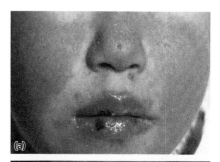
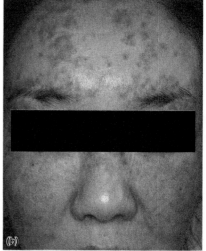

Fig. 12.1-1 Systemic lupus erythematosus (SLE). a: Butterfly rash and edematous erythema on the cheeks of a young woman. The skin lesion does not usually spread to the nasolabial groove and lips. Butterfly-shaped erythema. b: Butterfly rash from recurrence of SLE in a woman in her 30s. Such rashes may recur with aggravation of the SLE.

Shimizu's Dermatology, Second Edition. Hiroshi Shimizu.
© 2017 John Wiley & Sons, Ltd. Published 2017 by John Wiley & Sons, Ltd.

Table 12.1 Lesions of cutaneous lupus erythematosus.

Acute: progresses in a few days
Malar rash, lupus hair, palmar erythema, aphtha, maculopapular rash, etc.
Subacute (SCLE): progresses in a few weeks to a few months
Papulosquamous and annular-polycyclic lesions
Chronic: progresses over a long period of time
DLE, lupus profundus, chilblain lupus, nodular cutaneous lupus mucinosis, etc.

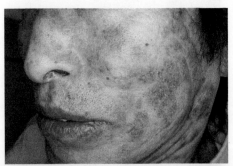
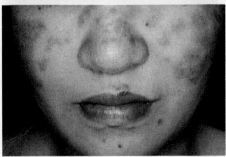

Fig.12.1-2 Systemic lupus erythematosus.

positive LE cells, decreased complements, and pancytopenia.
- The diagnostic criteria are those published by the American College of Rheumatology.
- The main treatment is oral corticosteroids.

Epidemiology
The onset tends to be between the ages of 20 and 50 years. There is a female preponderance (nine females to one male), and the majority of patients are women of child-bearing age.

Cutaneous features
Cutaneous findings are observed in more than 80% of cases. The four main symptoms of SLE, which are included in the diagnostic criteria (Table 12.2), are erythema on the cheeks, DLE, oral ulcers, and photosensitivity (Fig. 12.1). The frequencies of these symptoms are listed in Fig. 12.2.
- **Erythema on the cheeks** (see Fig. 12.1-1a,b): also called butterfly rash, this is the most characteristic eruption, seen in about 70% of cases. Among that 70%, the rash is the first symptom in 40% of cases. Edematous erythema spreads symmetrically on the cheeks, forming a butterfly pattern. Generally, it does not extend beneath the nasolabial groove. Blistering is rarely present. The rash is largely asymptomatic or is associated with mild subjective symptoms such as a slight burning sensation. It heals without scarring.
- **Discoid lupus erythematosus (DLE):** a skin manifestation, consists of sharply demarcated discoid erythema. The lesions are seen in 25% of patients with SLE, occurring on exposed sites such as the face, lips, and ears. Scales and crusts often form. (See next section.)
- **Palmar erythema:** this is seen in about 50% of SLE cases. Diffuse erythema occurs on the palms.
- **Alopecia:** this occurs diffusely on the scalp, resulting in short, thin, broken hairs at the hairline and uneven hair length (lupus hair). The alopecia often worsens during the active stage of SLE.
- **Enanthema:** this is seen in about 40% of SLE cases. Small hemorrhagic lesions with a red halo and small ulcers appear on the lips and the oral, rhinopharyngeal, and laryngeal mucosa. They may be found in DLE involving the mucous membranes.
- **Subcutaneous nodules:** nodules form on the face, buttocks, and upper arms as a result of inflammation

Table 12.2 1982 Revised criteria for classification of systemic lupus erythematosus.

Criterion		Definition
1.	Malar rash	Fixed erythema, flat or raised, over the malar eminences, but tending not to appear on the nasolabial folds
2.	Discoid rash	Raised erythematous patches with adherent keratotic scaling and follicular plugging; atrophic scarring may occur in older lesions
3.	Photosensitivity	Skin rash from unusual reaction to sunlight, revealed by patient history or physician observation
4.	Oral ulcers	Oral or nasopharyngeal ulceration, usually painless, observed by physician
5.	Arthritis	Nonerosive arthritis involving 2 or more peripheral joints, characterized by tenderness, swelling or effusion
6.	Serositis	a) Pleuritis: convincing history of pleuritic pain or rubbing heard by a physician or evidence of pleural effusion OR b) Pericarditis: documented by ECG or rub or by evidence of pericardial effusion
7.	Renal disorder	a) Persistent proteinuria greater than 0.5 g per day or greater than 3+ if quantitation is not performed OR b) Cellular casts: may be red cells, hemoglobin, granules, tubules or mixed
8.	Neurologic disorder	a) Seizures: in the absence of causative drugs or known metabolic disorder (e.g., uremia, ketoacidosis, electrolyte imbalance) OR b) Psychosis: in the absence of causative drugs or known metabolic disorder (e.g., uremia, ketoacidosis, electrolyte imbalance)
9.	Hematologic disorder	a) Hemolytic anemia: with reticulocytosis OR b) Leukopenia: less than 4,000/mm^3 total on 2 or more occasions OR c) Lymphopenia: less than 1,500/mm^3 on 2 or more occasions OR d) Thrombocytopenia: less than 100,000/mm^3 in the absence of causative drugs
10.	Immunologic disorder	a) Positive LE cell preparation OR b) Anti-DNA: antibody to native DNA in abnormal titer OR c) Anti-Sm: presence of antibody to Sm nuclear antigen OR d) False positive serologic test for syphilis known to be positive for at least 6 months and confirmed by *Treponema pallidum* immobilization or fluorescent treponemal antibody absorption test
11.	Antinuclear antibody	An abnormal titer of antinuclear antibody by immunofluorescence or an equivalent assay at any point in time and in the absence of drugs known to be associated with drug-induced lupus syndrome

The proposed classification is based on 11 criteria. For clinical studies, a person is said to have systemic lupus erythematosus if any 4 of the 11 criteria are present, serially or simultaneously at any time during observation (Tan EM, et al. The 1982 revised criteria for the classification of systemic lupus erythematosus. Arthritis Rheum 1982; 25: 1271-7).

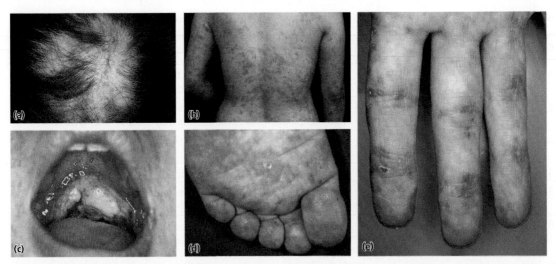

Fig. 12.1-3 Systemic lupus erythematosus (SLE). a: Diffuse alopecia caused by SLE. In this case, discoid lupus erythematosus (DLE) is present at the sites with alopecia. b: Edematous erythema and papules on the trunk during the acute stage. c: A large ulcer in the pharyngeal region. Large oral mucosal ulcers may be seen in SLE. d: Diffuse erythema on the sole and toes. e: Skin lesion on fingers caused by DLE. Tenderness may be present.

of subcutaneous fat. This type of LE is also called lupus erythematosus profundus (described later).

- **Other cutaneous symptoms:** erythema papulatum tends to occur on the dorsal hands during the acute stage.

Livedo, palpable purpura, bleeding in the nail folds, ulcers in the extremities (angiitis), petechia (thrombopenia), and Raynaud's phenomenon are seen.

Systemic symptoms

The systemic symptoms of SLE can be wide-ranging (see Fig. 12.2). The onset is an attack of fever, fatigue, arthralgia, and edema, accompanied by cutaneous symptoms (described above).

- **Arthralgia:** this is seen in more than 90% of SLE cases. The proximal interphalangeal joints, knees, shoulders, and elbow joints are most frequently affected. Joint destruction is not observed by X-ray examination.
- **Renal symptoms:** treatment is based on the diagnosis of lupus nephritis. The nephritic lesions are classified into types I–VI, based on the pathological findings, with the prognosis varying by type. Proteinuria, hematuria, nephrotic syndrome, and renal failure are seen.
- **Cardiac symptoms:** epicarditis, Libman–Sacks endocarditis, and myocarditis may occur.

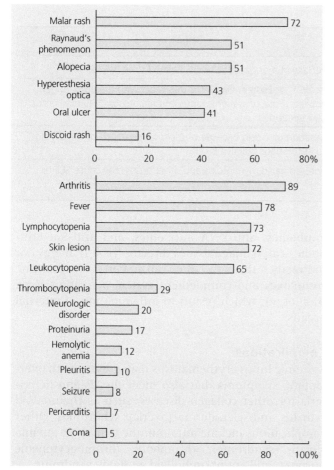

Fig. 12.2 Main eruptions caused by systemic lupus erythematosus and their frequency (% of cases).
Source: Hashimoto H, Miyamoto A (eds). Systemic lupus erythematosus. *Clinical Allergology*, 2nd edn. Nankodo, 1998.

- **Mental and neurological symptoms:** neurological manifestations such as convulsions, impaired consciousness, depression, and schizophrenia-like symptoms occur in about 20% of cases. It may be difficult to distinguish these from steroid-induced psychosis.
- **Lung symptoms:** pleuritis occurs in more than 50% of cases. Other symptoms include pulmonary hypertension, pulmonary hemorrhage, and pulmonary infarction.

Pathogenesis

The pathogenesis is complex but hereditary predisposition, viral infection, and other factors are thought to interact (Table 12.3). The production of antinuclear

MEMO 12–1 Drug-induced lupus erythematosus

Use of chlorpromazine, methyldopa, hydralazine, procainamide, isoniazid, and D-penicillamine may cause symptoms resembling mild SLE. Most cases improve by cessation of the causative drug; however, some cases progress to SLE. The differential pathological finding is anti-dsDNA antibody negative.

MEMO 12–2 Differentiating between SLE and DLE

Systemic lupus erythematosus is characterized by cutaneous and systemic involvement. Cutaneous lesions of DLE and subacute cutaneous lupus erythematosus may occur as symptoms of SLE; however, in some cases, only the cutaneous symptoms occur. SLE may be classified as intermediate LE, i.e., LE that satisfies only some of the SLE diagnostic criteria, or as cutaneous-limited LE, which has only the cutaneous lesions of LE.

Table 12.3 Factors associated with onset of SLE.

Factor	Finding
Genes	Familial prevalence, especially in monozygotic twins. Related to HLA-RD2
Viral infection	Immune reaction to retrovirus, or Epstein–Barr virus may react with the autoantigen. Clinical symptoms resembling those of systemic lupus erythematosus (SLE) may occur in human parvovirus B19 infection.
Immunology	Changes occur in fractionation of T cells because of the disappearance of the thymus, which results in elevated autologous reactive B cells.
Extrinsic	Procainamide, hydralazine, isoniazid, hydantoins and other drugs may cause SLE to become apparent.

antibodies, anti-DNA antibodies, and anti-Sm antibodies can damage tissues directly (type II allergy) or indirectly through the formation of immune complexes and complement system activation (type III allergy), which results in inflammation of internal organs.

Complications

Systemic lupus erythematosus may present with overlapping symptoms that also meet the diagnostic criteria for other collagen diseases, such as rheumatoid arthritis and scleroderma (overlap syndrome). Other complications include autoimmune hemolytic anemia (Evans syndrome), thrombotic thrombocytopenic purpura, and antiphospholipid antibody syndrome.

Pathology

The histopathological findings are diverse, since each eruption can present with different cutaneous features. Vacuolar degeneration of basal cells, infiltration of mononuclear cells in the periphery of appendages and blood vessels, and mucin deposition may be found. Keratotic plug formation may be seen in chronic cases. (See the section for DLE.) IgG, IgM, and C3 deposits may be seen in the cutaneous basement membrane zone of normal-looking skin by skin immunofluorescence microscopy labeling (lupus band test; Fig. 12.3).

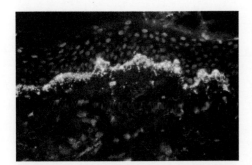

Fig. 12.3 Lupus band test. Normal skin in the unexposed area of a patient with SLE, observed by direct immunofluorescence. There is linear deposition of IgG (fluorescent green) in the epidermal basement membrane. The nuclei stain orange.

Laboratory findings

Pancytopenia and LE cells (i.e., phagocytosis by neutrophils of large nuclei) are seen. Biological false-positive (BFP) serological reaction is observed for syphilis. CRP is only slightly elevated, and it does not reflect the disease activity. The reduction of several complement factors (C3, C4, and CH50) may be seen. The reduction of C3 in particular reflects the disease activity. Autoantibodies such as antinuclear antibody may be detected (Table 12.4). Anti-double-stranded DNA antibody (dsDNA) reflects the specificity and activity of the disease.

Diagnosis

Skin biopsy and direct immunofluorescence (IF) are necessary for diagnosis. The diagnosis of SLE can be made when four or more of the 11 diagnostic criteria are met (see Table 12.2). A provisional diagnosis may be made even when the four diagnostic criteria are not met simultaneously, since other features may develop later. Careful observation is therefore required.

Treatment

Topical steroid is used for cutaneous symptoms. The first-line treatment option for SLE is oral steroids, and the initial doses are often determined by the type of renal symptoms. Administration of immunosuppressants such as cyclophosphamide and steroid pulse therapy may be done. Lifestyle guidance is important;

Table 12.4 Major autoantibodies found in SLE patients.

Name	Frequency	Feature
Antinuclear antibody (ANA)	95%	Frequently diffuse, speckled and peripheral
Anti-single-stranded DNA (ssDNA) antibody	60–70%	Disease specificity is low.
Anti-double-stranded DNA (dsDNA) antibody	60–70%	Disease specificity is high. Reflects the progress of disease
Anti-Sm antibody	20–30%	Disease specificity is high.
Anti-U1-RNP antibody	20–30%	Frequently found in cases with positive anti-Sm antibody
Anticardiolipin antibody	20%	Note that there may be the complication of antiphospholipid (antibody) syndrome.
Antihistone antibody	30–50%	Positive cases are frequently found in patients with drug-induced lupus erythematosus.
Anti-SS-A antibody	35–60%	Frequently found in the cases that accompany subacute cutaneous lupus erythematosus
Anti-SS-B antibody	20%	May secondarily cause Sjögren syndrome
Anti-Scl-70 antibody	25%	May be complicated by pulmonary hypertension
P-ANCA	25%	May be complicated with vasculitis

Sources: Wolff K et al. *Fitzpatrick's Dermatology in General Medicine*, 7th edn. McGraw-Hill Professional, 2007. Shiozawa S. *Principles and the Cause of Rheumatic Diseases*, 2nd rev. edn. Maruzen, 2005.

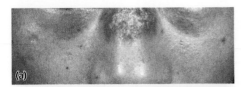

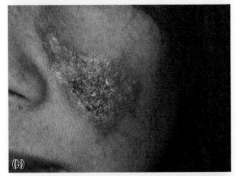

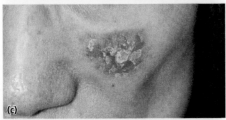

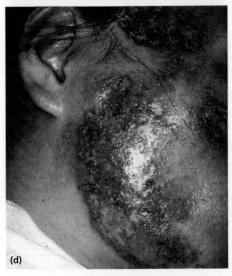

stress caused by direct sunlight exposure, overfatigue or cold temperature should be avoided. SLE tends to become aggravated during pregnancy.

Prognosis

Systemic lupus erythematosus is a chronic disease of remissions and relapses. The mortality rate from renal failure has been reduced by the availability of steroid and dialysis therapies, with the 5-year survival rate now exceeding 97%. Mortality rates from infection, central nervous system damage, and cardiac failure are high.

Discoid lupus erythematosus
Definition

Discoid lupus erythematosus (DLE) refers to LE involving the skin. Some patients with DLE may meet the criteria for SLE. In most cases of DLE, the skin is the only organ involved. Patients with SLE may have DLE lesions.

Clinical features

Multiple round to oval sharply demarcated erythematous lesions accompanied by scaling and follicular dilation develop (Fig. 12.4). Ulcers may form. These lesions heal with scarring and depigmentation. These tend to occur on sun-exposed sites, including the face, scalp, and auricular region, and on the lips and oral mucosa. When DLE is present in the scalp, irreversible scarring alopecia may develop. Multiple DLE lesions that develop below the neck are called disseminated DLE (Fig. 12.5).

Pathology

The characteristic findings are follicular plugging, epidermal atrophy, vacuolar degeneration and thickening of the basal membrane, dense focal infiltration in the periphery of appendages and blood vessels,

Fig. 12.4-1 Discoid lupus erythematosus (DLE). a: Affected nasal skin of a man in his 20s. The skin lesion consists of a sharply demarcated macule with a reddish-pink center. The periphery of the lesion has a brown discoloration and is accompanied by scaling. b: A sharply demarcated skin lesion accompanied by dilated hair follicles on the cheek of a woman in her 20s. The lesion is partly erosive. c: A lesion of DLE at a comparatively early stage on the cheek. d: A skin lesion present on the right cheek of a woman in her 30s. Multiple DLE lesions develop and gradually enlarge or coalesce into large plaques.

and mucin deposition in the dermis (Fig. 12.6). Linear deposition of immunoglobulins is found in the cutaneous basement membrane in most cases (positive lupus band test; see Fig. 12.3).

Laboratory findings
Lesions tend to involve the skin. Laboratory findings are generally normal. Progression to SLE is seen in some cases.

Differential diagnosis
Eruptions from lichen planus, sarcoidosis, mycosis fungoides, deep fungal infection, and mycobacterial infection may resemble those from DLE.

Treatment and prognosis
Patients with DLE should avoid sunlight, which tends to aggravate the condition. Topical steroids and tacrolimus are used; however, DLE is intractable. Squamous cell carcinoma may develop as a result of chronic DLE.

Lupus erythematosus profundus (LE profundus) (synonym: lupus panniculitis)
Definition and symptoms
Lupus erythematosus (LE) profundus is a subtype of chronic LE involving the subcutaneous fat tissues. Lesions occur as subcutaneous indurations with a diameter of 1–3 cm, which can be of normal color or erythematous, most frequently on the face, shoulders, upper arms, and buttocks (Fig. 12.7). DLE is often found on the surface of these sites. Concave lesions may develop during the course of LE profundus, and these heal with scarring and calcification. About half of cases are accompanied by SLE.

Pathology
Mucin deposition in the subcutaneous tissues and infiltration of mononuclear cells in the periphery of blood vessels are found, which gradually result in fibrosis. Deposition of immunoglobulins and complement factors may be seen on the blood vessel walls at lesional sites.

Treatment
When cosmetic problems are a concern, early oral or local injection of steroids is considered.

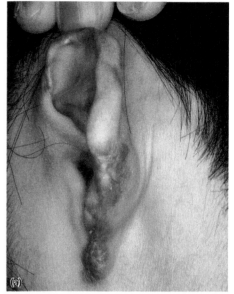
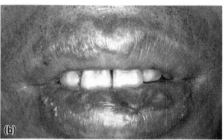
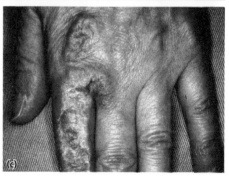

Fig.12.4-2 Discoid lupus erythematosus (DLE). a: DLE on the auricle, particularly noticeable on the lobule. The center of the lesion is scarred. b: DLE on the lips. Erythema and purple eruptions are present. It should be differentiated from lichen planus. DLE of the lips may induce squamous cell carcinoma. c: DLE on the dorsum of the hand and fingers.

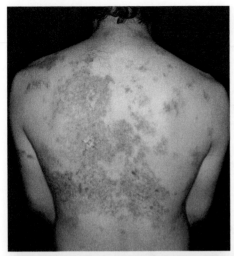

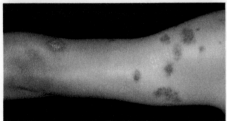

Fig. 12.5 Widespread discoid lupus erythematosus (DLE). Large areas on the trunk and arms are involved.

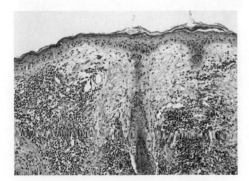

Fig. 12.6 Histopathology of discoid lupus erythematosus (DLE). There is a vascular degeneration in the basal cell layer, lymphocytic infiltration in the blood vessels and peripheral skin appendages, and severe edema and mucin deposition in the dermis. Neutrophils and eosinophils are rarely seen.

Chilblain lupus erythematosus

Also called chilblain lupus, this is a type of chronic erythematosus. Erythema that resembles chilblains occurs in the extremities, on the tip of the nose, and in the auricular region (see Chapter 13). The condition tends to aggravate in winter. Histopathological findings are similar to those for DLE.

Subacute cutaneous lupus erythematosus
Definition

Subacute cutaneous lupus erythematosus (SCLE) is characterized by eruptions whose course and duration are intermediate between those of chronic DLE and acute SLE.

Pathology

Multiple eruptions appear symmetrically on sun-exposed sites. Annular polycyclic SCLE, with erythema whose center displays color degradation (Fig. 12.8), and papulosquamous (psoriasiform) SCLE, which resembles psoriasis accompanied by mild scaling, are the two main subtypes. Both types heal without scarring and are recurrent. Although about half of patients with SCLE meet the diagnostic criteria of SLE, severe renal symptoms and central nervous system manifestations are rare. See the SLE section for the pathological findings.

Laboratory findings

Antinuclear antibodies are positive in 60–80% of cases. High frequencies of anti-SS-A antibodies (70–90% of cases) and anti-SS-B antibodies (30–50% of cases) characterize SCLE.

Treatment

The main treatments are topical or low-dose oral corticosteroids.

Neonatal lupus erythematosus (synonym: neonatal lupus syndrome)
Clinical features

Neonatal lupus erythematosus resembles the annular erythema that accompanies Sjögren syndrome, or SCLE-like annular eruptions with scaling in newborns in the first to third months after birth (Fig. 12.9). It heals within 6 months with mild abnormal pigmentation. Systemic symptoms (hepatosplenomegaly, thrombocytopenia) may occur. Careful attention is required for irreversible congenital cardiac block, which is found in 1–2% of cases.

Diagnosis and treatment

Neonatal lupus erythematosus is a passive type of autoimmune disease caused by autoantibodies placentally transmitted to the newborn from the mother with or without symptoms of SLE or Sjögren syndrome. Cutaneous symptoms are related to the anti-SS-A antibody. Sunlight avoidance and symptomatic therapies are the main treatment options. A pacemaker is often necessary for patients with cardiac block.

Nodular cutaneous lupus mucinosis

Papules and nodules occur on the back and upper arms. Nodular cutaneous lupus mucinosis is a subtype of chronic erythematosus. These lesions are caused by the deposition of mucin in large amounts in the dermis, and they often accompany SLE.

Bullous lupus erythematosus

Erythema multiforme-like edematous erythema occurs, mainly on the face and upper body, and single or multiple vesicles form (Fig. 12.10). The clinical features may resemble those found in dermatitis herpetiformis and epidermolysis bullosa acquisita (see Chapter 14). Autoantibodies against type VII collagen may be found.

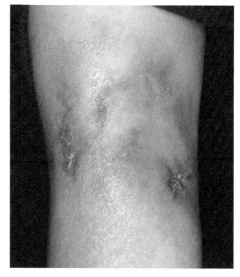

Fig. 12.7 Lupus erythematosus profundus. Large panniculitis in the skin of a patient with SLE. DLE eruptions are present on the skin surface.

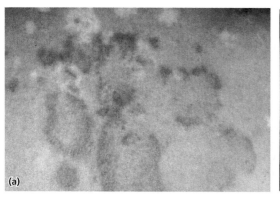
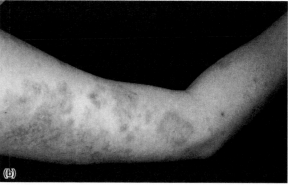

(a)   (b)

Fig. 12.8 Subacute cutaneous lupus erythematosus (SCLE). a: Annular polycyclic SCLE on the back. The center of the lesion heals centrifugally. This condition resembles the annular erythema of Sjögren syndrome. b: Papules with scaling.

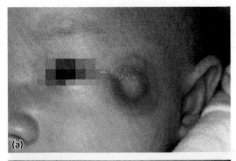

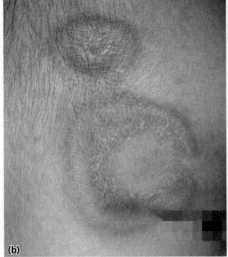

Fig. 12.9 Annular erythema in neonatal lupus erythematosus. a: Annular erythema on the cheek of an infant with neonatal lupus erythematosus. It begins as erythema of 5–10 mm diameter and gradually enlarges. The center of the lesion tends to regress; however, marked edema and elevation occur in the periphery. b: Two annular erythema on the face.

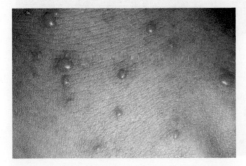

Fig. 12.10 Bullous lupus erythematosus. Bullous LE in a patient with SLE. Vesicles form not only on the LE erythema but also on the normal-looking skin.

Scleroderma

Scleroderma is characterized by sclerosis of the skin that follows a course of edema, sclerosis, and atrophy. It is divided into systemic sclerosis (SSc) and localized scleroderma. In SSc there is the involvement of internal organs, whereas in localized scleroderma the internal organs are not involved.

Systemic sclerosis (synonym: progressive systemic sclerosis (PSS))

- Skin induration and Raynaud's phenomenon first occur in the fingers and toes.
- Sclerosis manifests as systemic symptoms that involve multiple organs and blood vessels. Ankyloglossia, mask-like facies, esophageal blockage, sclerodermatous kidney, and lung fibrosis may occur.
- Anti-Scl-70 antibodies and anti-centromere antibodies may be positive.
- Vasodilators and steroids are used for treatment.

Classification

The LeRoy and Medsger system is mainly used for classification of SSc (Table 12.5). SSc is divided into two subtypes in this classification: diffuse cutaneous SSc (dcSSc) and limited cutaneous SSc (lcSSc). In the former, skin sclerosis occurs at proximal sites (e.g., the trunk and upper arms), the progress is quick and the symptoms tend to involve internal organs. In the latter, the lesions are seen only on areas distal from the elbows and the lesions in the internal organs are mild. The clinical features of the two subtypes are shown in Table 12.6.

Clinical features

Systemic sclerosis frequently occurs in adults aged 30–50 years old. The incidence is greater in women, with a ratio of three females to one male. The early symptoms are Raynaud's phenomenon and joint pain. After repeated aggravation during winter, hardening of the skin gradually spreads from the distal areas (e.g., fingers, toes, face) to proximal areas. SSc generally progresses over the course of a few years to several dozen years, and the progress basically follows the course of an edematous period followed by a hardening period and an atrophic period.

Fingers and toes

Raynaud's phenomenon is observed in nearly all cases. When the sclerosis progresses further, the fingers

Table 12.5 Classification of systemic sclerosis (SSc).

LeRoy and Medsger classification
Diffuse cutaneous: hardening of the skin enlarges from the elbows toward the proximal areas. Internal lesions may progress rapidly, and the prognosis is often poor. Cases positive for anti-DNA topoisomerase I (anti-Scl-70) antibody tend to be classified as this type. Limited cutaneous systemic sclerosis (LcSSc): hardening of the skin is seen only on areas distal from the elbows, and lesions in internal organs are mild. The prognosis is good. Most cases with positive anticentromere antibody are classified as this type.

Barnett classification
Type I: cutaneous symptoms are Raynaud's phenomenon and hardening of the fingers. Type II: hardening of the skin occurs on the extremities and face. Type III: hardening of the skin spreads to the trunk.

Table 12.6 Clinical symptoms of systemic sclerosis (SSc).

	Diffuse cutaneous (dcSSc)	Limited cutaneous systemic sclerosis (lcSSc)
Range of skin hardening	Enlarges from the elbow to the proximal areas	Limited to areas from the elbow to the fingertips
Progress	Comparatively rapid	Often slow
Cutaneous capillary blood vessels	Decreased	Telangiectasia (+)
Telangiectasia in the epionychium	(+)	(++)
Calcium deposition	(±)	(+)
Affected internal organs	Lungs, kidneys, esophagus	Lungs, esophagus
Antinuclear antibody	Anti-topoisomerase I antibody (Anti-Scl-70 antibody) Anti-RNA polymerase antibody	Anticentromere antibody (Anti-CENP-B antibody)

become pointed and occasionally swell (sausage fingers). The skin hardening can result in impaired finger extension, which makes it hard to put the palms together (prayer sign). When the sclerosis progresses further, the fingers become pointed (Madonna fingers), and small ulcers form on the finger pulps as a result of circulatory failure, which results in intractable scarring (digital pitting scars) (Fig. 12.11). These symptoms spread from the fingers to the upper arms (proximal scleroderma). Extended nail cuticle (>2 mm) and telangiectasia are observed on the nail plate. Telangiectasia, pigmentation, depigmentation, and calcium deposition are also found.

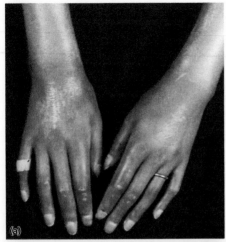

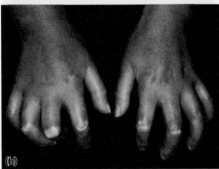

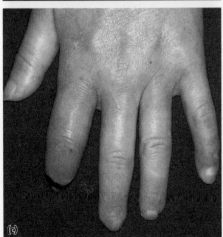

Fig. 12.11-1 Systemic sclerosis. a: There is intense sclerosis and impaired movement in the fingers. b: The sclerosis leads to reduced finger extension, a condition known as "prayer sign." c: The fingertips, particularly those of the index finger, are lost or shortened due to necrosis from impaired circulation.

Systemic sclerosis in the face (Fig. 12.11-2)

- **Mask-like facies:** wrinkles on the face disappear secondary to edema. The nose becomes pointed. Difficulty in opening the mouth occurs, which makes it appear small (microstomia), and radial wrinkles that are characteristic of this disorder form around the mouth.
- **Microglossia and ankyloglossia (tongue-tie):** there is difficulty in extending the tongue.

Systemic sclerosis in other organs

Symptoms caused by fibrosis and thickening of the tunica intima occur in other organs. The symptoms in other organs include arthralgia (swelling in the finger joints and tendon friction rubs), decreased esophageal peristaltic motion, reflux esophagitis, lung fibrosis, pulmonary hypertension, cardiac symptoms (myocardial ischemia, myocarditis), and renal symptoms (scleroderma renal crisis).

Pathogenesis

The primary event of this disorder is the hardening of collagen fibers from increased synthesis. The etiology is unknown but possible etiologic factors include immunology (increased activity of fibrocyte proliferation factors such as TGF-β and PDGF), genetics (polymorphism of the cytokines), microchimerism (small amounts of non-self cells that enter the patient through blood transfusion and are involved in the onset of the disorder), and environment.

Pathology

In the early stages of SSc, collagen fibrils increase or become mildly swollen in the mid to deep dermis. Edema and lymphocytic infiltration are present. As the lesions progress, atrophy in the epidermis and decrease or disappearance of appendages, deposition of collagen fibers parallel to the epidermis and deposition of mucin are observed. Direct immunostaining of skin tissues is generally negative for IgG deposition in SSc without complications.

Laboratory findings

Antitopoisomerase I antibodies (anti-Scl-70 antibodies), which is a finding specific to SSc, are seen in 40% of diffuse cutaneous SSc cases and 15% of limited cutaneous SSc cases. Anticentromere antibodies, which can be a marker for limited cutaneous SSc, are found in less than 3% of diffuse cutaneous SSc cases and 30–60% of limited cutaneous SSc cases. SSc is the only disorder that shows the discrete speckled pattern in the antinuclear antibody test. Other findings include anti-RNA polymerase antibodies, which are frequently found in severe cases in men.

Diagnosis and differential diagnosis

The diagnostic criteria for SSc are shown in Table 12.7. Biopsy of the skin sample taken from the extensor surface of the forearm is used for diagnosis. The modified Rodnan total skin thickness score (TSS) is frequently used in assessing the severity of the cutaneous symptoms. SSc in the edematous period should be carefully differentiated from mixed connective tissue disease. The following are related disorders that manifest skin lesions which resemble those of scleroderma.

- **Human adjuvant disease:** symptoms resembling those of scleroderma and collagen diseases occur in some individuals who have received silicon or paraffin injections or implants for cosmetic purposes.
- **Eosinophilic fasciitis:** this is described later.
- **Chronic GVHD:** see Chapter 10.
- **Scleroderma-like lesions caused by chemical substances:** chemical substances such as toluene and chloroethene, and drugs such as bleomycin may cause skin lesions similar to those from scleroderma.

Table 12.7 Preliminary criteria for classification of systemic sclerosis (SSc).

Major criterion
Proximal skin hardening (skin hardening from the fingertips or toes toward the proximal areas)

Minor criteria
1) Sclerodactyly (only of the digits) 2) Digital pitting scars or loss of substance of the finger pulps (pulp loss) 3) Bibasal pulmonary fibrosis
The diagnosis is made when the patient meets the major criterion or two of the three minor criteria (excluding lcSSc and pseudo-sclerodermatous disorder).

Adapted from the Subcommittee for Scleroderma Criteria of the American Rheumatism Association Diagnostic and Therapeutic Criteria Committee. Preliminary criteria for the classification of systemic sclerosis (scleroderma). *Arthritis Rheum* 1980;23:581–590.

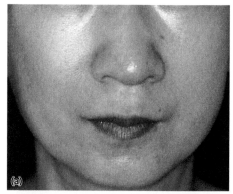
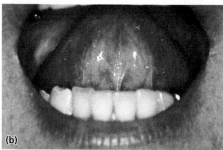
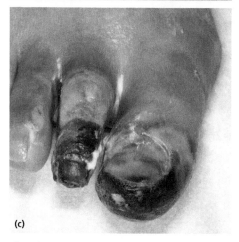

Fig. 12.11-2 Systemic sclerosis. a: Mask-like face. b: Microglossia. c: Ulceration and gangrene in the first and second digits.

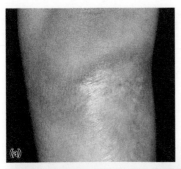

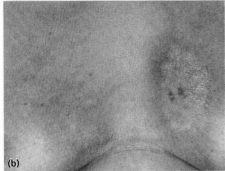

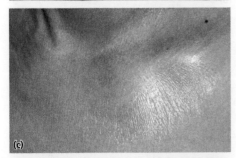

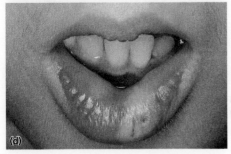

Fig. 12.12 Localized scleroderma (morphea). a: A sclerotic plaque of 10 cm diameter on the extensor surface of the forearm. The center of the lesion appears ivory-colored, with a glossy texture. A lilac ring with a faint erythema is present around the lesion. b,c: Morphea on the precordial region. d: Linear scleroderma (lip of a child).

Treatment and prognosis

Moderate doses of oral steroids are administered to treat early-onset skin sclerosis but care should be taken to avoid inducing scleroderma renal crisis. Prostaglandins may be administered for treating Raynaud's phenomenon and skin ulcers. It is important for the patient to warm the extremities and stop smoking. Administration of immunoglobulin and hematopoietic stem cell transplant may be done for severe cases. Poor prognosis is often caused by scleroderma renal crisis, and lung and cardiac symptoms.

Localized scleroderma
Definition and pathogenesis

Localized scleroderma is defined as sclerosis of the dermis, which occurs only in the skin. Systemic involvement does not occur. It is a disease with unknown etiology. Trauma induces the disorder in some cases. Infection by *Borrelia* bacteria has recently been reported in association with localized scleroderma.

Clinical features and classification

Localized scleroderma is divided into three subtypes based on the appearance of the lesions and the course of progress.

Morphea (circumscribed plaques)

Localized round or oval hardened lesions that are silvery at the center occur often on the trunk of the middle aged (Fig. 12.12). In the early stage, the lesions may be surrounded by a purplish-red halo called a lilac ring. Individual lesions vary from several millimeters to 30 cm in diameter. Morphea profunda, which is a deep type of morphea that affects mainly subcutaneous fat tissues, and bullous morphea with blisters are the subtypes of morphea.

Generalized morphea

This is morphea that occurs on the trunk of the middle aged; the lesions gradually multiply, spread, and merge. Joint pain and infrequent Raynaud's phenomenon may occur.

Linear scleroderma (scleroderma en bandes)

Linear scleroderma most frequently occurs in young children. It may be accompanied by facial hemiatrophy. Linear or band-like indurated lesions resembling morphea may occur on the body. Lilac rings are rarely seen. When the forehead is affected, it is called frontal linear scleroderma or morphea en coup de sabre (Fig. 12.13); the scalp may be involved, resulting in alopecia.

Pathology and laboratory findings
Localized scleroderma has similar histopathological findings to those of SSc. The abnormal laboratory findings present in SSc are not usually seen in localized scleroderma. Rheumatoid factor and antinuclear antibodies may, however, be present in generalized morphea.

Treatment
Steroids are topically applied or locally injected. Oral steroids may be administered for severe cases. For limited and stable lesions (no spreading tendency), surgery may be considered.

Eosinophilic fasciitis (synonyms: Shulman syndrome, diffuse fasciitis)
Eosinophilic fasciitis most commonly affects young and middle-aged men. Symmetrical skin sclerosis occurs on the distal extremities, often triggered by excess exercise (Fig. 12.14). The clinical features resemble those of SSc but there are three features that are used for differentiation: the hands and feet are not affected, increased eosinophils are found in peripheral blood and in skin biopsy, and linear depressed indurations occur along the superficial veins (groove sign). Moderate doses of oral steroids are administered.

Other collagen diseases

Dermatomyositis (DM)
- Heliotrope rash, Gottron's sign, poikiloderma, and edematous erythema appear, associated with telangiectasia in the nail folds.
- Proximal muscle weakness occurs. Elevated levels of CPK, aldolase, and urinary creatine reflect myositis.
- Dermatomyositis is associated with internal malignancy.
- Interstitial pneumonia may aggravate rapidly. The prognosis is poor.
- Steroids are the main treatment.

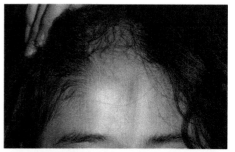

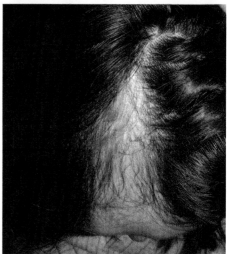

Fig. 12.13 Scleroderma en coup de sabre. Linear scleroderma with facial hemiatrophy. Alopecia and sclerosis on the head. It resembles the slash of a sword. Atrophy occurs in the hypodermic scalp.

MEMO 12–3 CREST syndrome

CREST syndrome is a subtype of SSc whose main features are carcinosis, Raynaud's phenomenon, esophageal dysfunction, sclerodactyly and telangiectasia. Positive anticentromere antibodies are the characteristic serological finding.

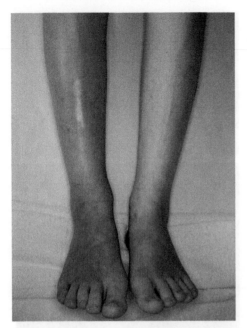

Fig. 12.14 Eosinophilic fasciitis. The skin on the lower legs is hardened and glossy. Skin hardening is not seen on the dorsa of the foot or toes.

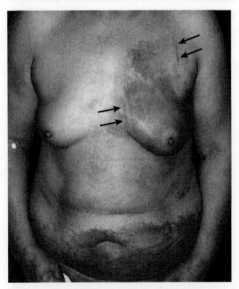

Fig. 12.15-1 Dermatomyositis (DM). Diffuse, edematous erythema accompanied by itching on the trunk. Flagellate erythema (arrows) caused by scratching is seen on the left precordial region.

Epidemiology

The condition most commonly occurs in adults aged 30–60 years, but it may also be seen in children. There is a female preponderance (a female-to-male ratio of 2:1).

Clinical features

Cutaneous symptoms

Edematous purplish-red patches on the face, especially the eyelids (heliotrope rash; in about 30% of cases), and flat elevated papules with scaling on the extensor surface of fingers and joints (Gottron's sign) are characteristic features (Fig. 12.15). In children, seborrheic dermatitis-like erythema on the cheeks and scalp often progresses to butterfly rash-like skin lesions (Fig. 12.16). Intensely itchy, dermatitis-like edematous erythema appears on the neck, trunk, and extremities, sometimes showing linear distribution on the trunk and extremities. The characteristic shape of the distributed eruptions is called the shawl sign or V-neck sign. Hyperkeratotic erythema may be seen on the sides of the index fingers, which is called mechanic's hand (Fig. 12.17). These eruptions cause abnormal pigmentation or depigmentation, skin atrophy, scaling, and telangiectasia over time (poikiloderma). Nail fold erythema and hair loss are also seen. Panniculitis resembling lupus erythematosus profundus and subcutaneous calcium deposition may be observed.

Muscular symptoms

Muscle pain (spontaneous pain, tenderness, gripping pain) and weakness symmetrically affect the trunk, the proximal muscle groups and the neck. Proximal muscle involvement causes functional difficulties such as in walking and climbing stairs. Weakness in the pharyngeal muscle group may lead to dysphagia, dysphonia, and respiratory disturbance.

Other symptoms

Arthralgia involving several joints, and fever and fatigue occur. Interstitial pneumonia and lung fibrosis may rapidly occur, which greatly influences the prognosis. Arrhythmia and cardiac failure may be present.

Dermatomyositis in children

Muscular symptoms are preceded by cutaneous symptoms that are often more severe than the muscular ones (see Fig. 12.16). Erythema occurs on the cheek, clinically resembling SLE. Subcutaneous and muscular calcium deposition is found in 10–20% of cases, frequently causing dyskinesia. Interstitial pneumonia is rarely seen. It may become chronic, or systemic angiitis may develop, which has a poor prognosis.

Classification and pathogenesis
Viral infection, autoimmunity, malignancy, and infection are thought to be involved in the pathogenesis of DM.

Complications
Internal malignancy may be seen in 30–40% of adult DM. The incidence is even higher when the patient is over age 50 or when severe edema and intense itching are present. There is frequent association with stomach, breast, and lung cancer, as well as with malignant lymphoma.

Pathology
Edema in the upper dermis and mild thickening of the cutaneous basement membrane (staining positive in PAS) are major findings in the early stages of DM. As the lesions progress, cutaneous atrophy, vacuolar degeneration of the basal cell layer, mucin deposition, telangiectasia, swelling of collagen fibers, lymphocytic infiltration, and increased numbers of histiocytes are observed. These histological features are similar to those seen in SLE. Immunoglobulins and complement deposition in the skin are rarely seen.

Laboratory findings
Non-specific inflammatory parameters such as leukocytosis and elevated erythrocyte sedimentation rate may be the only findings in the early stages. Rheumatoid factor and antinuclear antibodies are positive in 60–80% of cases. Myogenic enzymes such as CPK, aldolase, glutamic oxalic transaminase (GOT) and lactate dehydrogenase (LDH) are elevated, and creatine in urine and myoglobin are elevated due to myositis. Specific antibodies such as anti-Jo-1 (a type of anti-aminoacyl-tRNA synthetase), anti-PL-7, anti-Mi-2, and anti-p155 may be present (Table 12.8). Skin and muscle biopsy and MRI findings of the extremities are important for diagnosis.

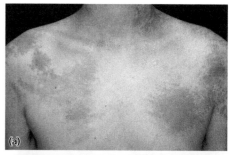
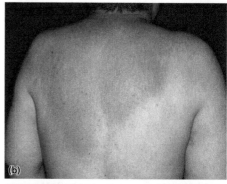
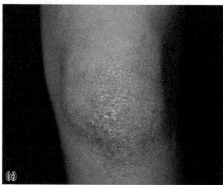
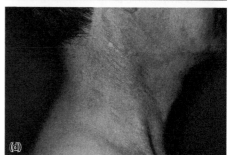

Fig. 12.15-2 Dermatomyositis (DM), Edematous erythema (a, b), Poikiloderma (c, d).

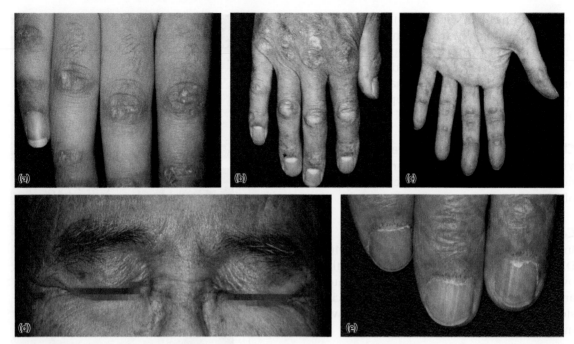

Fig. 12.15-3 Dermatomyositis (DM). a: Multiple, scattered, sharply demarcated keratotic papules of several millimeters in diameter on the extensor joints of DIP and PIP of fingers (Gottron's sign). b: Gottron's sign. c: Papules may occur on the flexor joints (reverse Gottron's sign). d: Intense edema and purplish eruptions on the eyelids (heliotrope rash). e: Telangiectasia of the nail folds.

 MEMO 12–4 Amyopathic dermatomyositis

Dermatomyositis without myositis but with typical cutaneous symptoms of dermatomyositis, such as Gottron's sign and heliotrope rash, is called amyopathic dermatomyositis. Systemic symptoms may occur rapidly, requiring careful observation. In recent years, it has been found that anti-CADM-140 antibodies are positive in about 20% of ADM cases.

Diagnosis

Dermatomyositis can be easily diagnosed by the characteristic cutaneous manifestations, muscular symptoms, and laboratory findings. In early stages, it is difficult to confirm the diagnosis based only on cutaneous features. The major diagnostic criteria are shown in Table 12.9.

Treatment

Systemic steroids are the main treatment. However, in cases complicated by malignancy, treatment should first be directed towards eradication of the cancer. Steroid pulse therapy may be given in severe cases. Immunosuppressants may also be administered.

Mixed connective tissue disease

- Symptoms of SLE, SSc, and PM/DM are seen. Anti-U1-RNP antibodies are positive.
- Raynaud's syndrome and swollen fingers are typical findings.
- Pulmonary hypertension may develop as a complication, and it greatly influences the prognosis.
- Controversy remains as to whether MCTD is an independent entity.

Chapter 12   Collagen diseases   **223**

Table 12.8 Major specific autoantibodies in collagen diseases and in related diseases.

Disease	Autoantibody
Systemic lupus erythematosus	Anti-dsDNA antibody (60–70%) Anti-Sm antibody (20–30%)
Systemic sclerosis	Anti-Scl-70 antibody (diffuse cutaneous 40%) Anticentromere antibody (limited cutaneous 30–60%) Anti-RNA polymerase antibody (6%)
Polymyositis/ dermatomyositis	Anti-Jo-1 antibody (30%) Anti-PL-7 antibody (5%) Anti-Mi-2 antibody (10–20%) Anti-p155 antibody (10–20%) Anti-CADM-140 antibody (ADM: 20%)
Mixed connective tissue disease	Anti-U1-RNP antibody (100%)
Overlap syndrome	Ku antibody (SSc + PM: 50%)
Sjögren syndrome	Anti-SS-A antibody (50–70%) Anti-SS-B antibody (20–30%)

Clinical features

Mixed connective tissue disease (MCTD) frequently occurs in women in their 40s. The typical clinical features are Raynaud's phenomenon and swelling in the dorsal aspect of the hands and fingers (sausage fingers; Fig. 12.18). Arthralgia is also seen. As a specific feature of this disorder, severe pulmonary hypertension occurs in less than 10% of cases. SLE-like symptoms such as erythema on the face and serositis, SSc-like symptoms such as stiffness of the fingers, lung fibrosis and esophageal hypokinesis, and PM/DM-like symptoms such as muscular weakness are often seen. Most cases of MCTD do not meet the diagnostic criteria of SLE, SSc or DM/PM. MCTD may progress to SLE.

Laboratory findings

Anti-U1RNP antibodies are positive; however, specificity is low. Unlike in SLE, CRP levels reflect the activity of MCTD. The serum complement titer is normal.

Treatment and prognosis

Systemic steroids are fairly effective. However, if MCTD is complicated by pulmonary hypertension, the prognosis may be poor.

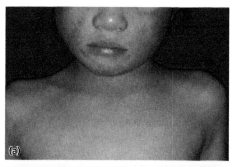
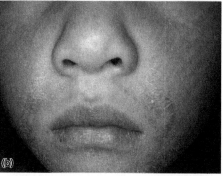
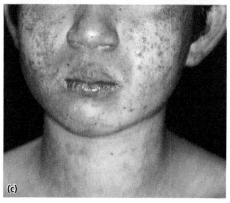

Fig. 12.16 Dermatomyositis (DM) in children. a: Diffuse erythema accompanied by scaling on the face and trunk. b,c: The cheeks are most commonly involved. The skin lesion clinically resembles the butterfly rash of SLE.

Table 12.9 Classification criteria for dermatomyositis and polymyositis.

Criteria
1 Skin lesions (a) Heliotrope rash (red-purple edematous erythema on the upper palpebra) (b) Gottron's sign: purplish-red erythema accompanied by hyperkeratosis and atrophy on the dorsa of the finger joints (c) Erythema on the extensor surface of extremity joints: slightly raised purplish-red erythema on the elbows or knees
2 Proximal muscle weakness (upper or lower extremities and trunk)
3 Elevated serum creatine kinase or aldolase level
4 Muscle pain on grasping or spontaneously
5 Myogenic changes in electromyography (short-duration, polyphasic motor unit potentials with spontaneous fibrillation potentials)
6 Positive anti-Jo-1 (histadyl tRNA synthetase) antibody
7 Non-destructive arthritis or arthralgia
8 Systemic inflammatory signs (fever: more than 37°C at the axilla, elevated serum CRP level or accelerated ESR of more than 20 mm/h by the Westergren method)
9 Pathological findings compatible with inflammatory myositis (Inflammatory infiltration of skeletal evidence of active regeneration may be seen.)
Diagnosis
Dermatomyositis: patients presenting with at least one clinical feature from the first criterion and four clinical features from the second through the ninth criteria
Differential diagnosis
Myositis caused by infections, drug-induced myopathy, myopathy resulting from endocrinopathy, muscular dystrophy, other congenital myopathies

Source: Japan Intractable Diseases Information Center (www.nanbyou.or.jp/)
CRP, C-reactive protein; ESR, erythrocyte sedimentation rate.

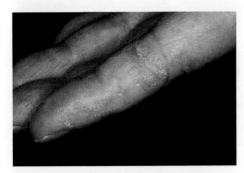

Fig. 12.17 Cutaneous symptom of dermatomyositis (mechanic's hand).

Overlap syndrome
Definition
This is the term used when clinical features meet the diagnostic criteria for two or more collagen diseases, such as SLE, DM/PM, SSc, rheumatoid arthritis or Sjögren syndrome. About 25% of patients with collagen diseases fall into this category. Many cases are SLE overlapping with SSc. In recent years, cases with multiple symptoms of collagen disease have tended to be diagnosed as overlap syndrome, even when the cases do not meet most of the diagnostic criteria. MCTD (see previous section) may be a type of overlap syndrome.

Laboratory findings
Systemic lupus erythematosus-specific antibodies (anti-dsDNA antibodies, anti-Sm antibodies), SSc-specific antibodies (anti-Scl-70 antibodies) and PM-specific antibodies (anti-Jo-1 antibodies) are often positive. Anti-Ku antibodies are positive when SSc and PM occur simultaneously (see Table 12.8).

Diagnosis and treatment

The symptoms of overlap syndrome meet the diagnostic criteria for various collagen diseases. When anti-U1-RNP antibodies are positive and the diagnostic criteria of MCTD are met, the disease is often diagnosed as MCTD. As a rule, the most significant symptom is treated according to the treatment guidelines for each collagen disease.

Antiphospholipid antibody syndrome (APS)

- Systemic thromboembolism occurs in arteries and veins as a result of autoantibodies against a complex of phospholipids and plasma proteins.
- Antiphospholipid antibody is a general term that includes anticardiolipin antibody and lupus anticoagulant.
- Spontaneous abortion, ischemic heart disease, distal cyanosis, lower leg ulceration, and livedo reticularis are present. It tends to accompany SLE.

Clinical features

Thromboembolism occurs in the dermal arteries and veins. The changes in veins cause livedo, thrombophlebitis or ulceration, all in the extremities, particularly the lower extremities; the lesions in the arteries cause subcutaneous nodules, ulceration or gangrene (Fig. 12.19). In cases of SLE complicated with APS, erythema on the cheek, DLE or photosensitivity may occur. In addition to cutaneous symptoms, the thrombotic tendency may result in pulmonary embolism, transient ischemic attack, cerebral infarction, Budd–Chiari syndrome, and myocardial infarction. Another typical finding is spontaneous abortion. Thrombus formed in the placenta reduces placental function. The fulminant form of APS may be fatal because of systemic thromboembolism that develops after a few days.

Pathogenesis

Antiphospholipid antibody is a general term that includes anticardiolipin antibodies (aPL), antiprothrombin antibodies, and several other antibodies. aPL antibody is roughly synonymous with anti-β-2-glycoprotein I antibody. Not all of these antibodies cause abnormal coagulation. The lupus anticoagulant (LAC) test is used to detect the presence of antibodies that cause abnormal coagulation. It is thought that the autoantibodies described above bind with the complex of phospholipids and plasma proteins, causing abnormal coagulation and vascular disorders.

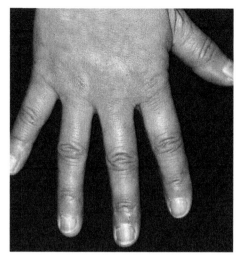

Fig. 12.18 Mixed connective tissue disease (MCTD).

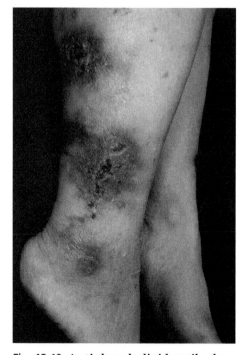

Fig. 12.19 Antiphospholipid antibody syndrome (APS). Intractable skin ulcer and purpura on the lower leg of a middle-aged postmenopausal woman. The ulceration results from circulatory disorder caused by angioma that is induced by antiphospholipid antibodies.

Laboratory findings

The activated partial thromboplastic time (APTT) prolongation is observed because of abnormal coagulation, but prothrombin time (PT) is normal.

Biological false-positive serological reaction is also seen. When the laboratory findings are similar to those described above, tests to detect aPL, b2GPI antibodies, and LAC are done in suspicion of APS. Decreased platelet sedimentation rate may be observed because of thrombus formation.

Diagnosis and treatment

When one of the typical clinical features (thromboembolism or spontaneous abortion) and one of the above-described laboratory findings (e.g., autoantibodies) are found together and then recur at least 12 weeks later, the disorder is diagnosed as APS (Miyakis S et al. *J Thromb Hemost* 2006;4(2):295–306). Anticoagulant therapy using heparin and warfarin potassium is effective for cases with thrombosis. Small doses of aspirin in combination with steroids are helpful in preventing spontaneous abortion.

Sjögren syndrome (synonym: sicca syndrome)

- This is an autoimmune disease that mainly targets exocrine glands such as the salivary and lacrimal glands. There is primary Sjögren syndrome (sicca syndrome) and secondary Sjögren syndrome.
- Purpura on the extremities and annular erythema are characteristic cutaneous features.
- Xerostomia, keratoconjunctivitis sicca, and distal renal tubular acidosis occur. Tooth decay is frequently found.
- Anti-SS-A and anti-SS-B antibodies are positive.
- Hashimoto's disease (chronic thyroiditis) and B cell lymphoma occur as complications.

Definition and classification

Sjögren syndrome is a chronic and progressive autoimmune disease of unknown etiology, which mainly targets the exocrine glands. Decreased production of saliva and lacrimal fluid is the main feature of the disease. When the characteristic symptoms of Sjögren syndrome are present and are unaccompanied by symptoms suggestive of other collagen diseases, it is referred to as primary Sjögren syndrome (sicca syndrome). Secondary Sjögren syndrome occurs in association with other collagen diseases such as SLE (Table 12.10).

Clinical features

Sjögren syndrome most commonly occurs in adults in their 30s to 50s and affects nine females for every male.

Cutaneous features

Annular erythema frequently occurs on the face. Single or multiple well-demarcated, slightly elevated annular erythemas of pink to purplish-red are seen, which are edematous and measure between 1 and 5 cm in diameter (Fig. 12.20). The lesions heal spontaneously within 2 weeks but can sometimes persist. Annular erythema is often seen in cases that are anti-SS-B antibody positive. Petechia with pigmentation, ecchymosis, and livedo occur mainly in the lower extremities, repeating for several years (hypergammaglobulinemic purpura). Angular cheilitis and asteatosis, which reflect dry skin, are also seen. Symptoms of angiitis such as palpable purpura and ulcers may be seen. Raynaud's phenomenon is observed in 10–20% of cases.

Table 12.10 Revised version of the European classification criteria for Sjögren syndrome (2002).

I. Ocular symptoms: a positive response to at least one of the following questions.
  1 Have you had daily, persistent, troublesome dry eyes for more than 3 months?
  2 Do you have a recurrent sensation of sand or gravel in the eyes?
  3 Do you use tear substitutes more than 3 times a day?

II. Oral symptoms: a positive response to at least one of the following questions.
  1 Have you had a daily feeling of dry mouth for more than 3 months?
  2 Have you had recurrently or persistently swollen salivary glands as an adult?
  3 Do you frequently drink liquids to aid in swallowing dry food?

III. Ocular signs – that is, objective evidence of ocular involvement defined as a positive result for at least one of the following two tests
  1 Shirmer's test, performed without anesthesia (≤5 mm in 5 min)
  2 Rose Bengal score or other ocular dye score (≥4 according to van Bijsterveld's scoring system)

IV. Histopathology: in minor salivary glands (obtained through normal-appearing mucosa) focal lymphocytic sialoadenitis, evaluated by an expert histopathologist, with a focus score ≥1, defined as a number of lymphocytic foci (which are adjacent to normal-appearing mucous acini and contain more than 50 lymphocytes) per 4 mm² of glandular tissue

V. Salivary gland involvement: objective evidence of salivary gland involvement defined by a positive result for at least one of the following diagnostic tests
  1 Unstimulated whole salivary flow (≤1.5 mL in 15 min)
  2 Parotid sialography showing the presence of diffuse sialectasias (punctate, cavitary or destructive pattern), without evidence of obstruction in the major ducts
  3 Salivary scintigraphy showing delayed uptake, reduced concentration and/or delayed excretion of tracer

VI. Autoantibodies: presence in the serum of the following autoantibodies   1 Antibodies to Ro (SSA) or La (SSB) antigens, or both

Source: Vitali C et al. Classification criteria for Sjögren's syndrome: a revised version of the European criteria pro-posed by the American-European Consensus Group. *Ann Rheum Dis* 2002;61:554–558.

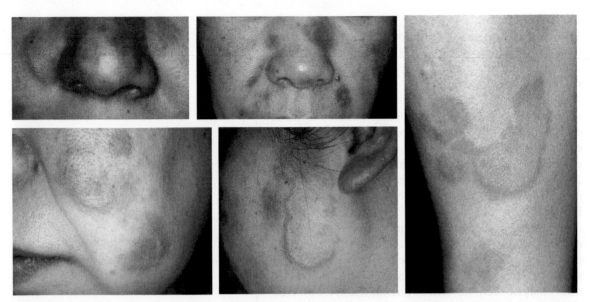

Fig. 12.20 Sjögren syndrome. It begins with elevated, edematous erythema 1 cm in diameter. The erythema gradually enlarges and becomes ring-shaped. It occurs multiply in most cases. The center of the erythema tends to heal, and there is severe infiltration at the periphery. Sjögren syndrome resembles the skin lesions seen in neonatal lupus erythematosus.

Eye symptoms

Discomfort of the eyes, photophobia, pain, itching, and lacrimal disorder occur because of the dry conjunctiva and diffuse keratoconjunctivitis sicca.

Oral symptoms

Dryness of the mouth, dysphagia, dry tongue, disorder of taste, and tooth decay occur.

Other mucosal symptoms

Dry or atrophic lesions are found in the nasal cavity, pharynx, larynx, bronchial tubes, external genitalia, and gastrointestinal mucosa.

Other symptoms

Interstitial pneumonia, renal symptoms (renal tubular acidosis), arthralgia, fever, fatigue, and depression occur.

Complications

Sjögren syndrome tends to accompany collagen diseases such as SLE and rheumatoid arthritis. Chronic thyroiditis (Hashimoto's thyroiditis), primary biliary cirrhosis, B cell lymphoma, and idiopathic thrombocytopenic purpura may occur as complications (Table 12.11).

Pathology

Unlike the annular erythema of SLE and SCLE, changes in the skin and vacuolar degeneration are rarely seen. The main symptom is dense lymphocytic infiltration in the peripheral blood vessels of the dermis. Skin biopsy of the purpuric lesions often shows infiltration of mononuclear cells in the peripheral blood vessels. Immunoglobulin deposition may be found in the blood vessels. Typically, the secretory glands are densely infiltrated by lymphocytes and plasma cells. Biopsy of minor salivary glands has prognostic value.

Laboratory findings

The Schirmer test, Rose Bengal test, and fluorescent dye test are performed to identify lacrimal tear gland abnormality. An apple-tree appearance may be observed by parotid gland radiography. Salivary gland dysfunction can be detected by parotid gland scintigram. Elevated levels of immunoglobulin and salivary amylase may be present. Antinuclear antibodies (80–90% of cases), rheumatoid factor antibodies (70%), anti-SS-A antibodies (50–70%), and anti-SS-B antibodies (20–30%) are often positive. Anti-SS-A antibodies tend to have high sensitivity for Sjögren syndrome, whereas anti-SS-B antibodies tend to be specific for this disorder.

Treatment

Treatment is largely symptomatic. Topical steroid is used for cutaneous symptoms. Mouthwash, treatment of periodontal disease, and administration of artificial saliva and tears for corneal protection are the main therapies.

Relapsing polychondritis

Relapsing polychondritis is an idiopathic disease with inflammation that occurs in the cartilaginous tissues. Autoimmune pathogenesis is hypothesized, because this disease is associated with SLE and rheumatoid arthritis. Auricular and nasal cartilage is most frequently affected,

Table 12.11 Major complications of Sjögren syndrome.

Other autoimmune diseases	SLE, rheumatoid arthritis, SSc, PN, PM/DM, primary biliary cirrhosis
Thyroid	Hashimoto's disease
Blood	Autoimmune hemolytic anemia, malignant lymphoma, hypergammaglobulinemia, macroglobulinemia, idiopathic thrombocytopenic purpura

PM/DM, polymyositis/dermatomyositis; PN, polyarteritis nodosa; SLE, systemic lupus erythmatosus; SSc, systemic sclerosis.

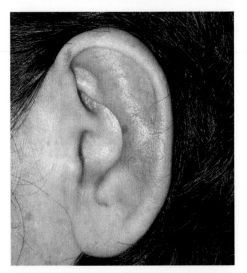

Fig. 12.21 Relapsing polychondritis.

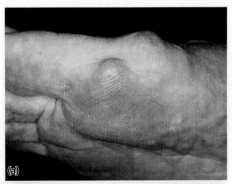

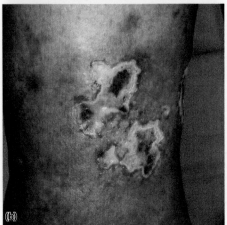

Fig. 12.22 Rheumatoid arthritis. a: Rheumatoid nodules. b: Ulceration from rheumatic vasculitis in the lower extremity.

and sharp pain occurs with swelling of the external ears or nose (Fig. 12.21). Cartilage disorders in other organs include arthralgia, eye symptoms, tracheostenosis, and valvular disorder. Oral steroids are effective.

Rheumatic diseases whose main symptom is arthritis

Rheumatoid arthritis (RA)
- This collagen disease causes sharp pain and swelling in the joints.
- Rheumatoid nodules and cutaneous lesions accompanied by vasculitis are found.
- Chronic inflammation occurs in the synovial membranes of joints. The articular cartilage and underlying bone are destroyed by synovial proliferation.

Clinical features
The skin features of RA are rheumatoid nodules and ulceration in the lower extremities; the ulceration accompanies cutaneous vasculitis (rheumatic vasculitis) (Fig. 12.22). The rheumatoid nodules, painless hard subcutaneous nodules of 0.5 cm to several centimeters in diameter, are found in 20–25% of patients with RA. Subcutaneous nodules frequently develop at sites where the skin is subjected to pressure, such as the extensor surfaces of the forearms and the occiput, knees, and hips. The lesions heal spontaneously in a few months. They persist for a long time and can sometimes rupture, resulting in secondary infection. Ulceration on the fingertips, gangrene, purpura, blistering, and livedo are associated with vasculitis.

Arthritis (synovial inflammation) starts with a symptom called morning stiffness, which appears symmetrically in the proximal interphalangeal joints. Destruction or dislocation of the joints may occur in the later stage, and swan neck, buttonhole, and ulnar drift deformities are seen in the fingers.

Symptoms in other organs include pericarditis, interstitial pneumonia, peripheral neuritis, and uveitis.

Pathology
Three-layered palisading granulomas are found at sites with rheumatoid nodules. Within the granuloma, there is fibrinoid degeneration of collagen fibers surrounded by palisading histiocytes as well as by inflammatory cells such as lymphocytes and plasma cells. In rheumatoid vasculitis, immune complex deposition is

seen on the vascular walls at lesional sites, and changes caused by leukocytoclastic vasculitis are often seen.

Laboratory findings

Rheumatoid factors (mainly IgM antibodies that react against abnormally produced IgG) are positive in 80–90% of cases. The value of matrix metalloproteinase-3 (MMP-3) is a useful index for assessing joint destruction. Anticitrullinated peptide (anti-CCP) antibodies have greater sensitivity and specificity than rheumatoid factors.

Diagnosis and treatment

The diagnostic criteria are shown in Table 12.12. In addition to D-penicillamine and methotrexate, biological agents may be used for cases with high disease activity.

Adult-onset Still's disease

- The three main symptoms are salmon-pink eruptions, intermittent and remittent fever, and arthritis.
- The laboratory findings are elevated erythrocyte sedimentation rate, leukocytosis, and marked increase in ferritin in the absence of rheumatoid factor.

Clinical features

Adult-onset Still's disease most frequently occurs in young women aged 16–35. Fever, arthritis, and specific cutaneous symptoms are found (Fig. 12.23). Salmon-pink eruptions occur mainly on the trunk and extremities. The lesions, several millimeters to centimeters in diameter, are asymptomatic and often unnoticed by the patient. The eruptions often occur concurrently with fever, and sometimes they are persistent.

Other features

Intermittent fever persists for more than a week, rising in the evening and at night and subsiding in the morning (evening spike). Arthritis occurs in the large joints (wrists, knees, feet, elbows) in all cases. Pharyngeal pain, lymph node enlargement, splenomegaly, and myalgia also occur.

Laboratory findings

Elevated erythrocyte sedimentation rate, strongly positive CRP, anemia, leukocytosis, and increases in complement titer are seen. The absence of antinuclear antibodies and rheumatoid factor differentiates this disease from other collagen disorders. Adult-onset Still's disease is characterized by elevated levels of serum ferritin, which indicates the disease activity.

MEMO 12–5 RS3PE syndrome

RS3PE is an abbreviation for "remitting seronegative symmetrical synovitis with pitting edema." The onset mechanism is thought to be similar to those of autoimmune disorders such as rheumatoid arthritis. Symmetrical arthralgia occurs. When antinuclear antibodies and rheumatoid factors are negative but pitting edema is seen on the extremities, this disorder is suspected.

Table 12.12 1987 revised criteria for the classification of rheumatoid arthritis.

1 Morning stiffness lasting at least 1 hour
2 Arthritis of 3 or more joint areas
3 Arthritis of hand joints (at least 1 area swollen in a wrist, MCP or PIP joint)
4 Symmetrical arthritis
5 Rheumatoid nodules
6 Serum rheumatoid factor
7 Radiographic changes

For classification purposes, a patient shall be said to have rheumatoid arthritis if he/she meets 4 of these 7 criteria. Criteria 1 through 4 must have been present for at least 6 weeks.

Source: American College of Rheumatology Classification Criteria of Rheumatoid Arthritis 1987.

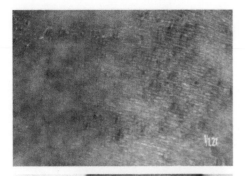

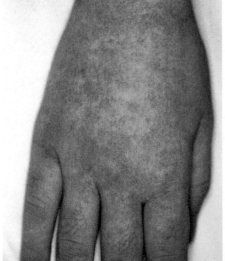

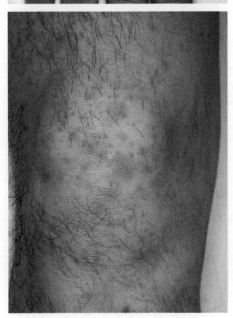

Fig. 12.23 Adult-onset Still's disease.

Diagnosis and treatment

The diagnostic criteria for adult-onset Still's disease are shown in Table 12.13. Oral steroid therapy is the mainstay of treatment. The effectiveness of treatment is measured by the CRP and serum ferritin values.

Juvenile idiopathic arthritis (JIA) (synonym: juvenile rheumatoid arthritis (JRA))

This is chronic arthritis that lasts 6 weeks or longer in patients under age 17. The etiology is unknown. JIA is the most frequent collagen disease in children.

Juvenile idiopathic arthritis is divided into systemic (Still's disease; the main symptoms are extracapsular), polyarticular (five or more joints are affected), and pauciarticular (accounting for about half of all children with JRA; four or fewer joints are affected).

In systemic JIA, intermittent and remittent fever and cutaneous eruptions (see previous section) are the main features. The arthritis is mild. Growth retardation, hepatosplenomegaly, and pericarditis are seen. Disseminated intravascular coagulation (DIC), which is fatal, may occur (macrophage activation syndrome). Arthritis resembling rheumatoid arthritis is the main symptom in both polyarticular JIA and pauciarticular JIA; other symptoms rarely occur. Rheumatoid nodules tend to occur in polyarticular JIA with positive rheumatoid factor.

Reactive arthritis (synonyms: Reiter's syndrome, Reiter's disease)

- Males aged 10–30 are most frequently affected. The disease is closely related to HLA-B27.
- Reactive arthritis occurs as a reaction to infections including urethritis. Polyarthritis, urethritis, and conjunctivitis are the three characteristic features.
- Erythema, pustules, and hyperkeratosis occur on the palms and soles. Circinate balanitis may be present.
- Most cases heal spontaneously within 6 months. It can be a complication of HIV infection.

Clinical features

Men in their 20s are most commonly affected. There is a strong male preponderance, with a ratio of 20 males to one female. Inflammatory symptoms such as urethritis or uterocervical inflammation (*Chlamydia trachomatis* in particular), and bacterial diarrhea precede

Table 12.13 Diagnostic criteria for adult Still's disease.

Major criteria
1 Fever (39°C or higher lasting 1 week or longer)
2 Joint symptoms (lasting 2 weeks or longer)
3 Typical eruptions
4 Increased leukocytes (10,000 or over, and 80% or more neutrophils)
Minor criteria
1 Pharyngeal pain
2 Swelling of the lymph nodes or splenomegaly
3 Liver dysfunction
4 Rheumatoid factors and antinuclear antibodies are negative.
Diagnosis is adult Still's disease if the patient meets at least two of the major criteria and the total of items is five or greater. Additional item: markedly elevated serum ferritin (i.e., five times the normal value or higher) is considered as one item added to the above items.
Items for exclusion: I. Infection (particularly sepsis and infectious mononucleosis) II. Malignant tumors (particularly malignant lymphoma) III. Collagen disease (particularly polyarteritis nodosa and malignant rheumatoid arthritis)

Source: Akihide Ota et al. *1995 Research Report*. Government Specified Autoimmune Diseases Research Group, Ministry of Health and Welfare, 1996, pp. 160–162.

reactive arthritis. One to 2 weeks after infection, arthritis, conjunctivitis, and cutaneous symptoms appear. Circinate balanitis (painless shallow erosion) occurs in about 30% of cases. Painless oral ulceration is also seen. Erythema, pustules, and hyperkeratosis on the palms and soles occur in about 15% of cases, and the lesions coalesce to form hyperkeratotic nodules (keratoderma blennorrhagicum). HIV infection should be suspected when the cutaneous lesions spread to the rest of the body. The conjunctivitis has an acute onset and is accompanied by burning sensation. Arthritis tends to occur in the knees, feet, and toe joints.

Laboratory findings
Most cases (about 90%) are HLA-B27 positive. The cutaneous lesions cannot be differentiated histopathologically from psoriasis. Calcification is observed in the calcanei, fingers, and phalanges by radiography.

Treatment
The treatment for cutaneous lesions of reactive arthritis is the same as that for psoriasis vulgaris. NSAIDs are used primarily for arthralgia. Most cases subside within 6 months but arthralgia may persist.

CHAPTER 13

Physicochemical injury and photosensitive diseases

An important role of the skin is to protect the body from extrinsic stimuli such as sunlight, heat, and cold. Melanin and the stratum corneum in the epidermis prevent DNA from being damaged by ultraviolet irradiation. Sweating and the cutaneous vasculature help maintain the body temperature. The stratum corneum and intercellular bridges protect the body from mechanical shock. However, the skin barrier function can be compromised when extrinsic stimuli exceed a certain level, resulting in injury such as electrical and/or chemical burns, frostbite, radiation damage, and solar dermatitis. This chapter introduces skin disorders and photosensitivity diseases with physicochemical causes.

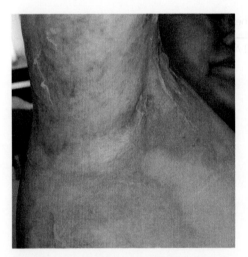

Fig. 13.1 Second-degree burn. Mix of superficial dermal burn (SDB) and deep dermal burn (DDB), caused by hot water.

Physicochemical injury

Burns

- Burns are injuries to cutaneous tissues caused by high temperature. The damage is classified according to the depth of the tissue injury into first-, second-, and third-degree burns.
- Burn size is measured by "the rule of nines" or "the rule of fives."
- The basic treatment is cooling. Systemic intensive care or escharotomy may be necessary for severe cases.
- The first infusion, if necessary, is lactate Ringer's solution. The volume of intravenous replacement therapy is determined according to the extent of the burn (e.g., by the Baxter method).

Clinical features and classification

The severity of a burn is evaluated by its depth and extent, as well as by the patient's condition.

Classification of burn by depth (Table 13.1)

The depth of a burn depends on the temperature of the heat source and the contact time. Burns are classified into first-, second-, and third-degree burns. However, the severity is difficult to determine

---

Shimizu's Dermatology, Second Edition. Hiroshi Shimizu.
© 2017 John Wiley & Sons, Ltd. Published 2017 by John Wiley & Sons, Ltd.

Table 13.1 Diagnosis of burn by depth and clinical features.

Diagnosis	Synonym	Clinical findings	Treatment	After-effects
First-degree burn	Epidermal burn	Painful erythema, edema	Topical medicine	Scarring (–)
Second-degree burn	Superficial dermal burn (SDB)	Painful blisters with clear fluid and red blister bottoms	Topical medicine dressing	Heals in about 2 weeks, scarring (–)
	Deep dermal burn (DDB)	Hypalgesic blisters with white bottoms	Debridement, skin graft	Heals in 3–4 weeks, scarring (+)
Third-degree burn	Deep burn (DB)	Grayish-white or brown carbonized skin Pain is usually absent	Debridement, skin graft	Scarring (+)

immediately after a burn. A burn may deepen with time after the incident.

- **First-degree burn (epidermal burn):** painful erythema and edema occur, healing in 3–4 days without scarring.
- **Second-degree burn (dermal burn):** intense burning sensation is present. Erythema is followed within several hours by erosions or tense blistering (Fig. 13.1). A second-degree burn is subclassified as a superficial dermal burn (SDB) or a deep dermal burn (DDB). SDB presents as painful blisters with an erythematous to pink base. There is mild damage to the dermis, and the injury heals without scarring in about 2 weeks. DDB affects the deep dermal layer and heals with scarring in 3–4 weeks. The base of a DDB blister is white and has reduced sensation. DDB often progresses to third-degree burn.
- **Third-degree burn (deep burn):** all the cutaneous layers and sometimes even deeper areas are damaged (Fig. 13.2). The skin appears grayish-white. Blistering is not present and the skin may appear brown. Necrotic tissue may be present with the formation of an eschar. Healing through the proliferation of the epidermis around the burn occurs, and skin grafts may be necessary.

A needle is sometimes used to examine the severity. The involved area is probed gently with a needle. If the area is painful, the diagnosis is second-degree burn; otherwise, the diagnosis is third-degree burn (Fig. 13.3). If hairs come out when pulled gently, the diagnosis is DDB or third-degree burn.

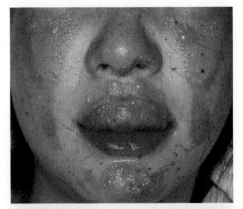

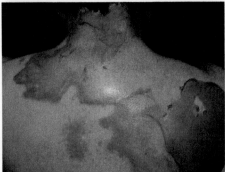

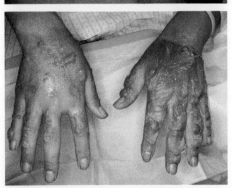

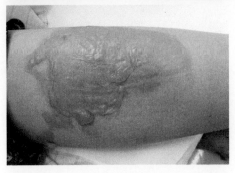

Fig. 13.2 First- and second-degree burns caused by explosion of a cigarette lighter.

Estimating burn extent

The "rule of nines" is generally used to determine the extent of burns in adults; the "rule of fives" or the Lund–Browder chart is used for children.

Evaluation of burn severity

Systemic intensive care is necessary in second-degree burns involving more than 10% of the body surface area in children or more than 15% in adults. Cases with a greater than 15% burn index score or with a greater than 80 prognostic burn index are treated as severe burns.

Pathogenesis

Burns are caused by exposure to high temperatures. They are common in infants and in children under age 10. Among the elderly or patients with diabetes, low-temperature burns caused by prolonged use of electric pads and air heaters have become increasingly prevalent (Fig. 13.4). In severe burns, metabolic changes and hypercytokinemia lead to an increase in systemic vascular permeability. This results in the leakage of plasma proteins and extracellular fluid causing multiple organ failure and shock.

Complications

Renal failure, pulmonary edema, disseminated intra-vascular coagulation (DIC), and multiple organ failure may arise as complications. Respiratory failure due to smoke inhalation and subsequent tracheal edema may also occur. Extensive burns are prone to infection (sepsis) and may induce peptic ulcer formation (Curling's ulcer) within a week after the burn incident. Squamous cell carcinoma is a complication of severe burns. In cases with hypertrophic scarring overlying joints, contracture may occur.

Treatment

Local treatment

The primary treatment for burns is cooling with running water for at least 30 min to relieve pain, inflammation, and edema. Topical steroids are used for first-degree burns.

In second- and third-degree burns, it is important to prevent infection. Blister puncture may be performed. Topical antibiotics, skin ulcer treatment drugs, and wound dressings may be used, depending

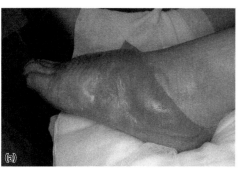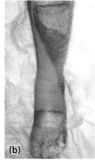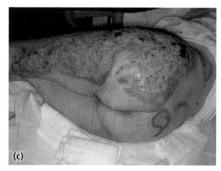

Fig. 13.3 Burns. a,b: Second-degree burns caused by hot water. Marked blistering is present. c: The epidermis has exfoliated with the stripping of clothes that were wetted by the scalding water. Third-degree burn is also present.

on the burn conditions. Sites with DDB and third-degree burns are debrided, and skin grafting may be considered.

The depth of the burn can be more clearly determined 2 weeks after the burn, as the passage of time often makes it possible to determine whether the affected site should be treated conservatively or whether surgical treatment is necessary. In extensive burns, debridement and skin grafting in the early stage are recommended. Cultured skin graft may be done. If severe edema impairs the blood supply, escharotomy (relaxing incision) is necessary to prevent necrosis.

Systemic treatment
Airway management and intravenous therapy are necessary in patients with severe burns. The Baxter method is a widely used infusion therapy (Table 13.2). Fluid balance is controlled by monitoring urine output, central venous pressure, and serum sodium and potassium concentrations. Systemic intensive care is done while paying attention to the development of sepsis, peptic ulcer, cardiac failure, pulmonary edema, or renal dysfunction.

Chilblains (pernio) and frostbite
- Chilblains and frostbite are cutaneous disorders caused by exposure to cold.
- Edema and erythema multiforme-like eruptions are caused by local vascular constriction.
- Avoidance of cold is the primary treatment. It is also important not to warm the affected sites rapidly.

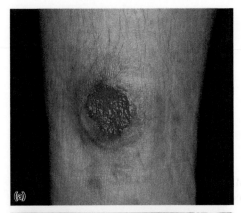

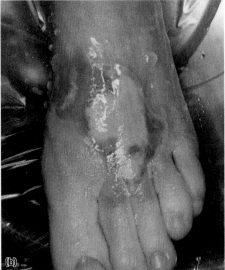

Fig. 13.4 Third-degree low-temperature burn. a: This burn was caused by a heated pad that was adhered to the skin for a long time during sleep. Although the burn seems small and superficial, it is deep and third degree. b: Third-degree burn caused by a hot water bottle during sleep. The patient has diabetes and diminished sensation in the peripheral nerves.

Table 13.2 Parkland (Baxter) formula.

Lactated Ringer's solution [4cc × %TBSA (total body surface area) × weight (kg)] is given for the first 24 h after the time of burn. Half the amount is given in the first 8 h. The rest is given in the subsequent 16 h.

Chilblains (pernio)
Clinical features

Chilblains (pernio) occur most commonly on the hands, fingers, feet, heels, auriculae, and cheeks (Fig. 13.5). The lesions are localized, bright-red to purplish-red edematous erythemas that are painful and itchy. Sometimes blisters or ulcers are present. Erythema multiforme-like eruptions may occur. They normally heal in 1–3 weeks.

Pathogenesis

Small arteries and veins become congested by repeated exposure to cold, and the congestion causes inflammation. Chilblains occur more often in early winter and early spring than in midwinter and are even seen in regions with warm temperatures. In addition to low temperature, moistness from perspiration and hereditary factors are closely associated with their occurrence. The onset mechanism is not clearly defined.

Treatment

Topical steroids, peripheral vasodilators, and vitamin E preparations may be given. Avoiding the cold, keeping warm, and massaging the chilblain-prone parts of the body are effective treatments.

Frostbite
Clinical features

Frostbite occurs secondary to acute freezing of tissues from exposure to extreme cold. Even a few seconds of exposure may be sufficient to cause it. The fingers, ears, and nose are most easily affected. It tends to occur in those who are not accustomed to the cold, and in the elderly. Severe cases of frostbite in winter mountain climbers and drunken individuals and from occupational accidents have been reported. The skin becomes white to purplish-red. Reduced sensory perception is accompanied by hypoesthesia. As frostbite progresses, blistering, ulceration, and necrosis occur. The depth classification for burns is used to determine the severity of frostbite (see Table 13.1).

Pathogenesis

Inadequate blood flow and thrombus formation (circulatory disorder) are caused when skin is exposed to the cold, leading to intercellular dehydration, destruction of cellular membranes (from tissue freezing), and blood vessel constriction. Frostbite most frequently occurs below −12°C. The duration of exposure and wind speed are factors in the occurrence and severity of frostbite. When the entire body surface is exposed to cold for a prolonged period, lethargy and death may occur.

Treatment
The affected sites are gradually warmed as an emergency treatment. Rapid warming and strong friction should be avoided. The sites are warmed with 40°C water for 20 min and kept clean and protected. Necrotic tissues may be debrided as in the treatment for burns. Intravenous vasodilators are useful in cases where the frostbite is related to circulatory disorder.

Chemical burn
During a chemical burn, the skin is damaged by acidic, alkaline or other corrosive compounds (Fig. 13.6). Acid induces coagulative necrosis. Crusts appear, and their color depends on the causative acid (brown for sulfuric acid, yellow for hydrochloric and nitric acids, and white for hydrofluoric acid). Alkaline substances tend to have long action, and the affected lesions tend to be deep. The affected sites should be immediately and thoroughly rinsed with running water. Neutralizing agents are not applied. The subsequent treatment is the same as for burns.

Electric burn
An electric burn results in skin damage caused by the conduction of an electrical current (Fig. 13.7). These burns, called "flash burns," occur at sites that are exposed to an electrical current, resulting in ulceration and necrosis caused by intense heat. Flash burns spread to become electric burns with dendritic reddening and ulceration. Lesions caused by metal present in electrodes that melts and fuses to the skin may be seen.

Radiodermatitis (synonyms: radiation dermatitis, radiation-induced dermatitis)
- In radiodermatitis, cutaneous lesions are caused by radiation. The condition is divided into acute radio-dermatitis, in which the lesions occur immediately after exposure, and chronic radiodermatitis, in which the lesions occur later.
- The treatments are the same as those for burns.

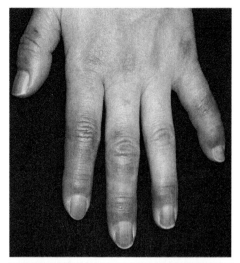

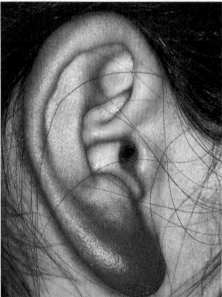

Fig. 13.5 Chilblains (pernio).

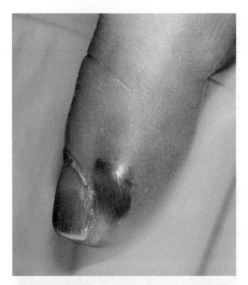

Fig. 13.6-1 Chemical burn.

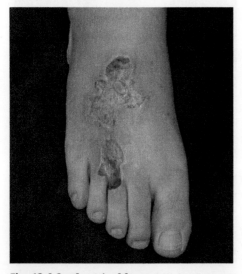

Fig. 13.6-2 Chemical burn.

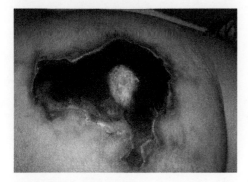

Fig. 13.7 Electric burn.

- Actinic keratosis and squamous cell carcinoma (radiation cancer) may develop. Surgical removal of the affected site is a treatment option.

Clinical features

Acute radiodermatitis

Acute radiodermatitis is caused by a single large exposure of irradiation. With a comparatively small amount of irradiation, erythema occurs several minutes after exposure and disappears within 2–3 days, followed by edema, dry skin (dry scaling), and exudative eczema (moist scaling). Ulceration and burn symptoms are caused by irradiation greater than 20 Gy. Fractionated X irradiation for treatment may cause the above-described symptoms when the total amount of irradiation exceeds 20 Gy (Fig. 13.8, Table 13.3).

Chronic radiodermatitis

Chronic radiodermatitis is commonly caused by a small amount of fractionated radiation at a single site (i.e., a total of 10 Gy or more in a 6-month period). It often occurs at sites where a malignant tumor was present and radiation therapy was repeatedly performed. It may also develop in the hands of medical professionals who deal with radiation (Fig. 13.9). There are four stages of chronic radiodermatitis: atrophy (atrophy, pigmentation, alopecia, and telangiectasia occurring 6 months after the irradiation incident), keratinization (the proliferation of horny cells), ulceration (intractable), and cancer (squamous cell carcinoma or basal cell carcinoma, occurring 15–20 years after irradiation).

Pathogenesis

Radiodermatitis is caused by exposure to X-rays and other radioactive materials. All types of radiation cause cutaneous lesions of different severity. In recent years, acute radiodermatitis caused by interventional radiology (IVR) has been gaining attention

Treatment

The treatments for acute radiodermatitis are the same as those for burns. For chronic radiodermatitis, the affected site is protected by ointment application and bandaging. Extrinsic stimulation should be avoided. Ulcers and tumors are removed and the site is repaired with tissue that has good blood circulation, such as with a pedicle flap procedure.

Table 13.3 Classification of acute radiodermatitis.

Severity	Major symptoms	Occurrence (after one irradiation)	One dose (Gy)	Total dose (Gy) (fractionated irradiation)	Clinical features
First degree	Early erythema	Immediately after to 24 h after irradiation	>2	<20	Transient erythema
	Main erythema, edema	A few days to 3 weeks	>10	20~30	Edematous erythema with burning sensation, transient hair loss
Second degree	Dry desquamation	3–6 weeks	>15	30~50	Mild poikiloderma, dry skin, scaling
Third degree	Moist desquamation	4 weeks or later	>18	50~70	Blisters, exudative eczema with erosions, permanent hair loss
Fourth degree	Ulcer, necrosis	6 weeks or later	>20	>70	When one dose exceeds 100 Gy, necrosis occurs within 2 weeks.

In fractionated irradiation, in particular, differences in symptoms greatly differ individually according to the source of radiation, the body part and extent of treatment, and the age of the patient.
Source: Fukuda H. *Nucl Med* 2003;40: 213–220.

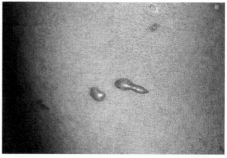
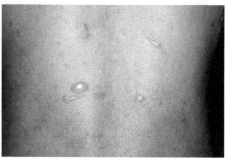

Fig. 13.8 Acute radiodermatitis.
Blistering after electron beam irradiation.

MEMO 13–1 Kerosene dermatitis

This dermatitis is caused by prolonged contact with kerosene. Kerosene dermatitis occurs when kerosene adheres to clothing for a long period. Characteristic fresh red erythema, edema, blistering, and erosion are seen at the site of contact, and the symptoms are similar to those of shallow second-degree burns. Steroids are a highly effective treatment. The treatment is the same as for burns.

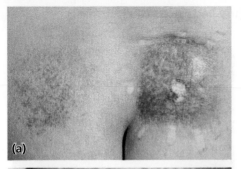

(a)

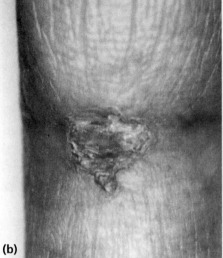

(b)

Fig. 13.9 Chronic radiodermatitis. a:
Chronic radiodermatitis on buttocks exposed
to therapeutic irradiation for uterine cancer.
Poikiloderma and ulcerations are seen in some
areas. The skin lesions are potential sites for
the development of squamous cell carcinoma.
b: Chronic radiodermatitis in a 62-year-old
male. Chronic radiation-induced actinic
keratosis is present on the flexor of a DIP joint.
This patient was diagnosed with tinea manus
about 30 years earlier and had been treated
with therapeutic soft X-ray irradiation.

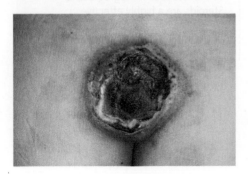

Fig. 13.10 Pressure ulcer, decubitus.

Pressure ulcer, decubitus
Clinical features
Pressure ulcers mostly occur in the sacrum, ischial
tuberosity, and ankles (Fig. 13.10 and Fig. 13.11).
Erythema, edema, induration, and eventually ulceration develop in areas subjected to constant pressure.
Ulcers may extend down to bone and may even
involve the joints, rectum or vagina. The ulcer may
have an undermined edge, and its base is moist and
covered by necrotic tissue and pus. Secondary infection such as from anaerobic fungi may result in sepsis.

Pathogenesis
Persistent pressure results in impaired vascular supply,
and subsequently skin necrosis. It commonly occurs in
bedridden individuals and in patients with spinal cord
injury. Perceptual dysfunction and undernutrition also
contribute to the occurrence of pressure ulcers. In
nursing care, the Braden scale is used to predict and
assess the risk of pressure ulcer.

Treatment
The primary treatment for pressure ulcers is the prompt
reduction of pressure to restore blood flow. Proper
wound bed preparation that promotes wound healing
is important. The affected site is cleansed and dressed
with the appropriate antibiotic ointments and dressing
materials. In the chronic stage, the affected site is
cleaned with water and necrotic tissue is removed.
Disinfectant tends not to be used unless there is apparent
infection. It is essential not to worsen the condition.

Factitial dermatitis (synonym: dermatitis artefacta)
Clinical features
Erythema, erosion, gangrene, and ulcers develop
mostly at sites within reach of the hands, such as the
extremities, chest, and face. Right-handed patients
tend to have dermatitis artefacta on the left side of the
body. Eruptions may present with different appearances according to the cause (e.g., fingernail scratch,
knife injury, misuse of drugs).

Diagnosis
Factitial dermatitis is characterized by factitious lesions.
Patients with mental stress, neurosis, depression, mental
disability or schizophrenia may cause self-harm to their
skin, nails or mucous membranes. Most patients deny

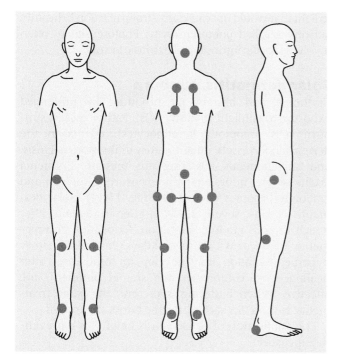

Fig. 13.11 Areas most likely to be affected by pressure ulcers. The most frequently involved areas are the sacral region, the ischial tuberosity and the bony areas of the skin, including the ankles, which tend to be subjected to pressure from the body weight during bed rest.

that the injury is self-inflicted. The specific types include trichotillomania (see Chapter 19) and onychotillomania. Akatsuki disease (Fig. 13.12), navel stones (Fig. 13.13), and pediculosis corporis resemble factitial dermatitis but are caused by chronic poor hygiene.

Treatment

Cutaneous symptoms should be treated appropriately. If necessary, referral to a psychiatrist may be needed; however, patients with this condition often refuse such treatment.

Photodermatosis

Sunlight, UV in particular, causes various changes on the skin. Lesions caused by various kinds of light are called photodermatoses. The solar dermatitis that normally occurs on anyone who is exposed to sunlight (suntan) and photoaging are photodermatoses. Abnormal skin reaction

MEMO 13–2 Munchausen syndrome

This is a factitious disorder based on the patient's desire to attract the attention of those around them. The patient makes up stories or pretends to have disorders such as factitial dermatitis. Some patients with factitial dermatitis have this disorder.

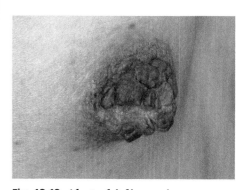

Fig. 13.12 Akatsuki disease in a woman in her 20s. There is marked deposition of keratin. This patient hardly ever washed her nipples for fear that she would contract a skin disease.

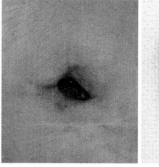 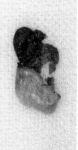

Fig. 13.13 Navel stone. This is so-called bellybutton lint. The patient consulted a doctor on what seemed to be a black tumor in the navel. When it was pulled out, there was a grimy mass of keratin. The patient had believed the superstition that the navel must not be washed.

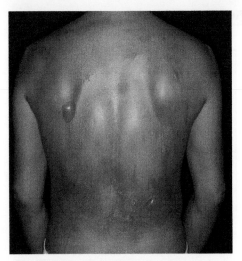

Fig. 13.14-1 Solar dermatitis, sunburn. a: Solar dermatitis caused by sleeping for 3 h on the beach. Blistering is marked. The cutaneous symptoms are equivalent to those of first-degree and second-degree burns.

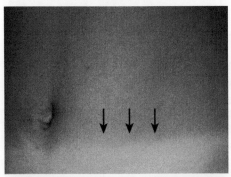

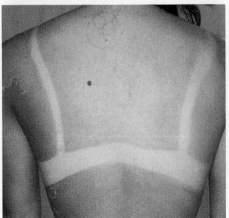

Fig. 13.14-2 Solar dermatitis, sunburn. Note the marked difference between skin that was covered by swimwear and skin that was exposed to direct sunlight.

to light that would not cause any strong reaction in healthy persons is called photosensitivity. Photosensitivity often involves specific intrinsic and extrinsic factors.

Solar dermatitis, sunburn

Erythema and blisters are produced by prolonged exposure to sunlight (mainly UVB). Pathologically, sunburn cells (apoptotic keratinocytes), edema in the dermal blood vessels, inflammatory infiltration, necrosis, and subcutaneous blistering are present. Erythema occurs several hours after the exposure to the sun and gradually becomes edematous (Fig. 13.14). Solar dermatitis is most severe 12–24 h after irradiation, after which there is gradual resolution. Exfoliation and pigmentation occur within several days. Postinflammatory hyperpigmentation may develop in some cases after healing. Cold compresses and steroid ointments are effective. When blistering is present, the same treatments as those for second-degree burns are applied.

The application of sunscreen is helpful as a preventive measure.

Photoaging

Photoaging is a general term for changes in the skin of healthy persons caused when the skin is chronically exposed to the sunlight, ultraviolet rays in particular. The conditions include wrinkling, solar elastosis, cutis rhomboidalis nuchae (see Chapter 18), senile lentigo, and Favré–Racouchot disease.

Photosensitivity (synonym: photosensitivity dermatoses)

- Photosensitivity dermatoses are cutaneous disorders that are caused or aggravated by exposure to sunlight.
- Both extrinsic (e.g., drugs; Table 13.4) and intrinsic factors (e.g., inherited and metabolic disorders) may be involved.
- Photosensitivity disorders may be caused by the direct action of drugs (phototoxic dermatitis) or by an immunological mechanism (photoallergic dermatitis).
- Xeroderma pigmentosum is an inherited photosensitivity dermatosis caused by the failure of DNA repair.

Pathogenesis

The two main causative factors of photosensitivity dermatoses are extrinsic chemicals and intrinsic factors. Disorders caused by intrinsic factors are described in other sections. This section describes photosensitivity disorders caused by extrinsic factors.

Extrinsic photosensitivity dermatoses are characterized by cutaneous inflammation caused by the excitation of chromophores from exposure to radiation (mainly UVA). Chromophores reach the skin either externally (skin lotion, perfume, tar) or internally (drugs, food) (Table 13.5). The mechanisms of inflammation are photoallergic (the excited substance becomes an allergen that induces inflammation via an immune hypersensitivity reaction) and phototoxic (the excited substance itself becomes toxic) (Table 13.6; see Fig. 13.5).

Photoallergic dermatitis
- Photoallergic dermatitis is a photosensitivity dermatitis caused by a type IV hypersensitivity reaction induced by sun exposure after topical application or intake of a drug.
- Erythema and blistering are the main symptoms.
- Chlorpromazine, thiazide drugs, and oral hypoglycemics are the main causative drugs.

Clinical features
Erythema and serous papules occur on sun-exposed sites, progressing to edema, blistering and erosion.

Pathogenesis
Chromophores that attach to the skin react to light of a certain wavelength (mostly UVA, but sometimes visible light) to become allergenic, or they may be converted into haptens, connect with endogenous proteins and become photoallergenic. After sensitization, a type

MEMO 13–3 Suntan and sunburn

Suntan is a term used for healthy tanning of the skin. Sunburn is used for the sunlight-exposed skin condition of reddening and irritation.

MEMO 13–4 Photosensitivity drug eruption

In addition to phototoxicity or photoallergy, drug intake may induce intrinsic photosensitivity diseases (e.g., porphyria, lupus erythematosus).

MEMO 13–5 MED, MRD, and MPD

The use of these terms has not been unified. They are defined in this book as follows.
- **MED (minimal erythema dose):** the minimum dose of UVB that causes erythema.
- **MRD (minimal response dose):** the minimum dose of UVA that causes erythema and papules.
- **MPD (minimal phototoxic dose):** the minimum UVA that, when irradiated with psoralen on the skin, causes erythema. MPD is used before various PUVA treatments. MED and MRD are easily confused in practice. They are sometimes described as UVB-MED and UVA-MED.

MEMO 13–6 Photocontact dermatitis

The skin comes into direct contact with the causative agent. Subsequent exposure to UV radiation changes the causative agent into a photoallergen, and eczema occurs only on the area exposed to sunlight. Similar to contact dermatitis, photocontact dermatitis is grouped into phototoxic (i.e., involving psoralen or bergapten) and photoallergic (i.e., involving ketoprofen).

Table 13.4 Main drugs that induce photosensitive dermatosis. (Blue font indicates frequently used drugs.)

Drug classification	Drugs
Psychoactive	Chlorpromazine HCl, promethazine HCl, diazepam, carbamazepin, imipramine HCl
Muscle relaxant	Afloqualone
Antihistamine	Diphenhydramine, mequitazine
Antibacterial agent	Ofloxacin, ciprofloxacin, lomefloxacin hydrochloride, sparfloxacin, fleroxacin, tosufloxacin tosilate hydrate, tetracycline HCl, doxycycline HCl hydrate
Antifungal agent	Griseofulvin, flucytosine, itraconazole
Antiinflammatory agent	Ketoprofen, tiaprofenic acid, suprofen, piroxicam, ampiroxicam, actarit, diclofenac sodium, naproxen
Antihypertensive agent	Hydrochlorothiazide, trichlormethiazide, meticrane, tripamide, furosemide, tilisolol HCl, pindolol, diltiazem HCl, nicardipine HCl, nifedipine, captopril, lisinopril hydrate
Antidiabetic	Tolbutamide, chlorpropamide, glibenclamide
Antipodagric	Benzbromarone
Antitumor agent	5-FU, tegafur, dacarbazine, flutamide
Lipid-lowering drug	Simvastatin
Prostatomegaly therapeutic agents	Tamsulosin HCl
Photochemistry therapeutic agent	8-Methoxypsoralen, trioxypsoralen, hematoporphyrin derivative
Vitamin	Etretinate, pyridoxine HCl, B_{12}
Antirheumatic agent	Sodium aurothiomalate, methotrexate

Based on Kamide R. Photosensitive dermatosis caused by extrinsic photosensitizing substance. In Tamaoki K (ed.) *New Dermatology,* vol. 16. Nakayama Shoten, 2003, pp. 293–300.

Table 13.5 Classification of photosensitive dermatosis and pages in which described.

Classification	Cause	Diagnostic name	Described on...
Extrinsic photosensitive dermatosis	Drug	Phototoxic dermatitis	Chapter 13
		Photoallergic dermatitis	Chapter 13
Intrinsic photosensitive dermatosis	Accumulation of chromophore in skin	Pellagra	Chapter 17
		Porphyria	Chapter 17
	DNA repair defect	Xeroderma pigmentosum (XP)	Chapter 13
		Cockayne syndrome	
		Bloom syndrome	Chapter 18
	Decrease of melanin	Oculocutaneous albinism (OCA)	Chapter 16
		Phenylketonuria	Chapter 17
	Unknown	Hydroa vacciniforme	Chapter 13
		Solar urticaria	Chapter 13
		Polymorphous light eruption	Chapter 13
		Chronic actinic dermatitis (CAD)	Chapter 13

Table 13.6 Phototoxic reaction and photoallergic reaction.

	Phototoxic reaction	Photoallergic reaction
Incidence	May occur in anybody	Immunologically mediated (Type IV) only
More than one exposure to agent required?	No	Yes
Onset of reaction after exposure to agent and light	Hours to 1 day	24–72 h
Clinical features	Exaggerated sunburn	Dermatitis
Distribution	Sun-exposed skin	Sun-exposed skin
Spread to unexposed areas?	No	Yes (possible)
Pathologic feature	Necrosis of epidermal cell (sunburn)	Spongiosis, eczema
Cross reaction caused by similar compounds?	Almost never	Yes (sometimes)
Amount of agent required for photosensitivity	Large	Small

IV allergic reaction is induced after the causative substance is reexposed to light (Fig. 13.15). This reaction requires prior sensitization; inflammation is not caused by the first exposure, nor does allergic reaction occur in everyone. A person who has been sensitized is prone to light-induced inflammation from exposure to even minute amounts of the causative substance.

Laboratory findings and diagnosis
- **Photo-patch test** (see also Chapter 5): the test substance is applied to the skin in two lines, as in the usual patch test. The minimum reaction dose (MRD) and minimal erythema dose (MED) are determined. After 24–48 h, half of the patch site is exposed to about half the amount of UV of the first MRD/MED exposure. The other half is left unexposed. The results are determined 48 h after exposure (Fig. 13.16).
- **Photo-drug test:** application of the suspected drug is discontinued for at least 20 days. A normal dose of a test drug is applied for 2 days. The diagnosis is photoallergic dermatitis if an eruption is produced by exposure to light.

Treatment
Intake of the causative substance and sunlight exposure should be avoided. The treatment is the same as that for contact dermatitis. A photosensitivity disease called "persistent light reaction," which is categorized as chronic actinic dermatitis (CAD), may remain after discontinuation of the causative substance.

> **MEMO 13–7 UDS value**
>
> The UDS (unscheduled DNA synthesis) test for XP indicates the potential degree of recovery from DNA damage under UV exposure, expressed as a percentage compared to normal controls. Cells are plated in a Petri dish and exposed to UV. When cultured in [3H] thymidine solution, damaged DNA is repaired, and the cells absorb [3H] thymidine.
>
> The amount of [3H] thymidine is measured by autoradiography and compared with normal cases; patients with XP have reduced UDS values.

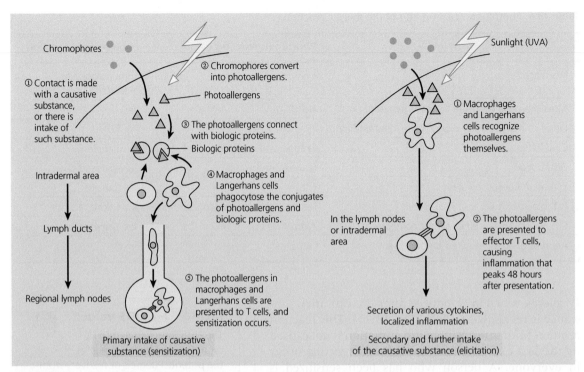

Fig. 13.15 Mechanism of photoallergic reaction. Secondary and further intake of the causative substance (elicitation).

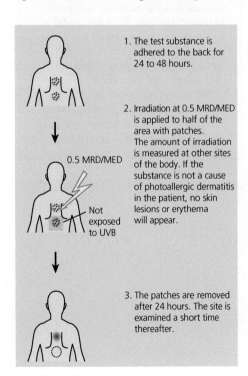

Fig. 13.16 Photo-patch testing.

Phototoxic dermatitis

- Phototoxic dermatitis may occur in anyone through the combination of a certain dose of drugs and sun exposure.
- It may even develop at the first irradiation (usually by UVA) and without any latency.
- The main causative drugs are psoralen, coal tar, and sparfloxacin.

Diagnosis and treatment

Sunburn-like symptoms characterized by erythema and edema and followed by exfoliation and pigmentation are mainly seen. Perfumes may cause both allergic contact dermatitis and phototoxic dermatitis (Berloque dermatitis). Intake of the causative substance and sunlight exposure should be avoided. The treatments are the same as those for contact dermatitis.

Solar urticaria

Definition, pathogenesis, and symptoms

Solar urticaria results from the existence of chromophores in the serum and a type I hypersensitivity reaction against an allergen that is intrinsically produced in skin by exposure to light. Several minutes after light exposure (mostly in the visible spectrum), extremely itchy urticaria occurs; however, it disappears within several hours. Anaphylactic shock may occur in rare cases.

Diagnosis and examinations

Solar urticaria is generally diagnosed from recurrent eruptions caused by exposure to sunlight or to artificial light. However, wheals may be produced or aggravated by light shielding in some cases; certain wavelengths in the light are thought to inhibit wheals. In young patients, differential diagnosis from erythropoietic protoporphyria may be necessary.

Treatment

Antihistamines are used as a symptomatic treatment. Sunbathing for a short period of time is recommended as a desensitization treatment. Immunosuppressants and plasma exchange have been reported to be effective in severe cases.

Chronic actinic dermatitis
Clinical features and pathogenesis

Chronic actinic dermatitis (CAD) most frequently occurs in adult males. It is characterized by chronic intractable dermatitis and slowly progressing lichenoid plaques on exposed areas of the body (Fig. 13.17).

In some cases, the lesions progress to erythroderma, leading to cutaneous lymphoma-like subcutaneous nodules, skin thickening or leonine facies. It is hypothesized that intrinsic antigens are produced by light exposure from an unknown mechanism. Photosensitivity disorders previously called "persistent light reaction," "actinic reticuloid" or "chronic photosensitivity dermatitis" are now categorized as forms of CAD.

Pathology

Eczematous lesions are the main symptom of CAD. As CAD progresses, lymphocytic infiltration and atypical cells are seen in all dermal layers and Pautrier microabscess-like lesions may occur in the epidermis (actinic reticuloid).

Laboratory findings, diagnosis, and treatment

The MED for UVB is greatly reduced. Reduced MRD and sensitivity to visible light may be present. For diagnosis, the skin is subjected to repeated UVB

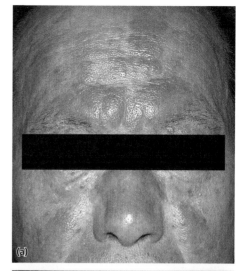
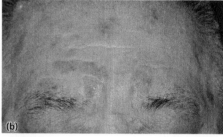
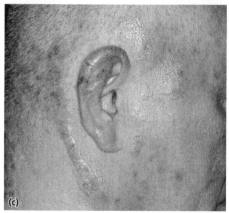

Fig. 13.17-1 Chronic actinic dermatitis. a: Intractable eczema presents as lichenified plaques that progress slowly. b: The skin lesions improved significantly after topical application of tacrolimus for several months. c: The skin lesions recurred after sun exposure.

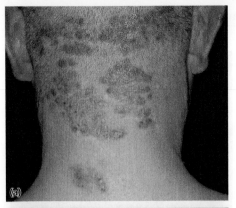

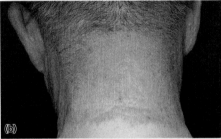

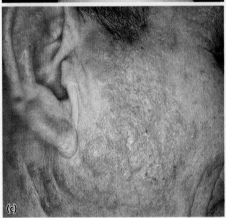

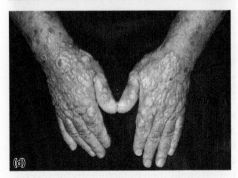

Fig. 13.17-2 Chronic actinic dermatitis (CAD). a: Chronic eczematous skin lesions accompanied by intense itching on the occipital region. b: A clearly demarked red plaque on the occipital region. Involvement of sunlight is suggested. c: Flatly elevated plaques on the cheek. d: Lichenoid plaque and prurigo nodularis on the dorsa of the hands.

exposure and if eczematous lesions appear then the diagnosis is CAD. Topical tacrolimus is helpful. Complete light shielding is essential. Topical steroids may be used. Oral steroids and immunosuppressants are effective in severe cases.

Polymorphous light eruption
Clinical features
Polymorphous light eruption occurs most commonly in women between the ages of 10 and 30. Itchy erythema and papular eruptions appear on sun-exposed sites in summer. Vesicles may also be found. They become chronic and gradually improve.

Diagnosis
Delayed-type hypersensitivity is thought to be a possible cause for this disorder; however, the cause is unknown. The MED and MRD are normal. The mechanism is also unknown.

Hydroa vacciniforme
- Hydroa vacciniforme is a rare intrinsic photosensitivity disease seen in infants and young children. The disease resolves spontaneously at puberty.
- Blisters with concave centers form at sun-exposed sites on the face and dorsa of the hands.
- The Epstein–Barr virus is involved. Lymphoma occurs in some cases and the prognosis is poor.

Clinical features and pathogenesis
Hydroa vacciniforme first appears in children between the ages of 2 and 3 years and spontaneously resolves at puberty. It occurs more often in males. Erythema and concave blisters develop after exposure to sunlight or UVB. Crust forms in 1–2 weeks, and the lesions heal with mild atrophic scars. They mostly occur on the face, auriculae, and dorsal hands (Fig. 13.18). The condition tends to aggravate during summer. Severe cases are accompanied by fever and hepatosplenomegaly. Some cases with poor prognosis may be accompanied by lymphoma with EB virus or hemophagocytic syndrome. Hydroa vacciniforme is thought to be an EB virus-involved disorder because the EB virus is found in the cutaneous eruptions.

Diagnosis and examinations
Hydroa vacciniforme is diagnosed by laboratory findings. Differentiation from porphyria is necessary.

The EB virus antibody titer often shows a test pattern that indicates previous infection. Sunlight avoidance and the application of strong sunscreen are helpful. For systemic symptoms, oral steroids may be considered.

Xeroderma pigmentosum

- Xeroderma pigmentosum (XP) occurs as a result of congenital failure in the DNA repair process. Photosensitivity and neurological symptoms occur.
- All types of XP are autosomal recessively inherited.
- Malignancy may occur as a complication with age.
- Complete avoidance of sunlight is necessary.

Classification and pathogenesis

Patients with XP have a congenital failure in repairing and eliminating DNA that is damaged by UV exposure. The failure results in severe photosensitivity and neurological symptoms. XP is classified based on the responsible gene and the unscheduled DNA synthesis (UDS) index into eight subtypes: groups A–G, and a variant group (Table 13.7). All types of XP are autosomal recessively inherited.

Group A is the most severe, while the variant group is the mildest. In the variant group, UDS is normal. However, there is failure of DNA modification after synthesis. It affects 1–1.5 persons per 100,000.

Clinical features

Abnormalities are not usually present at birth. However, intense and delayed sunburn reaction in 1–2-month-old infants may herald the onset of XP, especially in the group A subtype. Extremely intense and persistent sunburn reactions recur on sun-exposed sites such as the face and dorsae of the hands and forearms. Repeated sunburn reactions result in skin dryness and coarsening as well as poikiloderma with ephelides-like pigmented patches, hypopigmented macules, exfoliation, and telangiectasia (Fig. 13.19). Seborrheic keratosis, small ulcers, basal cell carcinoma, squamous cell carcinoma, keratoacanthoma, and malignant melanoma may develop (see Fig. 13.19g).

Ocular symptoms such as blepharitis, photophobia, dacryorrhea (excessive flow of tears), and conjunctivitis occur in childhood and progress to ectropion, blindness, and malignant tumor in the terminal stages.

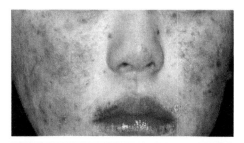
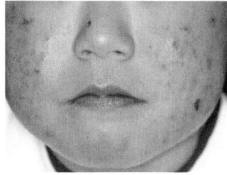
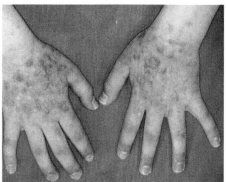

Fig. 13.18 Hydroa vacciniforme.

Table 13.7 Comparison between types of xeroderma pigmentosum.

Group	UDS (%)	Onset	Severity of skin manifestations	Neurological manifestations	Average age of skin cancer development
A	<5	Infancy	Severe	++	9.2
B	3–7	Infancy	Severe	+	
C	10–25	Infancy	Severe	−	10.5
D	25–50	Infancy	Moderate	++	35.5
E	40–60	Infancy and early childhood	Mild	−	41
F	10–20	Early childhood	Mild	−	47.7
G	<25	Early childhood	Mild	+	32
Variant	75–100	Early childhood (about 5 years old)	Mild	−	41

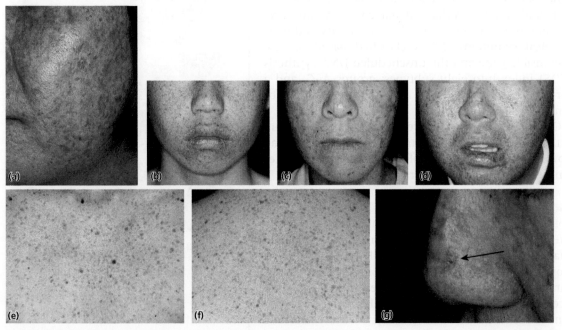

Fig. 13.19 Xeroderma pigmentosum (group D). a: Pigmentation is seen on the face of a woman in her 40s. b: Pigmentation mainly on the sun-exposed areas of a male in his teens. c: A woman in her 40s. She had experienced frequent basal cell carcinomas since her 30s. d: A man in his 20s. The disorder was accompanied by mental retardation and apraxia of gait. e,f: Pigmentation on the sun-exposed areas of the precordial region and upper back of the patient in (b). g: Basal cell carcinoma on the nasal dorsum of the patient in (d).

Neurological and motor development peak before age 10, and these abilities are progressively reduced. Hearing is impaired by around age 10 and cerebellar ataxia appears after that. Apraxia of gait and aspiration pneumonia often occur around age 20.

Xeroderma pigmentosum subtypes E, F, and G are often overlooked due to the mildness of their photosensitivity symptoms. The carcinogenic period is the third decade of life. Ocular and neurological symptoms are rarely found in these groups. Nevertheless, cutaneous and neurological symptoms in some cases of groups E, F, and G closely resemble those found in group A. In the variant group, MED is almost normal, but ephelides gradually appears after childhood. Although ocular and neurological symptoms are rarely seen, basal cell carcinoma or squamous cell carcinoma occurs in adulthood.

Laboratory findings and diagnosis
Xeroderma pigmentosum diagnosis is confirmed by the MED level (group A has a much lower MED and a delayed peak in reaction), measurement of UDS, genetic complementation test, and genetic testing.

Treatment
Group A, B, and C patients with severe cutaneous symptoms should avoid sunlight thoroughly by dressing appropriately, wearing eyeglasses with UV protection, placing UV-screening film on windows, applying shades to fluorescent lamps, and using sunscreen. Early detection and treatment of cutaneous malignancy are important. Neurological disorders are helped by regular speech and motor ability retention training.

CHAPTER 14

Blistering and pustular diseases

Blistering diseases are classified into inherited and acquired disorders. Congenital blistering diseases such as epidermolysis bullosa are caused by mutations in genes that encode several epidermal basement membrane structural proteins. Ultrastructural molecular sites where the mutant protein is expressed become fragile, resulting in blistering. Since the causative genes for epidermolysis bullosa have been identified, it has become possible to accurately diagnose the disease subtypes, provide genetic counseling, and offer prenatal diagnosis. Acquired blistering diseases such as pemphigus and bullous pemphigoid have an autoimmune etiology. Autoantibodies against epidermal structural proteins are produced, which leads to epidermal fragility and blistering. Pustular diseases are characterized by the presence of multiple sterile pustules. This chapter does not discuss blistering and pustular diseases caused by physical injuries (e.g., burns and frostbite) or infections (e.g., bacterial or viral).

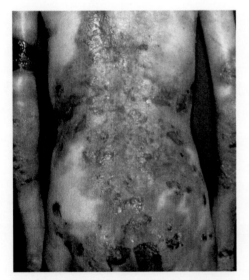

Fig. 14.1 What is epidermolysis bullosa?
Epidermolysis bullosa is a group of hereditary diseases in which even slight mechanical stimuli produces blisters, erosions, and ulcers. This photo shows dystrophic epidermolysis bullosa (RDEB, severe generalized).

Blistering diseases

Genetic blistering diseases

Epidermolysis bullosa (synonym: epidermolysis bullosa hereditaria)

- Shortly after birth, blisters, erosions and ulcers form at sites of friction in the neonate.
- Epidermolysis bullosa (EB) is classified according to the ultrastructural level of cleavage into EB simplex (in the epidermis), junctional EB (in the lamina lucida), and dystrophic EB (in the dermis). It is further subdivided based on the new international classification published in 2008 and on the basis of clinical features, inheritance patterns, and causative genes (Table 14.1, Fig. 14.1, Fig. 14.2).
- It is caused by mutation in genes that encode the structural molecules of the epidermal basement membrane.
- The basic examination is for protein abnormality by direct immunofluorescence of the patient's skin sample. If necessary, the cleavage location is determined and the genetic mutation is identified.
- Symptomatic therapies are the mainstay treatments for EB.

Shimizu's Dermatology, Second Edition. Hiroshi Shimizu.

Table 14.1 Classification of epidermolysis bullosa (EB).

Major classification	Minor classification	Target protein
EB simplex (EBS)	Localized	Keratin 5, keratin 14
	Dowling–Meara	Keratin 5, keratin 14
	Other generalized	Keratin 5, keratin 14
	EBS associated with muscular dystrophy	Plectin
	JEB associated with pyloric atresia	Plectin
Junctional EB (JEB)	Herlitz JEB	Laminin-332
	Non-Herlitz JEB	Type 17 collagen, laminin-332
	JEB associated with pyloric atresia	α6β4 integrin
Dystrophic EB (DEB)	Dominant	Type VII collagen
	Recessive, severe generalized	Type VII collagen
	Recessive, other generalized	Type VII collagen
Kindler syndrome	–	Kindlin-1

Adapted from Fine JD, et al. The classification of inherited epidermolysis bullosa (EB): Report of the Third International Consensus Meeting on Diagnosis and Classification of EB. *J Am Acad Dermatol* 2008;58:931–950.

Epidermolysis bullosa simplex (EBS)

- Blisters form at sites prone to friction, such as the hands and feet, with onset at birth or early childhood. These subside with age. Most cases are autosomal dominantly inherited.
- The prognosis is generally good.

Clinical features and classification

Shortly after birth, blisters of various sizes form at friction-prone sites, such as the hands, feet, elbows, and knees. There are three subtypes of EBS. In the localized type, blisters occur only in localized areas of the body. In the Dowling–Meara type, blisters occur on the whole body. A generalized type of EBS caused by mutation of the *K5* or *K14* gene has an autosomal dominant pattern of inheritance. The blisters are intraepidermal and heal without scarring. It tends to aggravate in summer as a result of heat. It subsides with age and generally has a good prognosis.

There are rare subtypes, including EBS with muscular dystrophy (EBS-MD) and EBS with pyloric atresia. These are caused by mutation of the plectin gene. They are autosomal recessively inherited.

MEMO 14–1 Epidermolysis bullosa simplex with mottled pigmentation

Blistering is almost the same as in localized EBS. However, there is the unusual presence of small pigmented patches of 2–5 mm in diameter on the lower abdomen, axillary fossae, and extremities. Epidermolysis bullosa simplex with mottled pigmentation is caused by the missense mutation P25L in the V1 domain of the *KRT5* gene encoding cytokeratin 5.

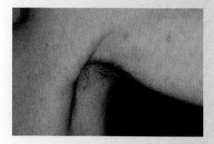

Epidermolysis bullosa simplex with mottled pigmentation.

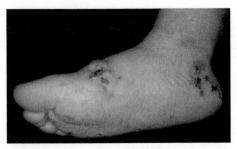

Fig. 14.3 Epidermolysis bullosa simplex (localized type). Blistering is localized on the hands and feet. Blistering is induced by friction, such as from long walks.

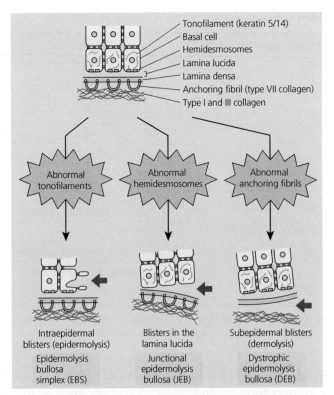

Fig. 14.2 The mechanism of epidermolysis bullosa and the location of minute cleavage formation.

Localized EBS
Blisters form only on the hands and feet. This is the mildest subtype. It was formerly called Weber–Cockayne type (Fig. 14.3).

Dowling–Meara EBS
Ring-shaped blisters form over the whole body. Mucosal erosion also occurs. In neonates, systemic blisters and death may occur (Fig. 14.4).

Other generalized-type EBS
This is a mild type of EBS with blisters on other parts of the body as well as on the hands and feet. It was formerly called Köbner type (Fig. 14.5).

Pathogenesis
Keratin 5 and 14 are involved in the formation of the cytoskeletal network in the basal cells (see Fig. 1.16). In EBS, the basal cells degenerate, and cleavages and blisters form in the epidermal basal cell layer. The

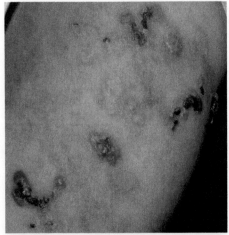

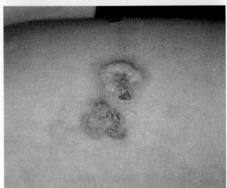

Fig. 14.4 Epidermolysis bullosa simplex (Dowling–Meara type). Blisters form ring shapes and heal without scarring.

severity of EBS depends on the location or type of mutation in K5 or K14, and on the type of mutated amino acids. The severity of the disorder is regulated by the function of the mutated keratin proteins. Plectin is present in hemidesmosomes and sarcolemmas of the muscle fascia. Mutation of plectin causes not only EBS but also muscular dystrophy or pyloric atresia.

Pathology

Separation within the cytoplasm of the epidermal basal cells leads to intraepidermal blistering (Fig. 14.6). In severe Dowling–Meara EBS, clumping of degenerated keratin fibers occurs, which can be observed by electron microscopy (Fig. 14.7).

Treatment

Symptomatic therapies are the mainstay treatments for EBS. Friction and warm temperatures should be avoided. Local therapies (e.g., the drainage of blisters and the application of petrolatum and dressings) are helpful. The cutaneous symptoms generally subside with age.

Junctional epidermolysis bullosa (JEB)

- This is caused by mutation in genes that encode the structural molecules of hemidesmosomes (laminin-332 or collagen 17). Systemic blisters occur in the lamina lucida.
- The mutations are autosomal recessively inherited. It is classified into severe Herlitz JEB and non-Herlitz JEB.
- The majority of patients with Herlitz JEB die within 1 year after birth. Non-Herlitz JEB has a better prognosis.
- JEB with pyloric atresia is an atypical type of JEB caused by genetic mutation in the integrin α_6 or integrin β_4 gene. The prognosis is poor.
- Symptomatic therapies are the mainstay of treatment for JEB. Genetic counseling and prenatal diagnosis may be conducted.

Clinical features

In Herlitz JEB, there is widespread blistering, erosion, and ulceration in newborns after birth. The lesions heal poorly, then recur and enlarge. Mucosal lesions and growth insufficiency of teeth and nails are seen. Herlitz JEB is fatal, with death resulting within 1 year after birth in almost all cases (Fig. 14.8).

Non-Herlitz JEB has a better prognosis, and patients may survive to reproductive age. Non-scarring alopecia,

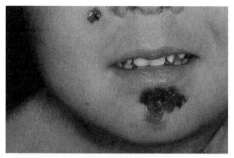
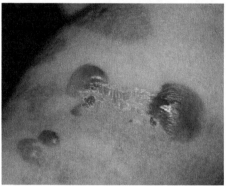
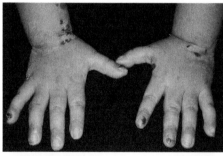
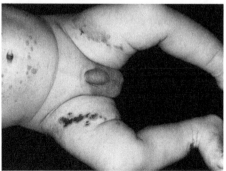

Fig. 14.5 Epidermolysis bullosa simplex (other, generalized type). Blistering occurs on the whole body surface. The clinical severity is between those of the Dowling–Meara and the localized types.

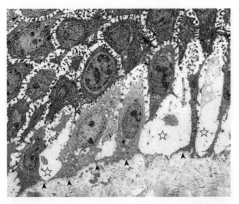

Fig. 14.6 Electron microscopic image of epidermolysis bullosa simplex. The arrows indicate the lamina densa. The cytoplasm of the basal cells (indicated by stars) on the basement membrane is disrupted, leading to blistering.

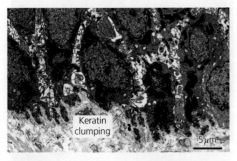

Keratin clumping

5 μm

Fig. 14.7 Aggregated keratin fibers seen in the Dowling–Meara type.

palmoplantar keratosis, nail deformity, and aplasia of dental enamel are present (Fig. 14.9). Nikolsky's sign is positive. JEB with pyloric atresia is an atypical type of JEB with systemic blisters and pyloric atresia. It is fatal soon after birth in many cases (Fig. 14.10).

Pathogenesis

The causative genes have been identified as those that encode the structural proteins of hemidesmosomes in the epidermal lamina lucida (see Figs 1.12, 1.13). Herlitz JEB is caused by the complete absence of laminin-332. Non-Herlitz JEB is caused by the reduction of laminin-332 or the complete absence of type 17 collagen (BP180). It has a better prognosis. JEB with pyloric atresia is an atypical type of JEB caused by

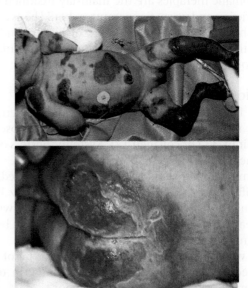

Fig. 14.8 Junctional epidermolysis bullosa, Herlitz type. Intractable, erosive ulcers cover the whole body surface. The ulcerations gradually enlarge.

MEMO 14–2 Lethal Herlitz junctional epidermolysis bullosa

The disease, once called "lethal Herlitz JEB," is now simply called "Herlitz JEB" because some patients are able to survive beyond 1 year of age.

MEMO 14–3 Laminin-332

Laminin-332 was previously called laminin-5. Laminin-332 consists of α3, β3, and γ2 chains, which are encoded by the *LamA3*, *LamB3*, and *LamC2* genes. Junctional epidermolysis bullosa occurs as a result of mutations in both alleles of any of the three genes.

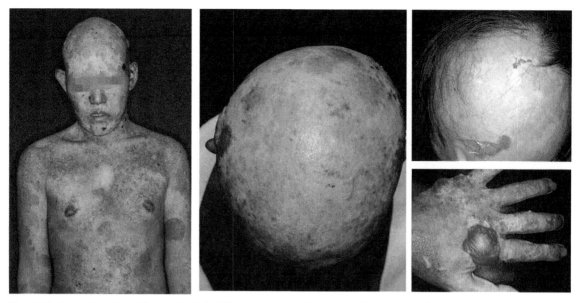

Fig. 14.9 Junctional epidermolysis bullosa, non-Herlitz type. Blistering and pigmentation occur on the whole body surface. Non-scarring alopecia also occurs on the scalp. Mutation in collagen type XVII is identified.

genetic mutation in the integrin α_6 or integrin β_4 gene. The genetic mutation leads to epidermal fragility and blistering.

Laboratory findings

It is most important to identify the basement membrane proteins that have been reduced or eliminated, such as laminin-332, collagen 17, and $\alpha6\beta4$ integrin. This is done by direct immunofluorescence. In JEB there is subepidermal blistering that can be observed by light microscopy. Blisters form between the plasma membrane of the basal cells and the lamina densa. The plane of separation at the lamina lucida can be visualized more clearly by electron microscopy (Fig. 14.11; see also Fig. 14.1).

Treatment

Treatments include minimizing friction and applying symptomatic treatments (ointments, dietary supplements). Genetic counseling and prenatal diagnosis may be offered to parents with a child with severe disease, such as Herlitz JEB.

Dystrophic epidermolysis bullosa (DEB)

- Systemic subepidermal blistering is found; it heals with milia (see Chapter 21) and scarring. Nikolsky's sign is positive.

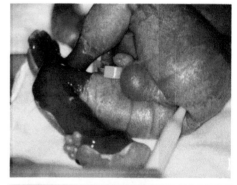

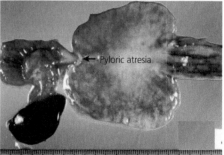

Fig. 14.10 Junctional epidermolysis bullosa associated with pyloric atresia. Aplasia cutis congenita-like ulceration of the skin and congenital pyloric atresia occur as complications. Mutation in the integrin $\beta4$ gene is identified.

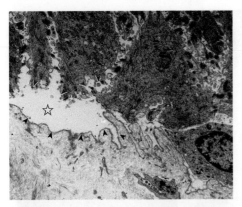

Fig. 14.11 Electron microscopic image of junctional epidermolysis bullosa. A blister (star) forms in the lamina lucida, between the plasma membrane of the basal keratinocytes (purple arrows) and the lamina densa (black arrows).

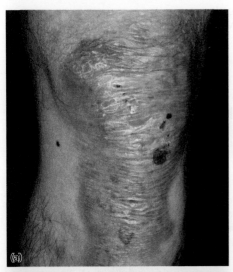

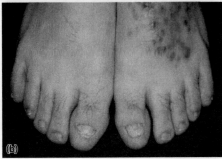

Fig. 14.12 Dystrophic epidermolysis bullosa (dominant type). a: Blistering and scarring occur on areas subjected to friction, such as the knees. b: Deformity in the toenails.

- DEB can be inherited in an autosomal dominant or recessive manner. The clinical symptoms of recessive DEB are severe. Coalescence of fingers and toes or squamous cell carcinomas occur in many cases.
- DEB is caused by abnormality in the anchoring fibrils that link the dermis with the lamina densa.

Clinical features and classification

Dystrophic epidermolysis bullosa is caused by mutations in the gene encoding type 7 collagen, which constitutes the anchoring fibrils (see Figs. 1.12, 1.13). Anchoring fibrils play the most important role in connecting the dermis and epidermis. Loss of anchoring fibrils or failure of their formation results in cleavage and blisters under the epidermis (see Fig. 14.1). DEB can be inherited autosomal dominantly (dominant DEB (DDEB)) or autosomal recessively (recessive DEB (RDEB)). The latter is further classified into two subtypes.

Dominant DEB

Dominant DEB is inherited in an autosomal dominant manner. This DEB subtype occurs in newborns and infants. Multiple blisters develop on the extensor surfaces of the extremities. The disease may cause esophageal atresia, or papules on the trunk. It heals with scarring (Fig. 14.12). Nail deformity is present. It tends to subside with age.

Recessive DEB–severe generalized

The most severe type of DEB, RDEB–severe generalized is caused by a total absence of type 7 collagen. It was formerly called Hallopeau–Siemens type. At birth or shortly thereafter, blisters and erosions appear on the extremities and trunk, with or without external influences. They heal with milia and scarring, which can result in mitten deformity of the extremities (Fig. 14.13). Lesions are also seen in the nails as well as the oral and esophageal mucosa, resulting in esophageal atresia and dysphagia. The symptoms do not subside with age. When patients reach adolescence, they often develop malignant skin tumors, particularly squamous cell carcinomas. It is extremely serious and may cause death in young patients.

Recessive DEB–generalized other

Type 7 collagen is reduced, but not completely absent. The severity of clinical symptoms varies (Fig. 14.14). Symptoms tend to be milder than for RDEB

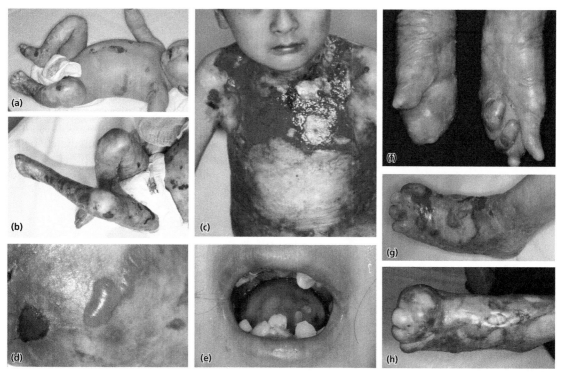

Fig. 14.13 Dystrophic epidermolysis bullosa (recessive, severe generalized type). a: Blistering and ulceration are relatively mild at birth. b,c: Intractable blisters form as the patient grows. d: Marked blistering is present on the whole body. e: Hypoplasia of the teeth is present. f,g,h: Adhesion is seen in the fingers and toes.

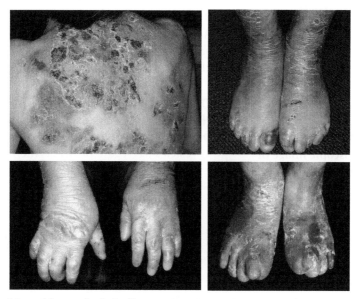

Fig. 14.14-1 Dystrophic epidermolysis bullosa (recessive, other generalized type). Scarring blisters, crusts, and adhesion occur in the fingers; however, these are milder than in the recessive, severe generalized type. Expression of collagen type VII is present but reduced.

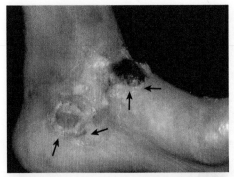

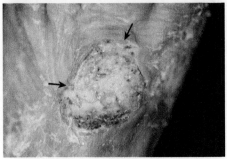

Fig. 14.14-2 Dystrophic epidermolysis bullosa (recessive, other generalized type). Cases with squamous cell carcinoma (arrows).

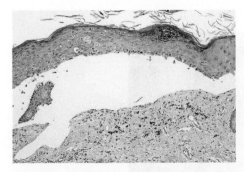

Fig. 14.15 Light microscopic image of dystrophic epidermolysis bullosa. Typical subcutaneous blistering and slight inflammatory cellular infiltration are present.

generalized type. Webbing of fingers and toes may occur, but not mitten deformity. It was formerly called non-Hallopeau–Siemens type.

Laboratory findings

It is most important to identify the decrease or disappearance of type 7 collagen by direct immunofluorescence. Subepidermal blistering is observed by light microscopy. Dissociation is observed immediately below the lamina densa by electron microscopy (Fig. 14.15, Fig. 14.16). Disappearance or hypoplasia of anchoring fibrils is observed.

Diagnosis

Diagnosis is done by findings obtained by clinical examination, electron microscopy, and immunofluorescence (IF). Identification of gene mutation may be necessary to differentiate RDEB from DDEB. For RDEB, prenatal diagnosis is made by fetal DNA analysis using amniocentesis or chorionic villus biopsy.

Treatment

Friction should be avoided and local therapies are used. Fluid and diet management are also important. Genetic counseling is offered to parents of children with RDEB. In recent years, new therapies, including synthetic type 7 collagen therapy, fibroblast cell therapy, and stem cell transplant, have been tried. Bone marrow transplantation therapies were done on patients with RDEB, and these have proven notably effective in some patients.

Other genetic blistering diseases
Hailey–Hailey disease (synonym: familial benign chronic pemphigus)

- Vesicles aggregate on an erythematous base in areas exposed to friction. The appearance resembles that of impetigo.
- It is autosomal dominantly inherited and occurs in adults in their 30s or 40s.
- It is caused by mutations in the *ATP2C1* gene encoding a calcium pump in the Golgi apparatus within keratinocytes.
- Histologically, there is acantholysis and villi formation. It is somewhat similar to Darier's disease (see Chapter 15).
- Topical steroid application is the main treatment.

Clinical features

Hailey–Hailey disease is autosomal dominantly inherited. It tends to manifest in adults, appearing as aggregated erythema and blistering in areas exposed to friction, such as the neck, axillary fossa, inguinal regions, and anus. The blisters rupture to form erosions. Crusts, pustules, pigmentation, and secondary infections resembling impetigo-like lesions may be present (Fig. 14.17). Itching is usually present. The lesions heal without scarring, but abnormal pigmentation may develop. The disease worsens in summer and subsides in winter. Other aggravating factors include friction, perspiration, infection, and UV radiation.

Pathology

Acantholysis of the epidermis leads to intradermal lacunae formation immediately above the basal layer. The dermal papillae, which are covered by basal cells in the single layer that is left in the lacunae, protrude and resemble villi. Dyskeratotic cells are occasionally found. Acantholytic cells in the lacunae are connected loosely to each other by a few desmosomes (Fig. 14.18).

Diagnosis

Hailey–Hailey disease is diagnosed by the clinical features and pathological diagnosis. It is also important to take a thorough family history. Genetic screening can identify pathogenic mutations in the *ATP2C1* gene.

Treatment

Topical application of steroids is useful. Bacterial and fungal infections may be present in many cases. Oral retinoids may be useful. Surgical ablation may be performed in intractable cases.

Ectodermal dysplasia–skin fragility syndrome

Skin fragility syndrome, an autosomal recessive inherited disease, is caused by abnormalities in the gene that encodes plakophilin 1, a desmosomal structural protein. Epidermal fragility, painful hyperkeratosis in the palms and soles, and abnormalities of hair, nails, and sweating are present.

Autoimmune blistering diseases

Pemphigus

- Pemphigus is an autoimmune disease caused by autoantibodies against desmoglein 1 and 3. Desmoglein 1 and 3 are structural components of desmosomes,

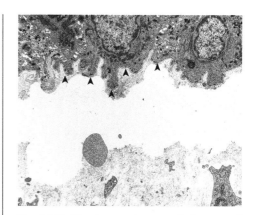

Fig. 14.16 Electron microscopic image of dystrophic epidermolysis bullosa. Anchoring fibrils are absent, and blistering is observed immediately beneath the lamina densa (arrows).

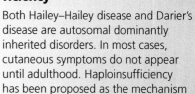

MEMO 14–4 Hailey–Hailey disease and haploinsufficiency

Both Hailey–Hailey disease and Darier's disease are autosomal dominantly inherited disorders. In most cases, cutaneous symptoms do not appear until adulthood. Haploinsufficiency has been proposed as the mechanism of onset.

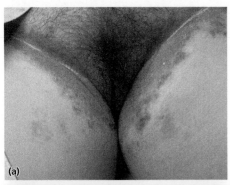

(a)

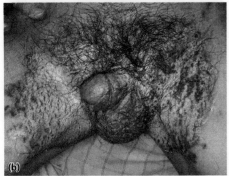

(b)

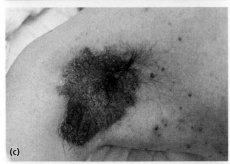

(c)

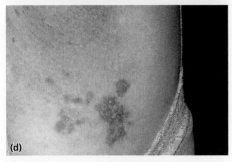

(d)

Fig. 14.17 Hailey–Hailey disease. a,b: Vesicles, erosions, impetigo, and pustules form in the groin. c,d: Axillary fossae. The blisters shown in photo (c) may appear, although only rarely.

which adhere the keratinocytes (see Fig. 1.14). Intraepidermal blisters with flaccid bullae form as a result of acantholysis.

- Pemphigus vulgaris and pemphigus foliaceus are the two major groups. Pemphigus most frequently affects the middle-aged and the elderly.
- The deposition of autoantibodies in the intercellular spaces (direct immunofluorescence), the presence of antidesmoglein antibodies (ELISA), and positive Nikolsky's sign are found.
- Oral steroids and immunosuppressants, and high-dose intravenous immunoglobulins are used.

Classification

Diseases with intraepidermal blistering (pemphigus group) are divided into two groups according to their pathogenesis: pemphigus vulgaris and pemphigus foliaceus. Pemphigus vegetans is a type of pemphigus vulgaris, whereas pemphigus erythematosus is a type of pemphigus foliaceus. The characteristics of each type are summarized in Table 14.2. Pemphigus vulgaris accounts for 60% of all pemphigus cases. Paraneoplastic pemphigus is also a disorder of this group.

Pathogenesis

In pemphigus vulgaris, autoantibodies against desmoglein 3 are produced. Because the basal cell layer is rich in desmoglein 3, the action of autoantibodies against desmoglein 3 causes keratinocytes to lose adhesion. The basal cell layer erodes and blisters. In pemphigus foliaceus, however, autoantibodies against desmoglein 1 (and not desmoglein 3) are produced. Acantholysis occurs in the upper epidermal layer. Because the basal cell layer is not rich in desmoglein 1, the action of autoantibodies against desmoglein 1 has little adverse effect on basal cell adhesion: The basal cell layer remains largely intact (Fig. 14.19).

Pathology

Dissociation of intercellular connections in the epidermis is called acantholysis. As dissociation progresses, epidermal cleavage and blistering occur. Keratinocytes become spherical from loss of intercellular connection within the blisters (acantholytic cells). In pemphigus vulgaris and pemphigus vegetans, acantholytic blistering occurs immediately above epidermal basal cells; in pemphigus foliaceus and pemphigus erythematosus, blistering occurs in the superficial epidermis, such as at sites immediately below the stratum corneum or in the granular cell layer. In pemphigus vegetans, besides the findings of pemphigus vulgaris, there is acanthosis and papillo-matosis with formation of eosinophil-filled pustules in the epidermis.

Laboratory findings

Autoantibodies against desmoglein 1 and 3 are detected by ELISA. Epidermal intercellular in vivo-bound IgG in lesional skin is identified by direct IF. IgG antiin-tercellular antibodies in the sera of patients are detected by indirect IF and ELISA (Fig. 14.20). The Tzanck test (see Chapter 5) is used only as a supplementary test. Elevated levels of eosinophils may be found in peripheral blood or in the blister contents.

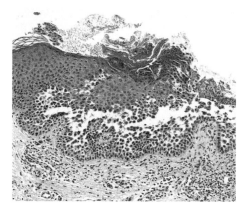

Fig. 14.18 Histopathology of Hailey–Hailey disease. Intraepidermal acantholysis.

Table 14.2 Types of pemphigus groups.

		Pemphigus vulgaris	Pemphigus vegetans	Pemphigus foliaceus	Pemphigus erythematosus
Age of onset		Middle age to elderly	Middle age to elderly	Middle age	Middle age
Frequent site of skin lesion		Whole body skin, oral mucosa	Intertriginous areas (e.g., axillary fossae)	Whole body skin	Oily areas of skin (e.g., face)
Clinical findings	Skin	Blisters, erosion	Blisters, erosion, papillary acanthosis, pustules	Erosion, lamellar exfoliation, crusts	Erosion, butterfly rash, seborrheic dermatitis-like skin lesion
	Mucosal lesions	++	+	−	−
	Nikolsky's sign	+	+	+	+
Pathological finding	Skin	Intraepidermal blisters (acantholysis)			
	Tzanck test	+	+	+	+
	Site of acantholysis	Lower epidermal layer (directly on basal cells)		Upper epidermal layer (granular cell layer)	
Targeted antigen		Only Dsg3, Dsg3 and Dsg1		Only Dsg1	
ELISA		Dsg1(+/−), Dsg3(+)		Dsg1(+), Dsg3(−)	
Immunofluorescence technique	Direct (skin lesion)	IgG(+) in the epidermal intercellular space, C3(+) positive			
	Indirect (serum)	IgG (+)			
Treatment		Steroids, immunosuppressants, high-dose intravenous immunoglobulin, plasmapheresis			

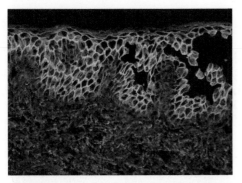

Fig. 14.20 Direct immunofluorescence of pemphigus foliaceus. Intercellular deposition of IgG is observed in the epidermis.

MEMO 14–5 Western blot and autoimmune blistering diseases

Identification of specific autoantibodies against the cutaneous proteins in the patient's serum can be done by this method. Extract from healthy epidermis or dermis is electrophoresed and then transferred onto a membrane. The membrane is incubated with the patient's serum and then with the labeled anti-human IgG.

MEMO 14–6 Transient acantholytic dermatosis

This disorder is also called Grover's disease. Itching pruritic papules and blisters with acantholysis occur on the trunk and extremities. It subsides within 3 months. The pathogenesis is unknown. Autoantibodies against skin are not present.

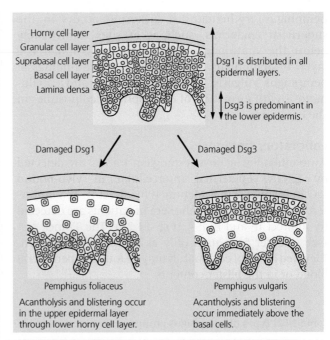

Horny cell layer
Granular cell layer
Suprabasal cell layer
Basal cell layer
Lamina densa

Dsg1 is distributed in all epidermal layers.

Dsg3 is predominant in the lower epidermis.

Damaged Dsg1

Damaged Dsg3

Pemphigus foliaceus
Acantholysis and blistering occur in the upper epidermal layer through lower horny cell layer.

Pemphigus vulgaris
Acantholysis and blistering occur immediately above the basal cells.

Fig. 14.19 Distribution of desmoglein 1 and desmoglein 3 in the epidermis, and the pathomechanism of pemphigus. Diseases with intraepidermal blistering are classified according to the desmoglein molecules that are impaired (see also Fig. 14.23).

Pemphigus vulgaris

- The disease most frequently occurs in the middle-aged and elderly. It tends to present with painful oral enanthema. Flaccid bullae and erosions are formed on the skin.
- To identify this disorder, the presence of autoantibodies against desmoglein 3, which causes the keratinocytes to adhere, is necessary.
- When only antibodies to desmoglein 3 are detected, the disease is membrane-dominant pemphigus vulgaris. When antibodies to desmogleins 1 and 3 are detected, the disease is the mucocutaneous type, with systemic blisters.
- Acanthosis and blisters occur immediately above the basal layer.
- Nikolsky's sign is positive.
- Oral steroids and immunosuppressants, and high-dose intravenous immunoglobulins are used.

Clinical features

It most frequently affects the middle-aged and the elderly. Erosions and ulcers develop in the oral mucosa in 70–80%

of cases. Subsequently, blisters of various sizes occur on normal skin (Fig. 14.21). This blistering may occur anywhere on the body but it tends to appear at sites prone to pressure and friction, such as the back, buttocks, and feet. The painful blisters easily rupture to form large erosions and crusts. When the blisters are pressed without breaking, the fluid contents extend to the peripheral normal skin around the blisters (blister diffusion phenomenon, or false Nikolsky's sign) and form erosions.

Erosions form in the oral cavity and esophageal mucosa, causing dysphagia. When the eruptions are widespread, electrolyte abnormalities resulting from loss of body fluid or hypoproteinemia may be present; this can be fatal when there is secondary infection. Associations of pemphigus vulgaris include thymoma and myasthenia gravis.

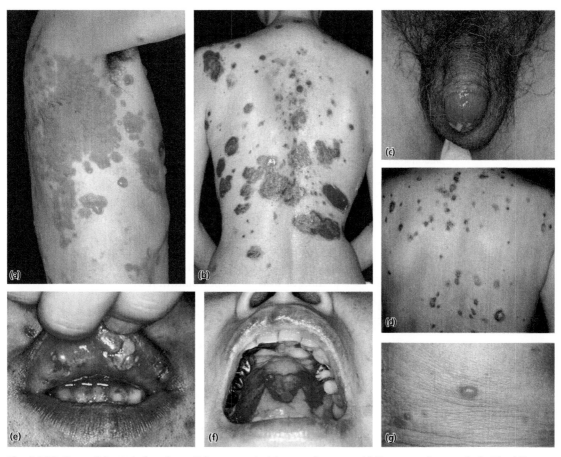

Fig. 14.21 Pemphigus vulgaris. a: Edematous itching erythema and blisters on the trunk. b: The blisters easily rupture and become erosive. c: Erosion on the membrane of the genitalia (glans penis). d: A mix of blisters, erosions, and crusts is present on the trunk. e,f: Intractable erosion on the lips and in the oral cavity. g: The skin appears healthy except for the blister.

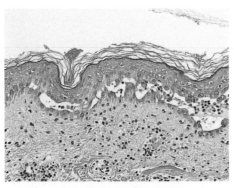

Fig. 14.22 Histopathology of pemphigus vulgaris. Acantholysis is observed immediately above the basal cells.

Table 14.3 Autoantibody against desmoglein detected by ELISA, and confirmed diagnosis.

ELISA		Diagnostic name
Anti-Dsg1 IgG antibody	Anti-Dsg3 IgG antibody	
−	+	Pemphigus vulgaris (mucosa predominant type)
+	+	Pemphigus vulgaris (mucocutaneous type)
+	−	Pemphigus foliaceus
−	−	Normal or Non-pemphigus

Pathology

Acantholysis causes intraepidermal blistering. Blisters often form leaving one basal layer at the base of the skin, resulting in a tombstone-like appearance (Fig. 14.22). Eosinophilic infiltration may be present in the blister and the dermal upper layer.

Diagnosis

To diagnose pemphigus vulgaris, it is necessary to detect antidesmoglein antibodies by IF or ELISA (see the previous section). The amount of antibodies in the serum reflects the severity of the pemphigus condition. When only antibodies to desmoglein 3 are detected, the disease is membrane-dominant pemphigus vulgaris, in which there is only minor blistering of the skin. When antibodies to both desmoglein 1 and 3 are detected, blistering is often seen in the oral mucosa and systemic skin (Table 14.3, Fig. 14.23).

Differential diagnosis

It is necessary to differentiate the disease from bullous pemphigoid, pemphigus foliaceus, dermatitis herpetiformis, impetigo contagiosa, drug-induced toxic epidermal necrolysis, bullous drug eruptions, erythema multiforme, and Stevens–Johnson syndrome.

Treatment

Systemic application of steroids is the first-line treatment. According to the severity, prednisolone at 0.5–1.0 mg/kg of body weight is administered daily. The dosage is tapered to a maintenance dose or until the condition has stabilized. Immunosuppressants may be used. In intractable cases, a large dose of intravenous immunoglobulin and plasma exchange may be considered. Local application of steroids or petrolatum may be used.

Pemphigus vegetans
Clinical features

Pemphigus vegetans is a subtype of pemphigus vulgaris. Its onset is characterized by the formation of vesicles and erosions that do not reepithelialize. Lesions are often accompanied by vesicles and pustules. There is a strong odor, and the disorder frequently occurs on areas exposed to friction, such as the axillary fossa, the umbilicus, and the periphery of the oculonasal and perioral regions (Fig. 14.24). Pemphigus vegetans can be subdivided into Neumann type or Hallopeau type. The Neumann type is marked by blistering and pemphigus vulgaris-like

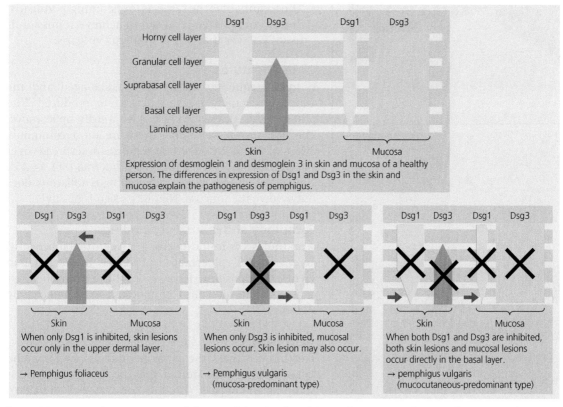

Expression of desmoglein 1 and desmoglein 3 in skin and mucosa of a healthy person. The differences in expression of Dsg1 and Dsg3 in the skin and mucosa explain the pathogenesis of pemphigus.

When only Dsg1 is inhibited, skin lesions occur only in the upper dermal layer.

→ Pemphigus foliaceus

When only Dsg3 is inhibited, mucosal lesions occur. Skin lesion may also occur.

→ Pemphigus vulgaris (mucosa-predominant type)

When both Dsg1 and Dsg3 are inhibited, both skin lesions and mucosal lesions occur directly in the basal layer.

→ pemphigus vulgaris (mucocutaneous-predominant type)

Fig. 14.23 Expression patterns of desmogleins in the skin and mucosa. The pemphigus type depends on whether the autoantibodies target desmoglein 1 or desmoglein 3 (see also Fig. 14.19).

erosions. In contrast, pustules are characteristic of the Hallopeau type, which has a better prognosis.

Differential diagnosis
Pemphigus vegetans should be differentiated from condyloma latum, condyloma acuminatum, chronic pyoderma, and deep mycoses.

Treatment
Treatment is the same as for pemphigus vulgaris.

Pemphigus foliaceus
- This most frequently affects the middle-aged and elderly. Fragile blisters, scaling, and erosion, accompanied by crusts, occur systemically. Lesions are not produced in the mucosa.
- Autoantibodies are produced exclusively against desmoglein 1.
- Acantholysis and blistering are seen in the superficial epidermis (in the granular cell layer).

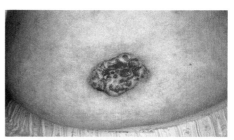

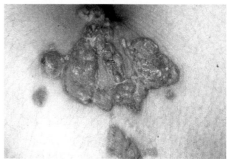

Fig. 14.24 Pemphigus vegetans.

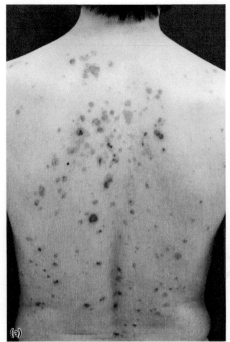

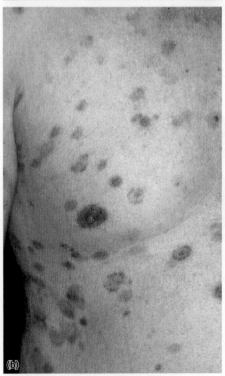

Fig. 14.25-1 Pemphigus foliaceus. a: Erosion on the back. b: Erythema and pigmentation on the chest.

- The treatment is the same as for pemphigus vulgaris. The steroid dosage required to achieve remission is usually lower than for pemphigus vulgaris.

Clinical features

It most frequently affects the middle-aged and the elderly. Extremely fragile vesicles are produced. The blistered skin dries quickly to give a leafy appearance. The face, head, back, and chest are most commonly affected. When the disorder progresses and spreads over the whole body, it resembles erythroderma (Fig. 14.25). Unlike pemphigus vulgaris, pemphigus foliaceus does not involve the mucosa. Nikolsky's sign is positive.

Pathology and laboratory findings

Acantholysis is found in and between the subcorneal layer and the epidermal upper layer. Intercellular in vivo IgG deposition is observed by immunofluorescence. Antidesmoglein 1 antibodies can be detected by ELISA.

Treatment

Treatment is the same as for pemphigus vulgaris. The initial dose of oral steroid may be less than that for pemphigus vulgaris (prednisolone at 0.5 mg/kg of body weight). Topical steroids are sufficient in some cases.

Pemphigus erythematosus (synonym: Senear–Usher syndrome)

Pemphigus erythematosus is a subtype of pemphigus foliaceus, and it occurs most commonly in the middle-aged and elderly. The clinical features resemble those of pemphigus foliaceus. Systemic lupus erythematosus (SLE)-like erythema appears on the cheek or seborrheic eczema-like eruptions appear on the face (Fig. 14.26). IgG deposition in the intercellular spaces and on the basal membrane is observed by direct immunofluorescence. Antinuclear antibody is positive, which implies an assocation with SLE; however, complications with SLE or progress into SLE are rarely found. The treatment is the same as for pemphigus foliaceus.

Paraneoplastic pemphigus

Erosions, ulceration, and crusts are present on mucous membranes in the oral cavity, pharynx, and lips. Pseudomembranous conjunctivitis may lead to blepharosynechia. In addition to flaccid bullae, skin lesions are of various forms, such as lichenoid and erythema multiforme-like eruptions. Autoantibodies against desmoglein 1 or 3 are detected by ELISA, and autoantibodies against multiple epidermal proteins including desmoplakin (250, 210, 190 kDa) are detected by Western blot. Most cases may occur as a secondary disorder of underlying lymphoproliferative diseases, of which about half of all cases are malignant lymphoma. Chronic lymphocytic leukemia and Castleman's disease may be in the primary lymphoproliferative diseases.

Drug-induced pemphigus

Drug-induced pemphigus encompasses diseases that cause lesions resembling pemphigus clinically and immunologically. It has symptoms of pemphigus foliaceus and various other clinical symptoms (Fig. 14.27). Autoantibodies against desmoglein 1 or 3 are often found.

Neonatal pemphigus

Neonatal pemphigus is seen in newborns of mothers with pemphigus. The mother's IgG autoantibodies pass into the placenta, affecting the newborn infant's skin. The clinical symptoms, and histological and immunohistological findings of pemphigus are transiently observed in neonatal pemphigus.

IgA pemphigus (synonym: intercellular IgA dermatosis)

Vesicles and pustules are present on the trunk and extremities, and they can become chronic. Some cases are clinically indistinguishable from subcorneal pustular dermatosis. IgG deposition in intercellular spaces is found. Histopathologically, IgA pemphigus can be divided into two subtypes: subcorneal pustular dermatosis, in which the lesions are localized below the stratum corneum, and an intraepidermal neutrophilic (IEN) type, in which cellular infiltration is seen in all layers of the epidermis.

Brazilian pemphigus foliaceus (synonyms: Fogo selvagem, Brazilian pemphigus foliaceus)

Brazilian pemphigus foliaceus is endemic to Brazil and certain other areas of South America. Autoantibodies recognize desmoglein 1, which is the same autoantigen present in pemphigus foliaceus

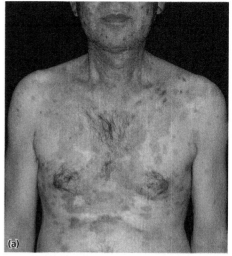

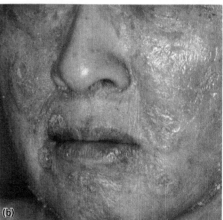

Fig. 14.25-2 Pemphigus foliaceus.
a: Erosions, erythema, and pigmentation on the chest. b: Exfoliation and erythema on the face. The blisters are thin and easily ruptured; tense blisters are rarely seen.

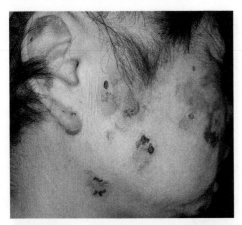

Fig. 14.26 Pemphigus erythematosus.
Erythema and erosions on the cheek. The lesions resemble those of pemphigus foliaceus.

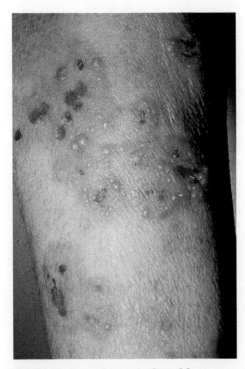

Fig. 14.27 Pemphigus induced by D-penicillamine. Erythema and vesicles are present. When induced by D-penicillamine, the skin lesions tend to persist even after the medication is discontinued.

and causes symptoms similar to those of pemphigus foliaceus in young patients. Transmission is thought to involve black flies.

Diseases with subepidermal blistering (pemphigoid group)

- These are autoimmune blistering diseases in which subepidermal blistering occurs as a result of autoantibody action against epidermal basement membrane structural proteins.
- Unlike the flaccid intraepidermal blisters of pemphigus, these subepidermal blisters are tense and do not rupture easily (Fig. 14.28).
- Hemorrhagic blisters and milia formation may be present.
- The disease is divided into bullous pemphigoid, linear IgA bullous dermatosis, epidermolysis bullosa acquisita, and others (Table 14.4).
- Immunofluorescence and ELISA are useful for diagnosis.
- The treatment options include corticosteroids and DDS (dapsone).

Bullous pemphigoid (BP)

- Bullous pemphigoid is an autoimmune blistering disease that frequently occurs in the elderly. The blisters are often tense.
- It is often accompanied by itchiness. It does not commonly involve the mucosa.
- It is caused by autoantibodies against type 17 collagen or the BP230 protein, which are the structural components of hemidesmosomes.

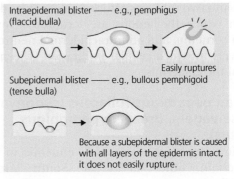

Intraepidermal blister —— e.g., pemphigus
(flaccid bulla)

Easily ruptures

Subepidermal blister —— e.g., bullous pemphigoid
(tense bulla)

Because a subepidermal blister is caused with all layers of the epidermis intact, it does not easily rupture.

Fig. 14.28 Difference between an intradermal blister and a subepidermal blister.

Table 14.4 Autoimmune blistering diseases that cause subepidermal blisters.

		Bullous pemphigoid	Herpes gestationis	Mucous membrane pemphigoid	Epidermolysis bullosa acquisita	Dermatitis herpetiformis (Duhring)	Linear IgA bullous dermatosis (LAD)
Age of onset		Elderly (youth in some cases)	Women 4 months pregnant to postpartum	Adults and elderly	Adults and elderly	Middle age	<10 or 40
Frequent site		Whole body	Abdomen, buttocks, extremities	Oral cavity, ocular mucosa	Intertriginous areas (e.g., elbows, knees)	Whole body (especially elbows, knees, buttocks)	Whole body
Clinical findings	Findings of skin	Tense blisters, edematous erythema, itching	Urticaria-like erythema, itching	Blisters, erosion, scarring	Erosion, blisters, scarring	Itching, erythema, urticaria-like wheal	Erythema, tense blisters, itching
	Mucosal infiltration	+	−	++	+	−	+
Pathological findings		Eosinophilic infiltration	Eosinophilic infiltration	Eosinophilic infiltration, low eosinophil count	Eosinophilic infiltration	Neutrophilic infiltration, microabscess	Neutrophilic infiltration
Autoantigen		Type 17 collagen	Type 17 collagen	Type 17 collagen, laminin 332	Type VII collagen	Epidermal transglutaminase	120 kDa-protein, 97 kDa-protein, type VII collagen
Immuno-fluorescence findings	Direct (pigmentation in vivo)	Linear deposition of IgG and C3 in the epidermal basement membrane zone (BMZ)	Linear deposition of C3 in the epidermal basement membrane zone; IgG may be negative	Linear deposition of IgG and C3 in the epidermal basement membrane zone	Linear deposition of IgG in BMZ	Granular deposition of IgA in the papillae of upper dermal layer	Linear deposition of IgG (sometimes C3) in BMZ
	Indirect (autoantibody in serum)	Detection of antibasement membrane antibody	Antiepidermal basement membrane antibodies are detected when complement is added	The antiepidermal basement membrane antibody titer is low or negative.	Autoantibodies that react to the epidermis side of skin processed with 1M NaCl are detected.	Anti-autoantibody not detected	Detection of anti-IgA antibody in BMZ
Treatment		Oral steroids, immuno-suppressant, DDS	Topical and oral steroids	Topical and oral steroids, immunosuppressants	Oral steroids, immunosuppressant, plasmapheresis	DDS, gluten-free diet	DDS, oral steroids

DDS, dapsone.

- The disease is characterized by subepidermal blisters and significant eosinophilic infiltration. IF and ELISA are useful for diagnosing BP.
- Oral steroids are administered.

Clinical features

The elderly are most commonly affected. Multiple large, severe subepidermal blisters form immediately

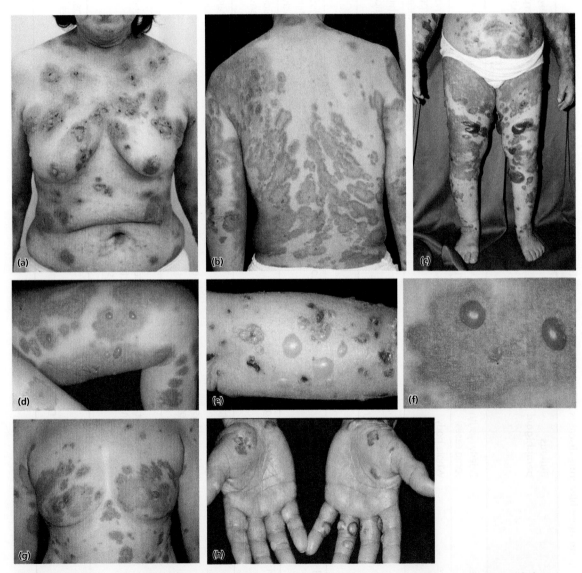

Fig. 14.29 Bullous pemphigoid. a: Precordial region. b: Back. The lesion resembles erythema multiforme. c: Large blisters are seen. d: Itching, edematous erythema, and tense bullae on the extremities. This is a typical skin manifestation of bullous pemphigoid. e: Upper arm. f: Comparatively large erythema and blisters. g: Chest. h: Palms.

below the epidermis. BP is often accompanied by urticarial plaques (Fig. 14.29) and, unlike pemphigus vulgaris, does not commonly involve the mucosa (about 20% of the mucosa is involved). BP may be complicated by internal malignancy.

Pathogenesis

Autoantibodies are produced against hemidesmosomal structural proteins, type 17 collagen and BP230 in the epidermal basement membrane, which leads to blistering (see Fig. 1.10). Autoantibodies against the NC16a domain of type 17 collagen in particular cause the blistering.

Pathology and laboratory findings

Subepidermal blistering in bullous pemphigoid is accompanied by eosinophilic infiltration (Fig. 14.30). Linear IgG and C3 deposition in the basement membrane zone of the lesions is observed by direct immunofluorescence (IF) (Fig. 14.31). Antiepidermal basement membrane antibodies in the sera of the patients are detected by indirect IF; autoantibodies against type 17 collagen are identified by ELISA. High IgE values and elevated levels of eosinophils are found in peripheral blood in some cases.

Diagnosis

Bullous pemphigoid is diagnosed on the basis of clinical and pathological features as well as by IF and ELISA (see Table 14.4). Linear IgG deposition at the skin basement membrane zone is seen in all patients with BP, which is a necessary criterion for diagnosis. Indirect IF using normal human split skin processed with 1M NaCl is conducted to distinguish BP from other subepidermal blistering diseases, such as epidermolysis bullosa acquisita (MEMO, see Chapter 14).

Treatment

Oral steroids (0.5 mg/kg/day) are administered in the acute phase. The dose is then tapered as the condition improves. Immunosuppressants such as cyclophosphamide, dapsone, tetracyclines, and nicotinamide may also be used. For elderly patients, dehydration and secondary infection should be prevented, and attention must be paid to the nutritional requirements of the affected individual. Topical steroid application may be sufficient in cases with mild symptoms. Administration of high-dose intravenous immunoglobulins or plasma exchange therapy may be performed in severe cases.

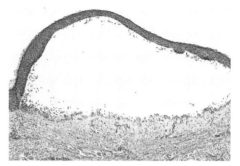

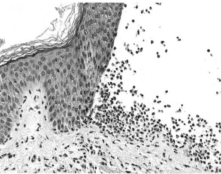

Fig. 14.30 Histopathology of bullous pemphigoid. A distinct subepidermal blister. Inflammatory cells including eosinophils are seen.

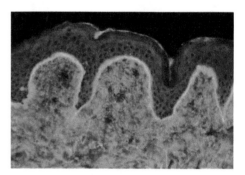

Fig. 14.31 Direct immunofluorescence of the skin of a patient with bullous pemphigoid. Linear deposition of IgG is observed in the epidermal basement membrane.

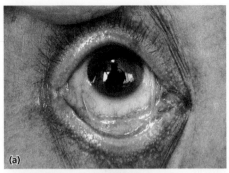
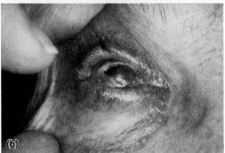
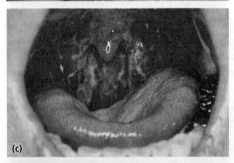
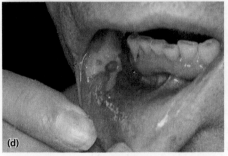

Fig. 14.32 Mucous membrane pemphigoid. a,b: Erosion in the eye and scarring occur. c,d: Erosion in the oral cavity.

Pemphigoid gestationis (synonym: herpes gestationis)

Clinical features

Multiple urticarial lesions appear on the abdomen (the umbilical region, in particular), buttocks and extremities, with vesicle formation at the periphery of the lesions. The onset occurs between the fourth month of pregnancy and immediately following delivery. The mucosa is rarely involved. Intense itching is present. Acute exacerbations may occur immediately before and after delivery.

Pathogenesis and epidemiology

Pemphigus gestationis is now regarded as a subtype of BP. It occurs in one in several tens of thousands of deliveries. Autoantibodies against type 17 collagen, which were once called HG factors, are present.

Diagnosis and differential diagnosis

Linear C3 deposition in the basement membrane zone of the lesions is observed by direct immunofluorescence. Autoantibodies against the NC16a domain of type 17 collagen are positive in ELISA. Itching is intense. Pemphigoid gestationis resembles dermatitis herpetiformis but it is distinguished by the absence of IgA deposition (see Table 14.4).

Treatment and prognosis

Topical steroids are mainly applied. In severe cases, oral steroids are administered. Pemphigoid gestationis disappears 2–3 months after delivery in most cases. It recurs in successive pregnancies at a rate of about 90%.

Mucous membrane pemphigoid (MMP) (synonym: cicatricial pemphigoid)

Blistering and erosions develop, mostly in the oral cavity and conjunctiva, resulting in scarring (Fig. 14.32). Lesions may occur in the genitalia, perianal region, pharynx, esophagus, and nasal mucosa. Prompt treatment is required if there is blepharosynechia or respiratory difficulty. Autoantibodies against type 17 collagen or laminin-332 are found.

Epidermolysis bullosa acquisita (EBA)

- The clinical features resemble those of bullous pemphigoid.

MEMO 14–7 Differential diagnosis between bullous pemphigoid (BP) and epidermolysis bullosa acquisita (EBA) using salt split-skin analysis

Differentiating between BP and EBA is often difficult because of the similarity in clinical and IF findings. Normal human split skin processed with 1M NaCl is used to differentiate between BP and EBA. When normal human skin is soaked in 1M NaCl for 48 h at 4°C, the epidermis and dermis separate at the level of the lamina lucida and artificial separation occurs. The patient's serum is then incubated with the salt split skin. In the case of BP, the serum reacts to hemidesmosomes on the epidermal side, whereas in EBA, the serum reacts to anchoring fibrils on the dermal side. Using this split-skin method, it is possible to distinguish between BP and EBA by the blistering location.

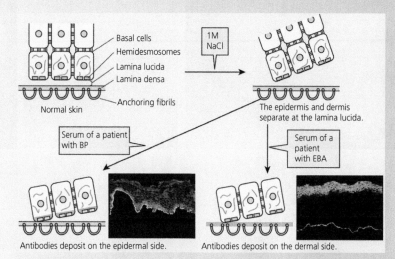

Differential diagnosis between bullous pemphigoid and epidermolysis bullosa acquisita using salt split-skin analysis.

- Subepidermal blisters form which leave milia upon healing.
- Autoantibodies against type 7 collagen, a structural component of anchoring fibrils, are produced.
- Steroids are administered orally. The disease is intractable.

Clinical features

In epidermolysis bullosa acquisita, erosions and tense blisters appear at sites prone to friction such as the knees, elbows, palms, and soles. Healing often leaves scarring and milia (Fig. 14.33). Erythema and blisters similar to those in bullous pemphigoid may appear in some cases. In progressive cases, cutaneous symptoms similar to dystrophic epidermolysis bullosa (nail deformity, coalescence of fingers and toes) may be present.

Pathogenesis

Autoantibodies against type 7 collagen, which is a structural component of anchoring fibrils that connect the epidermis and the dermis, are present, resulting in subepidermal blister formation.

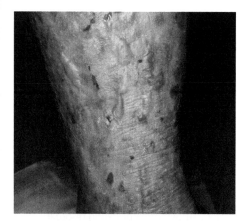

Fig. 14.33-1 Epidermolysis bullosa acquisita. Blistering, erosion, and ulceration occur, which may be partially accompanied by scarring.

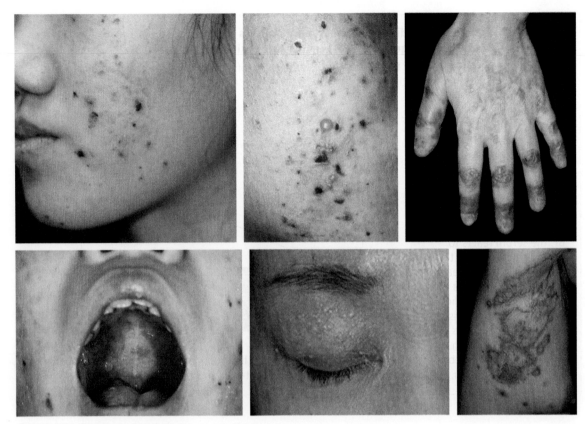

Fig. 14.33-2 Epidermolysis bullosa acquisita.

Laboratory findings

Linear IgG deposition is observed by direct immuno-fluorescence at the epidermal basement membrane zone of the lesions. Autoantibodies against type 7 collagen, a 290 kDa protein, are found by Western blot using the patient's serum.

Diagnosis and differential diagnosis

The absence of a family history of blistering formation is an important aid in diagnosis. It is essential to differentiate this disease from other blistering diseases, such as bullous pemphigoid, dystrophic epidermolysis bullosa, pemphigus, porphyria, drug-induced bullous eruptions, amyloidosis, and bullous lupus erythematosus. Indirect IF using normal human split skin processed with 1M NaCl (MEMO, see Chapter 14) and Western blot are useful.

Treatment

Epidermolysis bullosa acquisita is generally resistant to treatment. Oral steroids, immunosuppressants, and plasma exchange therapy are options for treatment.

MEMO 14–8 Antilaminin γ1 pemphigoid

This disorder was previously called anti-p200 pemphigoid. It is an autoimmune blistering disease with tense blisters that resemble the blisters of bullous pemphigoid. It features complications with psoriasis in about half of all cases, and autoantibodies deposit on the dermal side in direct IF using skin processed with 1M NaCl. It was clarified recently that the disease is an autoimmune blistering disorder associated with autoantibodies to laminin γ1, a 200 kDa basement membrane molecule.

Dermatitis herpetiformis

- This is characterized by extremely intense itching and irritation, chronically recurrent erythema, and vesicles. The vesicles tend to form circular patterns.
- Granular IgA deposition is found in the papillary dermis.
- Dermatitis herpetiformis is associated with gluten-sensitive enteropathy.
- Oral dapsone is effective.

Clinical features

Erythema and urticarial wheals occur, with vesicles arranged in a ring-shaped pattern at the periphery (Fig. 14.34). The severe itching causes the patient to scratch, resulting in crusts. The eruptions heal with pigmentary changes. Eruptions appear on the entire body, especially on the elbows, knees, and buttocks. The palms, soles, and mucosa are hardly affected.

Gluten-induced enteropathy is found in more than 90% of cases. As in celiac disease, atrophic changes in jejunal villi are found in dermatitis herpetiformis.

Pathogenesis

In recent years, it has been discovered that patients with this disease have IgA antibodies against tissue transglutaminase in the serum.

Pathology

Subepidermal blistering is present. Microabscesses are present in the dermal papillae as a result of neutrophilic infiltration (Fig. 14.35).

Laboratory findings

Granular IgA deposition is observed by direct IF in the dermal papilla. Anticutaneous autoantibodies are not seen in the patient's serum by IF. The patient's serum does not contain IgA class antitransglutaminase antibodies. The involvement of HLA-B8, DR3, and DQ2 in dermatitis herpetiformis has been found. Elevated levels of eosinophils are seen in the peripheral blood.

Diagnosis and differential diagnosis

Dermatitis herpetiformis is diagnosed on the basis of clinical features, such as intense itching, as well as subepidermal blistering and granular IgA deposition in the papillary dermis. The symptoms significantly improve with the use of dapsone; this fact has diagnostic significance. Dermatitis herpetiformis should be

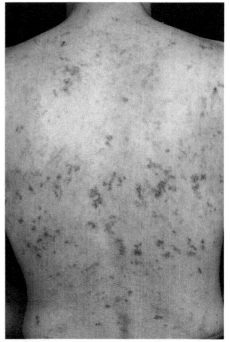
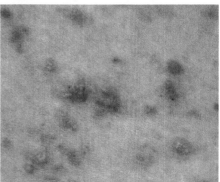

Fig. 14.34 Dermatitis herpetiformis.
Eczema and blisters accompanied by intense itching are present.

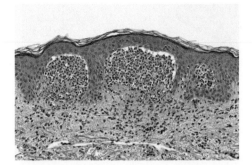

Fig. 14.35 Histopathology of dermatitis herpetiformis.

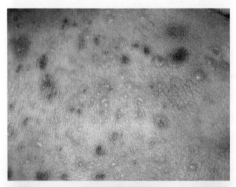

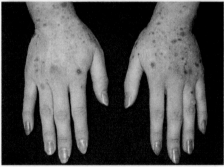

Fig. 14.36 Linear IgA bullous dermatosis.

distinguished from linear IgA bullous dermatosis, bullous pemphigoid, pemphigoid gestationis, and erythema multiforme.

Treatment
Dapsone is effective. A gluten-free diet and antihistamines are also useful.

Linear IgA bullous dermatosis
Clinical features
Linear IgA bullous dermatosis (LABD) is divided into childhood LABD, whose symptoms appear in children under the age of 10, and adult LABD, which occurs in adults aged 40 or older. Multiple tense blisters accompanied by intense itching are present over the entire body, as in dermatitis herpetiformis (Fig. 14.36). Lesions may also occur in the mucosa. The lesions tend to aggregate on the genitals and inner thighs in childhood LABD and heal spontaneously in some cases.

Pathogenesis and epidemiology
Linear IgA deposition in the epidermal basement membrane zone causes subepidermal blistering.

Pathology
Subepidermal blistering and neutrophilic infiltration are seen.

Laboratory findings and diagnosis
Linear IgA deposition at the epidermal basement membrane zone can be identified by direct IF. Antiepidermal basement membrane IgA autoantibodies may be detected in the patient's serum by indirect IF. In indirect IF using normal human split skin processed with 1M NaCl (MEMO, see Chapter 14), the epidermal side of the substrate may stain when the autoantibodies are directed against the 120 kDa and 97 kDa degraded forms of type 17 collagen, and the dermis side of the sample may stain when the autoantibodies are directed against type 7 collagen. The clinical features of both cases are not noticeably different.

Differential diagnosis
Linear IgA bullous dermatosis should be differentiated from dermatitis herpetiformis. In LABD, there are the following: a histopathological finding of linear patterns of IgA deposition; antibasement membrane IgA autoantibodies in serum in some cases; no

involvement of HLA-B8, DR3 or DQ2; involvement of the mucosa; and no gluten sensitivity.

Treatment
Oral dapsone is effective. When dapsone is ineffective, oral steroids may be used.

Pustular diseases

Palmoplantar pustulosis (synonym: pustulosis palmaris et plantaris (PPP))

- Multiple sterile pustules are distributed symmetrically on the palms and soles of middle-aged and elderly individuals. They can become chronic.
- Smoking, bacterial infection (tonsillitis), dental caries, and dental metal allergy are associated with PPP.
- Sternocostoclavicular ossification and pain may also develop.
- Topical steroid application, smoking cessation, and tonsillectomy are the main treatments.

Clinical features
Multiple vesicles form on the thenar and antithenar eminences of the palms and the arches of the feet, and become pustular. Erythema develops at the periphery of the lesions, which may coalesce into plaques (Fig. 14.37). Itching may be present. Punctate depressions and thickening occur frequently in the nails. Pustules recur in 2–4-week cycles and may progress in a chronic manner. They may appear on the knees, lower extremities, and scalp. In 10% of PPP cases, sternocostoclavicular ossification accompanied by chest pain develops as a complication.

Pathogenesis
The pathogenesis is unknown. PPP patients tend to have smoked at least a pack of cigarettes a day for more than 20 years. If focal infections (e.g., tonsillitis, dental caries) are found and treated, PPP may improve. Cases induced by bacterial allergic reaction and metal allergy have been reported. It is hypothesized that PPP is a localized type of pustular psoriasis.

Pathology
Sterile pustules in the epidermis contain neutrophils and degenerated epidermal cells. Mild cellular infiltration into the dermis is seen.

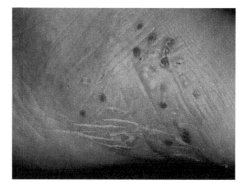

Fig. 14.37-1 Palmoplantar pustulosis (PPP).

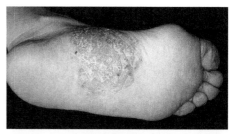

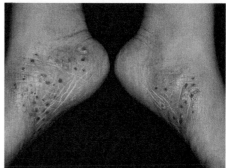

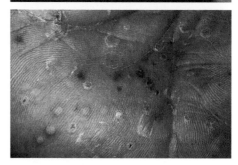

Fig. 14.37-2 Palmoplantar pustulosis (PPP). Multiple pustules aggregate on the hands and feet.

Laboratory findings

Elevated white blood cell count, antistreptolysin O titer, C-reactive protein, and erythrocyte sedimentation rate may point towards a focal infection such as tonsillitis.

In some cases, skin lesions are aggravated by pressure from massage of the tonsils. For confirmation of dental metal allergy, metal patch tests are conducted. Arthropathy and sternocostoclavicular ossification are also investigated.

Differential diagnosis

The disease should be distinguished from dyshidrotic eczema, tinea, pustular psoriasis, contact dermatitis, eosinophilic pustular folliculitis, and reactive arthritis (Reiter's syndrome).

Treatment

In most long-term smokers, the disorder improves with smoking cessation. Focal infectious diseases, if present, are treated. Prevention of tonsillitis and otological and dental treatments are important. Oral antibiotics are useful. Tonsillectomy may be performed. For skin lesions, topical steroids and activated vitamin D3 ointment are first-line treatments. PUVA therapy is also effective. Administration of oral retinoid, ciclosporin, methotrexate, and colchicine is considered in severe cases.

Subcorneal pustular dermatosis (synonym: Sneddon–Wilkinson disease)

Clinical features

Subcorneal pustular dermatosis occurs infrequently, but most commonly in women over age 40. Erythema and pustules appear in a ring-shaped or serpiginous pattern on the trunk and on sites exposed to friction. Pustules quickly dry, leaving crusts and scales (Fig. 14.38). Itching or systemic symptoms are not present, and the mucosa is not involved. The disease becomes chronic with recurrent aggravation and remission.

Pathogenesis, pathology, and differential diagnosis

The etiology of subcorneal pustular dermatosis is unknown in many cases. In some cases, IgA myeloma or ulcerative colitis may be present. Sterile pustules mainly containing neutrophils are found histopathologically

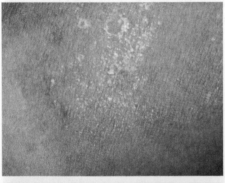
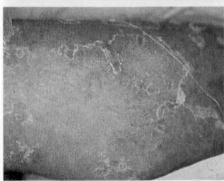
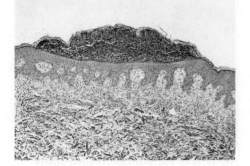

Fig. 14.38 Subcorneal pustular dermatosis.

beneath the stratum corneum. Kogoj's spongiform pustules, seen in pustular psoriasis, are not found.

Subcorneal pustular dermatosis is often indistinguishable from intracellular IgA dermatosis. Direct immunofluorescence is necessary for differential diagnosis. IgA deposition in the intercellular spaces is not found. Other disorders that require differentiation include fungal infections, pustular psoriasis, and impetigo contagiosa.

Treatment
Oral dapsone is effective. Retinoids and PUVA therapy are effective in some cases.

Eosinophilic pustular folliculitis (Ofuji) (EPF) (synonym: eosinophilic pustular dermatosis)

- Itching papules and pustules are produced. They aggregate, mainly in hair follicles.
- Male adults are the most commonly affected. The etiology is unknown. The disease is chronic, punctuated by recurrences and remissions.
- The pustules contain multiple eosinophils.
- The disease may accompany HIV infection.
- Indomethacin is effective.

Clinical features and pathogenesis
Eosinophilic pustular folliculitis most frequently occurs in men in their 20s to 30s. Sterile, follicular pruritic papules and small pustules occur and aggregate to form erythematous plaques that spread centrifugally (Fig. 14.39). The face, upper body, and extensor surface of the upper arms are the most severely affected regions; in some cases, eruptions resembling those of palmoplantar pustulosis can occur in the hands and soles where hair follicles do not exist. They leave abnormal pigmentation when they heal. EPF is a relapsing and remitting condition. The disease may accompany hematological malignancies or HIV infection. The cause is unknown.

Pathology, laboratory findings, differential diagnosis, and treatment
Eosinophils are found in large quantities in the pustules. Eosinophilic infiltration into the hair follicles and hair apparatus results in their destruction.

MEMO 14–9 SAPHO syndrome

S̲ynovitis, a̲cne, p̲ustulosis, h̲yperstosis and o̲steitis (SAPHO) syndrome is a relatively newly defined entity. Cutaneous symptoms include palmoplantar pustulosis, prominent acne, and psoriatic rash. Differentiation from psoriatic arthritis is necessary.

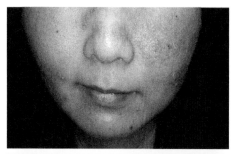
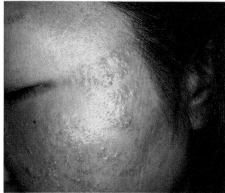
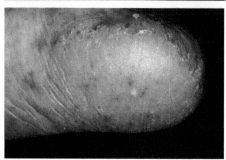

Fig. 14.39 Eosinophilic pustular folliculitis. Follicular papules and pustules aggregate, accompanied by itching.

Elevated levels of eosinophils are seen in the peripheral blood. Eosinophilic pustular folliculitis needs to be differentiated from tinea, candidiasis, folliculitis, acne, rosacea, and contact dermatitis. When it occurs on the hands and soles, differentiation from palmoplantar pustulosis is difficult. Indomethacin is very effective.

Acute generalized pustular bacterid (AGPB)

This condition is characterized by the appearance of acute sterile pustules on the trunk and extremities following an upper respiratory infection. Since the pathoetiology has not been clarified, there is controversy over whether acute generalized pustular bacterid is an independent clinical entity.

Infantile acropustulosis

The extremities of infants are affected. Infantile acropustulosis is a recurrent pustular disease characterized by multiple intensely itchy sterile pustules that resembles pustular psoriasis.

Refer to Chapter 15 for pustular psoriasis.

CHAPTER 15

Disorders of keratinization

The mechanisms of keratinization have been clarified in recent years. The genes responsible for many hereditary disorders of abnormal keratinization have been identified, but the pathogeneses of some disorders remain unknown. It is expected that these will be elucidated in the near future. Disorders of abnormal keratinization are classified as hereditary keratoses (e.g., ichthyosis, Darier's disease) and acquired keratoses. The acquired keratinization disorders are subclassified as inflammatory, whose main symptom is inflammation accompanied by itching (e.g., psoriasis, lichen planus), and non-inflammatory (e.g., clavus, callus). This chapter discusses typical disorders of keratinization, based on that classification.

Hereditary keratoses

Ichthyoses

Ichthyoses are clinical conditions in which the whole body skin dries and coarsens, resulting in scaling. The cause is abnormality in keratinization and exfoliation of the stratum corneum. The skin is covered with what appear to be fish-like scales. Patients with ichthyosis have a congenital abnormality in keratinization and scaling, and most cases are classified as hereditary keratoses. However, some may appear later in life as acquired conditions; these cases often accompany an internal malignancy. Ichthyoses are subclassified into 10 or more types based on the clinical features, the affected body parts, the causative genes, and the mode of inheritance. Note that the names were greatly revised when the new international system for subclassification was published in 2009 (Table 15.1).

Ichthyosis vulgaris
This is caused by mutations in the gene encoding filaggrin. Inheritance is semi-dominant.

Dryness and scaling of the skin are characteristic features. It is the mildest form of ichthyosis. The

Shimizu's Dermatology, Second Edition. Hiroshi Shimizu.
© 2017 John Wiley & Sons, Ltd. Published 2017 by John Wiley & Sons, Ltd.

Table 15.1 New international classification of ichthyosis (the terms in brackets are those used before revision).

I. Non-syndromic congenital ichthyosis
1 Ichthyosis with delayed onset (Symptoms are not seen at birth.) Ichthyosis vulgaris X-linked recessive ichthyosis (X-linked ichthyosis)
2 Congenital ichthyosis (Symptoms are present at birth.) Autosomal recessive congenital ichthyosis
Harlequin ichthyosis
Lamellar ichthyosis
Congenital ichthyosiform erythroderma (non-bullous congenital ichthyosiform erythroderma)
Keratinopathic ichthyosis
Epidermolytic ichthyosis (non-bullous congenital ichthyosiform erythroderma)
Superficial epidermolytic ichthyosis (ichthyosis bullosa of Siemens)
Other
Loricrin keratoderma
II. Syndromic ichthyosis (see Table 15.3)
Netherton syndrome Sjögren–Larsson syndrome Keratitis, ichthyosis and deafness (KID) syndrome Dorfman–Chanarin syndrome (neutral lipid storage disease with ichthyosis) Refsum syndrome Conradi–Hünermann–Happle syndrome Erythrokeratodermia variabili
III. Acquired ichthyosis
Malignant lymphoma, internal malignancy, sarcoidosis, etc.

Adapted from Oji V et al. Revised nomenclature and classification of inherited ichthyoses: results of the First Ichthyosis Consensus Conference in Soreze 2009. *J Am Acad Dermatol* 2010;63:607.

chance of having this disorder is 2–10%, which is extremely high.

The onset is in early childhood. Dryness and scaling of the skin are present, mostly on the extensor surfaces of the extremities and trunk. It subsides during summer.

Symptomatic therapies, including the application of moisturizer, are the main treatments.

Clinical features

The onset is in early childhood. It is progressive until the patients reach the age of about 10, the symptoms subsiding in adolescence in most cases. The skin dries, appearing pityroid and lamellar. The extensor surfaces of the legs and the back region are the most commonly affected; the flexure of joints in the extremities, and the axillary fossae, genitals, and trunk are unaffected (Fig. 15.1). Subjective symptoms and itching are rarely observed. The symptoms subside during the summer. Ichthyosis vulgaris often accompanies palmoplantar hyperlinearity and keratosis pilaris. Atopic dermatitis is strongly associated with ichthyosis vulgaris (see Chapter 7).

Pathogenesis

As a result of mutations in the filaggrin gene, which is found in the stratum corneum and is associated with epidermal moisturization, there is abnormal exfoliation of corneocytes and dryness and scaling of the skin (see Chapter 1). It is semi-dominantly inherited. The symptoms are severe in patients who have mutations in both alleles of the filaggrin gene.

Pathology

Hyperkeratosis and reduction or loss of the granular cell layer are found. Keratosis pilaris is often found.

Diagnosis and differential diagnosis

Diagnosis is done based on the distribution of eruptions, family history, and palmoplantar hyperlinearity. In other hereditary ichthyoses, onset is at birth, and the flexures of the joints in the extremities are often involved (Table 15.2). It was recently clarified that 20–50% of patients with atopic dermatitis have mutations in the filaggrin gene (Chapter 7). Most cases of dry skin seen in patients with atopic dermatitis are ichthyosis vulgaris.

Treatment

Symptomatic therapies are the mainstay treatments for ichthyosis vulgaris. Moisturizers and salicylic acid petrolatum are used topically.

X-linked ichthyosis (synonym: sex-linked ichthyosis)

This is caused by loss or marked reduction of steroid sulfatase, resulting in delayed exfoliation of the stratum corneum. It is X-linked recessively inherited. The symptoms are more severe than those of ichthyosis vulgaris. Eruptions occur not only on the extensor surfaces but also on the flexures of joints.

Clinical features

X-linked ichthyosis manifests shortly after birth and does not improve with age. The cutaneous symptoms are severe; the scales are large and dark brown (Fig. 15.2). The extensor surfaces and flexures of joints are both involved, and not only is the back involved, but so is the abdominal surface of the trunk. Comma-shaped corneal opacities may accompany the condition. As with ichthyosis vulgaris, X-linked ichthyosis aggravates during winter and subsides during summer.

Pathogenesis

X-linked ichthyosis is caused by mutations in the steroid sulfatase gene on the X chromosome. Steroid sulfatase is an enzyme that breaks down cholesterol sulfate, a substance that promotes intercellular adhesion in the stratum corneum (Chapter 1). The lack of steroid sulfatase causes accumulation of cholesterol sulfate, leading to delayed exfoliation of corneocytes and hyperkeratosis. X-linked ichthyosis is recessively inherited and occurs in males.

Pathology and laboratory findings

Hyperkeratosis is present. The granular and suprabasal cell layers are normal or mildly thickened, which differentiates X-linked ichthyosis from ichthyosis vulgaris. Follicular keratinization is rarely found. Absence or marked reduction of steroid sulfatase is observed in the stratum corneum, peripheral leukocytes, and fibroblasts. Estriol in the urine decreases in the mothers (carriers) of children with X-linked ichthyosis. Recently, it has become possible to visually examine

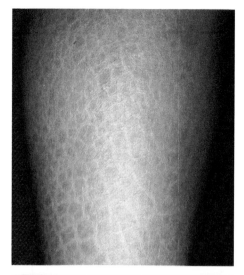

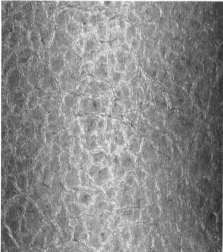

Fig. 15.1-1 Ichthyosis vulgaris. The skin dries and pityriasis-like lamellar exfoliation occurs.

Table 15.2 Comparison between types of ichthyosis.

		Ichthyosis vulgaris	X-linked ichthyosis	Harlequin ichthyosis	Lamellar ichthyosis	Congenital ichthyosiform erythroderma	Epidermolytic ichthyosis
Frequency		Common	Uncommon	Very rare	Rare	Rare	Rare
Inheritance pattern		SD	XR	AR	AR	AR	AD
Age of onset		Babyhood, infancy	At or shortly after birth	At birth	At birth	At birth	At or shortly after birth
Skin symptoms	Site	Extremities, trunk (back > abdomen), intertriginous sites, extensor surface > flexor surface	Abdomen > back, intertriginous sites, extensor surface = flexor surface	Whole body	Whole body	Whole body	Whole body
	Form	Fine scales	Large, dark brown scales	Extremely thick stratum corneum, fissures, ectropion of eyelids	Large, dark brown scales	Diffuse erythema, fine scales, ectropion of eyelids	Intense hyperkeratosis
Pathology		Hyperkeratosis and thinned granular cell layer, keratosis pilaris	Hyperkeratosis, almost normal granular cell layer	Marked hyperkeratosis	Hyperkeratosis	Hyperkeratosis with parkeratosis	Granular degeneration
Causative genes		FLG	STS	ABCA12	TGM1, ICHTHYIN, ALOXB12, ABCA12	TGM1, ABCA12, ALOXE3, ALOXB12, etc.	K1/K10

AD, autosomal dominantly inherited; AR, autosomal recessively inherited; XR, X-linked recessively inherited; SD, semi-dominantly inherited.

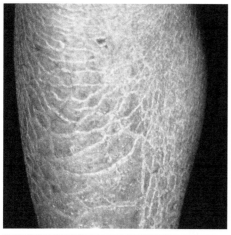

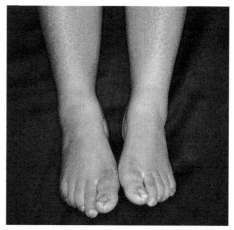

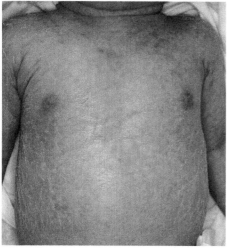

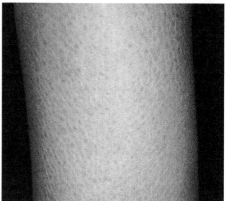

Fig. 15.1-2 **Ichthyosis vulgaris.**

Fig. 15.2 **X-linked ichthyosis.** Relatively large scales are present. The symptoms are more severe than those of ichthyosis vulgaris.

the steroid sulfatase gene in peripheral leukocytes by fluorescent in situ hybridization (FISH), which is useful in diagnosing X-linked ichthyosis.

Diagnosis and treatment

Ichthyosis vulgaris is differentiated from X-linked ichthyosis by the decrease of steroid sulfatase in the case of the latter. Treatments are the same as for ichthyosis vulgaris.

Harlequin ichthyosis (synonym: harlequin fetus)

The patient is covered with an extremely thick stratum corneum at birth. Deep cracks in the skin, ectropion of eyelids, protrusion of lips, and difficulty of opening the mouth are so severe that most patients die within

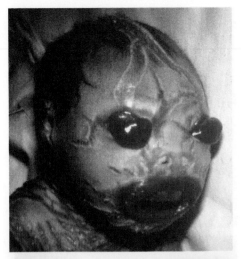

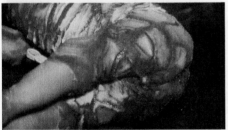

Fig. 15.3 Harlequin ichthyosis. There is marked hyperkeratosis on the whole body surface. Ectropion of the eyelids results in reddening above the eyes. Normal eyeballs are present underneath.

2 weeks after birth (Fig. 15.3). *ABCA12* has been identified as the causative gene. The ABCA12 protein is a major lipid transporter in lamellar granules. The lack of ABCA12 leads to a marked reduction of lipid content in the stratum corneum (Chapter 1), which causes harlequin ichthyosis. There is abnormality of the lamellar granules. It is autosomal recessively inherited. DNA-based prenatal diagnosis is clinically applied.

Lamellar ichthyosis

The scales in lamellar ichthyosis are clinically rough and large in most cases, dark brown, and plate-like or lamellar. Erythroderma (reddening or flush) is not very visible (Fig. 15.4). Patients may be born as collodion babies. Two to 3 days after birth, the collodion covering exfoliates. The concept of lamellar ichthyosis is for a group of clinically similar disorders and includes hereditarily varied types. In approximately half of all cases of lamellar ichthyosis, the cause is an absence of transglutaminase 1 (TGM1), which is involved in the formation of the cornified cell envelope (marginal band) (see Fig. 1.18 and Chapter 1). Cases caused by mutations in *ICHTHYIN*, *ALOXB12*, and *ABCA12* have been reported. Most of the cases are autosomal recessively inherited; however, some are autosomal dominantly inherited.

Congenital ichthyosiform erythroderma (CIE) (synonym: non-bullous congenital ichthyosiform erythroderma (NBCIE))
Clinical features

Many of the patients are born as collodion babies (see the preceding section). After exfoliation of the collodion covering, the whole body surface is covered with diffuse flushing (erythroderma) and fine scales (Fig. 15.5). Ectropion of eyelids sometimes occurs. Hyperkeratosis on the palms and soles may accompany CIE. There are minor changes in the symptoms according to the season. BCIE progresses until the age of 10, at which point it stops and subsides.

Pathogenesis

The concept of CIE covers a group of clinically similar disorders whose pathogenesis is often unknown. They are autosomal recessively inherited. Mutation in *TGM1* is the cause of some cases (see the preceding section); however, there are cases in which *TGM1* is normal. Complete lack of activity in *TGM1* causes lamellar ichthyosis, and partial lack of activity of *TGM1* causes CIE. Cases with mutation in *ABCA12* and *ALOXE3* have been reported.

Treatment
The same topical treatments as those for ichthyosis vulgaris are effective, as are oral retinoids. The skin should be kept clean to prevent secondary infection.

Epidermolytic ichthyosis (synonym: bullous congenital ichthyosiform erythroderma (BCIE))
Clinical features
Patients with epidermolytic ichthyosis are sometimes born as collodion babies. Diffuse flushing is found. Recurring blistering may occur at the parts that receive physical irritation during early childhood. The blistering abates with age, and hyperkeratosis becomes distinct. Severe keratinization becomes persistent in later childhood (Fig. 15.6). The thickly keratinized plaques are accompanied by flush and a characteristic odor. The whole body, including the flexures of joints and the extremities, appears erythrodermic and dark rose in color. Mutation in keratin 1 results in hyperkeratosis in the palms and soles, but the symptoms caused by mutation in keratin 10 do not involve the palms and soles. The prognosis is favorable.

Pathogenesis
The cytoskeleton (intermediate filaments) of suprabasal cells is composed of keratin 1 and keratin 10. Because of mutation in the keratin 1 or keratin 10 gene, abnormal keratin fiber formation, cytoskeletal distortion, and epidermal blistering occur, leading to secondary hyperkeratinization (see Fig. 1.16). Most cases are autosomal dominantly inherited.

Pathology
The stratum corneum and suprabasal cell layer thicken, keratin fibers aggregate and there are vacuolated cells containing large keratohyaline granules in the granular and suprabasal cell layers (granular degenerationl Fig. 15.7).

Diagnosis and treatment
Blistering is marked, particularly in newborns. It is necessary to differentiate epidermolytic ichthyosis from

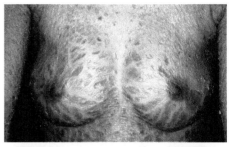
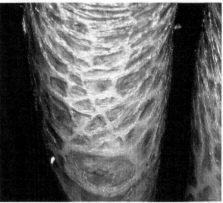

Fig. 15.4 Lamellar ichthyosis. Large, dark brown scales are characteristic of lamellar ichthyosis.

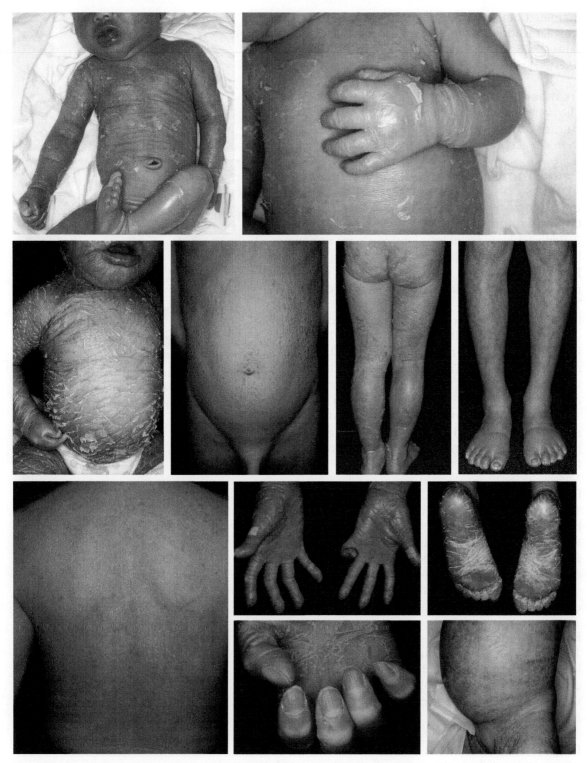

Fig. 15.5 Congenital ichthyosiform erythroderma. Erosive flushing and fine scales are seen on the whole body. Blistering does not occur.

epidermolysis bullosa, incontinentia pigmenti, and impetigo contagiosa by the pathological findings. The treatments are oral retinoids and topical moisturizers.

Superficial epidermolytic ichthyosis (synonym: ichthyosis bullosa of Siemens)

This is an autosomal dominant inherited disease caused by mutation in the keratin 2e gene expressed in the granular cell layers. Localized granular degeneration is histopathologically seen in part of the uppermost prickle layer and granular layer. Cutaneous symptoms resembling epidermolytic ichthyosis occur, but these are milder (Fig. 15.8).

Loricrin keratoderma

This is autosomal dominantly inherited. Loricrin keratoderma is a term for a keratinization disorder caused by mutation in the gene coding for loricrin, which is a structural component of the marginal band of corneocytes. The concept of loricrin keratoderma overlaps with those of keratosis palmoplantaris mutilans (Vohwinkel) and progressive erythrokeratoderma.

Ichthyosis syndrome

Ichthyosis syndrome is a general term for a rare congenital ichthyosis with the involvement of certain extracutaneous organs. Most of the cutaneous symptoms resemble those of congenital ichthyosiform erythroderma. The most frequently occurring types of ichthyosis syndrome are listed in Table 15.3.

Netherton syndrome

This is autosomal recessively inherited. It is caused by a mutation in the *SPINK5* gene, which encodes a serine protease inhibitor. The eruptions resemble congenital ichthyosiform erythroderma or atopic dermatitis (Fig. 15.9). Double-edged scales at the periphery of erythema are a characteristic clinical feature, and the disorder is also called ichthyosis linearis circumflexa. Scalp hair becomes knotted, short, and easily broken (bamboo hair). Disturbance in growth and mental retardation may accompany the disorder. Care should be taken when applying topical tacrolimus, because the agent is more readily absorbed in patients with this disorder, so the concentration of the agent in the patient's blood will be higher.

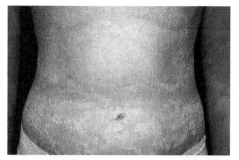
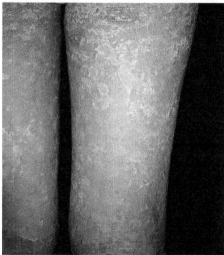
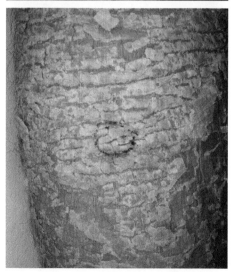

Fig. 15.6-1 Epidermolytic ichthyosis. Skin lesions accompanied by flushing and thick keratinization occur on the whole body surface.

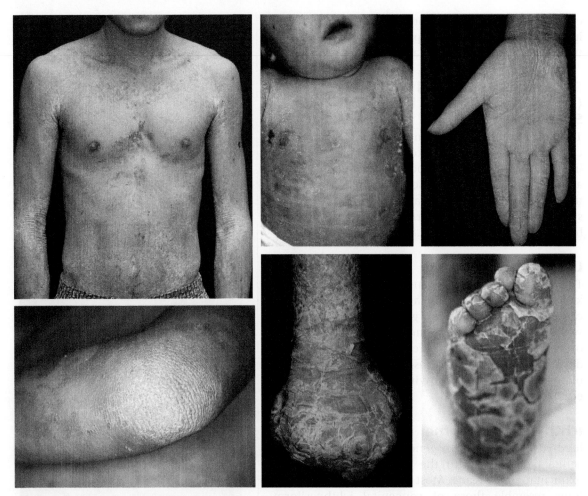

Fig. 15.6-2 Epidermolytic ichthyosis. Flushing appears on the whole body. Severe, dark keratinization with a dirty appearance occurs on the hands and feet (often in cases of mutation in the keratin 10 gene).

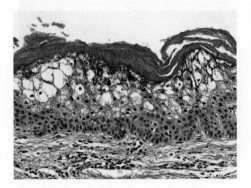

Fig. 15.7 Histopathology of epidermolytic ichthyosis. Granular degeneration occurs in the epidermis.

Sjögren–Larsson syndrome

This is autosomal recessively inherited. The main characteristics are congenital ichthyosis, spasmodic acroparalysis, and mild-to-moderate mental retardation (Fig. 15.10). There is abnormality in the gene that encodes fatty aldehyde dehydrogenase (*ALDH3A2*). Cutaneous symptoms are marked on the neck, lower abdomen, and flexures of the extremities.

Keratitis, ichthyosis, and deafness (KID) syndrome

This is autosomal dominantly inherited. KID syndrome is caused by mutation in the *GJB2* gene that encodes connexin 26. The main symptoms are keratitis, ichthyosis, and deafness. Papillomatous or prickle keratotic lesions occur mainly on the face and extremities. Hair loss and keratinization in the palms and soles occur (Fig. 15.11).

Dorfman–Chanarin syndrome (neutral lipid storage disease with ichthyosis)

This is a disorder with abnormality in the metabolism of neutral lipids. It is autosomal recessively inherited. The cause of the disorder is mutation in the *ABHD5 (CGI58)* gene. Triacylglycerol stored in the cytoplasm of various cells forms fat droplets. It is accompanied by ichthyosiform erythroderma and by other symptoms, including liver disorder, deafness, mental retardation, cataracts, and nystagmus (Fig. 15.12).

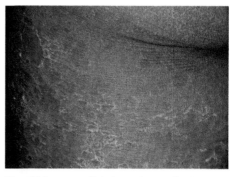

Fig. 15.8 Superficial epidermolytic ichthyosis. The clinical symptoms of flushing and hyperkeratosis are those of a mild case.

Table 15.3 Major ichthyosis syndromes.

Disease	Inheritance pattern	Eruptions	Other symptoms	Causative genes
Netherton syndrome	AR	Atopic dermatitis-like, ichthyosis linearis circumflexa, bamboo hair	Atopic condition, mental retardation, growth retardation	SPINK5
Sjögren–Larsson syndrome	AR	Congenital ichthyosiform erythroderma	Mental retardation, spasmodic acroparalysis	ALDH3A2 (FALDH)
KID syndrome	AD	Spinous hyperkeratosis of the face and extremities, hair loss, palmoplantar keratoderma	Hearing loss, keratitis	GJB2
Dorfman–Chanarin syndrome	AR	Congenital ichthyosiform erythroderma	Lipid droplets in leukocytes, hepatic, steatosis, cataracts, neurological manifestations	ABHD5(CGI58)
Refsum syndrome	AR	Ichthyosis vulgaris-like skin condition	Retinitis pigmentosa, polyneuropathy, cerebellar ataxia, inner ear deafness	PHYT,PEX7
Conradi–Hünermann–Happle syndrome	XD	Congenital ichthyosiform erythroderma (accompanied by atrophy)	Skeletal defects, cataract, punctate shadow at bone ends, quadriplegia	EBP
Rud syndrome	AR	Congenital ichthyosiform erythroderma	Seizure, mental retardation, low height, gonadal hypofunction	
Erythrokeratodermia variabili	AD	Keratotic lesions and migratory erythema	Hearing loss and cerebellar ataxia	GJB3,GJB4

AD, autosomal dominantly inherited; AR, autosomal recessively inherited; XD, X-linked dominantly inherited.

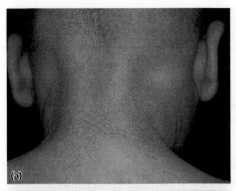

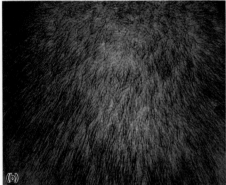

Fig. 15.9 Netherton syndrome. a: It is accompanied by atopic dermatitis-like eruptions and congenital ichthyosiform erythroderma-like eruptions. b: The scalp hair becomes knotted and easily breaks at the knots, resulting in short hair (bamboo hair).

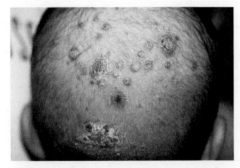

Fig. 15.11 KID syndrome. Hair loss and hyperkeratotic papules are seen.

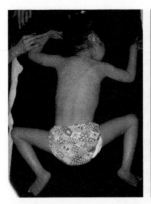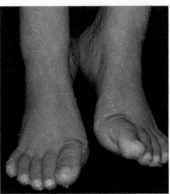

Fig. 15.10 Sjögren–Larsson syndrome. Congenital ichthyosiform erythroderma-like eruptions occur.

Refsum syndrome

This is autosomal recessively inherited. Refsum syndrome is a peroxisomal disorder that is caused by mutations in genes (e.g., *PHYT*) involved in the metabolism of phytanic acid in foods. Cutaneous eruptions resembling ichthyosis vulgaris occur in adolescence. The accompanying symptoms include rentinitis pigmentosa, cerebellar ataxia, multiple neuritis polyneuritis, and hearing loss. Increases in blood phytanic acid are found by peroxisomal disease diagnostic panel test.

Conradi–Hünermann–Happle syndrome

In addition to the symptoms of congenital ichthyosiform erythroderma with short stature, chondrodystropy and cataract are found. The disorder is a type of chondrodysplasia punctata. X-linked dominantly inherited, it is caused by mutation in the *EBP* gene. Males with this disorder tend to die in utero.

Erythrokeratodermia variabilis

See Chapter 15.

Acquired ichthyosis

Acquired ichthyosis occurs in association with a malignant tumor (e.g., malignant lymphoma), sarcoidosis and drug intake.

The clinical features resemble those of ichthyosis vulgaris, but acquired ichthyosis involves not only the extensor surfaces but also the flexor surfaces of the joints.

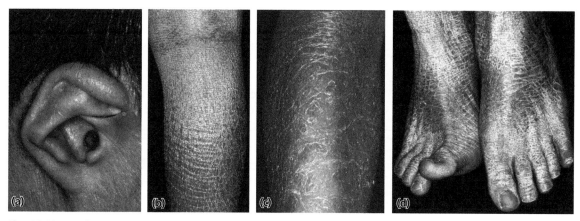

Fig. 15.12 Dorfman–Chanarin syndrome. Clinically, skin lesions similar to those of congenital ichthyosiform erythroderma are present.

Clinical features and pathology

Cutaneous eruptions resembling those of ichthyosis vulgaris occur. Not only are the extensor surfaces of the joints involved, but so are the flexor surfaces (Fig. 15.13). It also resembles ichthyosis vulgaris histopathologically.

Pathogenesis

Acquired ichthyosis may result from malignant tumors (e.g., malignant lymphoma (Hodgkin's disease in particular), leukemia, internal malignancy, Kaposi's sarcoma) or systemic disorder (e.g., sarcoidosis, hypothyroidism, Hansen's disease, tuberculosis, SLE, AIDS).

Diagnosis

Differentiation from other types of congenital ichthyoses is impossible only from the cutaneous symptoms or pathological findings. The clinical course and determination of the underlying disease are important for diagnosis.

Palmoplantar keratoderma (PPK)

Definition and classification

Palmoplantar keratoderma is a generic term for diseases that hereditarily cause hyperkeratosis in the palms and soles. It is subclassified by clinical features and patterns of inheritance (Fig. 15.14; Table 15.4). Genetic mutations are identified in some cases. Further

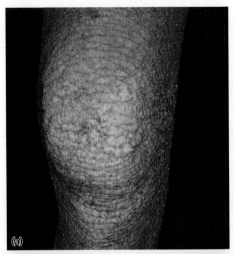

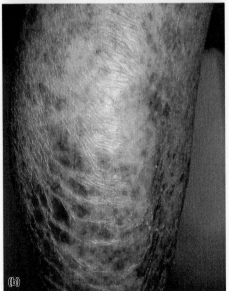

Fig. 15.13 Acquired ichthyosis. a: A case that accompanied Hodgkin's disease. b: A case that accompanied mycosis fungoides.

clarification is necessary for exact classification of palmoplantar keratoderma. The main types of palmoplantar keratoderma are discussed below.

Treatment

There is no effective treatment for any types. Oral retinoids and topical salicylic acid petrolatum and other moisturizers are used.

Unna–Thost palmoplantar keratoderma (synonym: diffuse non-epidermolytic palmoplantar keratoderma)

This is autosomal dominantly inherited. Localized diffuse lesions with a red halo form on the palms and soles of infants. Excessive sweating on the palms and soles is often observed. The dorsa of the hands and feet are not involved. Thickening of the stratum corneum and epidermis is seen. The genetic causes are thought to be various, and mutation in the keratin 1 gene is found in some cases.

Vörner palmoplantar keratoderma (synonym: diffuse epidermolytic palmoplantar keratoderma)

This is autosomal dominantly inherited. Differentiation from Unna–Thost palmoplantar keratoderma can be made by histopathological detection of granular degeneration; such differentiation is impossible from clinical findings. Mutation in the keratin 9 gene is found in most cases, and mutation in keratin 1 has also been reported.

Mal de Meleda

This is autosomal recessively inherited. Mutation in the *ARS B* (*SLURP-1*) gene is responsible for Mal de Meleda. This disease is often seen in offspring of consanguineous marriages. It hardly ever occurs in Asians. Hyperkeratosis accompanied by flush appears immediately after birth. Keratinization progresses and extends to the dorsae of the hands, feet, knees, and elbows, forming constriction rings as the patient ages. Mental retardation may occur.

Keratosis palmoplantaris transgrediens Nagashima

The symptoms are relatively mild, similar to those of Mal de Meleda. It is autosomal recessively inherited.

The *ARS B* gene is normal. The pathogenesis has not been identified.

Keratosis palmoplantaris linearis/striata

This is autosomal dominantly inherited. Band-like linear or round hyperkeratosis is present in the palms and soles. Mutations in the desmoglein 1, desmoplakin, and keratin 1 genes have been found in some patients.

Keratosis palmoplantaris mutilans (Vohwinkel)

Keratosis occurs in the palms and soles, which leads to strangulation obstruction or rupture in fingers and toes as a result of constriction rings (Fig. 15.15). Honeycomb-shaped keratinized plaques develop on the dorsae of the hands and feet, and on the elbows and kneecaps. Mutation in the loricrin gene has been reported.

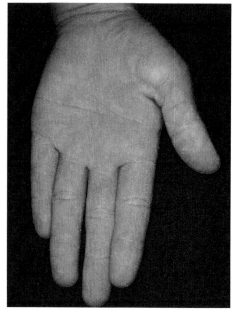

Fig. 15.14-1 Palmoplantar keratoderma.

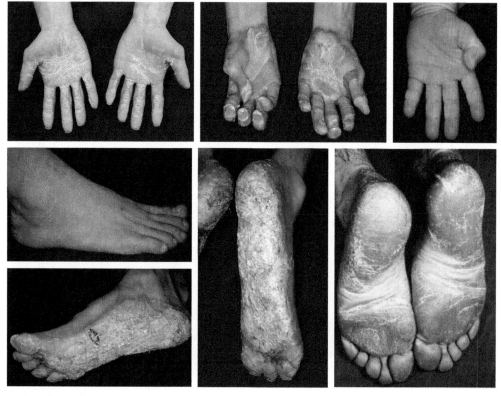

Fig. 15.14-2 Palmoplantar keratoderma. Keratinization of varying severity is present on the hands and feet. It is often difficult to determine the subtype by the clinical findings alone.

Table 15.4 Major types of palmoplantar keratoderma.

Disease	Inheritance pattern	Age of onset	Eruptions	Other symptoms
Unna–Thost keratoderma	AD	Babyhood, infancy	Diffuse keratotic eruption with a red halo in the periphery localized on the palms and soles	Hyperhidrosis on the palms and soles
Vörner keratoderma	AD	Babyhood, infancy	Unna–Thost keratoderma-like eruption	Granular degeneration (histologically)
Mal de Meleda	AR	Babyhood	Hyperkaratosis accompanied by flushing, spreading to the dorsum of hands and feet with age	Mental retardation
Dominant Mal de Meleda keratoderma	AD	Infancy, early childhood	Resembles eruptions in Mal de Meleda; however, keratosis and flushing are milder	
Keratosis palmoplantaris transgrediens Nagashima	AR	Babyhood, infancy	Mild keratosis on the dorsum of hands and feet	
Keratosis palmoplantaris linearis/striata	AD	Infancy, early childhood	Linear, band-like or round hyperkaratosis on the palms and soles	
Keratosis palmoplantaris mutilans (Vohwinkel)	AD	Babyhood, infancy	Honeycomb-shaped keratinization in the palms and constriction rings around the fingers	Loss of parts of fingers and toes may occur.
Punctate palmoplantar keratoderma	AD	Infancy, early childhood	Multiple, firm, punctate keratotic papules on the palms and soles	It may be accompanied by nail deformation.
Papillon–Lefevre syndrome	AR	Babyhood, infancy	The symptoms resemble those of Mal de Meleda.	Gingivitis, loss of teeth

AD, autosomal dominantly inherited; AR, autosomal recessively inherited.

Other hereditary keratoses

Darier's disease (synonyms: keratosis follicularis, Darier–White disease)

Keratotic papules of 2–5 mm in diameter appear, mainly on seborrheic and intertriginous areas. The papules coalesce to form plaques. The condition is aggravated by perspiration in summer. It is caused by a mutation in a calcium pump (SERCA2) within keratinocytes. It is autosomal dominantly inherited. The characteristic pathological findings are acantholysis, lacunae, corps ronds, and grains.

Clinical features

The onset of Darier's disease is generally between age 10 and 20. Multiple dark brown keratotic papules of 2–5 mm in diameter occur in the seborrheic and intertriginous areas, such as the neck, axillary fossae, sternal region, inframammary region, abdomen, and groin, and the papules coalesce to form plaques (Fig. 15.16). Itching is present. On perspiratory intertriginous areas, papules coalesce and papillary or condyloma-like proliferation occurs. The papules may be moist and foul-smelling. Bacterial or viral infection (e.g., Kaposi's varicelliform eruption) may occur secondarily. The characteristic clinical features are keratotic papules and punctuate depressions in the palms and soles. Small papules in the oral mucosa, nail plate fragility and sometimes nervous symptoms such as mental retardation are seen.

Pathogenesis

This is autosomal dominantly inherited. Darier's disease is caused by mutation in the *ATP2A2* gene, which encodes the SERCA2 calcium pump. That pump controls the calcium concentration in the cytoplasm of keratinocytes. Since calcium regulates the intercellular adhesion and differentiation of keratinocytes, the genetic mutation promotes keratinization and abnormal formation of desmosomes and keratin fiber complexes, leading to abnormal dyskeratosis and acantholysis.

Pathology

Darier's disease is characterized by dyskeratosis. Corps ronds (large round cells with basophilic pyknotic nuclei and bright cytoplasm) are found in the upper part of the suprabasal cell layer, and grains (long, thin,

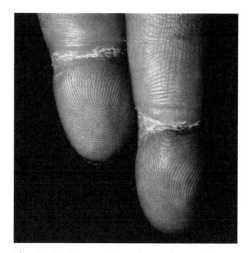

Fig. 15.15 Keratosis palmoplantaris mutilans (Vohwinkel).

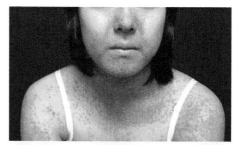

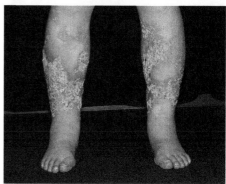

Fig. 15.16-1 Darier's disease. Dark brown, keratotic papules on the whole body.

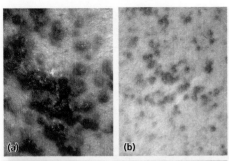

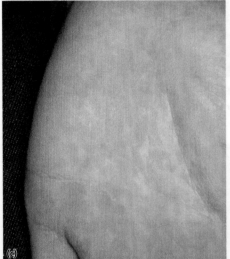

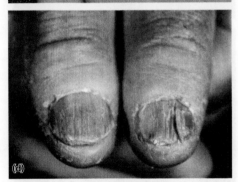

Fig. 15.16-2 Darier's disease. a,b: Keratotic papules. c: Verrucous keratinization on the palm. d: Changes of nail plates.

dark-staining cells) are found in the granular layer. There is acantholysis, its accompanying lacunae formation, and villi formation in which the dermal papillae extend upwards into the lacunae (Fig. 15.17).

Differential diagnosis

Darier's disease should be differentiated from Hailey–Hailey disease, acanthosis nigricans, and seborrheic dermatitis.

Treatment

The symptoms are improved temporarily by oral retinoid. Urea ointments are also useful. Secondary infections and sun exposure should be avoided.

Erythrokeratodermia

Localized keratotic lesions accompanied by flush may be produced in infancy; erythrokeratodermia is the generic term for these clinical conditions. There are various clinical features and causative genes (Fig. 15.18). The following are the major types of erythrokeratodermia.

Progressive symmetrical erythrokeratodermia

This is autosomal dominantly inherited. In some cases, mutation in the gene encoding loricrin has been identified. Localized, sharply circumscribed flushing and keratotic lesions are present. The extremities are most commonly affected. It often appears symmetrically. The lesions extend with time. The main treatment is oral retinoid.

Erythrokeratodermia variabilis

This is autosomal dominantly inherited. In some cases, mutation in connexin (*GJB3*, *GJB4*) has been identified. Localized, dark rose keratotic lesions appear on the face, trunk, and extremities of infants. The lesions often spread and coalesce. Sharply circumscribed, map-like erythema of several centimeters in diameter also appears. They recur at different sites, as if moving, in several minutes to days. The condition is usually asymptomatic. Hearing loss and cerebellar ataxia are seen in some cases. The main treatment is oral retinoid.

Ectodermal dysplasia and skin fragility syndrome

See Chapter 14.

Acquired keratoses

Inflammatory keratosis

Psoriasis

- This most frequently occurs in young and middle-aged men and women. Erythema and papules are accompanied by thick, silvery-white scales. Inflammation in the epidermis and accelerated turnover of epidermal cells are found.
- It is classified by clinical features into five types: psoriasis vulgaris, guttate psoriasis, pustular psoriasis, psoriatic erythroderma, and psoriatic arthritis.
- Auspitz phenomenon and Köbner phenomenon are characteristic features.
- The pathological findings are thickening of the epidermis, vasodilation in the papillary dermis, and neutrophilic infiltration directly under the stratum corneum (Munro's microabscess).
- The main treatments are application of activated vitamin D3 ointments and topical steroids, and PUVA and narrow-band UVB therapies. Ciclosporin, retinoids, and biologics such as monoclonal antibodies are used in severe cases.

Epidemiology and classification

Psoriasis occurs in 1–2% of Caucasians and about 0.02–0.1% of ethnic Japanese. Men outnumber women by 2 to 1. It most frequently affects persons in their 20s to 40s.

Psoriasis is classified by symptoms into five types: psoriasis vulgaris (mainly keratotic erythema accompanied by scaling), guttate psoriasis (scattered small lesions with a diameter of 1 cm or less), pustular psoriasis (mainly sterile pustular eruptions), psoriatic erythroderma, and psoriatic arthritis (psoriasis arthropathica) (Table 15.5). Some cases change from one type to another. Psoriasis vulgaris accounts for an overwhelming majority of all cases. Each type is described below.

Pathogenesis

The turnover from basal cell to corneocyte to exfoliation, which normally takes 28 days, takes only 4–7 days, because of enhanced proliferation of epidermal cells. The pathogenesis is unknown. Multiple factors may be involved.

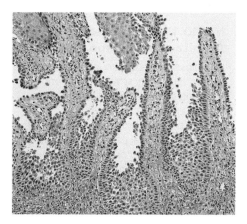

Fig. 15.17 Histopathology of Darier's disease. Acantholysis, fissures, and villi are seen.

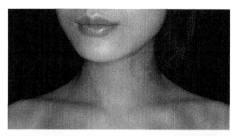

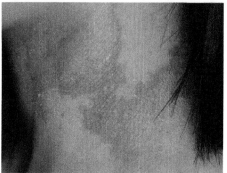

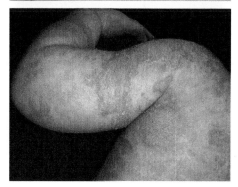

Fig. 15.18 Erythrokeratodermia variabilis. Sharply demarcated keratotic erythema.

MEMO 15–1 Laboratory findings on psoriasis: wax-fragment phenomenon, Auspitz phenomenon, Köbner phenomenon

When psoriatic eruptions are scraped with a fingernail, white scales that resemble wax flakes are seen. Exfoliation of the scales easily causes petechia; this is called Auspitz phenomenon. It is caused by the intrusion of dermal papillae immediately under the stratum corneum. Stimulation, such as scratching, may induce eruptions at normal sites of skin in patients with psoriasis (Köbner phenomenon).

Waxy silver-gray flakes and lamellar scales occur easily (wax-fragment phenomenon).

Petechia is caused by reduction in the granular layer and telangiectasia (Auspitz phenomenon).

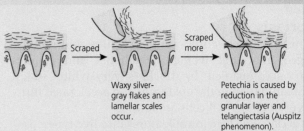

Laboratory findings on psoriasis: wax-fragment phenomenon, Auspitz phenomenon, Köbner phenomenon.

Table 15.5 Types and findings of psoriasis.

	Clinical findings	Pathological findings
Psoriasis vulgaris	Red papules become sharply demarcated erythema that is accompanied by silver-white scales. Scratching generates silvery-opaque scale. Auspitz phenomenon, Köbner phenomenon	Parakeratosis, Munro's microabscess, club-shaped epidermal rete ridges, capillary vasodilation
Guttate psoriasis	The same severity as psoriasis valgaris. The eruptions are up to 10 mm in diameter.	Munro's microabscess, club-shaped epidermal rete ridges, capillary vasodilation
Pustular psoriasis	Sterile pustules on erythema, fever, malaise	Kogoj's spongiform pustules
Psoriatic erythroderma	Diffuse flushing, fine scales on the whole body	
Psoriatic arthritis	Arthritis precedes or accompanies the psoriasis. Rheumatoid factors are negative.	Munro's microabscess, club-shaped epidermal rete ridges, capillary vasodilation

Genetic

Psoriasis is strongly familial, and multiple genes are involved. Many cases are familial, especially in Caucasians. HLA-Cw6 and HLA-B13 are associated with the occurrence. Involvement of disease susceptibility genes, including *PSORS1*, has been suggested.

Extrinsic

Physical irritation (e.g., injury, sunlight (Köbner phenomenon)), infections (hemolytic streptococcus), and drugs (lithium, β-blockers, calcium antagonists, interferon) have been identified as inductive factors (see also Table 10.1).

Immunological

Th1 immunoreaction occurs in the lesions. The lesions are thought to be formed by various cytokines (e.g., TNF-α) produced by lymphocytes, corneocytes, and endocapillary cells. The involvement of T cells (Th17) that produce IL-17 in chronic inflammation has been identified.

Pathology

Inflammation occurs most severely in the upper epidermal layer (Fig. 15.19). As the epidermal turnover is abnormally enhanced, epidermal cells forming the stratum corneum retain their nuclei (parakeratosis). Hyperkeratosis is present. Munro's microabscesses caused by infiltration of neutrophils are found directly below the stratum corneum. Because epidermal cells move to the stratum corneum before they produce keratohyaline granules, the granular layer disappears. The suprabasal cell layer thickens and the epidermal rete ridges become club-shaped and extend toward the dermis (regular acanthosis). The dermal papillae extend upwards to just below the epidermis, and there is proliferation and vasodilation of capillary blood vessels. Infiltration of lymphocytes is found at the periphery of blood vessels in the superficial dermis. In pustular psoriasis, multiple neutrophils infiltrate into the upper suprabasal cell layer, and epidermal cells are destroyed to form a spongiosis called Kogoj's spongiform pustule (Fig. 15.20, Fig. 15.21).

Laboratory findings

Köbner phenomenon and Auspitz phenomenon are present. Antistreptolysin O (ASO) titer is elevated in guttate psoriasis in which streptococcal infection is present. In pustular psoriasis and psoriatic erythroderma, elevated erythrocyte sedimentation rate, leukocytosis, hypocalcemia, and hypoproteinemia may be caused. In psoriatic arthritis, rheumatoid factors are usually negative.

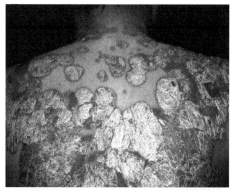

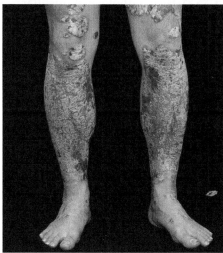

Fig. 15.19 Cases of psoriasis vulgaris. Erythema is accompanied by marked silvery-white scales.

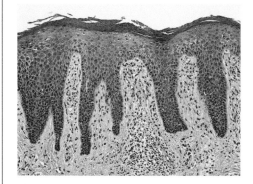

Fig. 15.20 Histopathology of psoriasis. There is hyperkeratosis and club-shaped extension of the epidermis (regular acanthosis).

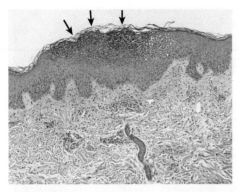

Fig. 15.21 Histopathology of pustular psoriasis (Kogoj's spongiform pustule (arrows)). Spongiosis with infiltration of neutrophils is seen in the suprabasal cell layer.

Diagnosis and differential diagnosis

Psoriasis is diagnosed by the characteristic clinical findings; however, a biopsy may be conducted for differential diagnosis. The diagnostic criteria are shown in Table 15.6. In pustular psoriasis, the pustules are sterile. To assess the severity of the case, the psoriatic area and severity index (PASI score) shown in Table 15.7 are mainly used.

Treatment and prognosis

The disease becomes chronic, with recurrent aggravation and remission. The main treatments are topical active forms of vitamin D3 ointments and steroids. Occlusive dressing therapy (ODT) may be used.

PUVA and narrow-band UVB therapies are also effective. Oral retinoids, ciclosporin, and methotrexate are used in severe cases. Oral steroids tend not to be used because they may induce pustular psoriasis. Recently, treatments using biologics such as

Table 15.6 Differential diagnosis of psoriasis.

Disease	Points for differentiation
Seborrheic dermatitis	The clinical findings resemble those of psoriasis, but the affected sites are relatively localized at seborrheic areas
Chronic eczema, nummular eczema	Various localized skin lesions including erythema, scales, papules, and blisters. Intense itching. The lesions are less clearly margined than in psoriasis.
Parapsoriasis	Pigmentation and atrophy are often present, and mild scaling occurs.
Pityriasis rosea (Gibert)	Psoriasis-like lesions appear after manifestation of the first eruption, and disappear in 1 or 2 months.
Mycosis fungoides	Clinical findings may resemble those of psoriasis. Histopathological infiltration of atypical lymphocytes to the epidermis (Pautrier's microabscess)
Syphilitic psoriasis	Psoriasis-like eruptions on palms and soles. History taking and serological test for syphilis are important.
Ankylosing spondylitis	Psoriasis-like eruptions in some cases; differentiation from psoriatic arthritis is important.

Table 15.7 Simplified table for calculating for PASI score (assessment of psoriasis severity).

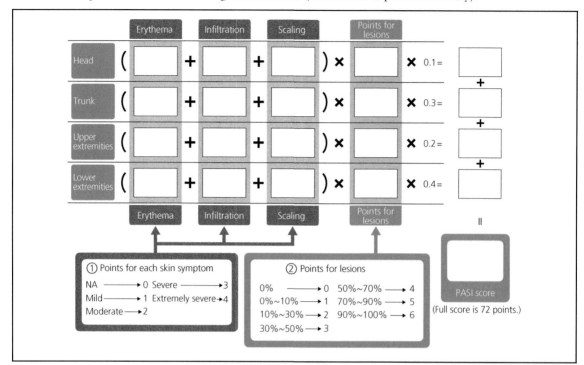

monoclonal antibodies (see Table 6.9) have been used in severe cases.

Psoriasis vulgaris

Rose pink papules appear and extend to coalesce gradually into sharply circumscribed erythematous plaques of 1 cm to several centimeters in diameter with thick silvery scales on the surface (Fig. 15.22). Psoriasis vulgaris is sometimes asymptomatic, but is often accompanied by itchiness. Areas that are subjected to external stimulation, such as the elbows, patellae, scalp (hairline in particular), and buttocks, are most commonly involved. The disorder may also occur in the intertriginous areas of obese people. Changes in the nails (coarse surface and punctate depressions) also occur frequently.

Guttate psoriasis

Keratotic erythemas of up to 1 cm in diameter occur multiply on the trunk and proximal sides of the extremities with a relatively acute course. Individual eruptions are the same as those of psoriasis vulgaris. It

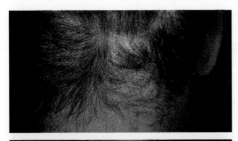

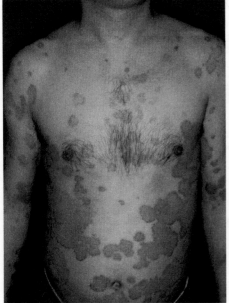

Fig. 15.22-1 Psoriasis vulgaris.

is often seen in children. Streptococcal infection in the upper respiratory tract or drugs can be causative factors. The condition tends to disappear within several months.

Pustular psoriasis

Sterile pustules are the main clinical feature. The disorder is subdivided into a generalized type and a localized type (Table 15.8). In the generalized type, fever, systemic fatigue and chills accompany erythema on which multiple sterile pustules occur and coalesce into larger "lakes of pus." The pustules rupture spontaneously to form erosions. Exudative fluid may cause hypoproteinemia, leading to marked systemic aggravation in some cases. It may occur in the course of psoriasis vulgaris, or it may develop suddenly without any history of psoriasis (Fig. 15.23).

Psoriatic erythroderma

Psoriatic skin lesions appear all over the body and become erythroderma (Fig. 15.24). Psoriasis vulgaris and pustular psoriasis often progress into psoriatic erythroderma. Hypoproteinemia, dehydration, and hypocalcemia often occur.

Psoriatic arthritis

In psoriatic arthritis, arthritis symptoms accompany the psoriasis (Fig. 15.25). Psoriatic arthritis is found in 10–15% of patients with psoriasis, and the severity of the arthritis often corresponds to the progression of the cutaneous symptoms. Most of the cases are those with symptoms resembling asymmetrical arthritis (i.e., single or multiple joints in the hand and foot are involved); however, there are cases resembling rheumatoid arthritis and ankylosing spondylitis. Arthritis proceeds without psoriatic skin lesions in many cases. There is an association with the *HLA-Cw6* gene.

Pityriasis rubra pilaris
Clinical features

Pityriasis rubra pilaris (PRP) frequently affects the palms and soles, the extensor surfaces of the extremities (elbows and knees in particular), and the thoracoabdominal region. The symptoms start with follicular hyperkeratotic papules of 1–2 mm in diameter, which coalesce to present sharply circumscribed, orange to red, irregularly shaped plaques to which scales are attached (Fig. 15.26). Multiple white keratotic papules also occur with a coarse, grater-like appearance. Diffuse keratosis is seen on the palms and soles. It is usually asymptomatic. Mild itchiness and painful fissures in the palms and soles may occur. Lesions sometimes become erythroderma with round patches of normal skin.

Pathogenesis and epidemiology

Although some suggest that abnormality in vitamin A metabolism is responsible for PRP, the etiology is unknown. There are peaks of occurrence at infancy and in the fifth and sixth decades of life; PRP is divided into a juvenile type and an adult type. About half of patients have the adult type. Juvenile PRP is sometimes autosomal dominantly inherited. Some cases accompanying HIV infection have been reported.

Pathology

The follicles are dilated and filled with keratin. The peripheral epidermis is thickened and there is parakeratosis in some parts. Complete keratinization alternates with incomplete keratinization. Neutrophils do not infiltrate into the epidermis, which is useful for differentiation from psoriasis. Vasodilation and lymphocytic infiltration are observed in the upper dermis.

Differential diagnosis

Pityriasis rubra pilaris should be differentiated from psoriasis, cutaneous T cell lymphoma, seborrheic dermatitis, drug eruption, ichthyosis, and contralateral progressive erythrokeratoderma.

Treatment and prognosis

Both types heal spontaneously, within a year for the juvenile type and within 2–3 years for the adult type. The symptomatic therapies are application of salicylic acid petrolatum ointments, topical steroids, and active forms of vitamin D3 ointments. Oral retinoids are also used.

Parapsoriasis

- This is a generic term for diseases that produce multiple psoriasis-like keratotic erythematous lesions.
- Parapsoriasis is classified into two types based on the cutaneous features: parapsoriasis en plaque and pityriasis lichenoides.
- It is usually asymptomatic. Lesions with erythema and scaling appear. New eruptions are present together with older ones.

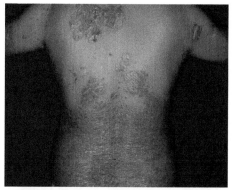
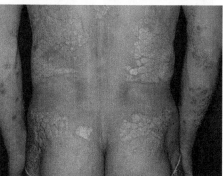
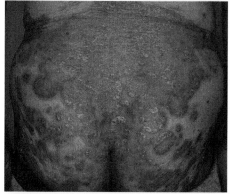
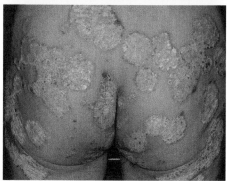

Fig. 15.22-2 Psoriasis vulgaris.

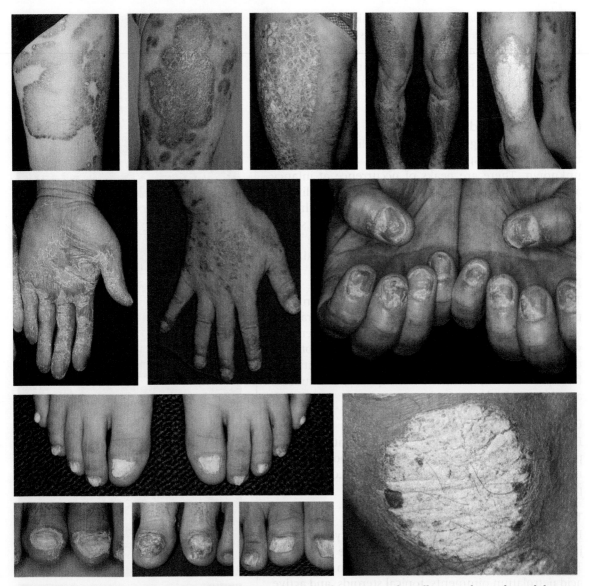

Fig. 15.22-3 Psoriasis vulgaris. Sharply demarcated, thick, silver-gray scales adhere to the surface of the erythematous plaques. Characteristic nail deformities.

- It progresses slowly over the course of several years.
- Topical steroids and PUVA therapy are the first-line treatments.

Classification

Parapsoriasis is classified into two types based on the clinical features: parapsoriasis en plaque and pityriasis lichenoides. The two types are further classified into subtypes (Table 15.9).

Table 15.8 Classification of pustular psoriasis.

		Classification	Clinical findings
Localized type	Localized pustular psoriasis		Pustules are localized around the plaques of psoriasis vulgaris.
	Pustular psoriasis with generalized skin lesions	Palmoplatar pustulosis (PPP)	Pustules are localized bilaterally on the thenar eminence and arch of the foot. See Chapter 14
		Acrodermatitis continua of Hallopeau	Often occurs secondarily after an exernal injury. Pustules and nail deformity occur on the tips of fingers or toes on one side of the body.
Generalized type	Generalized pustular psoriasis	von Zumbusch type	Multiple pustules suddenly occur with systemic symptoms. They tend to recur. Some cases progress from psoriasis vulgaris.
		Generalization of acrodermatitis continua	Rare
		Childhood generalized pustular psoriasis	Rare
		Impetigo herpetiformis	Pustules are generalized during the middle and last stages of pregnancy.
	Circinate annular form		Infants are most frequently affected. The systemic condition is good, but the lesions are intractable.

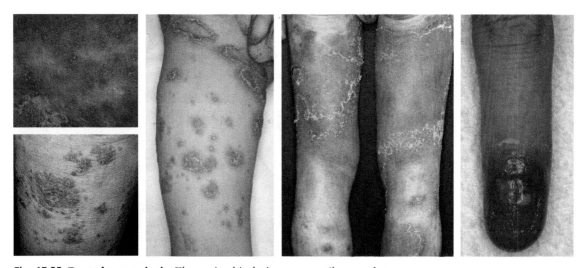

Fig. 15.23 Pustular psoriasis. The main skin lesions are sterile pustules.

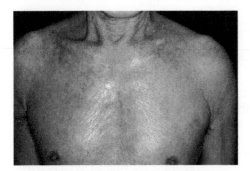

Fig. 15.24 Psoriatic erythroderma.

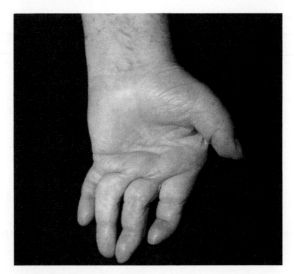

Fig. 15.25 Psoriatic arthritis.

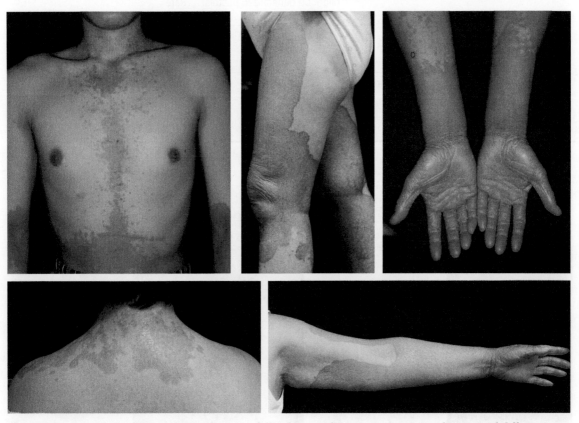

Fig. 15.26-1 Pityriasis rubra pilaris. There are follicular papules, orange psoriatic plaques and diffuse keratinization on the palms.

Pathogenesis

The pathogenesis is unknown. T cell infiltration at the epidermal-dermal junction is the main clinical feature; however, parapsoriasis varies from inflammatory disorders to conditions that precede mycosis fungoides.

Pathology

Parakeratosis and thickening of the epidermis are found. Notable lymphocytic infiltrates are seen in the epidermis and at the periphery of the blood vessels. Sometimes atypical cells are seen. In pityriasis lichenoides, vacuolar degeneration, spongiosis, dyskeratosis, leakage of erythrocytes, and ulceration may be found.

Differential diagnosis

It is necessary to differentiate parapsoriasis from psoriasis, seborrheic dermatitis, pityriasis rosea, and mycosis fungoides.

Treatment

Topical steroids and PUVA therapy are the first-line treatments. Large-plaque parapsoriasis may progress into mycosis fungoides or malignant lymphoma, so the clinical course should be observed regularly.

Parapsoriasis en plaque

Parapsoriasis en plaque most commonly affects middle-aged and elderly males. Pale pink, slightly scaling erythema with relatively clear borders is found on the trunk and extremities (Fig. 15.27). Although the name includes the term "en plaque," infiltration is not present. It is usually asymptomatic. Large-plaque parapsoriasis and small-plaque parapsoriasis are classified

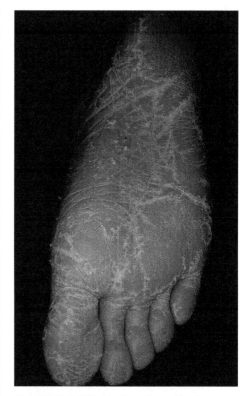

Fig. 15.26-2 Pityriasis rubra pilaris.

Table 15.9 Classification and features of parapsoriasis.

Parapsoriasis en plaque and pityriasis lichenoides
Clinical findings: pityroid scales and erythema appear. Itching is not present **Pathological findings**: lymphocytic infiltration in the dermo-dermal junctions • Large-plaque parapsoriasis: the eruption is 5 cm or more in diameter, accompanied by atrophy, and may be a precursor of mycosis fungoides in some cases. • Small-plaque parapsoriasis:the eruption is less than 5 cm in diameter.
Pityriasis lichenoides (guttate parapsoriasis)
Clinical findings: erythema of 1 cm or less in diameter, hyperkeratotic papules, old and new eruptions are present **Pathological findings**: lymphocytic infiltration to the epidermis, vacuolar degeneration, bleeding • Pityriasis lichenoides chronica (PLC) (previous guttate parapsoriasis): erythema with thin white scales, vesicles • Pityriasis lichenoides et varioliformis acuta (PLEVA): the main findings are severe inflammatory symptoms and ulceration.

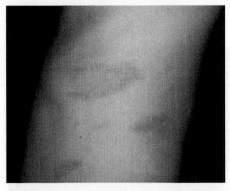

Fig. 15.27 Parapsoriasis en plaque. Mild, relatively sharply demarcated erythema is present.

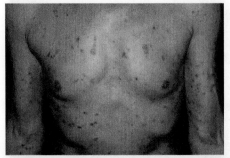

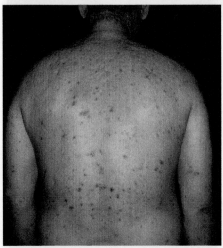

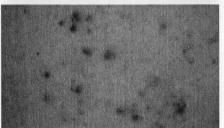

Fig. 15.28 Pityriasis lichenoides chronica (PLC). Old eruptions are rarely seen simultaneously with new ones on the lesion. Ulceration does not occur.

based on the size of the cutaneous eruptions. Large-plaque refers to lesions of 5 cm or more in diameter.

The large-plaque type is accompanied by mild atrophy, and 10–30% of the cases progress to mycosis fungoides. The small-plaque type often occurs as symmetrical multiple eruptions with pityroid scaling. Eruptions may fall along cleavage lines (digitate dermatosis).

Pityriasis lichenoides

Pityriasis lichenoides frequently occurs in young persons, and it tends to be limited to the trunk, thighs, and upper arms. The face and the palms and soles are not involved. Small keratotic papules of several millimeters to 1 cm in diameter continuously appear, and a distinguishing characteristic of the disorder is the presence of new eruptions concurrently with older ones. The eruptions heal with pigmentary changes and scarring. Pityriasis lichenoides is classified into the two types below based on the clinical course; however, there are many cases with the two types mixed or those that start as one type and progress to the other. Recurrent remissions and exacerbations are observed for many years in either case.

Pityriasis lichenoides chronica (PLC)

Erythema or small papules of up to 1 cm in diameter appear, to which white scales are attached (Fig. 15.28). The condition tends to be asymptomatic. The eruptions heal in several months. PLC was formerly called guttate parapsoriasis.

Pityriasis lichenoides et varioliformis acuta (PLEVA)

Multiple papules with crusts and ulceration accompanied by fever and fatigue occur (Fig. 15.29 and Fig. 15.30). The eruptions heal in several weeks and leave scarring. It was formerly called Mucha–Habermann disease.

Lichen planus (LP)

Flat-topped, elevated, grayish-blue to purplish-rose plaques form on the dorsa of the hands, on the extremities and in the oral mucosa. LP progresses slowly. It is often induced by drugs, hepatitis C, and dental metals. However, the cause is unknown. Köbner phenomenon is positive. White lines are seen on the surface (Wickham striae). Vacuolar degeneration is found histopathologically. Band-like infiltration of lymphocytes occurs in the superficial dermis.

Treatments include removal of the cause, application of topical tacrolimus, and topical steroids.

Clinical features

Lichen planus occurs in male and female adults. Polygonal or map-like, grayish-blue to purplish-red papules of 5–20 mm in diameter or flatly elevated, purplish-red erythema of coin size or smaller appear, often with a central concavity.

The erythema surface is either characteristically glossy or it has whitish scales attached. The eruptions may coalesce to form plaques (Fig. 15.31). Sometimes it is accompanied by intense itching. It often appears on the dorsa of the hands and extremities, and in the oral cavity and nails. In the oral mucosa, irregularly shaped infiltrative leukoderma, Wickham striae or erosive plaques are found. Intense pain may be present in some cases. Nail plate deformities, including ridges, thinning and pterygium, are seen (Fig. 15.32).

Pathogenesis

Cytotoxic reaction caused by $CD4^+$ T cells at the dermo-epidermal junction leads to dyskeratosis accompanied by impairment of basal keratinocytes, resulting in flatly elevated purplish-rose erythema or papules. It may be caused by drugs (antihypertensive agents, cerebral excitometabolic agents, antitubercular agents), hepatitis C or dental metals. Eruptions resembling lichen planus often appear after hematopoietic stem cell transplantation (MEMO, see Chapter 15).

Pathology

The pathological findings are hyperkeratosis that is not accompanied by parakeratosis, and wedge-shaped hypergranulosis, serrated extension of epidermal rete ridges, vacuolar degeneration and band-like lymphocytic infiltration in the papillae and lower papillary layer (Fig. 15.33). Degenerated corneocytes produced by the vacuolar degeneration are found in the superficial dermis (Civatte bodies). Melanophages are found in the dermis (incontinentia pigmenti histologica).

Laboratory findings and diagnosis

Lichen planus eruptions may appear when normal skin is rubbed or exposed to UVB (Köbner phenomenon is positive). Delicate grayish-white lines on the skin surface form a network on coalesced plaques (Wickham striae). Lichen planus is easily diagnosed by the clinical and pathological findings. History taking on drugs and

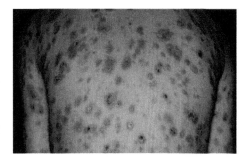

Fig. 15.29-1 Pityriasis lichenoides et varioliformis acuta (PLEVA). There are intense acute inflammatory symptoms, and old and new eruptions are present. These are accompanied by diffuse ulcers.

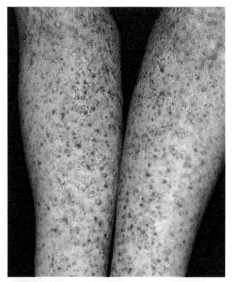

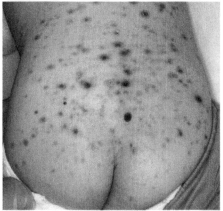

Fig. 15.29-2 Pityriasis lichenoides et varioliformis acuta (PLEVA).

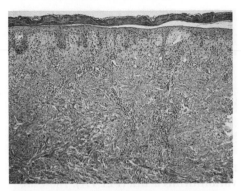

Fig. 15.30 Histopathology of pityriasis lichenoides et varioliformis acuta.
Vacuolar degeneration of basal cells and intense lymphocytic infiltration are observed.

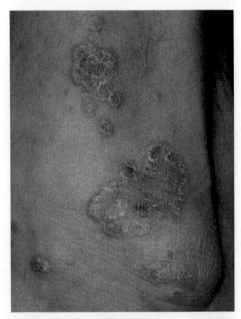

Fig. 15.31-1 Lichen planus. A typical case.

MEMO 15–3 Graft-versus-host disease (GVHD) and lichen planus

Lichen planus often occurs as a symptom of chronic GVHD after hematopoietic stem cell transplantation (see Chapter 10). GVHD results from destruction of host tissue caused by the immunological response of T cells, and the same mechanism is thought to be associated with the onset of lichen planus.

dental treatments is conducted to determine whether the lichen planus is induced by drugs or dental metal. Patch test is done if necessary.

Treatment and prognosis
The condition progresses chronically. The causative drug or other agent is determined and its use is discontinued. In drug-induced cases, eruptions often persist after discontinuation of use. Topical tacrolimus and steroids are used. Squamous cell carcinoma may occur from ulcerative lesions in the oral cavity and labial mucosa.

Lichen striatus
Clinical features and pathogenesis
Lichen striatus most frequently occurs in young children. Eruptions arrange in linear arrays or along cleavage lines, most frequently on the extremities on one side (Fig. 15.34). Lichen striatus begins as several light pink to dark rose papules 2–4 mm in diameter. The papules coalesce into linear or band-like eruptions about 1–2 cm in width. The condition is usually asymptomatic.

The etiology is unknown. Histopathologically, eczematous non-specific inflammation is observed.

Diagnosis, treatment, and prognosis
Differentiation from verrucous epidermal nevus, incontinentia pigmenti (second stage), verruca plana, and linear lichen planus is necessary. Most cases resolve after a few months. Topical steroids are used for treatment.

Lichen nitidus
Clinical features and pathogenesis
Lichen nitidus most commonly occurs in young people. Small papules of uniform size with a smooth, flat,

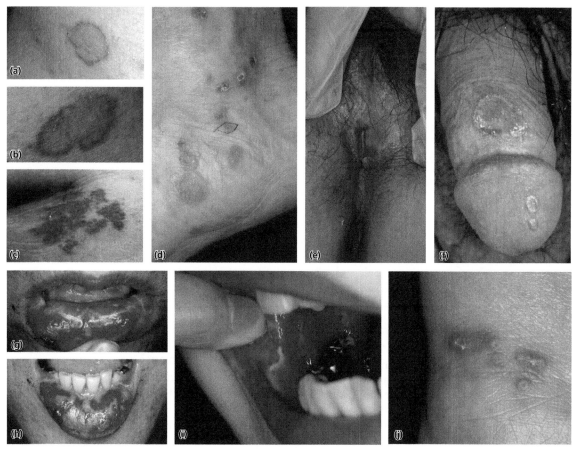

Fig. 15.31-2 Lichen planus. Various clinical features are seen. a,b: Lichen planus annularis. It is important to differentiate this from porokeratosis. Erythema at the periphery of the lesion is characteristic of lichen planus. c: Lichen planus pigmentosus. d: A typical case of lichen planus on the lower leg. e: It is necessary to differentiate this from lichen sclerosus. f: Multiple lichen planus on the foreskin and glans penis. g,h: Affected lips. i: Linear, white lichen planus near the molar teeth in the buccal mucous membrane. j: Typical lichen planus on the wrist.

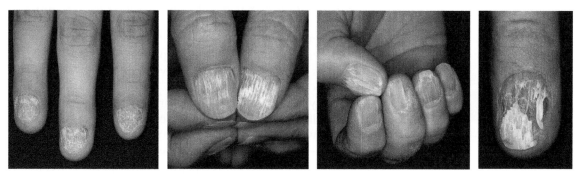

Fig. 15.32 Nail deformities in lichen planus. Atrophic changes to the nails.

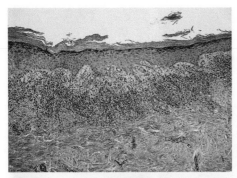

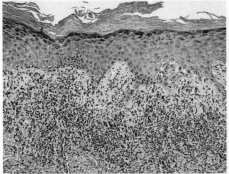

Fig. 15.33 Histopathology of lichen planus. Hyperkeratosis and hypergranulosis without parakeratosis characterize the disorder. Saw-toothed acanthosis, band-like lymphatic infiltration in the upper dermal layer and vacuolar degeneration in the basal layer are also seen.

glossy surface and a diameter of 1–2 mm occur. They can be scattered or aggregated (Fig. 15.35).

The eruptions do not coalesce or cause erythema; they are normal skin color to yellowish-white. Subjective symptoms such as itching are not present. The disorder frequently occurs on the lower abdomen, flexures of the extremities, and penis. Köbner phenomenon is observed in about 50% of all cases.

Pathology
Directly under the epidermal rete ridges that slightly extend from small papules, there are epithelioid cells, lymphocytes, and an infiltrative nest consisting of Langerhans giant cells. Vacuolar degeneration is also seen.

Treatment and prognosis
Most cases heal spontaneously in several months to a few years. If itchiness is present, topical steroids are used.

Pityriasis rosea (Gibert)
- This is transitory, inflammatory keratotic erythema of unknown etiology. It most commonly occurs in young men.
- Oval eruptions scatter mainly on the trunk, presenting as erythematous plaques with peripheral collarettes of scales. The long axes of the eruptions run parallel to the cleavage lines.
- The first eruption is called a herald patch.
- The disorder heals spontaneously in 1–3 months. Topical steroids are the first-line treatment.

Clinical features
Pityriasis rosea occurs frequently in men and women from the ages of about 10 to 40, especially in spring and autumn. Common cold-like symptoms precede the onset of some cases. About 50–90% of all cases begin as an eruption called a herald patch (Fig. 15.36). A round or oval light pink plaque with a diameter of 2–5 cm occurs, mainly on the trunk. The plaque is accompanied by scaling at the rim (collarette of the herald patch). Slightly yellowish central discoloration occurs with time. Two to 14 days after onset, multiple oval erythema of 1–2 cm diameter with peripheral scaling suddenly appear on the trunk and the proximal parts of the extremities. These eruptions vary in size, and the long axes run along

the Langer cleavage lines of the skin; a Christmas tree appearance is seen on the back. New eruptions continue to appear for several weeks. The eruptions spread from the trunk to distal areas; however, the palms, soles, and head are not involved. There are no severe systemic symptoms, except mild itching sometimes.

Pathogenesis
The cause is unknown. Hereditary predisposition and association with reactivation of HHV-6 and HHV-7 have been pointed out. Some eruptions induced by drugs or chemicals (e.g., metronidazole, arsenic) resemble those of pityriasis rosea.

Pathology
Thickening of the epidermis, spongiosis, parakeratosis, and intraepidermal infiltrates of mononuclear cells are found. These findings are non-specific.

Diagnosis, treatment, and prognosis
Pityriasis rosea should be differentiated from the diseases listed in Table 15.10. Symptomatic therapies are the main treatment options. Topical steroids and antihistamines are applied. The condition usually heals naturally in 1–3 months and seldom recurs.

Non-inflammatory keratosis

Clavus, corn
Clinical features and pathogenesis
A clavus, commonly called a "corn," is localized hyperkeratosis, usually caused by prolonged pressure (Fig. 15.37). It tends to occur on the sole from the pressure of walking. The center of the thickened stratum corneum sinks deep into the dermis (core), resembling the eye of a chicken or fish. Tenderness is present (Fig. 15.38).

Differential diagnosis
A clavus should be differentiated from a plantar wart (see Chapter 23). Plantar warts tend to occur multiply. By dermoscopy, petechia is often found in the scraped stratum corneum.

Treatment
Prolonged pressure should be avoided. Cushioned footpads are helpful. Salicylic acid is applied.

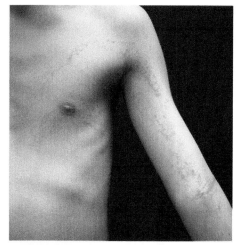
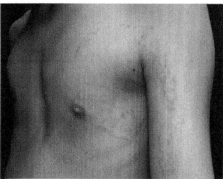

Fig. 15.34 Lichen striatus.

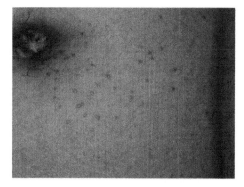

Fig. 15.35 Lichen nitidus. Small, scattered, multiple papules of a few millimeters in diameter and normal skin color or yellowish-white occur.

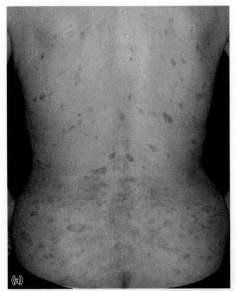

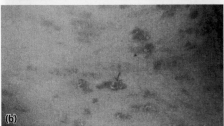

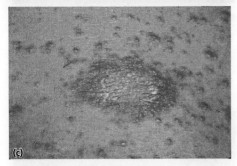

Fig. 15.36 Pityriasis rosea. a: The eruptions are distributed in a Christmas tree pattern. b: Pityriasis caused by pityriasis rosea. c: The first rash, called a herald patch.

Table 15.10 Diseases that are differentiated from pityriasis rosea.

Disease	Points of differentiation
Pityriasis versicolor	Flushing does not occur. *Malassezia furfur* is detected.
Seborrheic dermatitis	Seborrheic areas such as the head and face are most commonly involved.
Roseola syphilitica	Fewer scales are present. Eruptions also appear on the palms and soles. Serological test for syphilis is positive.
Guttate psoriasis	Silver-gray scales are present. Auspitz phenomenon and Köbner phenomenon are positive.
Drug eruption	History taking on drugs
Tinea corporis	Intense itching is present. *Trichophyton* fungi are detected by KOH method.

Callus, tylosis

A callus (tylosis) is also caused by prolonged pressure. The stratum corneum is even in thickness, and there is almost no tenderness (Fig. 15.39; see also Fig. 15.38). Sites that are repeatedly subjected to mechanical stimulation, including pressure and friction, and bony sites are involved. When the condition persists, fibrosis of the dermis may occur. The most common sites are between the second and third distal phalanxes (from penholding) and the dorsal region of the ankles (from sitting on the floor).

Keratosis pilaris (synonym: lichen pilaris)
Clinical features, pathogenesis, and pathology

Multiple follicular keratotic papules of 1–3 mm in diameter and of normal or light pink color occur on the extensor surfaces of the upper arms and thighs (Fig. 15.40). This condition is common in teenagers. In most cases, the onset is in early childhood, and the clinical features become distinct in adolescence. The papule surface is coarse, and there is no tendency of coalescence or enlargement. The condition is usually asymptomatic. Pathologically, the hair follicles are dilated and filled with keratin plugs and there is pili torti. Lichen pilaris tends to be hereditary, and it is assumed to be autosomal dominantly inherited. There are cases associated with ichthyosis vulgaris or atopic dermatitis.

Treatment and prognosis

Lichen pilaris heals naturally after adolescence. The symptomatic therapy is topical moisturizer or keratolytic agents, such as salicylic acid petrolatum.

Erythromelanosis follicularis faciei

Erythematous plaques occur symmetrically on the preauricular region and cheeks. Follicular keratotic papules form on the erythematous plaques (Fig. 15.41). The disorder is frequently seen in young men. Internationally, erythromelanosis follicularis faciei is defined as a subtype of keratosis pilaris. Keratosis pilaris on the extremities often accompanies this condition.

Lichen spinulosus

In lichen spinulosus, follicular papules with prickle-like projections aggregate and form plaques 2–5 cm in diameter. The neck, buttocks, and abdomen of young persons are most commonly involved. Histopathologically, it is identical to keratosis pilaris. The etiology is unknown, but cases occurring secondarily to AIDS and Crohn's disease have been reported.

Acanthosis nigricans (AN)

Plaques with a coarse dark brown surface occur on the neck and axillary fossae. The pathological findings are papillomatosis, hyperkeratosis, and pigmentation. Thickening of the epidermis (acanthosis) does not usually occur.

Clinical features

Dark brown papillary elevations with a coarse surface occur on the neck, axillary fossae, umbilical fossa, and groin. They have a velvety or rough-textured

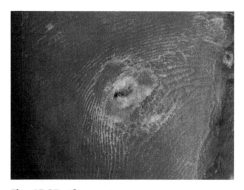

Fig. 15.37 Clavus, corn.

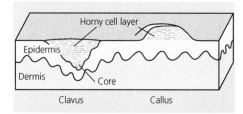

Fig. 15.38 Diagram of clavus and callus.

MEMO 15–4 Dorsal fibromatosis (synonym: knuckle pad)

Multiple keratotic elevated lesions of normal skin color to brown and 1–2 cm in diameter appear on the joints of fingers and toes. The changes occur as a reaction to repeated external force applied on the same spots.

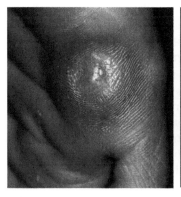
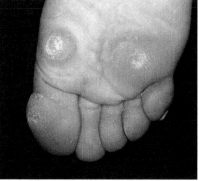

Fig. 15.39 Callus, tylosis.

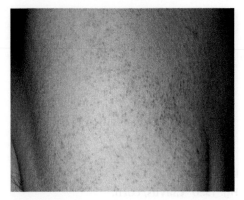

Fig. 15.40-1 Keratosis pilaris.

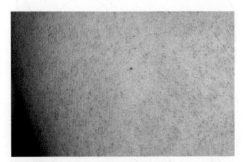

Fig. 15.40-2 Keratosis pilaris.

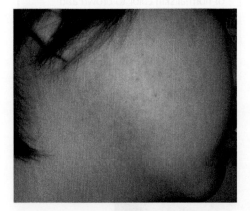

Fig. 15.41 Erythromelanosis follicularis faciei. Erythematous plaques caused by follicular keratotic papules are observed on the preauricular area and cheek.

appearance (Fig. 15.42). The disorder is divided into three types: malignant AN, accompanying an internal malignancy (stomach cancer in particular), obesity-associated AN, which was formerly called pseudo-AN, and syndromic AN (formerly called benign AN), accompanying hyperinsulinism or SLE. Obesity-associated AN has the highest percentage of cases.

In malignant AN, lesions tend to appear around the mouth.

Pathology
The main symptoms are papillomatosis, hyperkeratosis, and hyperpigmentation. Despite the name, thickening of the epidermis is not present in most cases.

Diagnosis and treatment
Diagnosis of AN can be confirmed by the clinical features. An eruption precedes or coincides with a malignant tumor in more than 70% of cases of malignant AN; diagnosis of AN may lead to the early discovery of cancer. The eruptions subside with treatment of the underlying disease or weight loss.

Confluent and reticulated papillomatosis
Grayish pigmented macules and keratotic papules occur on the trunk (inframammary region and upper abdomen, in particular), and coalesce to form a network of plaques (Fig. 15.43). The disorder occurs most frequently in men and women from adolescence to adulthood. It progresses slowly and is asymptomatic. The etiology is unknown, but association with *Malassezia* fungal infection has been suggested. Treatment is the topical administration of antifungal agents and the oral administration of minocycline.

Paraneoplastic acrokeratosis (synonym: Bazex syndrome)
Several months after psoriatic erythematous lesions appear symmetrically on the extremities, nasal apex, and auricle (Fig. 15.44), an internal malignancy becomes apparent. The syndrome occurs most commonly in men over age 40. The main malignant tumors caused by paraneoplastic acrokeratosis are squamous cell carcinomas in the esophagus, lungs, pharynx, and larynx. The keratotic lesions aggravate according to the progression of the malignant tumor.

Keratosis follicularis squamosa (Dohi)

Small black follicular spots occur symmetrically on the trunk, particularly on the hips, abdomen, and buttocks. Round or lamellar, grayish-white scales varying in size from 3 mm to 1 cm attach mainly to the black spots (Fig. 15.45 and Fig. 15.46). It is asymptomatic. The disorder occurs most frequently in adolescence.

Pityriasis circinata (Toyama)

This is an acquired dyskeratosis in which lesions occur on the hips, abdomen, and buttocks. The eruptions are round or oval, sharply circumscribed keratotic light pink plaques of 1 cm to several centimeters in diameter. Scaling, crêpe-surfaced, brown to grayish-white plaques form. Complications with internal malignancies have been reported.

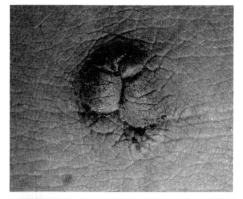

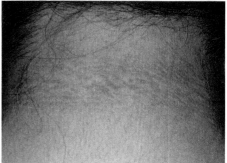

Fig. 15.42-1 Acanthosis nigricans.

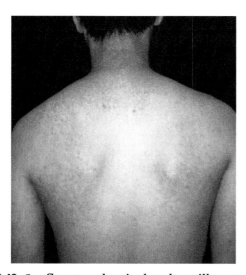

Fig. 15.43 Confluent and reticulated papillomatosis.

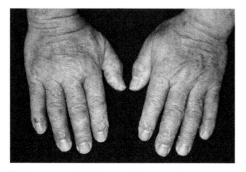

Fig. 15.44 Paraneoplastic acrokeratosis.

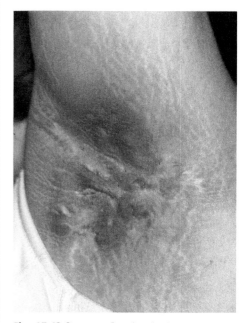

Fig. 15.42-2 Acanthosis nigricans.

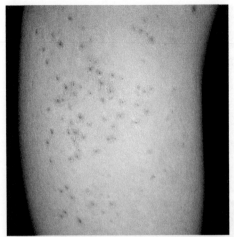

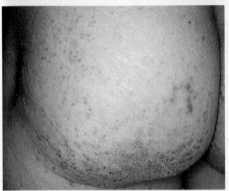

Fig. 15.45 Keratosis follicularis squamosa.

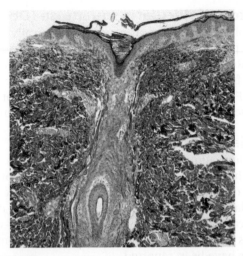

Fig. 15.46 Histopathology of keratosis follicularis squamosa.

Hyperkeratosis lenticularis perstans (synonym: Flegel's disease)

The disorder frequently occurs on the extremities of middle-aged men and women, especially on the dorsal surfaces of the hands and feet. Prickle-like, flatly elevated red to dark brown scaling papules of 1–5 mm diameter appear symmetrically. The disorder, whose etiology is unknown, progresses chronically.

CHAPTER 16

Disorders of skin color

Human skin color is mainly determined by melanin pigments, carotenes, and hemoglobin, with the melanins contributing the most. Racial differences in skin color result from differences in the kinds and amounts of melanin. Most diseases of abnormal pigmentation are caused by elevated or reduced melanin content; disorders involving skin color tend to be congenital or to be caused by autoimmune reaction or sun exposure.

When carotene, a precursor of vitamin A, is taken into the body, it accumulates in the stratum corneum and subcutaneous fat layer, resulting in yellowish skin color (carotenoid pigmentation). This chapter also discusses dermal deposition of extrinsic substances caused by tattooing or injury.

Although abnormalities of the blood vessels and hemoglobin may also cause changes in skin color, they are not included here.

Diseases of depigmentation

Oculocutaneous albinism (synonym: congenital albinism)

- There is congenital abnormality in melanin synthesis (see Fig. 1.20). Pigment in the skin, hair, and eyes is reduced or absent from birth.
- Nystagmus is often present.
- All types are autosomal recessive.
- Patients tend to be prone to malignant skin tumor, from high photosensitivity to sunlight.
- Use of sunscreen and eye protection is essential.

Classification

Oculocutaneous albinism (OCA) is classified by the causative genes into OCA1, OCA2, OCA3, and OCA4 (Table 16.1). It is also seen as a symptom of hereditary diseases, including Hermansky–Pudlak syndrome and Chédiak–Higashi syndrome.

Pathology

Melanocytes are normal in number and size; however, immature melanosomes (stages I, II, and III) are observed by electron microscopy (Fig. 16.1).

Table 16.1 Major types of oculocutaneous albinism (OCA).

OCA type 1	Tyrosine-related
1A	Complete lack of synthesis of tyrosinase (formerly tyrosinasenegative type)
1B	Dysfunction of tyrosinase synthesis (formerly yellow mutant type)
1mp	Minimal-pigment albinism
1ts	Temperature-sensitive
OCA type 2	P protein-related type (formerly tyrosinase-positive type)
OCA type 3	TRP-1 related
OCA type 4	MATP-gene type
HPS type	Hermansky-Pudlak syndrome
CHS type	Chédiak-Higashi syndrome

Shimizu's Dermatology, Second Edition. Hiroshi Shimizu.
© 2017 John Wiley & Sons, Ltd. Published 2017 by John Wiley & Sons, Ltd.

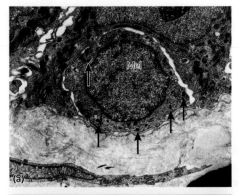

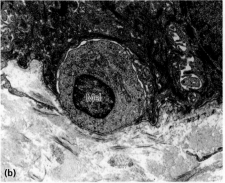

Fig. 16.1 Electron microscopic image of a melanocyte (Mel) from a healthy person (a) and from a patient with oculocutaneous albinism (OCA1A) (b).
a: In a melanocyte from a healthy person, the cytoplasm contains large amounts of mature, blackish, stage IV melanosomes (arrows). The melanocytes transport melanosomes to neighboring keratinocytes.
b: In oculocutaneous albinism, most melanosomes are immature, not progressing beyond stage II. Mature melanosomes are not seen in the cytoplasm.

Diagnosis and examination

The maturity of melanosomes in melanocytes should be observed by electron microscopy. In the most severe OCA1A cases, there are only immature melanosomes, i.e., they lack melanin deposition (stage I or II). Identification of the affected gene is necessary for determination of subtype.

Treatment

Use of sunscreen is essential from birth, in order to protect the skin from UV-related cancer and skin aging. Tinted contact lenses or sunglasses are used to protect the eyes and correct the vision.

Types of oculocutaneous albinism
OCA1

This type is caused by a tyrosinase gene mutation (see Fig. 1.20). OCA1 is classified into subtypes that include OCA1A, in which tyrosinase activity is completely lost from such mutation, and OCA1B, in which some tyrosinase activity remains. All OCA1 subtypes are autosomal recessively inherited.

When melanin is not synthesized, as is the case in OCA1A, the skin appears white to pink, and the hair is white from birth (Fig. 16.2). The skin easily sunburns (solar dermatitis), and sun-exposed areas of the body are prone to malignant tumors (e.g., basal cell carcinoma, squamous cell carcinoma, malignant melanoma). The iris and choroid membrane are blue, and the ocular fundus is pink; the eyes appear blue when lit edge-on, and pink when lit head-on (pink-eye). Patients have a characteristic facial expression of squinting and looking out of the corner of the eyes, from photophobia and impaired eyesight that cannot be corrected. Horizontal nystagmus may be present. When melanin is scant but present, pigment may gradually appear in hair and skin as the patient grows, although it is impossible to distinguish these cases from OCA1A at birth.

OCA2

OCA2 is caused by a mutation in the P protein gene on chromosome 15. It is autosomal recessive. The role of P protein has not been clarified, but the protein is thought to regulate pH in melanosomes and decrease in this regulatory function of melanosomes is thought to be caused by mutation in the P protein gene.

Pigment may be largely or completely absent at birth; it is impossible to distinguish OCA2 from OCA1 only by the clinical symptoms. In OCA2 the eye color is bluish-gray and the hair is pale yellow to blonde; both come to contain more pigment as the patient ages.

OCA3

OCA3 is caused by genetic mutation in TRP-1 (tyrosinase-related protein 1), which controls melanin synthesis. It tends to occur in patients of African descent. The skin color is reddish-brown, and the hair is light reddish-brown to red. Eye symptoms do not usually occur.

OCA4

OCA4 is caused by abnormality in the membrane-associated transporter protein (MATP). MATP is a transporter protein on the surface of the melanosome membrane. In Japan, OCA4 is the second most common OCA subtype, after OCA1. Pigment is present in the skin in small amounts. The hair is light yellow in many cases; however, there are some cases in which the hair is brown (Fig. 16.3). The eyes are blue, gray or reddish brown.

Hermansky–Pudlak syndrome

Some causative genes that are thought to be associated with intracellular protein transport have been identified in Hermansky–Pudlak syndrome (HPS). HPS is classified by the causative genes into the four subtypes of HPS1, HPS2, HPS3, and HPS4. It is autosomal recessively inherited. Pigment appears in the skin and hair to some extent (Fig. 16.4). Pulmonary fibrosis or granulomatous colitis may occur as a complication from deposition of ceroid-lipofuscin. There is a hemorrhagic tendency in HPS, which manifests as susceptibility to gingival hemorrhage.

Chédiak–Higashi syndrome (CHS)

Abnormality of the lysosomal trafficking regulator gene (LYST) on chromosome 1 (1q42) disturbs the normal function of microtubules. It is autosomal recessively inherited. The main symptoms are partial albinism from melanocyte trafficking failure, and photosensitive disorder. The hair is red and the skin color is cream, although sun-exposed areas such as the face become dark red because of solar dermatitis. Neutrophilic immune compromise often

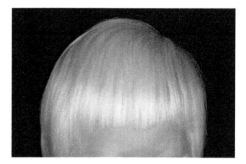

Fig. 16.2 Oculocutaneous albinism (OCA1A) in a girl. The hair will be white throughout her lifetime from lack of melanin production. A mutation in the tyrosinase gene was identified. Tyrosinase mutation (+).

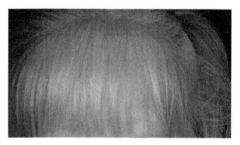

Fig. 16.3 Oculocutaneous albinism (OCA4). This patient had white hair at birth; however, pigmentation gradually appeared in the hair with age. Her hair is now blonde. MATP mutation (+).

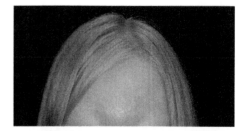

Fig. 16.4 Hermansky-Pudlak syndrome (HPS). This patient had blonde hair and a fair complexion; however, more pigment gradually appeared as she grew. There was a hemorrhagic tendency in this case. Symptoms such as pulmonary fibrosis and intestinal catarrhs often appear after the patient reaches a certain age.

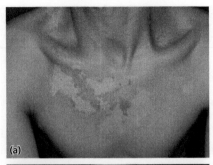

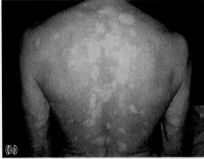

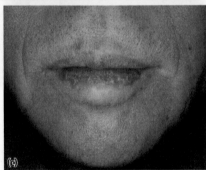

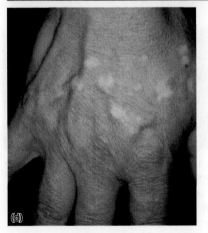

Fig. 16.5-1 Vitiligo vulgaris on various sites. a: Chest. b: Back. c: Lips. d: Sharply demarcated depigmented macules occur on the dorsum of the hands.

leads to bacterial infection. Histopathologically, giant lysosome granules (peroxidase-positive) are found in the peripheral leukocytes. Symptomatic therapies are performed for infection. Hematopoietic stem cell transplantation may also be conducted. The prognosis is often poor, because lymphoproliferative diseases or hemophagocytic syndrome occur.

Vitiligo vulgaris

- Because melanocytes are reduced or lost, hypopigmented patches (leukoderma) occur.
- Autoimmunity against melanocytes or melanin is thought to cause vitiligo vulgaris; however, the precise pathogenesis is unknown.
- Topical steroids and PUVA therapy are the first-line treatments.

Classification

Vitiligo vulgaris is classified into focal, segmental, generalized, and universal types. Vitiligo vulgaris in which leukoderma distribution is not associated with cutaneous innervation is called generalized vitiligo vulgaris. When unilateral leukoderma runs parallel to cutaneous nerves, it is called segmental vitiligo vulgaris. When leukoderma localizes around the mouth and the fingers and toes, it is called acrofacial vitiligo.

Clinical features and epidemiology

Vitiligo vulgaris often occurs in men and women from about age 20. The incidence has been calculated as between 1% and 2% of the population. Familial cases account for 1–2% of all cases. Sharply circumscribed complete leukoderma occurs. There is a slight increase in pigmentation at the periphery of the eruptions. The lesions are irregular in shape and size, and they often coalesce (Fig. 16.5). Gray hair is seen around the leukoderma. It is asymptomatic. Generalized vitiligo vulgaris occurs most frequently on areas prone to mechanical stimulation, such as the seborrheic areas and the extremities, lumbar region, abdomen, intertriginous areas, face, and neck. Affected areas are often symmetrical and tend to enlarge. Segmental vitiligo vulgaris occurs unilaterally on certain innervated areas. The face is often affected.

Pathogenesis and complications

The cause has not been identified. Autoimmunity against melanocytes and melanins and abnormal peripheral nerve function are thought to be involved. Graves' disease, chronic thyroiditis (Hashimoto's thyroiditis), Addison's disease, pernicious anemia, and diabetes may develop as complications.

Pathology
In the early stages, there is melanocyte degeneration with reduced or lost dopa response and lymphocytic and histiocytic infiltration in the dermal upper layer. In the final stages, melanocytes are lost and melanin granules are absent in the basal layer.

Differential diagnosis
The disease should be differentiated from piebaldism, nevus depigmentosus, senile leukoderma, Vogt–Koyanagi–Harada disease, melanoleukoderma, pityriasis versicolor, and Hansen's disease.

Treatment
PUVA and narrow-band UVB therapies, and topical medicine such as steroids, activated vitamin D3, and tacrolimus are effective. Leukoderma on the face and fingers can be concealed by special cosmetics to alleviate psychological distress. Skin graft of healthy skin to the affected area (vacuum-assisted: Fig. 16.6) may be conducted.

Piebaldism (synonym: partial albinism)
Definition
Piebaldism is characterized by localized leukoderma with leukotrichia on the forehead and frontal region of the head. Few melanocytes are found around the areas of leukoderma and white hair. It is a rare, congenital, autosomal dominant disease.

Clinical features
Triangular or diamond-shaped leukotrichia and leukoderma are seen on the forehead and frontal region of the head (white forelock) at the time of birth. These do not enlarge or shrink with age. Contralateral geographic vitiligo occurs on the extremities and trunk. Small, pigmented patches often occur within the leukoderma.

Pathogenesis and pathology
Piebaldism is caused by abnormality in the *KIT* gene. In fetal development, melanoblasts migrate from the neural crest to the epidermis to anchor

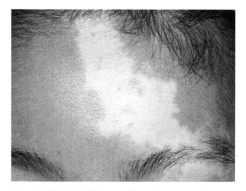

Fig. 16.5-2 Vitiligo vulgaris on various sites. On the forehead.

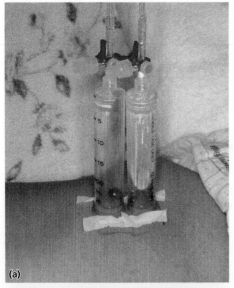

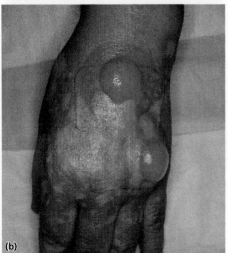

Fig. 16.6 Suction blister treatment of vitiligo vulgaris. a: Vacuum aspiration is applied on normal skin to artificially produce a suction blister. b: Vacuum aspiration is applied on skin with vitiligo vulgaris to produce a suction blister. The covering of the vitiligo vulgaris blister is removed and replaced with the covering of the normal skin blister.

and differentiate into melanocytes. The *KIT* gene is associated with the migration and anchoring of melanoblasts. Abnormality occurs in half of each receptor, leaving an area on which melanoblasts do not anchor and resulting in leukoderma. Histopathologically, melanocytes are lacking at the sites with leukotrichia and leukoderma.

Diagnosis and treatment

Diagnosis is made by history taking of autosomal dominant expression, and white forelock and small pigmented patches on leukoderma. Waadenburg–Klein syndrome, whose symptoms are similar to those of piebaldism, is accompanied by heterochromia iridis, facial dysplasia, and congenital deafness. Skin graft and cultured pigmented cell transplantation have been reported to be effective.

Sutton nevus (synonyms: leukoderma acquisitum centrifugum Sutton, leukoderma Sutton)

Definition, pathogenesis, and clinical features

Sutton nevus has nevocellular nevus (lentigo) at the center, surrounded by oval leukoderma (Fig. 16.7). Leukoderma occurs in children and in young men and women on the trunk, face, and neck. Vitiligo vulgaris may develop as a complication. Autoimmunization occurs against melanin at the center of the lentigo, and immunoreaction occurs against melanin at the periphery of the lentigo; this is thought to be the mechanism of Sutton nevus. Leukoderma may also be produced at the periphery of a malignant melanoma, angioma, blue nevus, neurofibroma, and seborrheic keratosis; this is called Sutton's phenomenon.

Pathology

Degenerated or destroyed nevus cells and melanocytes, with dense lymphocytic and macrophagic infiltration, are found at the periphery.

Treatment and prognosis

Leukoderma enlarges centrifugally. At the same time, the central nevus discolors, flattens, and eventually disappears. As the nevus disappears, the leukoderma heals spontaneously. Excision of the central nevus often induces spontaneous healing of the leukoderma.

Vogt–Koyanagi–Harada disease (synonym: Vogt–Koyanagi–Harada syndrome)

- Vogt–Koyanagi–Harada disease is caused by autoimmunization against melanocytes. Inflammation occurs in the uvea, skin, auris interna, and meninges.
- Uveitis, leukoderma, leukotrichia, and alopecia occur.
- Oral steroid therapy is the main treatment. The treatments for vitiligo vulgaris are applied for cutaneous lesions.

Clinical features

Vogt–Koyanagi–Harada disease progresses rapidly, and the main symptom is eye lesions. Cutaneous lesions appear during recovery, after remission of inflammation (about 2 months after onset) (Fig. 16.8). Melanocytes are destroyed and poliosis is found in 90% of cases. The eyebrows, eyelashes, and hair become white from pigment loss, and alopecia may occur. Irregularly shaped, diffuse cutaneous leukoderma is found on the face and trunk. The cutaneous leukoderma is often found around the eyes (Sugiura's sign) and in the sacrum.

There are three stages: prodromal, eye disease, and recovery. In the prodromal stage, the symptoms resemble those of the common cold, including headache, fever, dizziness, and eye pain, persisting for 5–7 days. During this stage, the patient may have hyperaphia of the skin and scalp hair. In the eye disease stage, acute bilateral uveitis and serous retinal dialysis develop. These symptoms persist for 1–2 months and then gradually subside. The main symptoms of the recovery stage are those of the prodrome stage and the eye disease stage. Loss of uveal melanocytes results in light red color of the entire fundus oculi.

Pathogenesis

Vogt–Koyanagi–Harada disease should be grouped with autoimmune diseases, because of the autoimmune reactions against melanocytes, tyrosinase, and TRP-1. HLA-DR4 is highly associated with the disease.

Treatment

High-dose oral steroids are used as early as possible. Steroid pulse therapy and immunosuppressants are also used. The treatments for vitiligo vulgaris are applied for the cutaneous lesions.

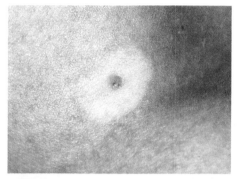

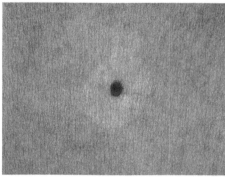

Fig. 16.7 Sutton nevus. Sharply demarcated leukoderma appears around the nevus cells.

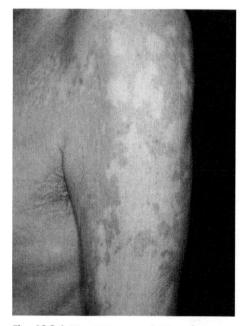

Fig. 16.8-1 Vogt-Koyanagi–Harada disease. Irregularly shaped leukoderma is sporadically seen.

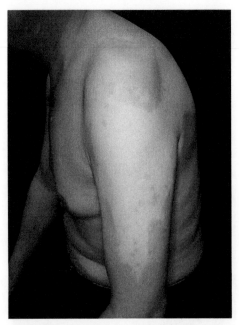

Fig. 16.8-2 Vogt–Koyanagi–Harada disease.

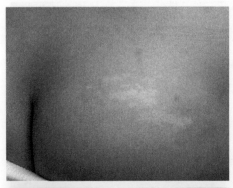

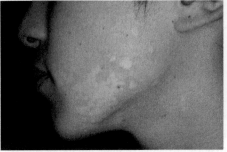

Fig. 16.9 Nevus depigmentosus.

Idiopathic guttate hypomelanosis (synonym: senile leukoderma)

Sharply circumscribed, round or irregular-shaped leukoderma of 3–4 mm diameter appear diffusely on the trunk and extremities in the third decade of life, increasing in number with age. Histopathological findings show a reduction in the number of activated melanocytes and melanosomes, and dysfunction in melanocytes and melanosomes from melanocytic senescence.

Nevus depigmentosus

Nevus depigmentosus is caused by congenital dysfunction of melanocytes at localized areas. The number of melanocytes is not abnormal. Incomplete hypopigmented patches are seen on the back and buttocks at birth or shortly thereafter (Fig. 16.9). The patches vary in shape and distribution from solitary and irregular to multiple and band-like. Size, distribution, and number of nevus depigmentosus patches remain constant throughout life.

Leukoderma pseudosyphiliticum

Leukoderma pseudosyphiliticum most commonly occurs on the lumbar regions and buttocks of men in their 20s and 30s whose skin is naturally dark, in Asians in particular. Multiple, sharply circumscribed, incomplete hypopigmented patches 1–2 cm in diameter occur, often coalescing to become reticular. It is asymptomatic. Leukoderma pseudosyphiliticum resembles syphilitic leukoderma but the two can be differentiated: syphilitic leukoderma tends to occur on exposed sites, and the standard serological test for syphilis is positive.

Hyperpigmentation

Ephelides
Clinical features

Multiple round, smooth-surfaced brown patches about 3 mm in diameter occur on sun-exposed areas of the face, neck, and forearms (Fig. 16.10). Ephelides darkens with sun exposure (especially exposure to UVR) in summer and tends to fade in winter. It worsens with age until puberty, lightening thereafter.

Pathogenesis and pathology

Ephelides tends to run in families. Genetic polymorphism of the melanocortin 1 receptor (MC1R) is involved. Ephelides is autosomal recessively inherited in severe cases of xeroderma pigmentosum. Melanocytes are activated, and they markedly increase in the basal keratinocytes. Melanocytes in patients with ephelides have well-developed dendritic spines and enhanced function; however, the number of melanocytes does not change.

Diagnosis and treatment

Differentiation from lentigo, Peutz–Jeghers syndrome, xeroderma pigmentosum, and progeria is necessary. Sunscreen is useful for blocking UVR.

Melasma
Clinical features

Melasma tends to occur in women in their 30s or older. It is rare in men. Sharply demarcated light brown patches occur, mainly on the cheeks and usually symmetrically. The patches may spread to the forehead and around the mouth, but they are not found around the eyes. Melasma patches are irregular in size and shape. The disorder is aggravated by UVR in summer, and it subsides in winter (Fig. 16.11). Pregnancy may trigger the onset (chloasma gravidarum).

Pathogenesis and pathology

Changes in the secretion of sex hormones and adrenocortical hormones, and chronic irritation by UVR are thought to activate melanocytes and cause melasma. Histopathologically, there is an increase in melanin granules, mainly in the basal cell layer. Melanophages may be found in the dermis.

Diagnosis and differential diagnosis

Differentiation from nevus of Ota and acquired bilateral nevus of Ota-like macule (see Chapter 20) is important. Melasma can be differentiated from these: in melasma, the skin tone of the lesions is not bluish, because of increased melanin in the basal cell layer, and the periphery of the eyes is affected. Melasma and acquired bilateral nevus of Ota-like macules may be found concurrently.

Treatment

The causal factors, such as use of contraceptives and exposure to UVR, are discontinued. Chloasma

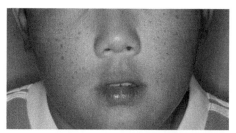
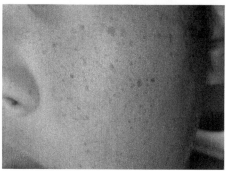

Fig. 16.10 Ephelides.

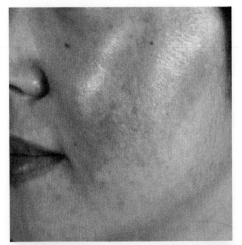

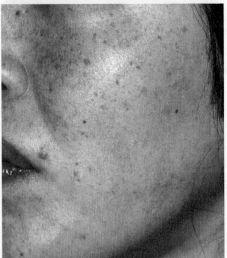

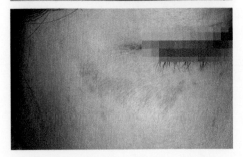

Fig. 16.11 Melasma, chloasma. Brown spots on the cheeks.

gravidarum occurs during pregnancy and subsides several months after delivery. Topical hydroquinone and sunscreen are used. Laser treatment must be avoided because it causes increase in pigments.

Riehl's melanosis (synonym: melanosis faciei feminina)

A diffuse, vaguely circumscribed grayish-purplish-brown network of pigment deposition appears, most commonly on the face of middle-aged women. Riehl's melanosis may be accompanied by follicular keratotic papules. In most cases, inflammatory symptoms such as flush and itching precede pigmentation.

The cause is recurrent contact dermatitis on the face. The antigens in most cases are cosmetic products containing tar pigment. Most of these products are no longer produced, because of restrictions on cosmetics components. Histopathologically, melanophages are observed in the upper dermal layer.

Friction melanosis (synonym: towel melanosis)
Definition and clinical features

Prolonged and vigorous use of nylon towels or brushes may stimulate the skin mechanically, resulting in pigmentation. Friction melanosis occurs frequently in adults. A network pattern or diffuse brown pigmentation is seen in the skin above the clavicular region, neck, ribs, and vertebral region (Fig. 16.12). Subjective symptoms such as itching are not present.

Pathogenesis and pathology

Melanosomes sink into the dermis from mechanical stimulation and inflammation. Increases in melanophages in the upper dermis lead to friction melanosis (histological pigmentary incontinence). Amyloid deposition is found in some cases.

Treatment

The skin color gradually returns to normal by discontinuation of the mechanical irritation.

Dyschromatosis symmetrica hereditaria
Definition, pathogenesis, and clinical features

Multiple brown patches and hypopigmented patches 3–8 mm in diameter occur on the extremities, including the dorsae of the hands and feet, coalescing into reticular forms (Fig. 16.13). Generally, the more distal the pigmentation, the more severe are the symptoms. The patches are flat and smooth. Ephelides-like pigmented patches tend to occur on the face. The onset is age 6 or younger in most cases. Inheritance is autosomal dominant, and the cause is mutation of the double-stranded RNA-specific adenosine deaminase (*ADAR1*) gene. It progresses with age until adulthood, when it becomes apparent. It occurs most commonly in Asians.

Diagnosis and differential diagnosis

Dyschromatosis symmetrica hereditaria can be diagnosed by the characteristic cutaneous features and familial incidence. It should be differentiated from acropigmentatio reticularis, a similar autosomal dominant disease with reticular pigmentation in the distal extremities. Acropigmentatio reticularis is distinguished by the fact that the pigmented patches are concave and there are no hypopigmented patches.

Treatment

Special concealing cosmetics are useful. Dermabrasion may be conducted for pigmented patches.

Senile lentigo (synonym: solar lentigo)
Definition and clinical features

Senile lentigo appears in almost all men and women middle aged and older. Round brown patches of various sizes occur on sun-exposed areas of the face, the dorsae of the hands, and the extensor surfaces of the arms. The patches are relatively clearly circumscribed. Mild scaling may be present (Fig. 16.14). Some lesions may progress to seborrheic keratosis (see Chapter 21).

Treatment

Alexandrite or ruby laser therapies and cryotherapy are conducted.

Addison's disease

Secretion of ACTH and MSH from the anterior lobe of the hypophysis is enhanced by reduced secretion of adrenocortical hormones, and this causes pigmentation by stimulating melanocytes (Fig. 16.15). Pigmentation is seen on the entire body. The palms, knees, elbows, areola mammae, axillary fossae,

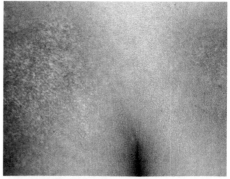
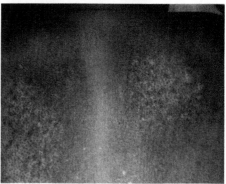

Fig. 16.12 Friction melanosis. Diffuse, reticular, brown pigmentation occurs on the trunk, particularly on the back. The eruptions are blackish papules of several millimeters in diameter. On histopathology, amyloid deposition is observed.

MEMO 16–1 Hydroquinone

Hydroquinone acts on cells that have high tyrosinase activity, including melanocytes, and acts as a skin-lightening agent by inhibiting the cell's bioactivity and tyrosinase. Topical drugs with 2–5% hydroquinone content are generally used.

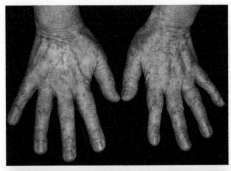

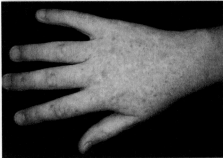

Fig. 16.13 Dyschromatosis symmetrica hereditaria. Multiple brownish macules of 3–8 mm diameter occur on the dorsum of the hands. They coalesce to present a reticular pattern. Depigmentation is also seen.

and genitalia are most severely affected. The pigmentation is also found on areas that normally have less pigmentation than the skin, such as the tongue, the gingiva, and the oral mucosa; this is useful for diagnosis.

Pigmentatio petaloides actinica

Multiple sharply circumscribed, brown, petal-shaped or spiny patches of several millimeters to 1 cm in diameter occur on the shoulders and upper back (Fig. 16.16). The multiple patches often occur in persons with light complexion 1–3 months after intense sunburn, such as from a beach outing.

Erythema dyschromicum perstans

Multiple small erythematous lesions occur on the trunk and extremities of non-Caucasians, and these soon turn into grayish-white to grayish-blue patches of 1–3 cm diameter. Erythematous elevation is seen at the periphery in some cases (Fig. 16.17). Itching may be present; however, it is asymptomatic in most cases and develops slowly. The pathogenesis is unknown. Drug eruptions and lichen planus may resemble erythema dyschromicum perstans.

Diseases caused by extrinsic deposition

Carotenemia
Definition, pathogenesis, and clinical features
The blood carotene concentration is elevated, resulting in carotene deposition in the stratum corneum and subcutaneous fat tissues. This yellows the skin (Fig. 16.18). The coloration is marked in the palms and soles, whose stratum corneum is thick. The color may appear on the face; however, it does not occur in the sclera or other mucous membranes, and it rarely becomes generalized. It is asymptomatic. Coloration tends to appear when the carotene concentration in the blood remains at 0.5 mg/dL or over for about 1–2 months. Carotenemia is caused by high intake of carotene-containing foods (citrus fruits, pumpkins, carrots, spinach, seaweed, corn, egg yolks, butter), by liver dysfunction (carotene concentration in the blood increases when carotene fails to be metabolized

into vitamin A) or by hyperlipidemia (carotene concentration tends to increase because of carotene's liposolubility).

Diagnosis and treatment
Jaundice is differentiated from aurantiasis cutis by yellowed sclera, itching, and bilirubin level. Aurantiasis cutis heals spontaneously in 2–3 months when intake of the causative food is restricted.

Argyria
Definition, pathogenesis, and clinical features
Argyria results from deposition of silver in the skin. This occurs from the use of silver medical supplies (silver needles, sutures, dental fillings) or prolonged intake of silver-containing foods. Silver compounds deposit in the sweat glands and elastic fibers, giving the skin a bluish-gray hue. The condition tends to occur in exposed areas such as the face, neck, and forearms.

Diagnosis, treatment, and prognosis
Fine brown granular masses are found histopathologically. Silver can be observed by micro X-ray fluorescence. There is no effective treatment for argyria, except to refrain from intake of silver.

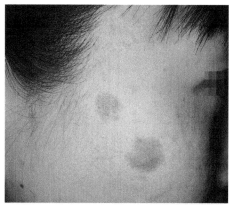
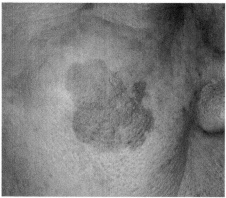

Fig. 16.14 Senile lentigo. Sharply demarcated brown patches appear. They may partially elevate and progress to seborrheic keratosis in some cases.

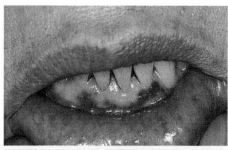
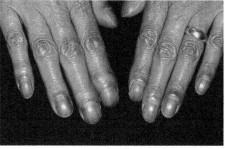

Fig. 16.15 Addison's disease.

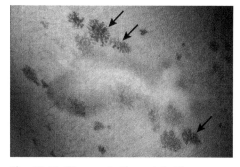

Fig. 16.16 Pigmentatio petaloides actinica. This skin lesion occurred after PUVA therapy for vitiligo vulgaris (center of photo).

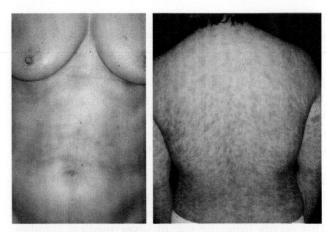

Fig. 16.17 Erythema dyschromicum perstans, ashy dermatosis. Grayish-blue patches and erythematous eruptions are seen around the patches.

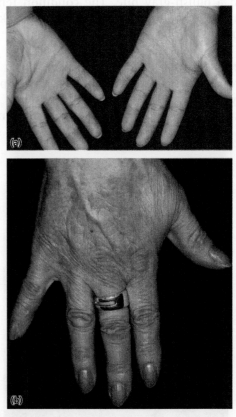

Fig. 16.18 Carotenemia. a: Color changes are seen in the hands. b: Multiple brown pigmented macules of 2–10 mm diameter occur on the dorsum of hand. The macules coalesce to form reticular patterns. Hypopigmented macules are also seen.

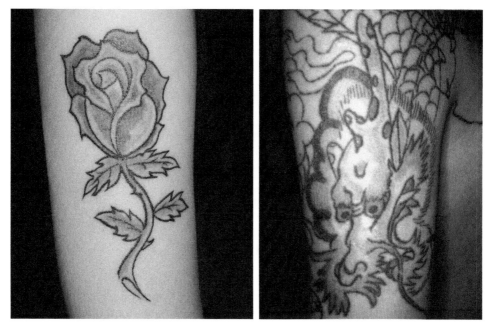

Fig. 16.19 Tattoo. Pigments of various colors have been injected.

Systemic complications of argyria include pulmonary fibrosis, pneumonitis, hepatotoxicity, and myopathy.

Tattoos

Tattoos are images or text artificially created in the skin by injection of pigment or ink (Fig. 16.19). When foreign matter penetrates the dermis accidentally as the result of a fall or the like, it is called traumatic tattoo (Fig. 16.20). Pigmented granules tend to remain in the dermal upper layer; however, some are phagocytosed by macrophages and carried in the lymph flow to deposit in the lymph nodes. Allergic reactions against the injected pigment or photosensitivity may occur as complications. Laser therapies are useful in removing tattoos of certain colors.

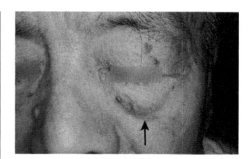

Fig. 16.20 Traumatic tattoo.

CHAPTER 17
Metabolic disorders

Congenital or acquired abnormality in biosynthesis and metabolic pathways can cause qualitative and quantitative abnormalities in bodily substances. Diseases caused by such abnormalities are called metabolic disorders.

Metabolic abnormalities in amyloids, mucins, lipids, nucleic acids, porphyrins, vitamins, and electrolytes, for example, cause various cutaneous disorders.

Table 17.1 Classification of cutaneous amyloidoses.

Disease	Deposited amyloid (precursor protein)
Localized cutaneous amyloidoses	
Primary localized cutaneous amyloidoses	
Lichen amyloidosis	AD (keratin?)
Macular amyloidosis	AD
Nodular cutaneous amyloidosis	AL (immunoglobulin L-chain)
Anosacral cutaneous amyloidosis	AD
Secondary localized cutaneous amyloidosis	AD
Systemic amyloidoses	
AI amyloidosis	AL
AA amyloidosis	AA (serum amyloid A)
Familial systemic amyloidosis	ATTR (transthyretin), etc.
Hemodialysis-related amyloidosis	Aβ2M (β$_2$-microglobulin)

Amyloidoses

- These disorders are caused by deposition or accumulation of amorphous glycoproteins, called amyloids, in the tissue or intercellular spaces.
- Amyloids consist of various precursor substances whose compositions differ according to the type of disease.
- Localized cutaneous amyloidosis occurs only in the skin; systemic amyloidosis affects systemic internal organs (Table 17.1).

Classification and pathogenesis

Amyloids deposit and accumulate in the tissue and intercellular spaces, inducing dysfunction in the whole body or specific organs. Amyloids are glycoproteins that have a fibrous structure called a β-sheet. They are not seen in normal metabolism. They consist of various precursors, such as immunoglobulin L-chains, β2 microglobulin, and keratin. In each disease, the amyloids have a different composition. Cutaneous amyloidoses are classified as shown in Table 17.1.

Pathology and laboratory findings

Amyloids stain light pink with eosin in H&E staining, light red with PAS and orange-red with Congo red, and they appear green to yellow in polarizing microscopy. The deposition of tangled elongated fibers of 7–15 mm in length is observed by electron microscopy. Localized cutaneous amyloidosis does not readily stain with

Shimizu's Dermatology, Second Edition. Hiroshi Shimizu.

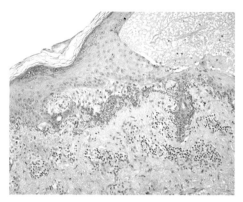

Fig. 17.1 Histopathology of amyloidosis. Amyloids stain reddish brown in direct fast scarlet staining.

Congo red; instead, direct fast scarlet (orange) and dylon staining (reddish brown) are used (Fig. 17.1; see Table 2.1). Detection of Bence Jones proteins (monoclonal immunoglobulin L-chains) in the urine and detection of M proteins by electrophoresis of the serum have diagnostic value for systemic amyloidosis.

Treatment and prognosis

Topical steroids with ODT (see Chapter 6) are effective against localized cutaneous amyloidosis. Systemic amyloidosis accompanied by myeloma has a poor prognosis. Many patients die from renal dysfunction or heart failure.

Localized cutaneous amyloidoses
Lichen amyloidosis

Lichen amyloidosis frequently occurs on the extensor surfaces of the lower legs, and on the forearms and back. Multiple, flat-surfaced, smooth, light-brown papules 2–10 mm in diameter appear and may aggregate (Fig. 17.2). Intense itching is present in most cases. Pathologically, the stratum corneum and epidermis thicken diffusely, melanin granules increase in the basal layer, and amyloid accumulates in the dermal papillae. Topical steroids and oral histamines are effective.

Macular amyloidosis

Punctate or reticular pigmentation occurs, most commonly on the scapular region and back of middle-aged women (Fig. 17.3). Chronic rubbing of the skin with nylon towels causes friction melanosis (see Chapter 16). Amyloids may deposit in the skin.

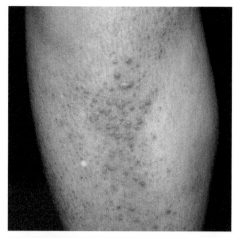

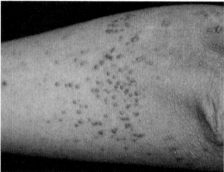

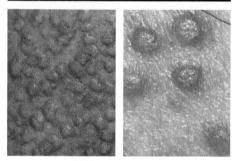

Fig. 17.2 Lichen amyloidosis. Multiple light brown papules appear and aggregate, accompanied by intense itching.

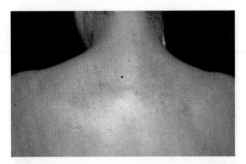

Fig. 17.3 Macular amyloidosis.

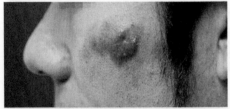

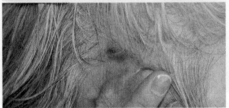

Fig. 17.4 Nodular cutaneous amyloidosis.

MEMO 17–1 Familial primary localized cutaneous amyloidosis

This is a rare condition of itchy hereditary eruptions resembling lichen amyloidosis. In recent years, it has been clarified that the disorder is caused by a mutation in the oncostatin M receptor b (*OSMR*) gene.

Friction melanosis is thought to be strongly associated with macular amyloidosis.

Nodular cutaneous amyloidosis

Multiple or single firm nodules of normal skin color to reddish-brown and several millimeters to several centimeters in diameter occur on the face and trunk (Fig. 17.4). The amyloids are derived from AL (immunoglobulin L-chains), and the disorder is accompanied by plasma cell infiltration. Complications such as diabetes and Sjögren syndrome are often found. About 7% of cases progress to AL amyloidosis. Amyloidosis cutis nodularis atrophicans, which occurs on the lower abdomen of middle-aged women as yellowish-brown atrophic nodules, is a subtype of nodular cutaneous amyloidosis.

Anosacral cutaneous amyloidosis

This occurs in the perianal region of the elderly. It is clinically characterized by pigmentation accompanied by hyperkeratosis. Chronic pressure from sitting is thought to be related to this condition. Amyloid deposition is seen histopathologically.

Secondary localized cutaneous amyloidosis

Deposition of amyloids is observed in the dermal papilla in association with various skin disorders. Underlying skin disorders include nevocellular nevus, tumors of sweat glands, calcified epithelioma, dermatofibroma, seborrheic keratosis, actinic keratosis, basal cell carcinoma, Bowen disease, porokeratosis, discoid lupus erythematosus, and lichen simplex chronicus.

Systemic amyloidoses
AL amyloidosis (synonyms: primary systemic amyloidosis, immunocytic amyloidosis)

AL amyloidosis occurs frequently in men and women in their 60s. It is known to be associated with plasma cell dyscrasia (such as multiple myeloma), in which abnormal immunoglobulin-related amyloid light chain (AL) is produced. Shiny yellowish-white papules occur, most frequently on the eyelids and other parts of the face and the neck. It is called pinch purpura because purpura readily occurs with slight trauma. Generalized scleroderma-like stiffness in the fingers and nail deformity are present (Fig. 17.5a,b). Amyloid deposition is found among the collagen fibers in the epidermis and outer membranes of the blood vessels at sites around the eruptions. Such deposition is also seen in the systemic organs, such as the gastrointestinal tract, cardiac muscles and skeletal muscles, where it causes various symptoms (Fig. 17.5c). Lesions develop in the oral cavity and laryngeal mucosa, resulting in macroglossia and hoarseness. Bence Jones proteins are excreted in the urine in some cases (a finding of myeloma). Treatments are mainly made for plasma cell dyscrasia. The prognosis is poor.

Reactive (AA) amyloidosis

The precursor protein of AA amyloidosis is the serum amyloid A (AA) protein. The disorder is caused secondarily by a chronic inflammatory disease or an infectious disease, such as rheumatoid arthritis, SLE or tuberculosis. Skin lesions rarely form.

Familial systemic amyloidosis

The typical familial systemic amyloidosis is familial amyloid polyneuropathy, which is caused by amyloidogenic transthyretin. This disorder is autosomal dominantly inherited. Amyloid deposition in various organs, including the nerves, stomach and heart, causes dysfunction.

Dialysis-related amyloidosis (synonym: β2-microglobulin amyloidosis)

This occurs in those who undergo prolonged hemodialysis. β2-microglobulin, which is not readily removed by hemodialysis, deposits as amyloid. The intercarpal synovial membranes, joints, heart, blood vessels, digestive tract, and kidneys are affected. Erythema, papules, purpura, and subcutaneous nodules are the main cutaneous symptoms. Macroglossia is also observed (Fig. 17.6).

Mucinoses

Definition and pathogenesis

Mucinosis is a general term for diseases in which mucins (glycoproteins in mucus) deposit in the skin. The mucins, produced by fibroblasts, consist of complexes of mucopolysaccharides (glycosaminoglycans) and core proteins. The mucin stains positive with Alcian blue and colloidal iron, and it stains blue with toluidine blue. The main types of mucopolysaccharides found in the

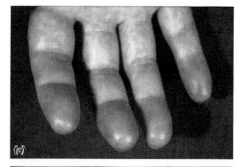
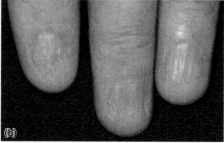
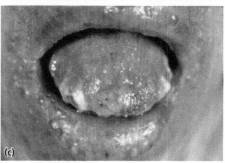

Fig. 17.5 AL amyloidosis. a: Amyloid deposition in the fingers results in hardening of the skin that resembles systemic scleroderma. b: Nail deformity is caused by amyloid deposition in the nail matrix and nail beds. c: Macroglossia. The tongue is markedly firm and swollen from amyloid deposition.

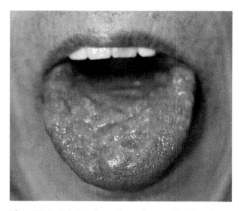

Fig. 17.6 Dialysis-related amyloidosis.

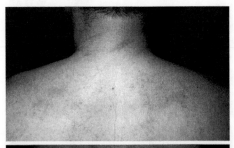

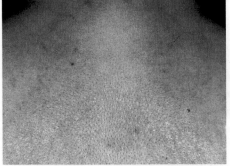

Fig. 17.7 Scleredema. Marked hardening of the skin on the neck and upper back.

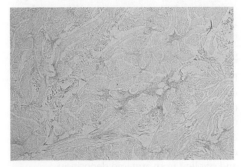

Fig. 17.8 Histopathology of scleredema. Deposition of mucin.

dermis are hyaluronic acid, dermatan sulfate, chondroitin sulfate, and keratan sulfate.

Abnormal deposition of mucin among collagen fibers results in swelling and separation of those fibers, and edematous skin. Mucin deposition is often found histopathologically in collagen diseases and is induced by thyroid dysfunction, diabetes or tumor; it results in characteristic cutaneous eruptions.

Systemic deposition of mucopolysaccharides caused by hereditary abnormality in lysosomal enzymes is called mucopolysccharidosis (Table 17.2).

Scleredema (synonym: scleredema adultorum)

Scleredema is often induced by acute infectious disease. Stiffness occurs in the skin, especially on the face, neck, shoulders, upper back and, in some cases, the upper extremities and the trunk (Fig. 17.7). The induration is non-pitting and hard. It is asymptomatic in the early stages; however, mild mobility impairment appears gradually. The distal portions of the extremities are not involved. The epidermis of the lesions thickens. Mucins deposit among dermal collagen fibers (Fig. 17.8). Differentiation from diabetic scleredema is important; when scleredema is suspected, diabetes should be tested for. Scleredema heals spontaneously in several months to several years.

Generalized myxedema

Generalized myxedema often occurs when there is decreased thyroid activity. Mucin deposition is found in the skin of the whole body, and edema is found in the face and extremities in particular. The skin is cold, dry, and white. When pinched, the skin is soft and no marks are left (non-pitting edema). The disorder is characterized by the facial features, The entire face swells, the nose widens, and macroglossia and lip swelling are present. The scalp hair and the hairs in the lateral one-third of each eyebrow become thin and fragile.

Pretibial myxedema

The frontal tibia and the dorsa of the foot are most commonly involved. Light pink to brownish plaques, subcutaneous induration, and nodules occur. Dilated follicles and hirsutism are present. Pretibial myxedema often occurs when the patient has hyperthyroidism or after treatment for hyperthyroidism.

Table 17.2 Classification of cutaneous amyloidoses.

Classification and disease	Clinical features							Inheritance pattern	Deficient enzyme
	Short stature	Characteristic facial features	Bone malformation	Joint contractures	Splenohepatomegaly	Corneal opacification	Intelligence impairment		
MPS IH Hurler's disease	++	++ / +	++ / +	+ / +	+ / +	+	++ / +	AR	α-l-iduronidase
MPS II Hunter's disease	±	+	+	+	+	−	− / ~ / ±	XR	L-iduronate sulfatase
MPS III Sanfilippo syndrome	±	+	+	±	+	−	++	AR	Sulfatase, etc.
MPS IV Morquio disease	++ / +	−	++ / +	+	±	± / ~ / +	−	AR	Galactose-6-sulfatase
MPS VI Maroteaux–Lamy syndrome	++	++	++	+	+	+	−	AR	β-galactosidase
MPS VII Sly syndrome	− / ~ / +	− / ~ / +	± / ~ / ++	− / ~ / +	− / ~ / +	− / ~ / +	− / ~ / +	AR	β-glucuronidas
MPS IX Hyaluronidase deficiency	+	+	±	−	−	−	−	AR	Hyaluronidase

AR, autosomal recessively inherited; MPS, mucopolysaccharidosis; XR, X-linked recessively inherited.

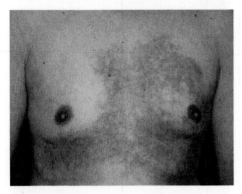

Fig. 17.9 Reticular erythematous mucinosis.

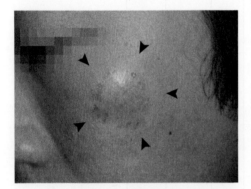

Fig. 17.10 Follicular mucinosis. The skin lesion is accompanied by relatively sharply demarcated, reddish infiltration of 3–4 cm in diameter, and alopecia.

Lichen myxedematosus (synonyms: scleromyxedema, papular mucinosis)

Soft, yellowish papules 1–3 mm in diameter aggregate and coalesce on the face, hands, and fingers, the extensor surfaces of the forearms and other parts of the extremities, presenting an orange peel-like appearance. Single or diffuse papules may be found. Thyroid dysfunction is not generally found. A primary disease such as multiple myeloma, plasma cell dyscrasia, diabetes, collagen disease, or liver dysfunction is frequently involved.

Reticular erythematous mucinosis (REM)

Reticular erythema without clear subjective symptoms occurs on the trunk of middle-aged women (Fig. 17.9). It is characterized by mucin deposition in the dermis and significant infiltration of mononuclear cells in the periphery of blood vessels.

Follicular mucinosis

Papules of normal skin color to rose pink aggregate, coalescing into elevated plaques, mainly on the scalp and face (Fig. 17.10). Alopecia often accompanies this. Edema and mucin deposition are seen in the outer root sheaths and sebaceous glands. Vacuolar degeneration of follicles and lymphatic infiltration also occur. Follicular mucinosis is classified into cases that heal naturally and cases that become chronic. Some of the latter cases accompany malignant lymphoma.

Xanthomas

Definition

Lipid-laden foamy histiocytes aggregate on the skin or mucous membranes to form yellowish lesions (Figs. 17.11–17.14). This condition usually accompanies a systemic abnormality of lipid metabolism; however, there are some cases without lipemia (non-lipemic xanthomatosis). Xanthoma is divided by clinical features into the several subtypes described below. There are other subtypes, including tuberoeruptive xanthoma and palmar xanthoma.

Pathology

Xanthoma presents histologically as an aggregation of foam cells in the dermis (Fig. 17.15). Touton giant cells may be found.

Treatment

The hyperlipemia should be treated first. In treatment for xanthelasma palpebrarum that does not accompany hyperlipidemia, medicines for hyperlipidemia are still sometimes effective. Eruptive xanthoma disappears within a few weeks after the hyperlipidemia is corrected; however, tuberous xanthoma and xanthelasma palpebrarum require several months to completely resolve, and tendon xanthoma requires several years. Surgical removal may be performed for refractory cases or cases with cosmetic problems.

Tuberous xanthoma

Tuberous xanthoma occurs mostly on the extensor surfaces of the elbows and knees, and on the joints of the hands and feet. Firm, reddish to yellowish nodules of 5 mm to several centimeters in diameter occur (see Fig. 17.11). The condition accompanies cholesterolemia (type II hyperlipidemia).

Tendon xanthoma

The Achilles tendons and the tendons of the hands, legs, and knees become tumorous. It may be accompanied by restricted movement of the joints. The condition accompanies hypercholesterolemia (type II).

Plane xanthoma

Flat or slightly elevated yellowish lesions occur. The lesions may occur at the creases of the palms in cases with type III hyperlipidemia (xanthoma striatum palmare). It is classified into cases accompanied by hyperlipoproteinemia and cases that occur secondary to cutaneous symptoms (see Fig. 17.12).

Xanthelasma palpebrarum

The inner canthus of the upper eyelids becomes flatly elevated. About half of all cases accompany hypercholesterolemia (type II, type III) (see Fig. 17.13).

Eruptive xanthoma

Multiple small yellowish papules 5 mm or smaller in diameter appear on the buttocks, the back, and the extensor surfaces of the extremities. Itching is generally present. Eruptive xanthoma accompanies hypertriglyceridemia (types I, IV, V) (see Fig. 17.14). It may occur secondary to diabetes.

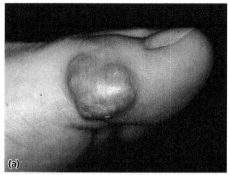

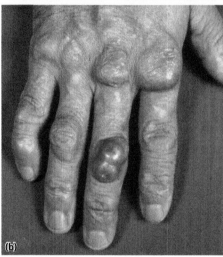

Fig. 17.11 Tuberous xanthoma. a: A lesion on the left pollex. b: Lesions on the metacarpophalangeal joints and proximal interphalangeal joints. Redness is seen in some of the affected sites.

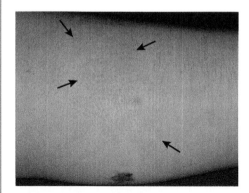

Fig. 17.12 Plane xanthoma that occurred secondarily after lymphedema on the upper arm. There are vaguely demarcated yellow plaques.

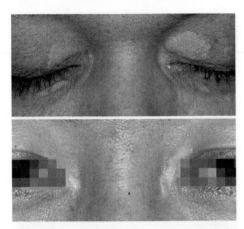

Fig. 17.13 Xanthelasma palpebrarum.
Flatly elevated yellow plaques occur on the inner canthus of the upper and lower eyelids, accompanied by mild infiltration.

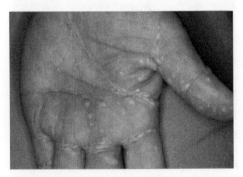

Fig. 17.14 Eruptive xanthoma.

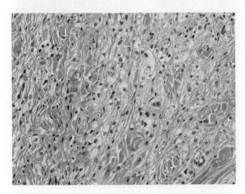

Fig. 17.15 Histopathology of xanthoma.
Foamy histiocytes that have phagocytosed fat droplets are observed in the dermis.

Electrolyte abnormalities

Zinc deficiency syndrome (synonym: acrodermatitis enteropathica)

- This is a zinc deficiency whose main symptoms are dermatitis, alopecia, and diarrhea.
- The main types are an autosomal recessively inherited congenital type (acrodermatitis enteropathica) and an acquired type that is caused by the administration of parenteral central venous nutrition.
- Erythema and erosions form on the distal portions of the extremities, and on the genitalia and orifices (the periphery of the eyes and mouth, the nares, and the auditory meatus), presenting clinical features similar to psoriasis, seborrheic dermatitis, and candidiasis.

Clinical features

The eruptions tend to occur symmetrically on the distal portions of the extremities, the genitals, and the facial orifices (the periphery of the eyes and mouth, nares, and auditory meatus) (Fig. 17.16). Acrodermatitis enteropathica begins with papules, small blisters or erythema accompanied by pustules, and progresses to erosions and crusts. Annular scaling is clinically observed, resembling psoriasis, impetigo contagiosa, seborrheic dermatitis, candidiasis, and necrolytic migratory erythema. Nail deformity and perionychia occur. Alopecia occurs in almost all cases, appearing on the occipital and temporal regions of the head first, and then spreading to the entire scalp and eyebrows. Diarrhea and vomiting recur.

Pathogenesis

The congenital type is autosomal recessively inherited. It is caused by mutations in the *SLC39A4* gene (*ZIP4*), which codes for a specific protein for transporting zinc. The onset is during the weaning period (acrodermatitis enteropathica). Acquired zinc deficiency is caused mainly by prolonged parenteral central venous nutrition, excision of the digestive tract, inflammatory enteric diseases or anorexia nervosa. The required daily zinc intake is 7–15 mg for adults, and 3–5 mg for infants. The disorder sometimes occurs in 2–3-month-old infants because of zinc deficiency in breast milk despite normal zinc content in the mother's serum. It may be induced by D-penicillamine taken by the mother.

Laboratory findings and diagnosis

Serum zinc levels are low (less than 70 mg/dL), the ratio of serum zinc to copper is low (less than 0.7) and zinc levels in urine are low in patients. The alkaline phosphatase level in the blood is also low, because of the low zinc level.

Treatment

Sufficient supply of zinc is essential. The cutaneous conditions improve in 3–7 days after the start of treatment.

Hemochromatosis (synonym: bronze diabetes)

- Excessive accumulation of iron in the body leads to organ failure from deposition of hemosiderin (an iron-binding protein) in various organs. It is caused hereditarily or by anemia, liver dysfunction, excessive intake of iron preparations or excessive transfusions.
- It is characterized by three main symptoms: diffuse, brownish-blue-gray pigmentation on the skin, cirrhosis, and diabetes. Abnormality is not seen in the central nervous system.
- Iron and elevated ferritin are found in the serum by blood test.
- Phlebotomy and iron chelator administration are the main treatments.

Clinical features

Diffuse, brownish-blue-gray pigmentation occurs in the skin as a result of marked deposition of hemosiderin, ferritin or melanin (Fig. 17.17). The sun-exposed areas of the body, such as the face, dorsal hands, extensor surfaces of the forearms, and genitals, are most severely affected. Atrophy and dryness are present. Axillary and pubic hair may become sparse. The symptoms progress gradually. Liver dysfunction almost always accompanies the cutaneous symptoms. Impaired hepatic function, hepatomegaly, and cirrhosis are found. Without proper treatment, the liver cirrhosis may progress to hepatocellular carcinoma. Complications include diabetes and cardiac failure.

Classification and pathogenesis

Hemochromatoses are divided into hereditary (autosomal recessively inherited) and secondary. Most hereditary hemochromatoses are caused by abnormality in

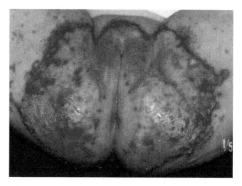

Fig. 17.16-1 Zinc deficiency syndrome. A large area of impetigo-like erythema around the external genitalia. Blisters and pustules form in some parts.

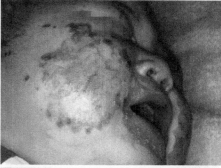

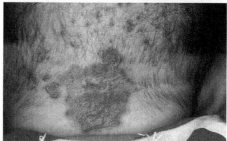

Fig. 17.16-2 Zinc deficiency syndrome.

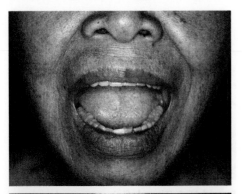

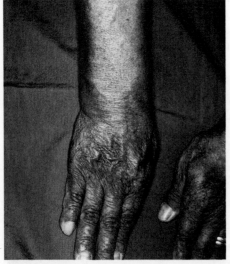

Fig. 17.17 Hemochromatosis.

the *HFE* gene; overabsorption of iron from the intestinal tract and iron metabolic dysfunction in the endothelial system are present. Secondary hemochromatosis may be caused by the following:

- anemia accompanied by ineffective erythropoiesis (e.g., sideroblastic anemia, hemolytic anemia)
- liver disease (e.g., alcoholic cirrhosis)
- excessive oral intake of iron (e.g., high intake of red wine, excessive intake of iron preparations)
- blood transfusion in large volumes.

Pathology

Hyperpigmentation of the skin is caused by increased dermal melanin and dermal hemosiderin within macrophages, seen as melanophages and siderophages. Iron deposits in the deep dermis. Dermal atrophy and pigmentation are present. Marked iron deposition can be found at the periphery of the sebaceous glands (Fig. 17.18).

Laboratory findings and diagnosis

Serum iron, transferrin saturation and serum ferritin values increase from iron excess. Unsaturated iron binding capacity (UIBC) is decreased. A liver biopsy is conducted for differential diagnosis.

Treatment

Phlebotomy is the first line of treatment. When phlebotomy is not possible, an iron chelator (deferoxamine) is administered. Symptomatic therapies are performed for organ failure.

Menkes kinky hair disease

- This disease is an X-linked recessive disorder of copper metabolism.
- It is characterized by kinky hair and reduced skin pigmentation.

Clinical features

Congenital lack of a copper-dependent enzyme that is essential for the synthesis of melanin and keratin leads to reduced skin pigmentation immediately after birth. Hair is whitish and fragile (kinky hair). Babies with Menkes kinky hair disease are born underweight and demonstrate convulsions and other neurological symptoms shortly after birth. Psychomotor retardation, muscular hypotonia, poor sucking, and low body temperature are present. Abnormality in the blood vessels in the whole body, osteoporosis, and urinary tract infection are also present.

Pathogenesis
Mutation in the gene that codes for copper-transporting ATPase (*ATP7A*) causes malabsorption of copper in the intestinal tract, resulting in copper insufficiency in the body. It is an X-linked recessive disorder; boys are most commonly affected.

Treatment
Parenteral copper salt is effective in mild cases. The gene responsible for Menkes kinky hair disease has been identified; this may be useful for gene therapies.

Calcinosis cutis
Calcinosis cutis is a condition in which calcium deposits in large amounts to form firm, yellow to white papules or nodules. When the deposition is in the stomach, kidneys, lungs or muscles, or when it is in/under the skin and hypercalcemia or hyperphosphatemia is present, the cause is hyperergasia of the accessory thyroid (tumor, chronic renal failure), excessive intake of vitamin D, myeloma multiplex or metastatic bone disease. Calcinosis cutis may appear as a symptom in systemic sclerosis and dermatomyositis, even in cases with normal serum calcium level (Fig. 17.19). There are also idiopathic cases:,e.g., scrotal calcinosis cutis (Fig. 17.20).

Calciphylaxis
Calciphylaxis occurs in patients with chronic renal failure who have prolonged hemodialysis and hyperergasia of the accessory thyroid, such as after receiving minor physical trauma. An intensely painful ulcerous lesion rapidly enlarges (Fig. 17.21). Histopathologically, calcification in the small arteries is found. The prognosis is generally poor.

Vitamin deficiencies

Pellagra
- It is caused by a lack of niacin (nicotine acid, nicotinic acid amide).
- The main symptoms are dermatitis, diarrhea, and dementia.

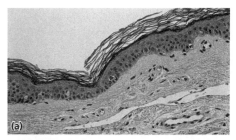

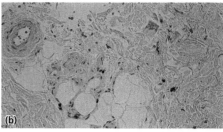

Fig. 17.18 Histopathology of hemochromatosis. a: Melanin deposition is observed in the epidermal basal keratinocytes. b: There is iron deposition in the dermis (the portions stained blue).

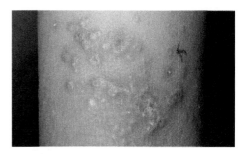

Fig. 17.19 Calcinosis cutis on the extensor surface of an infant's forearm. Multiple papules of several millimeters in diameter are caused by calcium deposition. Some rupture and coalesce, discharging their contents.

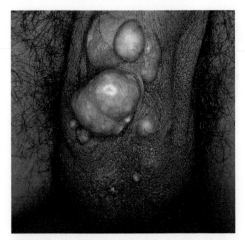

Fig. 17.20 Calcinosis cutis on the scrotum.

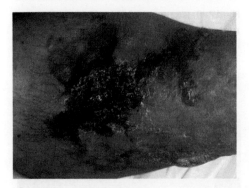

Fig. 17.21 Calciphylaxis.

MEMO 17–2 Hartnup's disease

In this rare, autosomal recessive disorder, niacin deficiency occurs as the result of inhibited uptake of tryptophan. Abnormality in the neutral amino acid transporter that is coded by the *SLC6A19* gene is the cause. Cutaneous symptoms similar to those of pellagra occur in infancy. Oral administration of niacin is the treatment.

• It most frequently occurs in recipients of isoniazid (INH), and in alcoholics and those who have had a gastrectomy or who have poor eating habits.
• Supplementation of niacin is the main treatment.

Definition and symptoms

The disorder is caused by lack of niacin (nicotine acid, nicotinic acid amide). Pellagra is characterized by the "3Ds" of dermatitis, diarrhea, and dementia; however, there now tend to be few cases with all three symptoms together. The cutaneous symptoms are burning sensation and intensely itchy photosensitive dermatosis. Sunburn-like eruptions appear on sun-exposed areas of the body, which develop into reddish-brown erythema, blistering, and erosions. The skin roughens. Sharply circumscribed, dark-brown pigmentation and atrophy are present (Fig. 17.22). Eruptions on the frontal neck region are called Casal's necklace. Angular cheilitis, stomatitis, and glossitis occur.

Diarrhea, esophagitis, nausea and vomiting occur as gastrointestinal symptoms. Psychoneurotic symptoms including peripheral neuropathy, depression, delirium, and hallucinations may occur.

Laboratory findings and diagnosis

The total nicotinic acid in the blood is low. The amount of N1-methyl nicotinamide, a metabolic product of niacin, quantitated in the urine for 24 h is low. Pellagra should be carefully differentiated from other photosensitive dermatoses.

Treatment

Administration of nicotinic acid amide, dietary improvement, and avoidance of exposure to light are useful.

Biotin deficiency

Biotin deficiency is caused by a lack of this water-soluble vitamin, which is a coenzyme necessary for gluconeogenesis, amino acid metabolization, and biosynthesis of fatty acids (Fig. 17.23). Cutaneous symptoms that resemble zinc deficiency syndrome occur, and exfoliative dermatitis-like lesions are produced on the face and in the intertriginous areas. Atrophy in the lingual papillae, loss of appetite, tremors, and muscular pain are present. It can occur in patients who undergo prolonged central venous nutrition or in newborns. Biotin deficiency occurs autosomal recessively in infants because of congenital abnormalities and deficiencies in enzymes associated with biotin (biotin dependency).

Vitamin C deficiency (scurvy)

Vitamin C (ascorbic acid) is essential for hydroxyproline production, which in turn is necessary for the synthesis of collagen types II and III. Deficiency leads to fragility of the blood vessels and the hair tissues. Follicular keratotic papules and purpura are characteristic symptoms, and gingival hemorrhaging and swelling of the gums occur.

There may be systemic symptoms, such as fatigue and bone fracture. These are promptly improved by vitamin C supplementation.

Porphyria

- Porphyria is a general term for diseases caused by the deposition of intermediate products such as porphyrins in the liver or skin, as a result of congenital or acquired impairment of an enzyme essential for heme synthesis.
- It is divided into hepatogenous porphyrias and myelogenous ones.
- The main cutaneous symptom is photosensitivity accompanied by blistering.

Classification and pathogenesis

Porphyrin is a general term for molecules that have a porphyrin ring, which is an intermediate metabolite synthesized in the process of heme biosynthesis from glycine and succinyl-CoA. Eight enzymes are involved in heme biosynthesis. Abnormalities in the enzymes cause deposition of porphyrins (Fig. 17.24). Metabolic enzymes such as P450 occur as hemoproteins in the liver and are synthesized into the heme of hemoglobin. That is, there are hepatogenous porphyrias and erythropoietic (myelogenous) porphyrias. These are further subclassified. The major subtypes are shown in Table 17.3.

Porphyrins induce cutaneous and neurological symptoms. They become activated by light energy, which produces reactive oxygen that causes cytotoxicity and results in the cutaneous symptoms of photosensitive diseases. δ-Aminolevulinic acid (δ-ALA) passes through the blood–brain barrier and acts neurotoxically.

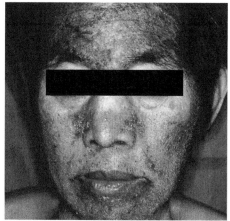
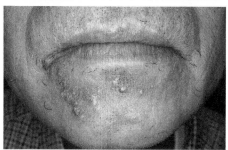
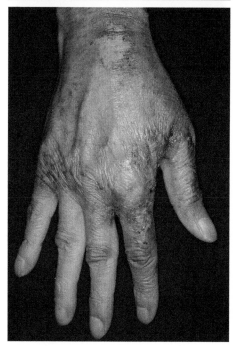

Fig. 17.22 Pellagra. Erythema and dark brown pigmentation on sun-exposed areas. Poor diet is the cause.

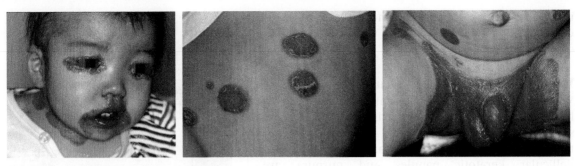

Fig. 17.23 Biotin deficiency.

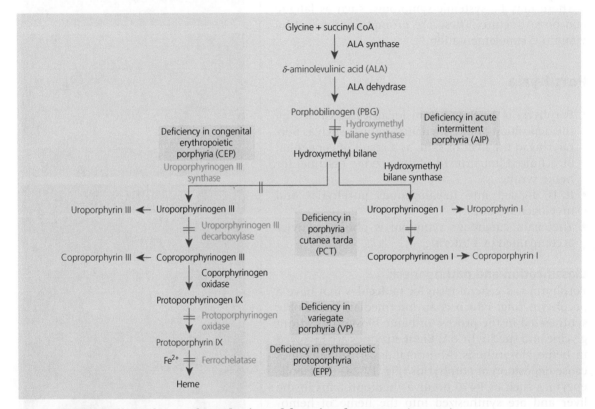

Fig. 17.24 Metabolic pathway of porphyrin and functional enzymes (arrows).

Congenital erythropoietic porphyria
Clinical features

Congenital erythropoietic porphyria (CEP) appears shortly after birth, first as photosensitivity (blistering, pustule formation, ulceration) and later as scarring. Wine-colored urine and purplish-black feces are observed. The intermediate products

Table 17.3 Major types of porphyria.

Porphyria		Photosensitivity	Causative enzyme	Inheritance pattern	Erythrocytes			Urine		Feces		
					URO	CP	PP	URO	CP	URO	CP	PP
Erythropoietic porphyrias	Congenital erythropoietic porphyria (CEP)	+	UROS	AR	++	++	−	++	++	++	++	−
	Erythropoietic protoporphyria (EPP)	+	FECH	AD	−	−	++	−	−	−	−	++
Hepatic porphyrias	Acute intermittent porphyria (AIP)	−	HMBS	AD	−	−	−	+	+	−	−	−
	Variegate porphyria (VP)	+	PPOX	AD	−	−	−	+	+	−	++	++
	Porphyria cutanea tarda (PCT)	+	UROD	AD in familial PCT	−	−	−	++	++	+	+	−

CP, coproporphyrin; FECH, ferrochelatase; HMBS, hydroxymethylbilane synthase; PP, protoporphyrin; PPOX, protoporphyrinogen oxidase; URO, uroporphyrin; UROD, uroporphyrinogen decarboxylase; UROS, uroporphyrinogen III synthase.

deposit in erythrocytes, teeth, and bones. They fluoresce red under Wood's lamp. Hemolytic anemia causes splenomegaly.

Pathogenesis
It is autosomal recessively inherited. Uroporphyrin I and coproporphyrin I are produced in large amounts in the hematopoietic tissue as a result of congenital absence of uroporphyrinogen III synthase (UROS) (see Fig. 17.24).

Uroporphyrin I and coproporphyrin I deposit in the skin and hemoglobin, where they absorb light energy and destroy cellular membranes. Uroporphyrin and coproporphyrin are found in blood, urine, and feces.

Erythropoietic protoporphyria
Clinical features
Mild photosensitivity, heat sensation, pain, flushing and edema or urticaria manifest in children age 10 or younger. Moderate hemolytic anemia occurs. Protoporphyrin deposited in the liver is crystallized and excreted in the bile; mild liver dysfunction and gallstones are present.

Pathogenesis
Erythropoietic protoporphyria (EPP) is autosomal dominantly inherited. It is caused by congenital abnormality in the ferrochelatase (*FECH*) gene. Protoporphyrin IX is not transformed into heme and deposits in the erythron of the bone marrow, causing EPP (see Fig. 17.24). Protoporphyrin is elevated in the blood and feces, but not in the urine.

Acute intermittent porphyria (AIP)
This disorder, too, is autosomal dominantly inherited, and it most frequently occurs in women of adolescent age or older. Reduced activity of hydroxymethylbilane synthase (HMBS) leads to the deposition of porphobilinogen and δ-aminolevulinic acid. Cutaneous symptoms are not seen but neurological symptoms, peripheral nervous symptoms, and abdominal symptoms are present.

Variegate porphyria
Variegate porphyria (VP) is an autosomal dominantly inherited hepatic porphyria caused by abnormality in protoporphyrinogen oxidase (PPOX). It is clinically similar to porphyria cutanea tarda (described below).

Porphyria cutanea tarda (PCT)
Clinical features
Blistering is caused by injury and sun exposure on the face and dorsal hands during the spring and summer. It resolves with moderate scarring, atrophy, and pigmentation; the course recurs (Fig. 17.25). Reddening of urine, abdominal symptoms resembling those of AIP, hypertrichosis of the face, and liver dysfunction may occur.

Pathogenesis
Uroporphyrinogen decarboxylase (UROD) activity decreases, and uroporphyrin deposits in the liver and skin (see Fig. 17.24). The condition is induced by hepatitis C, chronic alcohol consumption, hemodialysis or drugs such as estrogen, hexachlorobenzene, iron preparations or sulfonylurea drugs. PCT is sometimes autosomal dominantly inherited. Familial cases have been reported. It most frequently occurs in women of middle age and older.

Pathology
Subepidermal blistering is found. Endothelial cells are damaged. PAS-positive substances are detected in the peripheral blood vessels.

Laboratory findings
There are elevated levels of uroporphyrins in the urine and coproporphyrins in the feces. Elevated serum iron and serum ferritin values are often observed. It should be noted that hepatitis C or hepatic carcinoma is often present as a complication.

Treatment
Cessation of alcohol consumption, shading from light, phlebotomy, administration of an iron chelating agent, liver support therapy, and oral sodium hydrogen carbonate are effective.

Skin manifestations associated with diabetes

Diabetes induces various cutaneous symptoms. Major disorders are discussed below.

Diabetic gangrene
Gangrene occurs on the toes, soles, and fingers. It is associated with underlying diseases such as microangiopathy

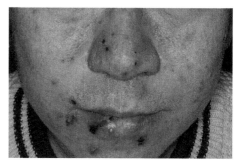

Fig. 17.25-1 Porphyria cutanea tarda.
Blisters, mild scarring, atrophy, and pigmentation occurred at all these sites. The symptoms recurred when the sites were exposed to the sun.

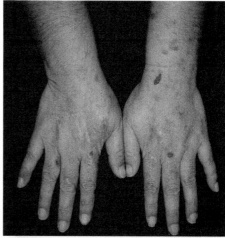

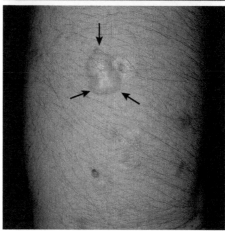

Fig. 17.25-2 Porphyria cutanea tarda.
Blister (arrows).

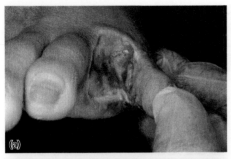

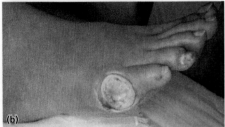

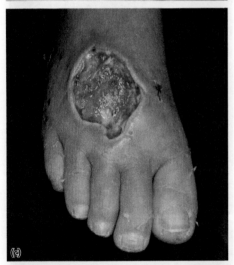

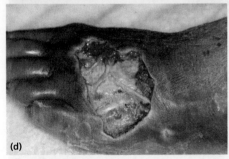

Fig. 17.26 Diabetic gangrene. a: Ulceration occurring secondarily after tinea pedis. b,c: Ulceration resulting from shoe sores. d: Advanced diabetic gangrene in a foot. The aponeurosis is exposed by the deep ulcer.

> **MEMO 17–3 Clear cell syringoma**
>
> The symptoms are similar to those of syringoma (see Chapter 21). The lesions contain clear cells rich in glycogen. Diabetes is frequently associated with this disorder.

> **MEMO 17–4 Necrobiosis lipoidica: can it occur without diabetes?**
>
> Necrobiosis lipoidica used to be understood as a skin lesion caused by diabetes, hence the name "diabetic necrobiosis lipoidica." However, some cases without diabetes have recently been described. Even so, reports have found a close association between the two. This textbook includes it in the diabetes section.

and arterial sclerosis. Minor injuries lead to secondary infection that induces ulceration. Necrotic foci occur secondarily to ulceration, and these become intractable (Fig. 17.26). Vasodilators, skin ulcer treatment drugs, and surgical treatments including debridement and amputation are conducted. Arteriosclerosis obliterans in the main artery is surgically treated (see Chapter 11).

Diabetic scleredema (synonym: scleredema diabeticorum)

Scleredema occurs on the back and nuchal region (Fig. 17.27). Acute infection does not occur in diabetic scleredema as a prodrome, nor is there spontaneous healing.

Diabetic xanthoma

Eruptive xanthoma occurs commonly on the extensor surfaces of the extremities and buttocks. When hyperglyceridemia is resolved by diabetic treatment, the xanthoma also subsides in several weeks.

Necrobiosis lipoidica

The frontal tibiae of adult women are most commonly affected. Irregularly shaped, sharply circumscribed, atrophic and yellow to tan plaques of 5–10 cm diameter occur. The periphery is purplish-brown, accompanied by telangiectasia (Fig. 17.28). The histo-pathological findings are similar to those for granuloma annulare. It may also occur on the thighs and hands. Necrobiosis lipoidica has been reported to occur in 0.3% of diabetes patients. It progresses chronically (MEMO, see Chapter 17).

Bullosis diabeticorum

Tense blisters appear suddenly on the lower legs or fingers and toes. Microangiopathy is thought to be the cause of bullosis diabeticorum. Because the reduced sensory perception of diabetic patients tends to make them less sensitive to high temperatures, differentiation from second-degree burn is necessary.

Dupuytren's contracture (synonym: palmar fibromatosis)

Cord-like induration occurs on the palms, the ulnar side in particular. Fibrous thickening of the aponeuroses is present. As it progresses, flexion contracture occurs in the fingers and becomes painful. It may occur on the soles (plantar fibromatosis). It tends to affect patients with alcohol dependence, diabetes or epilepsy. The pathogenesis is unknown but genetic factors are suggested, because about half of cases are familial. Aponeurectomy and rehabilitation are conducted.

Generalized granuloma annulare

Aggregated, solid, light-pink papules or infiltrating erythema occurs (see Chapter 18). Glucose intolerance is frequently seen.

Eczema, dermatitis, and pruritus

The seborrheic and intertriginous areas are the most commonly affected. If diabetes is not treated appropriately, eczema and dermatitis tend to recur. Sebum reduction and dry skin are also present, and they result in pruritus (see Chapter 8).

Opportunistic infection

Cutaneous infectious diseases, including various opportunistic infections, occur and become refractory. These include candidiasis, tinea, furunculosis, subcutaneous abscess, cellulitis, perionychia, necrotizing fasciitis, and non-clostridial gas gangrene.

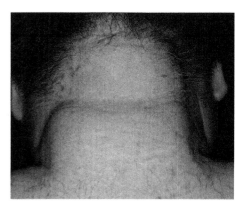

Fig. 17.27 Diabetic scleredema in the nucha. This is a markedly firm, large, plate-like plaque.

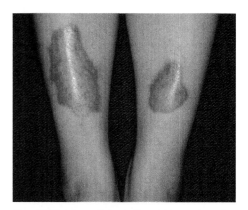

Fig. 17.28 Necrobiosis lipoidica. Sharply demarcated, irregularly shaped, atrophic plate-like plaques on the tibial anterior regions.

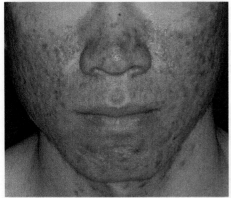

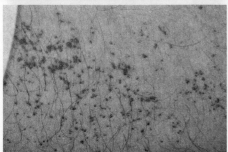

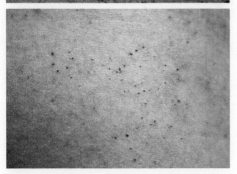

Fig. 17.30 Fabry's disease in a male in his 20s. Multiple red papules 2–3 mm in diameter are present on the face and trunk, accompanied by telangiectasia (angiokeratoma).

Other metabolic disorders

Fabry's disease (synonym: angiokeratoma corporis diffusum)

This is an X-linked recessive disorder. The pathogenesis is absence or marked reduction of α-galactosidase (α-gal A) activity caused by genetic mutation (Fig. 17.29 and Fig. 17.30). Female carriers may develop symptoms of varying severity. Trihexosylceramide fails to be degraded because of a lack of α-galactosidase, resulting in deposition in blood vessels, causing dysfunction (Fig. 17.31). Multiple angiokeratomas, small reddish or black papules of a few millimeters to 1 cm in diameter, occur (see Chapter 21), mostly on the abdominal and lumbar regions ("bathing trunk" distribution). The lesions appear at infancy and increase with age. Lymphedema in the extremities and oligohidrosis are also present. It is characterized by paroxysmal pain in the distal portions of the extremities and abdominal pain (Fabry crisis). Progressive corneal opacification, cerebrovascular disorder, renal failure, and heart failure are present. Recombinant human α-galactosidase is used in enzyme replacement therapy. A carbon dioxide laser is used for treating the angiokeratomas.

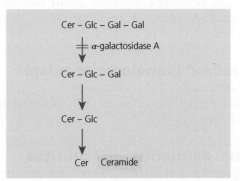

Fig. 17.29 Mechanism of Fabry's disease. Trihexosylceramide (Cer-Glc-Gal-Gal) deposits in the kidneys and vascular tissue from lack of α-galactosidase A activation.

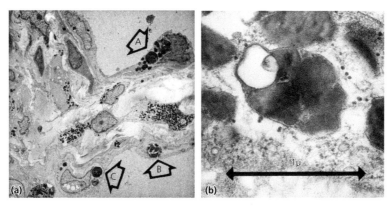

Fig. 17.31 Electron microscopic view of the dermis in Fabry's disease. a: Low-power magnification. Arrows indicate the following: A. Vascular endothelial cell. B. Macrophage. C. Neurocyte. b: High-power magnification. Trihexosylceramide is observed as black deposition with high electron density in the cytoplasms of various cells.

Kanzaki's disease (synonyms: angiokeratoma corporis diffusum (Kanzaki), Schindler disease (type II))

This is a lysosomal storage disorder. Enzyme deficiency results from mutation in the α-N-acetyl galactosaminidase gene. It is autosomal recessively inherited. The cutaneous symptoms resemble those of Fabry's disease: small multiple angiokeratomas occur on the whole body, particularly on the lumbar region (Fig. 17.32). Oligohidrosis, minor sensory nerve failure in the extremities and hearing impairment are present. The prognosis is good.

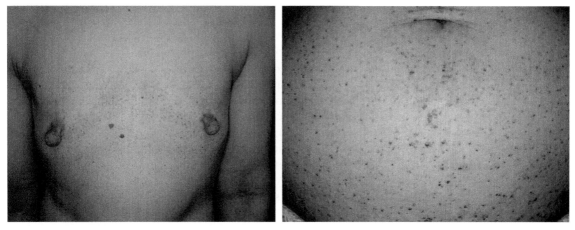

Fig. 17.32 Kanzaki's disease in a woman in her 40s. Multiple angiokeratoma 2–3 mm in diameter occurred on the chest and abdominal region. It is impossible to differentiate Kanzaki's disease from Fabry's disease only by the clinical features of the eruptions.

Tophus

Tophus occurs in gout patients when hyperuricemia is left untreated for a long time. Multiple nodules of 5–30 mm diameter occur on the auriculae, finger and toe joints, elbows, knees, and Achilles tendons. It is generally painless. The skin becomes tense and thin, with a yellowish-white tone in subcutaneous areas. When the skin is broken, a chalk-like substance containing uric acid crystals is expelled. Tophus heals with scarring after ulceration. Histopathologically, amorphous deposition of needle-like crystals (monosodium urate crystals) with voids and foreign body giant cells is found. Monosodium urate crystals are identified by alcohol-fixed specimen.

Lipoid proteinosis (synonym: hyalinosis cutis et mucosae)

Hyaline-like substances deposit in the skin and membranes. Small papules that resemble a string of pearls occur on the margins of the eyelid as a characteristic symptom. Wart-like nodules and papules form on the elbows, and white nodules form in the oral cavity. Nodules in the glottis cause hoarseness. Cases caused by autosomal recessively inherited mutation in the extracellular matrix protein 1 (*ECM1*) gene have been reported.

Phenylketonuria

This autosomal recessively inherited disorder is caused by mutations in the phenylalanine hydroxylase (*PAH*) gene, which codes for an enzyme that metabolizes phenylalanine into tyrosine. Reduced skin pigmentation, brownish hair color, and mental developmental delay result from the reduced tyrosine. In Japan, Guthrie newborn mass screening is conducted for phenylketonuria; the incidence is 1 in 70,000. Initiation of a phenylalanine-restricted diet within 1 month after birth, continued for life, prevents mental retardation. The skin and hair color return to normal by dietary supplementation of tyrosine.

CHAPTER 18
Disorders of the dermis and subcutaneous fat

The dermis and subcutaneous tissue hold and support the epidermis. If the tissue is injured, the entire structure of the skin may be greatly affected, even though the surface of the skin itself might show only minor changes. This chapter discusses diseases that predominantly affect the dermis and subcutaneous tissue.

Disorders of the dermis

Cutaneous atrophy

Striae distensae (synonyms: striae atrophicae, stretch marks)
- Slightly concave, linear cutaneous atrophy follows the cleavage lines.
- The thighs and lower abdomen are most commonly affected.
- Oral steroids may be the inducing factor. Striae occur when skin undergoes rapid growth or stretching, especially in pregnancy (striae gravidarum) and adolescence.

Clinical features
Striae are linear atrophy several millimeters in width and 10 cm or more in length. They run in a roughly parallel pattern. The striae are commonly known as "stretch marks." The color is rose pink in the early stages (striae rubra), becoming grayish-white later on (striae alba). Fine wrinkles appear following the lines of cleavage (Fig. 18.1). The long axis of the striae follows the lines of cleavage. Rapid growth in adolescence often causes striae in the lateral thighs, buttocks, and breasts. Striae gravidarum is seen in more than 90% of all pregnancies. It occurs on the lower abdomen, breasts, and buttocks around the

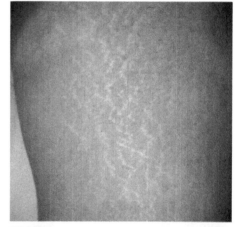
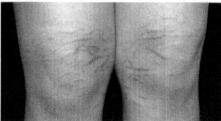

Fig. 18.1 Striae atrophicae ("stretch marks").

Shimizu's Dermatology, Second Edition. Hiroshi Shimizu.
© 2017 John Wiley & Sons, Ltd. Published 2017 by John Wiley & Sons, Ltd.

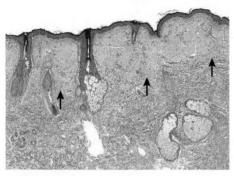

Fig. 18.2 Histopathology of skin aging. The epidermis is atrophic. The elastic fibers and collagen fibers in the upper dermis tear in a club shape (arrows).

---

sixth month of pregnancy. Oral steroids, Cushing's syndrome, severe infections or diabetes may induce striae.

Pathogenesis

Steroid (glucocorticoid) inhibits fibroblast activity (collagen production). Connective tissue collapses when external pressure or excessive extension occurs, and the result is striae and atrophy. Increases in endogenous steroids are thought to be associated with striae during adolescence or pregnancy.

Treatment and prognosis

There are no effective treatments. The symptoms subside with age; nonetheless, the changes are irreversible and do not disappear completely.

Skin aging (synonyms: senile skin atrophy, solar elastosis)

- Any changes in the skin that occur with age are called skin aging. Prolonged sunlight exposure is associated with such aging.
- Overall functional degeneration and atrophy of the skin are the main features.
- Deep rhombus striae that occur in the nuchal region are called cutis rhomboidalis.

Clinical features

Any changes in the skin that occur with age are called skin aging. The skin becomes thin and yellowish, and slackens on the whole body. Large folds of skin form on the face, neck, and joints. Dry skin occurs, followed by pityroid scaling. Asteatotic eczema and pruritus cutaneous may also occur. Because of atrophy, the skin becomes a glossy pale yellow or brown. Skin aging is remarkable on sun-exposed areas (photoaging) (see Chapter 13). Outdoor workers show marked changes caused by skin aging. Deep wrinkles are seen, particularly in the nuchal region (cutis rhomboidalis nuchae).

Pathology

Atrophy and thinning of the dermis occur. Reduction of collagen fibers is marked (Fig. 18.2). The elastic fibers are ruptured, and solar elastosis is observed by the Elastica-van Gieson method. The sweat glands and seborrheic glands decrease in size and number, and subcutaneous fat tissue decreases.

White fibrous papulosis of the neck (Shimizu)
Clinical features
Small round or oval papules 2–4 mm in diameter and white to light yellow occur on the neck region of the elderly (Fig. 18.3). Sharply circumscribed eruptions occur on follicular and non-follicular sites. They do not coalesce. Thickening of the collagen fibers is histopathologically observed in the upper dermal layer (Fig. 18.4). The pathogenesis is age-related dermal degeneration.

Epidemiology
White fibrous papulosis of the neck may occur in any race.

Lichen sclerosus (LS) (synonym: lichen sclerosus et atrophicus)
Clinical features
White, flat-topped papules 2–3 mm in diameter appear and aggregate, forming firm white plaques. Later, the plaques shrink and take on a crepe-like appearance (Fig. 18.5). Comedo-like keratotic plugs characterize LS. LS may be accompanied by itching and pain. Roughly 80% of cases occur on the genitals of patients middle-aged and older or patients younger than about age 10. There is a female preponderance (5–15 females to one male). In women, the lesions often occur on the labia majora, clitoris, and anal region, distributing in the shape of a figure 8. In men, LS often occurs on the penis, and atrophy may result in urethral stricture. Lesions may occur on the trunk, including the back, and on the forearms. Blisters may form. LS may be accompanied by alopecia areata and vitiligo.

Pathogenesis
The pathogenesis is unknown; however, hereditary factors, endocrine abnormality or immunological mechanisms may be involved. Autoantibodies against extracellular matrix 1 (ECM1) have been found in patients' sera.

Pathology
In the dermal upper layer, collagen fibers are homogeneous and edematous, leading to the reduction of cellular components. As the condition progresses, band-like lymphatic infiltration is seen in the dermis. There is hyperkeratosis and the formation of keratin plugs in some cases (Fig. 18.6).

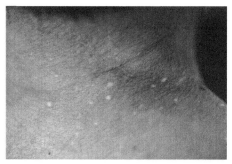
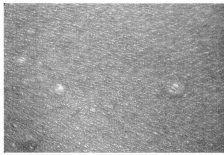
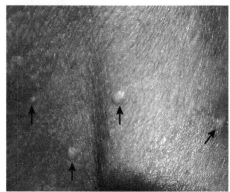

Fig. 18.3 White fibrous papulosis of the neck. Small, multiple white papules of 2–4 mm in diameter appear on the neck.

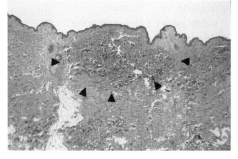

Fig. 18.4 Histopathology of white fibrous papulosis of the neck. Fibrosis in the upper dermis (arrows).

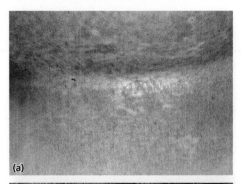

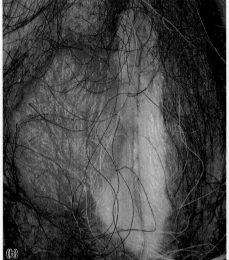

Fig. 18.5 Lichen sclerosus et atrophicus.
a: White plaques on the precordial region.
b: A lesion (white) on the labia majora of
an elderly woman. The lesion has partially
progressed to squamous cell carcinoma
(elevated red).

**MEMO 18–3 Lichen
sclerosus of the external
genitalia**

Lichen sclerosus in the female external
genitalia used to be called kraurosis
vulvae, and that in the penis used to
be called kraurosis penis or balanitis
xerotica obliterans.

Treatment and prognosis

Young children respond to topical steroids, and LS often
resolves spontaneously. LS in adults often becomes
chronic and intractable. When the genitalia are affected,
it progresses to squamous cell carcinoma in several percent of all cases. Careful follow-up is necessary.

Werner syndrome (synonym: adult progeria)

- This typifies diseases of premature aging. Aging
  occurs in systemic tissue at adolescence.
- It is caused by mutations in the *WRN* gene. It is autosomal recessive.
- Characteristic symptoms are skin atrophy, scleroderma-like changes, intractable ulcers, gray hair,
  and alopecia.

Clinical features

Most of the reported cases have been in Japan. The
patients stop growing around adolescence. Atrophy
and scleroderma-like changes with telangiectasia of
the whole body, gray hair, and alopecia occur around
the age of 20 (Fig.18.7a). The atrophy occurs not only
in the dermis but also in the subcutaneous fat tissues
and muscles. Radial wrinkles appear around the
mouth, and the nose becomes thin and pointy from
atrophy, giving the face a bird-like appearance.
Calcinosis cutis often occurs.

Hyperkeratosis and intractable ulceration are seen
on the sole (Fig. 18.7b). In addition to the skin changes,
there is a high-pitched voice in the early stage, and
cataracts, diabetes, osteoporosis, and gonadal hypo-
function in the later stages, leading to arterial sclerosis
and malignant tumors, including sarcoma (Table 18.1).

Pathogenesis

Werner syndrome is caused by a mutation in the gene
encoding WRN, on chromosome 8. The WRN protein is
a type of RecQ-like helicase that plays an important role
in repairing DNA damage or abnormality from replication. The mechanism of premature aging is unknown;
however, it is thought that chromosomal instability is
increased by incapacitation of the repairing gene.

Differential diagnosis

Differential diagnosis from other premature aging syndromes (see Table 18.1) and systemic sclerosis must
be made.

Prognosis

Most patients are short-lived, with an average age of 46 years, as a result of myocardial infarction, cerebral apoplexy, aggravated diabetes, and malignant tumors.

Rothmund–Thomson syndrome (synonym: congenital poikiloderma)

This is autosomal recessive. One of the causative genes is *RECQL4* on chromosome 8. In infancy and childhood, the skin atrophies, reticular or diffuse erythema occurs on the face and juvenile cataract appears. Photosensitivity is present in one-third of cases. In adulthood, head and body hair becomes sparse, and keratinization occurs on sun-exposed areas. There is impaired development of nails (Fig. 18.8). Internal malignant tumors (osteosarcomas, in particular) accompany roughly 30% of cases. The prognosis is good in the absence of malignancy. Like Werner syndrome, Rothmund–Thomson syndrome may be categorized as a type of premature aging syndrome.

Dysplasia

Ectodermal dysplasia

This term is a catch-all for congenital diseases of the hair, teeth, nails, and sweat glands that cause abnormal formation of ectodermal tissue. It is classified into more than 150 subtypes according to the combinations of dysplastic components and complications. The main diseases caused by ectodermal dysplasia are listed below.

Anhidrotic (hypohidrotic) ectodermal dysplasia

The main symptoms are thinning of the hair, anhidrosis, and abnormality in dental formation (Fig. 18.9). Many cases are X-linked recessively inherited, caused by a mutation in the *EDA1* gene. It may also be caused by a mutation in the *EDAR* gene, in which case it is autosomal recessively or dominantly inherited. The whole body skin is thin and dry from the absence or marked reduction of sweat gland complexes. The patient is prone to heatstroke. Decreased lacrimation and dryness of the oral and nasal membranes lead to keratoconjunctivitis, stomatitis, purulent rhinitis, and hoarseness. It is possible for patients to have a normal life as long as they avoid living environments with high temperatures.

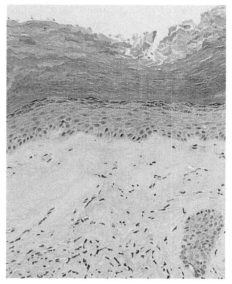

Fig. 18.6 Histopathology of lichen sclerosus et atrophicus. Hyperkeratosis, loss of epidermal rete ridges, homogenization of collagen fibers in the upper dermis, edema, and lymphocytic infiltration occur.

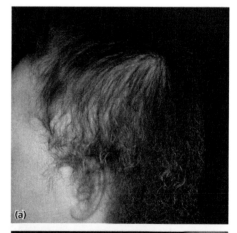

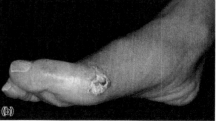

Fig. 18.7 Werner syndrome. a: Thin and sparse scalp hair. b: Ulcer on the foot.

Table 18.1 Major congenital premature aging syndromes.

Disease	Inheritance pattern	Causative gene	Clinical features and findings	Prognosis
Werner syndrome	AR	WRN	Onset is in the 20s. High-pitched voice, systemic skin atrophy, bird-like facial appearance	Lifespan of 40–50 years
Rothmund–Thomson syndrome	AR	RECQL4	Erythema on the face, photosensitivity, and poikiloderma occur in infancy. Cataract occurs in early childhood.	Good
Progeria (Hutchinson–Gilford syndrome)	AR	LMNA	Marked bird-like facial appearance, joint contractures, and slowed growth occur in infancy.	Lifespan of 10–20 years
Acrogeria (Gottron)	Partially AD	Partially COL3A1	Localized atrophy at the ends of the extremities, nose, and auricle. Some cases of vascular EDS are included	Good
Cockayne syndrome	AR	CSA, CSB	Photosensitivity, short stature and premature facial aging occur in early childhood. Cases that accompany xeroderma pigmentosum have been reported.	Lifespan of 10–20 years
Hallermann–Streiff syndrome	AR	GJA1	Congenital cataract, bird-like facial appearance, oligotrichia, atrophy	Relatively good
Wiedemann–Rautenstrauch syndrome	AR	?	Premature facial aging, oligotrichia, and atrophy occur at birth	Mortality in babyhood or infancy

AD, autosomal dominantly inherited; AR, autosomal recessively inherited; EDS, Ehlers–Danlos syndrome.

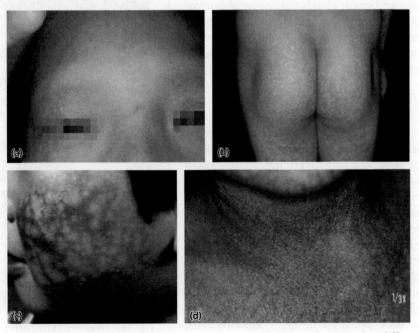

Fig. 18.8 Rothmund–Thomson syndrome. a: Thin and sparse body hair. b: Reticular, diffuse erythema on the buttocks. c: Reticular erythema on the cheek. d: Lesions on the precordial region.

Hidrotic ectodermal dysplasia, Clouston syndrome

Deformity of the nail plates, thinning of the hair, and palmoplantar keratoderma are the three major symptoms. However, some cases demonstrate only deformity of nail plates. Linear patterns form in the nail plates, which thicken and suffer from growth retardation. It is an autosomal dominant disease caused by a mutation in the *GJB6* gene encoding connexin 30 (see Chapter 1).

Aplasia cutis congenita

This is a disorder seen at birth with absence of a part of the skin, subcutaneous tissue, and bone in some cases. It often occurs at the top of the head as a sharply circumscribed atrophic plaque, erosion or ulcer (Fig. 18.10). Aplasia cutis congenita is localized hypoplasia that occurs during intrauterine development.

Cutis verticis gyrata

Hyperplasia of the scalp results in skinfolds at the top of the head. It occurs most commonly in boys. The folds are 1–2 cm wide, highly elastic, and mobile. Normal hair growth is present in the groove portions, but not in the elevated portions (Fig. 18.11). Cutis verticis gyrata is classified into a primary form and a secondary form that accompanies nevoid abnormalities (e.g., nevus cell nevus, connective tissue nevus) or systemic diseases (e.g., acromegaly). Plastic surgical repair may be conducted.

Pachydermoperiostosis (MIM, 167100) is a hereditary disease in which cutis verticis gyrata can be seen with Hippocratic nails (clubbed fingers), osteohypertrophy, and thickened skin change. It is autosomal dominant.

Perforating dermatosis

Elastosis perforans serpiginosa
Clinical features

Small, bilaterally symmetrical, reddish-brown keratotic papules 2–10 mm in diameter are produced in linear or circular arrangement on the neck region, extremities, and upper trunk, giving the skin a serpiginous appearance (Fig. 18.12). The skin surrounding the papules becomes atrophic.

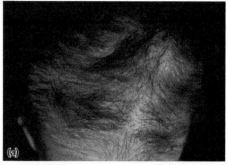
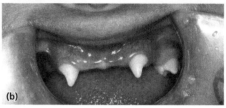

Fig. 18.9 Anhidrotic (hypohidrotic) ectodermal dysplasia. a: Thin and sparse scalp hair. b: Dental dysplasia.

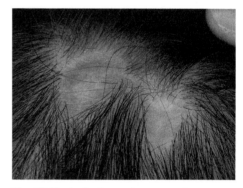

Fig. 18.10 Aplasia cutis congenita. Alopecia cicatricans on the parietal region of the scalp.

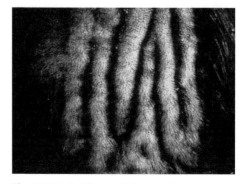

Fig. 18.11 Cutis verticis gyrata.

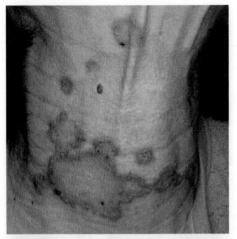

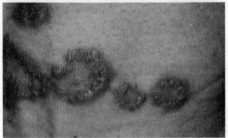

Fig. 18.12 Elastosis perforans serpiginosa in a patient with Wilson's disease who was taking D-penicillamine.

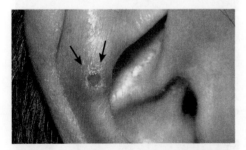

Fig. 18.13 Chondrodermatitis nodularis chronica helices. A painful nodule.

Pathogenesis

Transepidermal elimination results from elimination of degenerated elastic fibers in the upper dermal layer through the epidermis. It may appear idiopathically in young men. It tends to accompany abnormalities of the dermis, such as those of pseudoxanthoma elasticum, Marfan syndrome, Ehlers–Danlos syndrome, Rothmund–Thomson syndrome, and Down syndrome. It may also be caused by intake of D-penicillamine.

Pathology

Degenerated elastic fibers accumulate in the dermal upper layer, on which the epidermis proliferates to enwrap the abnormal fibers into the dermis. Thickening of the epidermis and foreign body granuloma in the dermis occur.

Reactive perforating collagenosis

Multiple firm, brownish-red nodules of roughly 1 cm diameter with keratotic plugs occur on the face and trunk. Transepidermal elimination results from elimination of degenerated elastic fibers, which is caused by trauma, in the upper dermal layer through the epidermis. Underlying disorders such as diabetes or renal failure are often found. Intense itching is present. Köbner phenomenon may be positive.

Chondrodermatitis nodularis helicis (synonym: chondrodermatitis nodularis chronica helicis)

Painful keratotic nodules of roughly 1 cm diameter occur in the helices, particularly their upper parts (Fig. 18.13). Degeneration and inflammation occur in the cartilage and elastic fibers of the ear because of extrinsic stimulation, such as from sunlight, injury or the cold. Transepidermal elimination results from elimination of degenerated elastic fibers through the epidermis. The condition occurs most frequently in men of middle age and older. This disorder should be differentiated from seborrheic keratosis, basal cell carcinoma, and squamous cell carcinoma. The main treatments are topical and local injection of steroids and surgical excision.

Granulomatous disorders

Sarcoidosis

- This is a systemic granuloma of unknown pathogenesis.

MEMO 18–4 What is perforating dermatosis?

Perforating dermatosis is a general term for skin lesions resulting from epidermal excretion of decomposed skin components. Perforating dermatosis is subclassified as shown in the table below, based on the excreted material and the affected body part. These diseases tend to occur in patients with chronic renal failure or diabetes. Epidermal excretion of decomposed skin components may be seen in some cases of granuloma annulare (see Chapter 18).

Disease	Material excreted through the skin
Elastosis perforans serpiginosa	Elastic fibers
Reactive perforating collagenosis	Collagen fibers
Chondrodermatitis nodularis helicis	Collagen fibers (with degeneration of cartilage)
Kyrle's disease	Keratin, keratinocytes
Perforating folliculitis	(from follicular sites) collagen fibers, elastic fibers

---

- The skin symptoms are specific lesions (granulomatous lesions) and reactive non-specific lesions (inflammatory reactive lesions such as erythema nodosum).
- Bilateral hilar lymphadenopathy (BHL) and uveitis are included in this category.
- Angiotensin converting enzyme (ACE) activity in the serum is elevated, hypercalcemia is present, and tuberculin test is negative.
- Topical and oral steroids are the first-line treatments.

Definition, pathogenesis, and epidemiology

Sarcoidosis is an inflammatory disorder with granulomas of unknown pathogenesis. It involves multiple organs. Epithelioid cell granuloma is found histopathologically. It most frequently occurs in individuals in their 20s and in their 50s or older. The pathogenesis is unknown, but complex interactions are thought to be responsible. The three main factors are:

- heredity (e.g., HLA-A1 has been reported as a hereditary factor in Europe and the USA)
- environment (e.g., in recent years, association with the cell wall-deficient bacterium *Propionibacterium acnes* has been attracting attention)
- immunology (e.g., activation of Th1 cells and histiocytes, and increases in IL-2 levels).

Cutaneous symptoms

Skin lesions are seen in approximately 25% of sarcoidosis cases. The lesions consist of specific ones caused by epithelioid cell granulomas and non-specific ones caused by inflammatory reactions.

MEMO 18–5 Sarcoidosis and erythema induratum

Erythema induratum may occur as inflammations of a reactive form of panniculitis in sarcoidosis patients. Such patients sometimes develop granulomas in the subcutaneous fat tissues, often on the extensor surface of the lower legs. The specific lesions of sarcoidosis are impossible to distinguish clinically from erythema induratum and are called erythema nodosum-like eruptions of sarcoidosis.

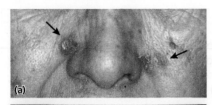

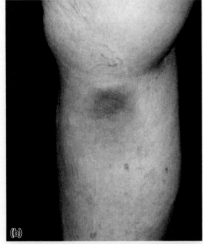

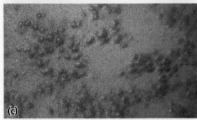

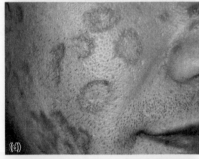

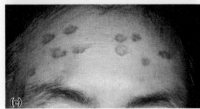

Fig. 18.14-1 Sarcoidosis. a–c: Nodular sarcoidosis. d,e: Plaque sarcoidosis.

Specific skin lesions

The major subtypes are described below. Multiple subtypes are often found simultaneously.

- **Nodular sarcoidosis (Fig. 18.14-1a–c):** this is the most frequent type. The face, particularly around the nose, the extremities, and the center of the trunk are most commonly affected. Multiple papules and erythemas occur, ranging in color from light pink to dark red and in diameter from 3 to 30 mm. Small papules are often produced on the lower legs.
- **Plaque sarcoidosis (Fig. 18.14-1d,e):** flat-topped infiltrative plaques with an elevated rim and an atrophic center occur, most frequently on the face.
- **Diffuse infiltrative sarcoidosis (Fig. 18.14-2a,b):** dark red, diffuse, infiltrative plaques occur symmetrically, mainly on the nose, cheeks, ears, fingers, and toes. It is asymptomatic. Areas that are prone to frostbite are frequently involved (lupus pernio). Clinical findings resemble those of chilblains, but diffuse infiltrative sarcoidosis is not associated with the seasons. It is intractable.
- **Subcutaneous sarcoidosis:** this most commonly appears in the extremities, as palpable, elastic, subcutaneous induration of 3–30 mm in diameter.
- **Scarring infiltrative sarcoidosis (Fig. 18.14-2c,d):** this tends to occur on areas that are prone to injury, such as knees and elbows. Epithelioid cell granuloma occurs on a preexisting scar that was caused by injury, for example. This is specific to sarcoidosis and has diagnostic value.
- **Erythema nodosum-like eruptions:** the lesions resemble erythema nodosum, except that epithelioid cell granulomas are found histopathologically. They heal spontaneously in many cases.
- **Sarcoidosis in other organs:** other types of sarcoidosis are lichenoid sarcoidosis, ichthyosis-like eruptions and ulcerative, leukodermal, verrucous, and erythematous types.

Non-specific lesions

Erythema nodosum (MEMO, see Chapter 18), pruritus or erythema multiforme may also occur as a non-specific eruption.

Systemic symptoms

There are many asymptomatic cases with early symptoms of fever and fatigue which may be a cause of unexplained fever. Epithelioid cell granulomas form in various organs. The lungs, eyes, and heart are often involved.

- **Pulmonary lesion:** BHL and lung parenchymatous infiltration occur, and pulmonary fibrosis develops as it progresses. Non-productive cough and dyspnea are found in about half of cases.
- **Eye lesion:** granulomatous anterior uveitis occurs.
- **Cardiac lesion:** heart block and other heart disorders may cause unexpected death. Heart lesions are a frequent cause of death in sarcoidosis.
- **Sarcoidosis in other organs:** liver dysfunction, arthritis, muscular lesions, bone cyst, symptoms in the central and peripheral nervous systems, and parotiditis may occur.

Pathology

Non-caseating epithelioid cell granuloma (sarcoidal granuloma) is characteristically observed (Fig. 18.15). Slight infiltration of inflammatory cells is seen at the periphery of granulomas (naked granuloma). There are inclusion bodies, such as Schaumann bodies and asteroid bodies, in the giant cells of granuloma, but these are not specific for sarcoidosis and may occur in other granulomatous reactions.

The Schaumann bodies have a basophilic round lamellar structure with calcium deposition. The asteroid bodies have a radiated, acicular structure with a central core. In addition to granulomatous lesion, foreign substances such as silica are found in scarring infiltration.

Diagnosis and differential diagnosis

Sarcoidosis is diagnosed basically from clinical and histopathological findings and elimination of other disorders. Differential diagnosis from other cutaneous disorders such as granuloma annulare, annular elastolytic giant cell granuloma, necrobiosis lipoidica, Melkersson–Rosenthal syndrome, lupus miliaris disseminatus faciei, rosacea, mycobacterial infection, and malignant tumor is necessary. Skin biopsy must be done. Tissue culture test and polymerase chain reaction (PCR) analysis are performed if necessary.

Treatment

About two-thirds of sarcoidosis cases resolve spontaneously. Oral steroids are effective for cases with progressive lung, heart, eye or nerve lesions. Topical steroids are used for the cutaneous symptoms.

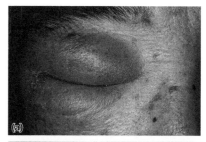
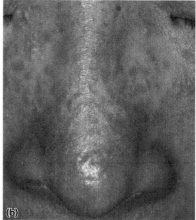
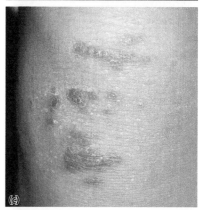
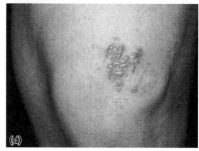

Fig. 18.14-2 Sarcoidosis. a,b: Diffuse infiltrative sarcoidosis (lupus pernio). c,d: Scarring infiltrative sarcoidosis.

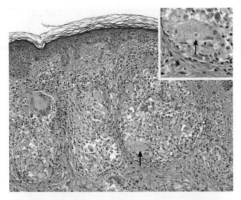

Fig. 18.15 Histopathology of sarcoidosis. Non-caseating granuloma is characteristically observed. The arrows show the asteroid body.

MEMO 18–6 Syndromes associated with sarcoidosis

A disorder that manifests fever, facial nerve paralysis, anterior uveitis, and parotid bubo is called Heerfordt syndrome. That with fever, BHL, erythema induratum, and joint pain is called Lofgren syndrome.

Granuloma annulare

- This is a doughnut-shaped eruption with an elevated rim.
- Histopathologically, there is the formation of a palisading granuloma.
- Granuloma annulare (GA) is classified by the shape and distribution of eruptions into four subtypes.
- When GA generalizes to the whole body, diabetes mellitus may be involved.

Clinical features and pathology

Small, firm, doughnut-shaped papules appear, mainly on the dorsa of the hands and feet. They spread centrifugally to distribute in circular arrangements (Fig. 18.16). The papules are normal skin color to light pink. The circle of papules has a concave center. Scaling or subjective symptoms are not present. Histopathologically, degenerated collagen fibers at the center are radially surrounded by histiocytes, lymphocytes, and giant cells (palisading granuloma) (Fig. 18.17). Acid mucopolysaccharides deposit in the lesion in the central area of incomplete necrosis.

Pathogenesis

The mechanism of GA has not been fully clarified. Impaired peripheral circulation, diabetes, insect bites, UV radiation, and injury may induce GA. Cases induced by infectious disorders such as hepatitis B and HIV have been reported.

Treatment

Granuloma annulare tends to resolve spontaneously. After a skin biopsy, the biopsy lesion often disappears. As local therapies, topical steroids, PUVA therapy, and cryotherapy are conducted. If diabetes mellitus is involved, it is treated.

MEMO 18–7 Granuloma annulare classified by clinical features

- **Localized granuloma annulare:** this subtype is the most common. Lesions tend to localize at a single site, such as the dorsal hands and finger joints. About half of cases heal spontaneously within 2 years after onset.
- **Generalized granuloma annulare:** multiple lesions of small contralateral or dispersed granuloma annulare occur, most frequently on the trunk and distal extremities of middle-aged women. Diabetes is often found as a complication.
- **Perforating granuloma annulare:** this is a papule with a centralized concavity that may ulcerate and crust. Dermal excretion of degenerated collagen fibers occurs.
- **Subcutaneous granuloma annulare:** with palpable, subcutaneous nodules of normal skin color, this commonly occurs in early childhood. It often occurs on the scalp and frontal tibiae.

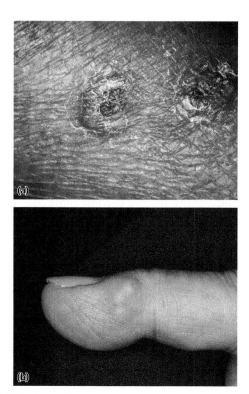

Fig. 18.16-2 Granuloma annulare. a: Perforating granuloma annulare. b: Subcutaneous granuloma annulare.

Annular elastolytic giant cell granuloma (AEGCG) (synonyms: actinic granuloma, elastophagic giant cell granuloma)

A granulomatous lesion whose main components are elastic fiber-phagocytosing giant cells occurs, most frequently in middle-aged women. A large, circular erythematous eruption with an elevated rim and central depigmentation occurs on exposed areas, such as the face, neck region, and extremities (Fig. 18.18). It may resemble annular erythema. The lesion heals spontaneously in many cases. AEGCG is a widely known subtype of GA.

Melkersson–Rosenthal syndrome (synonym: cheilitis granulomatosa)
Clinical features

Men and women in their 20s are most frequently affected. When all three main symptoms are present together (swelling of the lips, fissured tongue (scrotal tongue, lingua plicata), and facial nerve palsy), it is called Melkersson–Rosenthal syndrome. Cheilitis

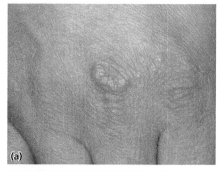
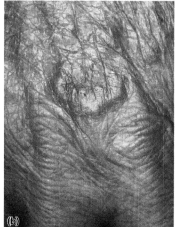
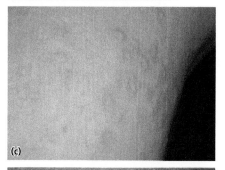
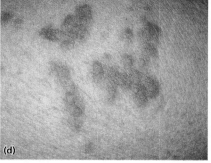

Fig. 18.16-1 Granuloma annulare.
a,b: Localized granuloma annulare.
c,d: Generalized granuloma annulare.

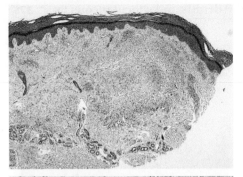

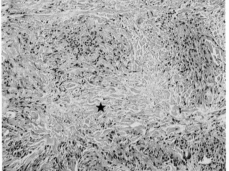

Fig. 18.17 Histopathology of granuloma annulare. Collagen fiber degeneration and mucin deposition are observed at the center (star). Palisading epithelioid cell granuloma forms at the periphery.

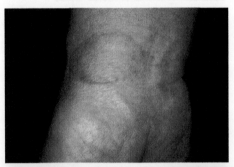

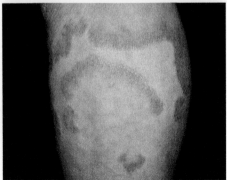

Fig. 18.18 Annular elastolytic giant cell granuloma.

granulomatosa is the term for cases with only swelling of the lips, which are frequently seen.

- **Swelling of the lips:** swelling occurs suddenly in the lips, particularly the upper lip, as the earliest symptom in most cases of cheilitis granulomatosa (Fig. 18.19). The buccal mucosa may also be involved. Although subjective symptoms such as pain are not present, the swelling persists for several hours to several days. It recurs, leading to rubber-like stiffness.
- **Lingua plicata:** swelling occurs in the tongue at the same time as the lips are affected. The folds in the surface of the tongue become marked.
- **Facial paralysis:** preceding or concurrent with the swelling of the cheeks, peripheral facial paralysis suddenly occurs on one cheek. Recurrences and remissions are repeated. The condition is chronic.

Pathogenesis and pathology

The cause is unknown but dental metal allergy and sarcoidosis reaction are suspected. Lymphatic edema in the dermis, and lymphoid and histiocytic infiltration are histopathologically found in the early stages. As it progresses, inflammatory granulomatous lesions consisting of lymphocytes, epithelioid cells, and Langhans giant cells occur.

Treatment

Oral antihistamines and oral or locally injected steroids are useful as symptomatic therapies.

Granuloma gluteale infantum

Multiple relatively firm, flatly elevated reddish-brown nodules appear on areas where an infant has contact with the diaper (e.g., perianal region and buttocks). The nodules are round and 1–4 cm in diameter. Erosions or ulcers may be present. The lesions are also found in elderly diaper users. It is thought to be caused by prolonged extrinsic stimulation by feces, urine or candidiasis. Histopathologically, acanthosis and infiltration of various cells in the dermis are seen. The condition spontaneously improves within a few months after removal of the irritants.

Hereditary connective tissue disease

Ehlers–Danlos syndrome (EDS)

- This is a congenital disease of the connective tissue. Most cases are autosomal dominant.

- Hyperextensible skin, fragility of the skin and blood vessels, and excessive mobility of joints and ligaments are the main symptoms.

Clinical features, classification, and symptoms

Ehlers–Danlos syndrome is classified into more than 10 subtypes by the clinical features, pattern of inheritance, causative gene, and biochemical abnormality (Table 18.2). It is caused by mutations in the genes encoding collagen types I, III, and V. Many cases are autosomal dominantly inherited.

The skin is soft and stretches excessively, despite appearing normal; when stretched and released, the skin immediately returns to its former appearance. The skin is easily torn by extrinsic force or injury. A hemorrhagic tendency is particularly strong in vascular EDS, the most severe type. The skin of the patient is thin and translucent, and the blood vessels are visible. Atrophic scars called cigarette paper scars caused by repeated injuries appear at sites that are subject to extrinsic irritation, such as the knees. In the terminal stages, the skin hangs sac-like from the body. In areas subjected to strong extrinsic forces, such as the heels, subcutaneous fat enters the torn collagen fibers of the dermis and develops into lump tumors. The joints of the digits, elbows, and knees hyperextend, exceeding 180° of bending in the direction opposite the flexure direction. They become valgus (Fig. 18.20). Deformity and dislocation of the joints often occur. Congenital

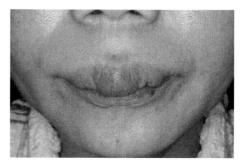

Fig. 18.19 Cheilitis granulomatosa.

Table 18.2 Types of Ehlers–Danlos syndrome (EDS).

Newly established	Traditional	Causative molecule	Inheritance pattern
Classical	Gravis (EDS type I)	Type V collagen, type I collagen	AD
	Mitis (EDS type II)	Type V collagen, type I collagen	AD
Hypermobility	EDS type III	Type III collagen, Tenascin-X	AD, AR
Vascular	Arterial-ecchymotic (EDS type IV)	Type VII collagen	AD
Kyphoscoliosis	Ocular-scoliotic (EDS type VI A, VI B)	Lysine hydroxylase	AR
Arthrochalasia	Arthrochalasis multiplex congenita (EDS type VII A, VII B)	Type I collagen	AD
Dermatosparaxis	Human dermatosparaxis (EDS type VII C)	ADAMTS2	AR
Other	Periodontitis (EDS type VIII)		AD
	Progeroid EDS	B4GALT7	AR

AD, autosomal dominantly inherited; AR, autosomal recessively inherited.

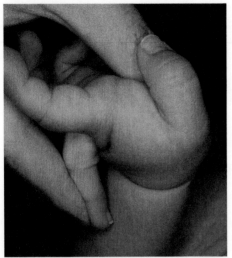

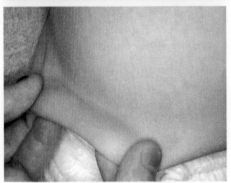

Fig. 18.20 Ehlers–Danlos syndrome. Overextension of the skin occurs.

MEMO 18–8 Abraham Lincoln and Marfan syndrome

Some have speculated that the 16th president of the USA, Abraham Lincoln, suffered from Marfan syndrome, because he was tall and had long fingers and a funnel chest.

dislocation of the hip joints and scoliokyphosis are present. Bleeding under the skin and in the ocular fundus, cardiac anomaly and mitral valve prolapse, aneurysm, lens deviation and severe myopic astigmatism occur in the later stages of life, from fragility of the blood vessels.

Diagnosis and treatment

Histopathologically, collagen fibers are decreased and disrupted. Diagnosis is done based on the clinical symptoms. Identification of the gene mutation is done if necessary. There are no ultimate treatments for EDS, only symptomatic therapies. Pregnancy and delivery by patients with EDS may cause uterine rupture or massive bleeding.

Marfan syndrome

- This is a congenital disease of the connective tissue. Skeletal abnormalities, eye symptoms, and cardiovascular impairment are the main symptoms.
- It is autosomal dominant, caused mainly by mutation in the fibrillin-1 (*FBN1*) gene.
- Striae atrophicae occur on the chest as a cutaneous symptom. Abnormal elastic fibers are eliminated from the epidermis and elastosis perforans serpiginosa is often present.
- The major symptoms are arachnodactyly, skeletal deformity of the chest, annuloaortic ectasia, and lens deviation.

Clinical features

Severe striae appear on the chest and thighs as cutaneous symptoms. Elastosis perforans serpiginosa is present, in which abnormal elastic fibers produced in the patient's upper dermal layer are eliminated. The patients are abnormally tall, with a markedly elongated lower body relative to the upper body. The extremities and digits are thin and long (arachnodactyly). Deformities occur in the chest (funnel chest or pigeon breast) and spine, and hypertension and dislocation of the joints occur. Mitral valve prolapse often occurs as a result of reduced elasticity of the cardiovascular system. Aortic valve incompetence and dissecting aortic aneurysm are easily caused by annulo-aortic ectasia. Death may result.

Since Marfan syndrome is caused by abnormality in the fibrillin-1 gene, deviation occurs in the crystalline lens, because the zonules of Zinn, which support that lens, are composed of fibrillin. Severe myopia may be caused by elongation of the eyeball in the anteroposterior direction.

Pathogenesis

Marfan syndrome is caused by a mutation in the *FBN1* gene on chromosome 15. Fibrillin-1, a protein component of the extracellular matrix, is essential to elastic fiber synthesis. The condition is autosomal dominant but it is caused by sporadic mutation in about 30% of cases. There have been some cases caused by mutation in the *TGFBR2* gene.

Diagnosis and differential diagnosis

Marfan syndrome is diagnosed comprehensively based on the clinical features and family history. The Ghent criteria may be used. In recent years, use of angiotensin II receptor blockers has been reported as an effective treatment for the cardiovascular problems.

Pseudoxanthoma elasticum (PXE)

- This is an autosomal recessively inherited disease in which abnormality in elastic fibers occurs. It is caused by a mutation in the *ABCC6* gene.
- Yellow or orange papules aggregate on the neck region and axillary fossae. Dermal laxity progresses with age. It is asymptomatic.
- Eye symptoms and vasoconstriction occur. Women outnumber men by two to one. Although the cutaneous symptoms appear in early childhood, the condition is generally found in adolescence or later because it is without subjective symptoms. Slightly yellowish papules aggregate and form characteristic plaques with a cobblestone appearance, most frequently symmetrically on the lateral region of the neck, axillary fossae, and flexor surfaces of joints. The skin is soft and saggy. Skin wrinkling becomes marked with age (Fig. 18.21). Elastosis perforans serpiginosa may be present.

Wrinkling of the chin in young patients is characteristic of this disorder. Angioid streaks in the retina result from degeneration and calcinosis of Bruch's membrane, which exists between the retina and choroids and contains abundant elastic fibers. Angioid streaks in the retina are seen in 85% of adult patients. Punctate pigmentation is found in the retina (peau d'orange).

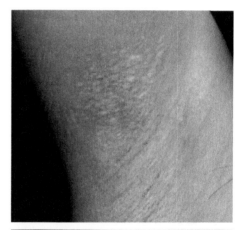

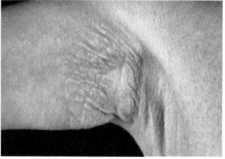

Fig. 18.21 Pseudoxanthoma elasticum. The skin of the axillary fossae becomes soft and saggy, resembling cobblestones.

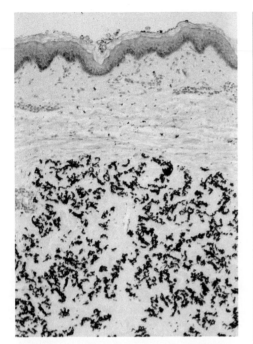

Fig. 18.22 Histopathology of pseudo-xanthoma elasticum (von Kossa stain). Calcium deposition stains brownish-black with von Kossa.

As it progresses, retinal detachment or blindness occurs. Degeneration and calcinosis of the elastic layer of the arteries occur, and intermittent claudication, angina, cardiac infarction, and gastrointestinal bleeding are often present.

Pathogenesis
Pseudoxanthoma elasticum is autosomal recessive and caused by mutation in ABCC6, a member of the ATP binding cassette (ABC) family. Carriers of PXE mutations are found in high frequency. The histories of families with PXE sometimes show modes of inheritance similar to those of autosomal dominant disorders.

Pathology
Swelling and disruption occur in the elastic fibers in the middle to deep dermal layers, accompanied by calcium deposition (Fig. 18.22). Histopathological changes similar to those found in the skin lesions are often found in other parts of the skin.

Treatment and prognosis
Early, preventive treatments for eye and vascular lesions are important. The skin lesions may be surgi-cally removed for cosmetic reasons.

Disorders of the subcutaneous fat

Panniculitis

Erythema nodosum (EN)
- Red nodules accompanied by tenderness occur, most commonly on the extensor surfaces of the lower extremities. They do not ulcerate.
- This is an inflammatory reaction whose inducing factors include upper respiratory infection, drug eruption, Behçet's disease, and sarcoidosis.
- Inflammation is histopathologically found in the septum of subcutaneous fat tissue.
- It should be differentiated from erythema induratum.
- Conservative therapies such as bed rest and cooling are the first-line treatments. When induced by an infection, antibiotics are administered. NSAIDs and potassium iodide are also useful. Oral steroids may be used for severe cases.

Clinical features

Adult women are most commonly affected. After a precursor of upper respiratory infection, a few symmetrical, vaguely margined, light pink erythema occur, sometimes accompanied by fever and fatigue. There is arthralgia. The erythema occurs predominantly on the extensor surfaces of the lower legs (Fig. 18.23). The erythema varies in size from 1 to 10 cm. The eruptions are slightly elevated and indurated. Tenderness and spontaneous pain are present. Ulceration does not occur. In progressive cases, the same type of eruptions may develop on the thighs, upper extremities, and trunk. New eruptions continue to appear for 2–6 weeks.

The eruptions change color from dark red to yellow to blue over the course of 2–4 weeks, and mild scaling occurs before healing without scarring.

Pathogenesis

Erythema nodosum is often induced by infectious allergy to bacteria, fungi or viruses. It often appears secondarily after upper respiratory or gastrointestinal infection caused by the *Streptococcus pyogenes* bacterium. Other disorders that may cause EN include Hansen's disease (erythema nodosum leprosum), tuberculosis, toxoplasmosis, and chlamydiosis. EN may be accompanied by Behçet's disease, inflammatory gastrointestinal diseases or sarcoidosis. Primary diseases that are frequently associated with EN are listed in Table 18.3. However, it may occur sporadically without any underlying disease.

Pathology

In the early stages of EN, lymphocytes and neutrophils infiltrate the dermis and subcutaneous fat tissue, the fatty septum in particular; the condition is septal panniculitis. Generally, there are no findings of vasculitis or degeneration of fat cells. Granulomas that contain giant cells develop in the later stages.

Diagnosis and differential diagnosis

Clinical features of tenderness, pathological findings, and precursory infectious disease are diagnostic. The primary disease should be identified. Disorders that require differentiation from EN include erythema induratum, sarcoidosis, Sweet syndrome, cellulitis, lupus erythematous profundus, and polyarteritis nodosa.

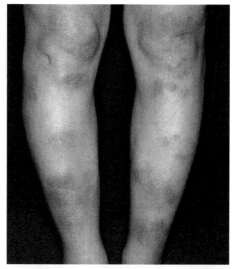

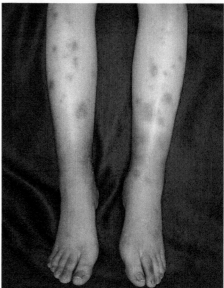

Fig. 18.23-1 Erythema nodosum.
Multiple erythema accompanied by severe tenderness on the extensor of the lower legs.

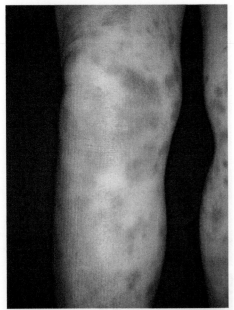

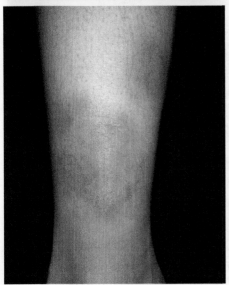

Fig. 18.23-2 Erythema nodosum.

Table 18.3 Infection, underlying disease, etc. that cause erythema nodosum.

Bacterial infection	*Streptococcus, Yersinia, Salmonella, Campylobacter, Chlamydia, Mycoplasma*
Mycobacterial infection	Tuberculosis, leprosy
Viral infection	Infectious mononucleosis, hepatitis B, herpes simplex
Other infection	Tinea, toxoplasma
Drug	Sulfa drugs, oral contraceptives, potassium iodine agents
Malignant disease	Malignant lymphoma (Hodgkin's disease, etc.), leukemia
Inflammatory bowel disease	Ulcerative colitis, Crohn's disease
Other	Sarcoidosis, Behçet's disease, reactive arthritis (Reiter's syndrome)

Treatment

Erythema nodosum is a disorder that heals spontaneously. Bed rest is required. The lower extremities are kept cool and elevated. Any primary diseases are treated. In cases with intense inflammation, oral NSAIDs, potassium iodide, and steroids are administered.

Erythema induratum (EI) (synonyms: erythema induratum Bazin, nodular vasculitis)

- Erythema induratum occurs most frequently on the lower legs of women. It is clinically similar to EN but acute inflammatory findings are not present. It is often accompanied by ulceration, and heals with scarring. Tenderness may be present.
- Histopathologically, lobular cellulitis is seen.
- When tubercle bacillus allergy (tuberculid) is identified, therapy for tuberculosis should be given.

Clinical features

Erythema induratum tends to occur on the lower legs of middle-aged and elderly women. Obesity or chronic venous insufficiency (see Chapter 11) are often found. Vaguely marginated, diffuse and slightly elevated dark-red erythemas and subcutaneous nodules occur (Fig. 18.24). Indurations may coalesce to become plate-like or ulcerated. The skin lesions may occur singly or multiply. When multiple, eruptions from each stage are concurrent.

The induration disappears with scarring in 1–2 months. EI often recurs for many years. The tenderness in EI is not as intense as that in erythema nodosum.

Pathogenesis

Erythema induratum used to be regarded as tuberculid, i.e., an allergic reaction to tubercle bacilli or to the metabolites of such bacilli (see Chapter 26). Nevertheless, there were cases in which tuberculosis did not present, and steroids were effective as a treatment. Therefore, EI has come to be thought of as nodular panniculitis that occurs with circulatory failure as the underlying disease. Even so, the DNA of the tubercle bacillus was recently reported to be detected by PCR assay of skin biopsies in about 80% of cases. The association of the tubercle bacillus with the occurrence of EI has been under discussion. At present, it is useful to consider disorders with the above-described clinical symptoms as EI, and to divide them into two subtypes: one associated with tuberculosis (Bazin) and one not associated with tuberculosis (non-Bazin, nodular vasculitis). EI sometimes occurs in association with hepatitis C.

Pathology

Necrosis of fat tissue and epithelioid cellular infiltration are seen mainly in the fat lobular tissue (lobular panniculitis). In the chronic stage, caseating necrosis and epithelioid cell granuloma with infiltration of Langhans giant cells and lymphocytes are found. Vasculitis of the subcutaneous fat tissue is often present (see Fig. 2.23).

Diagnosis and examinations

It is necessary to identify tuberculosis infection by QuantiFERON RTB-2G (see Chapter 26), chest X-ray, skin biopsy, PCR test or tuberculin test. It is not rare for positive results of the skin biopsy PCR test to be obtained after several tests.

Differential diagnosis

The disorder should be differentiated from EN, thrombophlebitis migrans, polyarteritis nodosa, and ulcerations from other causes. EN is differentiated by its bright red color, spontaneous pain, acute, intense inflammatory reaction, and lesions that do not ulcerate

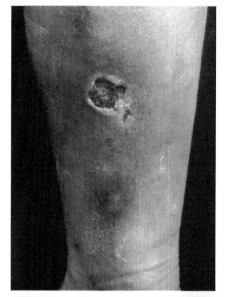
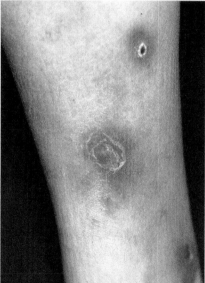
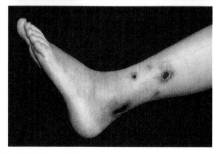

Fig. 18.24 Erythema induratum. Erythema and ulceration are accompanied by induration.

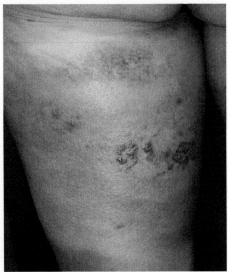

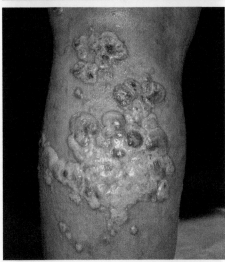

Fig. 18.25 Eosinophilic cellulitis.

spontaneously and whose main histopathological component is the septum of the fat tissue.

Treatment

If tuberculosis is present, therapy should be given. Tubercular lesions subside with treatment in a few months in most cases. Erythema induratum that is not caused by tuberculosis is intractable and progresses slowly. Bed rest for the lower extremities and prevention of stasis are effective. NSAIDs and potassium iodide are administered orally. Oral steroids are effective in severe cases.

Eosinophilic cellulitis (synonym: Wells syndrome)

Itchy edematous erythema, blisters or blood blisters suddenly appear on the extremities, induced by infections or insect bites (Fig. 18.25). Marked eosinophilic infiltration is seen in the dermis to subcutaneous fat tissues. Eosinophilic degeneration of collagen fibers, called flame figures, is present. Elevated levels of eosinophils are seen in the peripheral blood. Topical or oral corticosteroids are effective in the treatment of eosinophilic cellulitis.

Poststeroid panniculitis

This occurs a few days after high-dose steroids are tapered or stopped. Infants who are receiving treatment for rheumatic fever or leukemia are often affected. Multiple subcutaneous nodules of 5–50 mm diameter occur on the upper body, including the cheeks and neck. They are normal skin color or light pink. The lesions on

---

MEMO 18–9 Weber–Christian disease

A disorder whose clinical features were those of lobular panniculitis but with systemic symptoms such as fever and subcutaneous nodules on the extremities and trunk used to be called Weber–Christian disease. Currently, the disorder is not recognized as an independent disease. The conditions are thought to be those of erythema induratum, lupus erythematosus profundus, panniculitis caused by enzyme deficiency or pancreatitis, cutaneous symptoms of hemophagocytic syndrome (cytophagic histiocytic panniculitis) or subcutaneous panniculitis-like T cell lymphoma (see Chapter 22).

the cheeks tend to heal with scarring. It is necessary to reschedule the reduction of steroid administration.

Cold panniculitis

Vaguely marginated subcutaneous nodules accompanied by erythema and cool sensation occur, mainly where the cheeks and extremities are exposed to cold air or ice. The lesions appear a few days after such exposure. Newborns and infants are most commonly affected. Warming the affected area resolves the symptoms within a few weeks without scarring.

Traumatic panniculitis

This is an inflammatory reaction caused by damage to fat cells after injury. A painful erythematous plaque or nodule accompanied by palpable infiltration forms, most frequently in the breasts of obese women. In the case of lesions on the lower legs, minor injury may cause small movable subcutaneous nodules of several millimeters in diameter (encapsulated fat necrosis).

Subcutaneous fat necrosis of the newborn

Several days to 1 month after birth, plate-like subcutaneous indurations of various sizes occur on the buttocks and thighs, where fat is distributed. This is known to be panniculitis induced by minor injury at the time of birth, forceps delivery or dystocia. It may be accompanied by hypercalcemia. It generally heals in 2–3 months without scarring but slight fatty atrophy may be left.

Other panniculitis

There are other forms of panniculitis, including sclerosing panniculitis (see Chapter 11), lupus erythematous profundus (see Chapter 12), morphea profunda (see Chapter 12), subcutaneous granuloma annulare, necrobiosis lipoidica (see Chapter 17), factitial panniculitis, panniculitis from enzymopathy, and cytophagic histiocytic panniculitis.

Lipodystrophy

An abnormal increase or decrease (lipoatrophy) in subcutaneous fat tissues is termed lipodystrophy. It can be understood as a synonym for lipoatrophy, because lipodystrophy with abnormally increasing

MEMO 18–10 Hypereosinophilic syndrome

Hypereosinophilic syndrome is a disorder with unknown etiology that satisfies the following conditions:

- elevated levels of eosinophils (1500/mL or higher) are seen in the peripheral blood for more than 6 months
- causes for increased eosinophils, such as parasitic infection or allergy, are not found
- internal organ failure, such as hepatosplenomegaly or heart failure, is present.

Light pink eruptions appear on the extremities, and the symptoms, such as purple macules and blisters, sometimes resemble those of eosinophilic cellulitis.

MEMO 18–11 Panniculitis caused by enzymopathy

- α1-Antitrypsin deficiency, α1-antichymotrypsin deficiency: this is a rare congenital disease. Enhanced decomposition and panniculitis with fever and nodules may be caused by decreases in proteolytic enzyme-inhibiting substances.
- Pancreatic panniculitis: increase of lipase and amylase in serum may lead to panniculitis in patients with pancreatitis. Pancreatitis is an important underlying disease in patients with panniculitis.

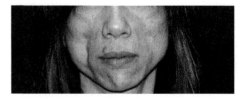

Fig. 18.26-1 Acquired localized lipodystrophy. Marked lipodystrophy on the cheeks. An idiopathic case with unknown cause.

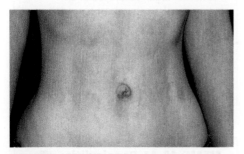

Fig. 18.26-2 Acquired localized lipodystrophy.

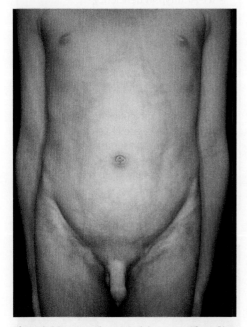

Fig. 18.27 Lipodystrophia centrifugalis abdominalis infantilis. Lipodystrophy occurs on both sides of the lower abdomen and groins.

subcutaneous fat tissue is rare. It can be classified into systemic versus partial, and into congenital versus acquired. Major subtypes are described below.

Generalized lipodystrophy
Congenital generalized lipodystrophy

This is a rare autosomal recessively inherited disorder caused by abnormality in the *AGPT2* or *BSCL2* gene. With absent or reduced fat in the whole body from the time of birth, muscles appear sharply defined. Hyperlipemia, hyperinsulinemia, enlargement of internal organs, and insulin-resistant diabetes occur as complications.

Acquired generalized lipodystrophy

Girls are more commonly affected than boys. It may manifest after precursors such as dermatomyositis and febrile diseases. Fat disappears in several months to several years, sometimes in several weeks. Bulimia and insulin-resistant diabetes occur as complications.

Acquired localized lipodystrophy

This localized deterioration of fat tissues occurs by extrinsic stimulation or after panniculitis (Fig. 18.26). The disorder, whose etiology is unknown, often occurs idiopathically. Lipoatrophy sometimes occurs at the injection site of insulin, steroids, iron preparations or vaccinations (postinjection panniculitis). Lipodystrophy may occur after panniculitis associated with collagen diseases (lupus erythematosus profundus, dermatomyositis, and scleroderma). In recent years, HIV-associated lipodystrophy, which occurs as lipoatrophy or fat increase several months after administration of anti-HIV drugs, has been drastically increasing.

Lipodystrophia centrifugalis abdominalis infantilis (synonym: centrifugal lipodystrophy)

This is a localized lipodystrophy that occurs most frequently on the groin or axillary fossae of infants (Fig. 18.27). The etiology is unknown but genetic involvement is suspected, because there are familial cases. It is a rare disorder. Most patients are Asian girls. Painless erythemas progress into sharply defined concavities that enlarge centrifugally, and the blood vessels underneath the skin are visible. Within 7 years after onset, the depressions stop expanding, and they subside in two-thirds of all cases.

CHAPTER 19
Disorders of the skin appendages

This chapter discusses disorders of the skin appendages: the sweat glands, sebaceous glands, hair follicles, and nails. When these are affected by intrinsic or extrinsic factors, cosmetic appearance and the ability to regulate the body temperature are affected. This chapter focuses on diseases whose main lesions occur in the skin appendages (see Chapter 1 for the functions of the skin appendages).

Disorders of the sweat glands

Miliaria (synonym: sweat retention syndrome)
- Commonly called heat rash, it is caused by obstruction of the eccrine sweat ducts.
- Skin care is the main treatment.

Clinical features and classification
Miliaria is classified by the location of the obstructed sweat ducts into miliaria crystallina, miliaria rubra, and miliaria profunda (Fig. 19.1).

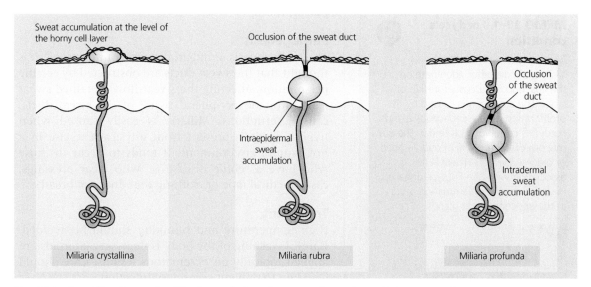

Fig. 19.1 Classifications of miliaria, and the obstructed portion of the sweat duct.

Shimizu's Dermatology, Second Edition. Hiroshi Shimizu.
© 2017 John Wiley & Sons, Ltd. Published 2017 by John Wiley & Sons, Ltd.

Fig. 19.2 Miliaria crystalline.

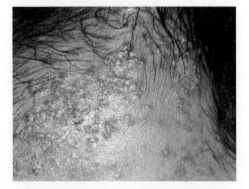

Fig. 19.3 Miliaria rubra after fever.

MEMO 19–1 Fordyce's condition

Multiple yellowish small papules 1–2 mm in diameter aggregate on the lips, buccal mucosa, foreskin or labia. The condition is caused by the proliferation of free sebaceous glands. Fordyce's condition is found in the oral mucosa of about 80% of middle-aged or older individuals. There is no association with Fox–Fordyce disease, in which chronic inflammation occurs in the apocrine sweat glands.

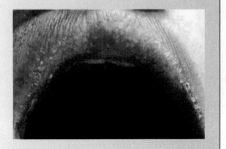

Miliaria crystalline

The sweat ducts are obstructed in or directly under the stratum corneum, producing superficial transparent vesicles of several millimeters in diameter. Flushing is not present. The vesicles soon dry and become thin, white scales. They heal in 1 day to several days without itching or inflammation. They commonly occur on the face of newborns; however, they may appear accompanying fever in adults (Fig. 19.2).

Miliaria rubra

This frequently occurs in an environment with high temperature and humidity, or in infants, the obese, and persons with hidrosis (Fig. 19.3). Inflammation occurs from obstruction of the sweat ducts in the granular cell layer region, and rose pink papules of 1–2 mm in diameter are produced. It is accompanied by flushing and intense itching. The trunk, extensor surfaces of the extremities, neck region, and axillary fossae are most commonly affected. It often becomes eczematous or pustular (miliaria pustulosa).

Miliaria profunda

The sweat ducts are destroyed at the dermoepidermal junction. After recurrence of miliaria rubra, multiple white, flat papules without itching occur with perspiration.

Pathogenesis

The pathogenesis of miliaria is poorly understood. It is thought that the sweat ducts are obstructed by eccrine perspiration, affecting the sweat flow. Retained sweat leaks into the peripheral tissue of the sweat ducts, causing eruptions. Miliaria is easily caused when hyperhidrosis is present from physical exercise in a hot, humid environment. It tends to occur in those who have a febrile disease or who wear dressings, casts, medical tape or clothing that does not breathe.

Treatment

High temperature and humidity should be avoided. Careful washing of the body is necessary. Steroids are applied topically on eczematous lesions. Care should be taken to prevent secondary infection.

Bromhidrosis/osmidrosis
Definition, classification, and clinical features

Bromhidrosis (osmidrosis) is a general term for abnormal body odor arising from the sweat glands.

Eccrine bromhidrosis and apocrine bromhidrosis are the main types.

Eccrine bromhidrosis
Eccrine sweat may have a distinct odor from intake of drugs or foods such as garlic and spices. Bromhidrosis in the feet is caused by bacterial action on sweat-softened keratin.

Apocrine bromhidrosis
Osmidrosis axillae, commonly called armpit odor, is the well-known type. Bromhidrosis of the genitalia is also caused by apocrine sweat. The sweat itself is odorless; the odor results when fatty acids are decomposed by superficial bacteria. The apocrine glands begin to develop at puberty. Perspiration increases with physical exercise and nervousness.

Treatment
The skin should be kept clean to reduce bacterial flora and apocrine sweat of the axilla. The application of antiperspirants or deodorants, and shaving are effective. Laser, surgical or electrolysis depilation may be performed as a permanent cure. However, many patients who complain of offensive odor do not actually have the odor; the complaints may represent paranoia and phobia (osmidrophobia).

Fox–Fordyce disease (synonym: apocrine miliaria)
Clinical features
This occurs in women in their 20s. Follicular papules 2–3 mm in diameter and normal skin color or rose pink aggregate on areas distributed with apocrine sweat glands, such as axillary fossae, areolas of nipples, and genitals. They are accompanied by intense itching and aggravate with physical exercise or nervousness. They become chronic, and lichenoid or secondary infections such as suppurative hidradenitis may be caused by rubbing or scratching.

Pathogenesis
When the sweat ducts of apocrine sweat glands are obstructed, apocrine sweat exudes into the epidermis.

Treatment and prognosis
Topical steroids and oral histamines are used for the itching, which is intractable. Surgical excision as for osmidrosis axillae may be done.

MEMO 19–2 Symmetrical lividity (synonyms: symmetrical lividities of the soles of the feet, symmetrical lividities of the palms and soles)

Edematous erythema occurs symmetrically on the palms and soles. It is induced by sweating, and often occurs in young individuals.

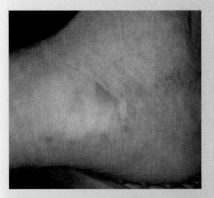
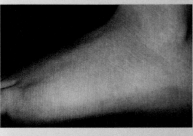
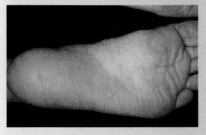

Hyperhidrosis

Definition and symptoms

Hyperhidrosis, caused by enhanced perspiration from the eccrine glands, is classified into the subtypes described below.

Generalized hyperhidrosis

This occurs physiologically in hot, humid environments, during exercise or from sympathetic hypertonia. It also occurs in patients with hyperthyroidism, diabetes, hypoglycemia, infections, neurological disease (e.g., Parkinson's disease), malignancies or other primary disease, or it may be induced by drugs (e.g., antipyretics, steroids, psychotropic agents), pregnancy or obesity. Idiopathic generalized hyperhidrosis without any particular cause also exists.

Localized hyperhidrosis

This occurs in the palms, soles, axillary fossae, face, and elsewhere. Most cases aggravate with physical exercise or nervousness. Perspiration that exceeds evaporation may occur even at rest, affecting quality of life.

- **Palmoplantar hyperhidrosis:** hyperhidrosis palmaris et plantaris may accompany atopic conditions or palmoplantar keratosis.
- **Hemihyperhidrosis:** this is seen in patients with partial paralysis or Parkinson's disease. The hyperhidrosis occurs on one side of the body from impairment of the peripheral nerves on that side.

Diagnosis and treatment

Many hemihyperhidrosis cases are easily diagnosed. Starch-iodine test is used for mild cases. Antiperspirants containing aluminum chloride and antianxiety medications are used. Iontophoresis using tap water and a local injection of botulinus toxin are useful. Sympathetic nerve block is done for intractable cases; however, perspiration in other parts of the body often increases (compensatory sweating/reflex sweating).

Anhidrosis

This is a condition with scant or absent perspiration (Fig. 19.4). The skin is dry and coarse. Scaling and mild itching occur, and fever may be produced by exercise from lack of perspiration. Anhidrosis is classified into systemic (anhidrotic (hypohidrotic) ectodermal dysplasia; see Chapter 18) and localized (neurological disorder). Diseases suspected of causing anhidrosis are shown in Table 19.1.

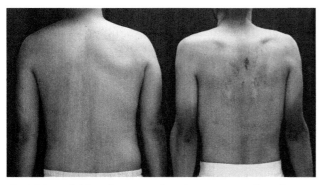

Fig. 19.4 Anhidrosis. Sweat function test (starch-iodine test). The patient on the left shows no color changes on his back, from which it is understood that he has markedly decreased perspiration.

Table 19.1 Diseases thought to cause anhidrosis.

Cause of anhidrosis	Disease producing the dysplasia
Congenital absence of sweat gland function	Hypohidrotic ectodermal dysplasia, congenital insensitivity to pain with anhidrosis (CIPA)
Metabolic disorder	Hypothyroidism, dehydration, thermic fever, Fabry's disease, Kanzaki's disease, diabetes
Neurological disorder	Disorders of the hypothalamus and spinal cord, alcoholic neuritis, leprosy, acquired idiopathic generalized anhidrosis (AIGA)
Obstruction of sweat pores and ducts	Ichthyosis, seborrheic dermatitis, atopic dermatitis, erythroderma, psoriasis
Atrophy or damage of the sweat glands	Scleroderma, Sjögren syndrome, skin aging and the like

Disorders of sebaceous glands

Acne vulgaris
- Most adolescent men and women (>90%) experience acne vulgaris. Comedones, folliculitis, papules, and pustules are produced.
- Agents and factors such as the *Propionibacterium acnes* bacterium, the *Demodex folliculorum* mite, endocrine secretion, and stress are associated with the occurrence.
- Lifestyle guidance and administration of topical retinoids and antibiotics are effective.

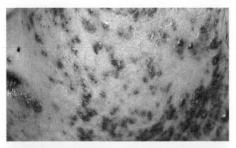

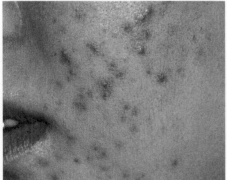

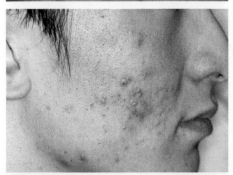

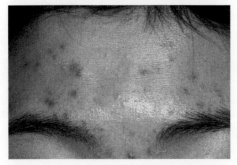

Fig. 19.5 Acne vulgaris. Multiple follicular inflammatory papules occur on oily areas of the face, such as the cheeks and forehead. Comedones are also seen.

Clinical features

Follicular inflammatory papules occur, most commonly on the seborrheic areas of the face, back, and precordial region of men and women from the ages of about 10 to 40 (Fig. 19.5). Pustules, cysts, and nodules may occur in this chronic inflammatory disorder. The papules worsen at puberty. The initial eruption, called a comedo, is classified as open (the follicles are open; "blackheads") or closed (small yellowish-white nodules in the skin; "whiteheads"). Keratotic plugs formed in the follicles cause the disorder without inflammation or subjective symptoms. Closed comedos often progress to erythematous papules or pustules (inflammatory eruptions), and nodules form in severe cases. Acne vulgaris is characterized by intermingled eruptions of different stages. Scarring may occur after healing. The following are atypical types of acne.

- **Neonatal acne:** small inflammatory papules appear on the face of newborns at about 2 weeks of age and spontaneously disappear in 2–3 months. Hormones derived from the mother are thought to cause the disorder. Neonatal acne is found in 20% of healthy babies.
- **Acne conglobate:** multiple severe acne lesions, scars, and nodules aggregate on the face and back. Acne conglobate can be classified as a subtype of chronic pyoderma (see Chapter 24).
- **Steroid-induced acne:** small, uniform follicular papules appear on the chest about 2 weeks after the use of steroids. Topical immunosuppressants sometimes cause eruptions similar to those of acne conglobate.
- **Acne demodecica:** this is caused by the *Demodex folliculorum* mite. Intractable acne that occurs often in adult women may be caused by this mite.
- **Acneiform drug eruption:** see Table 10.1.

Pathogenesis

The main pathogenesis involves hormonal imbalance, abnormal sebum retention and keratinization, and bacterial infection (Fig. 19.6). Along with these main factors, hereditary factors, the patient's age, diet, stress, and extrinsic factors such as cosmetics are complicatedly associated with the onset.

- **Hormonal imbalance:** androgen in the blood increases according to pubertal endocrine changes, and the function of the sebaceous glands is enhanced by adrenogenic dihydrotestosterone (DHT). Accordingly, sebum retention and bacterial proliferation readily occur.

- **Overproduction of sebum:** hormonal imbalance, described above, causes overproduction of sebum. Abnormal keratinization and bacterial infection tend to occur as the result of oversecretion of sebum and the decomposition products of the sebum.
- **Abnormal keratinization:** when sebum components are decomposed by bacteria, free fatty acids are produced; stimulated by this phenomenon, the infundibulum induces keratinization. The infundibulum is obstructed by keratin as a result of poor hygiene or hereditary factors (retention hyperkeratosis), which induces further retention of sebum and leads to the initial eruption (comedo).
- **Bacterial infection:** *Propionibacterium acnes* bacteria resident in the infundibulum break down triglycerides in the sebum, producing free fatty acids that destroy the hair follicles and lead to inflammation. The bacteria themselves also cause destruction of follicles and inflammation.

Pathology

Acne vulgaris is characterized by enlargement of the sebaceous glands and follicular keratinization. Cystic dilation occurs in follicles, and destruction of the follicular walls causes inflammatory reaction.

Differential diagnosis

Acne vulgaris must be differentiated from milium, sebaceous gland hyperplasia, rosacea, rosacea-like dermatitis, miliaria rubra, lupus miliaris disseminatus faciei, and verruca plana. Thorough history taking is important.

Treatment

Guidance on hygiene, diet, and the like is the primary treatment. Observance of a regular schedule of sleeping and eating, and avoidance of cosmetics (cold cream and foundation, in particular) are helpful. Washing the face and maintaining regular bowel movements are important. The application of topical retinoids is the basic first-line treatment. Administration of topical sulfa drugs is helpful for comedos, and topical or oral antibiotics are used for inflammatory eruptions. Chemical peeling may be helpful in some cases. Local injection of steroids may be done when nodules or scarring are formed.

Rosacea
Definition and pathogenesis

Rosacea is a chronic inflammatory disease that causes diffuse reddening and vascular dilation on the face,

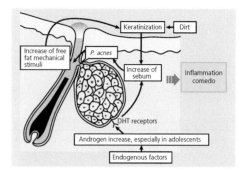

Fig. 19.6 Mechanism of acne vulgaris.

MEMO 19–3 Adapalene

The topical retinoid adapalene selectively combines with the retinoic acid receptor to prevent inflammatory and non-inflammatory eruptions by inhibiting the keratinization of epithelial cells of follicles and the formation of comedos.

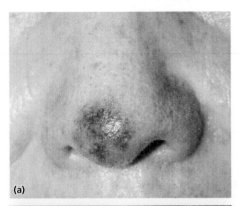

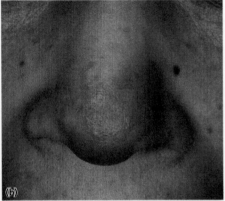

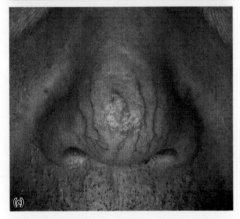

Fig. 19.7 Rosacea erythematosa on the tip of the nose. a: A male patient in his 20s. b: A female patient in her 30s. c: A male patient in his 30s. Telangiectasia is remarkable.

the nose in particular, of middle-aged and older men and women. The condition may last several months or longer. Acne-like papules and pustules may be produced.

Clinical features

Rosacea is classified into four subtypes by the clinical symptoms and affected parts. Rosacea frequently occurs in middle-aged and older women but severe cases are found more commonly in men.

Erythematotelangiectatic rosacea, first-stage rosacea

Transient reddening appears on the tip of the nose and on the cheeks, glabella, and chin. It progresses gradually to become persistent and accompanied by telangiectasia and seborrhea (Fig. 19.7). Hot and cold weather, sunlight, and alcohol consumption aggravate it. Subjective symptoms such as itching, hot flashes, and irritability are present.

Papulopustular rosacea, second-stage rosacea

As rosacea progresses, follicular papules and pustules resembling acne vulgaris occur in addition to the symptoms of first-stage rosacea, and seborrhea becomes intense (Fig. 19.8). The lesions spread to cover the face.

Phymatous rosacea, third-stage rosacea

The papules aggregate and coalesce to become tumorous. The surface of the nose becomes rough and reddish purple. The skin appears orange peel-like with open follicles (Fig. 19.9).

Ocular rosacea

Swelling around the eyes, conjunctivitis, and keratitis occur. In about 20% of cases, ocular rosacea precedes cutaneous symptoms.

Pathogenesis

Involvement of sunlight, mental stress, intake of alcohol or spicy food, liver dysfunction, and infection by the *Demodex folliculorum* mite are suspected but the pathogenesis remains unclear.

Treatment and prognosis

Rosacea progresses gradually and tends to be intractable. Spicy foods, excessive sun exposure, and stress should be avoided. Laser irradiation is performed on the telangiectasia. The treatments for acne rosacea are the same as those for acne vulgaris. Topical metronidazole, imidazoles, and tretinoin may bring improvement. Steroids should never be used. Laser therapy, cryotherapy, and surgical treatment are conducted for rhinophyma.

Rosacea-like dermatitis (synonyms: perioral dermatitis, steroid-induced dermatitis)

- Prolonged application of steroids to the face induces rosacea-like erythematous papules, diffuse flushing, and acne. Perioral dermatitis is also known to be caused by topical steroid therapy.
- After discontinuation of steroids, the treatments for acne vulgaris are given.

Clinical features

Rosacea-like dermatitis, which most commonly occurs in middle-aged women, is a typical side effect of topical steroids. Erythema, telangiectasia, papules, pustules, diffuse flushing, and scaling occur on sites where steroids have been applied. These symptoms are accompanied by itching and burning sensation (Fig. 19.10). Localized rosacea-like dermatitis around the mouth is called perioral dermatitis.

Pathogenesis

Epidermal atrophy and vasodilation, as side effects of prolonged topical steroid use, are the basic symptoms. It has been reported that topical steroids induce over-expression of TLR2 in corneocytes that have already been stimulated by inflammation and, as a result of the activated natural immunity system, the TLR2 contributes to the occurrence of rosacea-like dermatitis.

Treatment

Steroids are immediately discontinued, after which rebound phenomenon occurs. Reddening and swelling aggravate, and the erosions may persist for several weeks to several months. The same treatments as those for acne vulgaris are given. Topical tacrolimus is effective but it should be used carefully because it sometimes aggravates the disorder. Topical steroids are tapered off instead of being stopped immediately only when the rebound is severe.

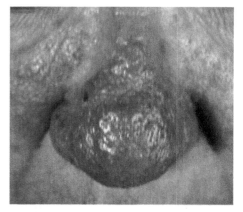

Fig. 19.8 Acne rosacea in a male patient in his 50s.

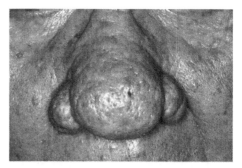

Fig. 19.9 Rhinophyma in a male patient in his 60s. The skin lesion becomes tumor-like and the hair follicles dilate. The skin takes on the appearance of orange peel.

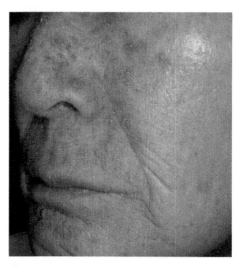

Fig. 19.10-1 Rosacea-like dermatitis. Eruptions occurred after continuous application of topical steroid for 1 month. Diffuse flushing, exfoliation, itching, and burning sensation occurred.

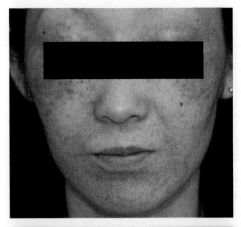

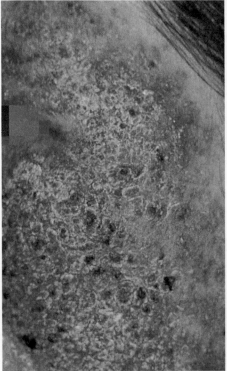

Fig. 19.10-2 Rosacea-like dermatitis as a side effect of topical steroids.

Lupus miliaris disseminatus faciei (LMDF) (synonym: acne agminata)

- Multiple small papules of 2–5 mm in diameter and the color of normal skin or redder occur on the face, particularly the lower eyelids. The disorder is asymptomatic.
- The histology is epithelioid cell granuloma with central necrosis. An association with tuberculosis has been excluded.
- Tetracycline is administrated in small doses.

Clinical features

Lupus miliaris disseminatus faciei occurs in both sexes equally, with most patients being in their 20s and 30s. Multiple small papules with central necrosis 2–5 mm in diameter and the color of normal skin or redder occur symmetrically on the face, especially on the lower eyelids, cheeks and the sides of the nose, accompanied by pustules (Fig. 19.11). The disorder is nearly asymptomatic or with mild itching. Small yellowish-white nodules are observed by diascopy. These heal with concave scarring 1 year to several years after onset. The scars often become indistinct eventually.

Pathogenesis and pathology

Lupus miliaris disseminatus faciei was first thought to be a form of tuberculid, but association with tuberculosis has been ruled out. The mechanism is predominantly thought to be a granulomatous reaction against hair follicle tissues or their contents. It is thought to be a subtype of rosacea with granuloma. Biopsies from well-established lesions reveal epithelioid granuloma with central necrosis.

Differential diagnosis

Syringoma, milium, acne vulgaris, and sarcoidosis should be differentiated from LMDF.

Treatment

Tetracycline and dapsone are administered in small doses.

Disorders of the hair

Alopecia areata

- Round, sharply margined hair loss suddenly occurs.
- Hair regrows spontaneously in several months in most cases. Cases with multiple alopecia areata

may progress to alopecia totalis or alopecia universalis.
- Topical steroids and PUVA therapy are the first-line treatments.

Clinical features

Alopecia areata most commonly occurs in young people. Besides occurring in the scalp, alopecia areata may occur in the eyebrows, beard areas, and extremities. Alopecia areata is quite common, affecting up to 1% of the population. Sharply margined hair loss occurs suddenly without prodromes or subjective symptoms (Fig. 19.12). The hair roots in the lesion are small and the proximal shafts are thin, which makes the shape of the hair look like an exclamation mark (exclamation point hair). Alopecia areata is usually round or oval, single or sometimes multiple, alopecia of 2–3 cm in diameter. Alopecia on the occipital and temporal scalp (ophiasis) is intractable. The alopecia patches may coalesce, progressing to complete scalp hair loss (alopecia totalis) in some cases (Fig. 19.13). Cases in which hair on the whole body is affected are called alopecia universalis. Slight depression and coarseness in nails may occur.

Pathogenesis

Hair matrix cells are impaired temporarily for unknown reasons. Theories include nutritional failure, heredity, and mental stress but the pathogenesis is unclear. Some cases are accompanied by autoimmune thyroid deficiency, vitiligo, and atopic dermatitis. Autoimmune involvement is suspected.

Pathology

In the lesion, there is infiltration of CD4[+] T cells and the appearance of Langerhans cells in the hair follicles at the anagen stage. Expression of MHC class II in hair bulb epitheliocytes, and deposition of C3, IgG, and IgM in the hair follicular basement membrane are observed. There is possible involvement of autoimmunity. The affected hair follicles form abnormal atrophic hair that falls out.

Differential diagnosis

Trichotillomania and alopecia cicatricans are distinguished from alopecia areata. Trichotillomania, which produces short, breakable, hard hair in the lesion, occurs most commonly in children; however, there is no diseased hair in trichotillomania, and the hair

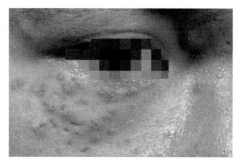

Fig. 19.11-1 Lupus miliaris disseminatus faciei (LMDF). Small multiple papules of normal skin color or red and 2–5 mm in diameter occur symmetrically on the face. Some heal with scarring.

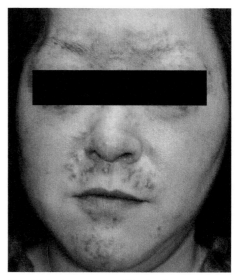

Fig. 19.11-2 Lupus miliaris disseminatus faciei.

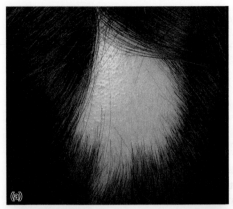

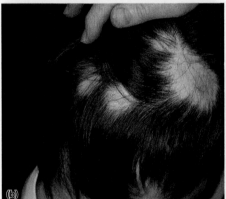

Fig. 19.12 Alopecia areata. a: Sharply demarcated hair loss occurs. In active alopecia areata, the hairs around the lesion easily come out. b: Regrowth of hairs is observed in some places.

MEMO 19–4 Finasteride

Finasteride is an oral antiandrogen agent used for male-pattern baldness. It inhibits 5α-reductase II, which converts testosterone to dihydrotestosterone. Care should be taken in the use of finasteride, because it lowers serum PSA levels; alopecia starts to progress after discontinuation of finasteride.

---

around the lesion does not come out easily. In alopecia cicatricans, fibrosis and pigmentation are present in the scalp at the lesion. Alopecia areata also should be distinguished from systemic lupus erythematosus (SLE) and alopecia caused by syphilis.

Treatment

Alopecia areata resolves spontaneously in several months, although in some cases it may be intractable or recurrent. Cases with multiple alopecia lesions tend to recur. Juvenile-onset alopecia, alopecia complicated with atopic dermatitis, and alopecia with wide-ranging hair loss are often refractory. Topical steroids or carpronium chloride are used. For intractable cases, localized immune therapies such as SADBE (squaric acid dibutylester), PUVA therapy, and cryotherapy are given. It is important to address the patient's distress about hair loss. Antianxiety medications may be used if necessary. For acute exacerbation of alopecia, oral therapies using steroids or ciclosporin are considered.

Male-pattern baldness (synonyms: androgenic alopecia (AGA), alopecia prematura)
Clinical features

Male-pattern baldness occurs in about half of adult men. Hair loss with vellus hair at the frontal region of the head or with vellus hair on the top of the head occurs. These patterns may appear separately or simultaneously. The Norwood–Hamilton Scale is used to classify the progress and pattern of the baldness. The diameter of the vellus hair is smaller than that of normal hair. The density (hairs per unit area) also is reduced.

It progresses to complete hair loss. The pathogenesis of female-pattern baldness, diffuse hair loss mainly at the parietal region of the scalp in women in menopause and after, is the same as that of male-pattern baldness.

Pathogenesis

Patients usually have a familial history of baldness. Elevated sensitivity of hair follicles to androgen (dihydrotestosterone, in particular) begins at some point. The anagen phase is shortened, hairs at the telogen phase decrease in number, the hair follicles contract and vellus transformation occurs. The thin, sparse vellus hair produced in androgenic alopecia becomes less densely distributed, eventually progressing to alopecia.

Treatment
Administration of oral finasteride, an antiandrogenic agent, is effective (MEMO, see Chapter 19). Topical minoxidil is effective in some cases.

Congenital alopecia
Congenital atrichia, alopecia, and oligotrichia are observed in the following conditions.

Alopecia universalis congenita
This is autosomal recessive. Hair may be present at birth but it falls out between several months after birth and puberty until no hair remains on the body. The involvement of the hairless (*hr*) gene has been identified as a cause in some cases of certain subtypes.

Hypotrichosis congenita
Normal hair is present at birth but alopecia gradually leads to thin, sparse hair (Fig. 19.14).

Other congenital atrichia and alopecia
Atrichia and congenital alopecia are associated with congenital ectodermal defect, dermatothlasia, Werner syndrome, Rothmund–Thomson syndrome, and Netherton syndrome. Odontogenesis imperfecta, abnormal nail plates, palmoplantar keratosis, and anhidrosis often occur as complications. For details of each disorder stated above, refer to the section describing it.

Trichotillomania
Patients with trichotillomania, who tend to be in their late childhood, pull out their own hair. The patients may deny this behavior. Vaguely circumscribed, irregularly shaped, incomplete alopecia is present. Both short and broken remaining hairs and newly produced hairs are observed in the same alopecia areas, which are within reach of the hand, often on the frontal and temporal scalp on the dominant hand side. The patient's psychological background, personality, and domestic environment may trigger trichotillomania; cooperation with a psychiatrist is necessary for treatment.

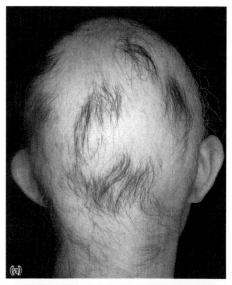

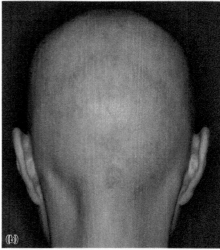

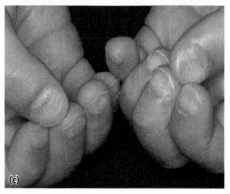

Fig. 19.13 Alopecia totalis. a,b: Complete alopecia on the head. c: Multiple small concavities in the nails.

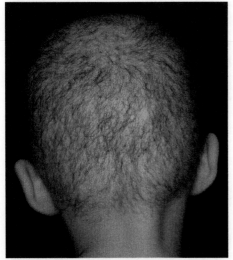

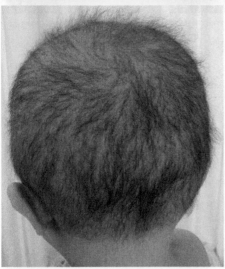

Fig. 19.14 Congenital hypotrichosis in a girl. This patient has thin, sparse hair (oligotrichia). She has never had a haircut, but the hair does not grow beyond this length.

> **MEMO 19–5 Telogen effluvium and anagen effluvium**
> - **Telogen effluvium:** hairs in the anagen phase are pushed into the telogen phase by mental stress, surgery or delivery, and diffuse hair loss occurs a few weeks to several months after. It is a reversible change, and hair growth recovers in several months to 1 year.
> - **Anagen effluvium:** differentiation and proliferation of hairs in the anagen phase are inhibited by chemotherapy, for example. Hair loss occurs in a short period of time. It is a reversible change.

Scarring alopecia

As a result of scarring caused by injury or by heat or radiation burn, the hair follicles are irreversibly destroyed, leading to alopecia. Scarring alopecia may occur in patients with discoid lupus erythematosus (DLE) or sclérodermie en coup de sabre. Reconstructive surgery is necessary.

Disorders of the nails

Color changes of the nail plates

Melanonychia

Melanonychia may be caused by increases in the number of nail matrix melanocytes (from nevocellular nevus, inflammation, mechanical pressure, malignant melanoma, Addison's disease or drugs, e.g., 5-FU, bleomycin, hydroxyurea). When the skin of the nail fold region is also affected, it is called Hutchinson's sign and has a high likelihood of indicating a malignant melanoma (Fig. 19.15). Blackening of the nail can be seen from subungual hemorrhage; however, many cases of subungual hemorrhage are differentiated from other disorders by dermoscopy. Longitudinal linear hemorrhage of a few millimeters in width (splinter hemorrhage) can be seen on the nail in healthy individuals; however, care should be exercised in diagnosis, because similar hemorrhages sometimes occur in patients with hereditary hemorrhagic telangiectasia (Osler's disease) or infectious endocarditis.

Yellow nail

This is caused by nutritional deficiency or infection of the nails, or by aurantiasis cutis or jaundice. When yellowing of the nails occurs in patients with lymphoma or chronic respiratory disorders, it is called yellow nail syndrome, which may be induced by D-penicillamine or tetracycline (Fig. 19.16).

Green nail

This opportunistic infection is caused by the *Pseudomonas aeruginosa* bacterium and tends to accompany tinea unguium and candida onychomycosis (Fig. 19.17).

Leukonychia

These white punctate patches in nails may be caused by localized incomplete keratinization from injury (Fig. 19.18). They are harmless. White nails accompany the hypoalbuminemia that is seen in nephrosis and cirrhosis (Muehrcke's nail), as well as accompanying diabetes, anemia, systemic sclerosis, arsenic poisoning, onychomycosis, and onycholysis.

Abnormal formation of the nails

Nail clubbing

This disorder is also called clubbed finger or Hippocratic nail. The entire nail plate bulges like the glass face of a watch. The distal fingers and toes enlarge in drumstick shape (Fig. 19.19). Clubbing is caused by mucopolysaccharide deposition in the soft tissue of the distal fingers and toes. It occurs in chronic cardiopulmonary diseases (pulmonary emphysema, lung cancer, bronchiectasis, congenital heart disease), hyperthyroidism, and inflammatory bowel disease. It may appear as a symptom of pachydermoperiostosis (see Chapter 18) running in families.

Spoon nail

Spoon nail is associated with iron deficiency anemia or thyroid dysfunction, lichen planus, psoriasis, fungal infection, extrinsic injury, and chemical substances. The nail plates become thin, with spoon-like concavity with raised edges (Fig. 19.20). Fingers are more severely affected than toes. It may be seen in

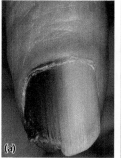
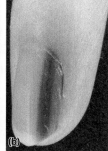
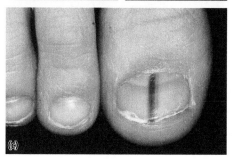

Fig. 19.15 Melanonychia. a: The nail is partially pigmented. Deformity is seen at the tip. Melanoma is suspected in this case. b: The fingernail of a 25-year-old woman. The symptoms rapidly progressed in the previous 6 months. Melanoma is presented in situ histologically. c: Nevus cell nevus in the nail matrix.

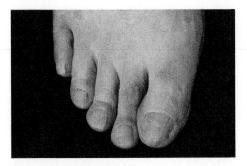

Fig. 19.16 Yellow nail.

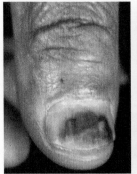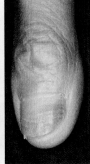

Fig. 19.17 Green nail.

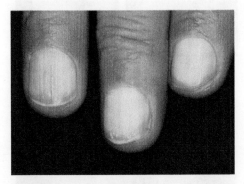

Fig. 19.18 Leukonychia.

otherwise normal infants and healthy individuals whose work requires intensive use of the fingertips.

Onycholysis

The nail plate detaches from the nail bed at the periungual area. Desquamation occurs, but the nails do not fall out. The causes may be infectious diseases including candida onychomycosis, injury or chronic stimulation, nail polish, or inflammation in the periungual skin of the nail plate region caused by detergents, systemic diseases such as hyperthyroidism, peripheral circulatory failure or drug-induced disease.

Onychomadesis, nail shedding

The nail plate detaches at proximal sites of the nail root, which is the end opposite that in onycholysis desquamation, and the nail exfoliates. It may occur sporadically or be caused by injury, perionychia, psoriasis, lichen planus, syphilis or erythroderma. Nail shedding occurs when the transverse groove in the nail becomes severe.

Pachyonychia

The nail plate thickens, or hyperkeratosis occurs under it. Thickening of the nail is also caused by hindered growth. Congenital cases are caused by mutation in the genes that code for keratins 6, 16, and 17 (pachyonychia congenita; Fig. 19.21). When the nail is thickened and curved, it is called onychogryphosis, which is often seen in the big toe of the elderly.

Longitudinal groove

Linear grooves run longitudinally in the nail plate. They are seen as senile changes. The condition may progress to onychorrhexis, in which nails tend to split

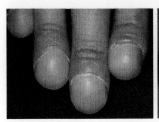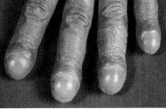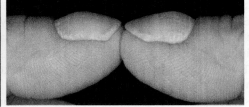

Fig. 19.19 Clubbing. The entire nail plate bulges like the glass face of a watch. The distal fingers enlarge in drumstick shape.

longitudinally. Longitudinal grooves are caused by injury, eczema, scleroderma, and anemia.

Transverse groove

Grooves cross the nail as a result of nail growth impairment from failure in the nail matrix. The width of the grooves shows the duration of the disease, and the depth shows the severity of the growth impairment. When the cause is localized (injury, etc.), so are the affected nails. However, when the cause is intrinsic, the grooves occur in all nails (Beau's lines). Possible causes include febrile or infectious diseases and diabetes, pregnancy and delivery, zinc deficiency, and drug use.

Nail pitting

Multiple, small, needle-like indentations occur on the nail plate. This is caused by psoriasis and alopecia areata (Fig. 19.22), or it may occur under normal conditions.

Onychoschizia

Fine, scaly, lamellar separation occurs at the tip of the nail, causing fragility. It is thought to be caused by low moisture content in the nail plate. It often occurs in winter. It is most frequently caused by nail polish application but may also be induced by systemic diseases such as SLE.

Ingrown nail

The sides of the nail grow into the nail fold, leading to swelling, reddening, and inflammation with a granulomatous appearance. The condition is accompanied by tenderness (Fig. 19.23). In severe cases, a secondary infection such as paronychia occurs, causing formation of reactive granuloma. It is commonly caused in the big toes by pressure from shoes or by excessive toenail clipping. When it occurs secondarily after nail deformity caused by fungi of the genus *Trichophyton*, the primary disease is treated. Avoidance of extrinsic pressure and maintenance of cleanliness are the first-line treatments but corrective procedures using wires and surgery may be necessary for intractable cases (Fig. 19.23d).

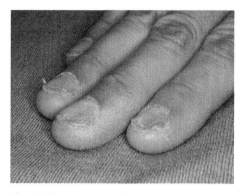

Fig. 19.20 Spoon nail.

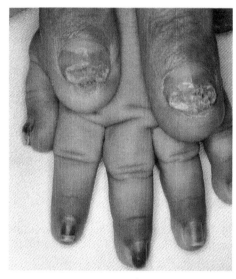

Fig. 19.21 Pachyonychia congenita. Deformity of the nail plate occurs in the mother's nails (upper) and in the child's nails (lower).

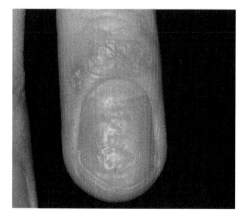

Fig. 19.22 Pitting in a patient with alopecia areata.

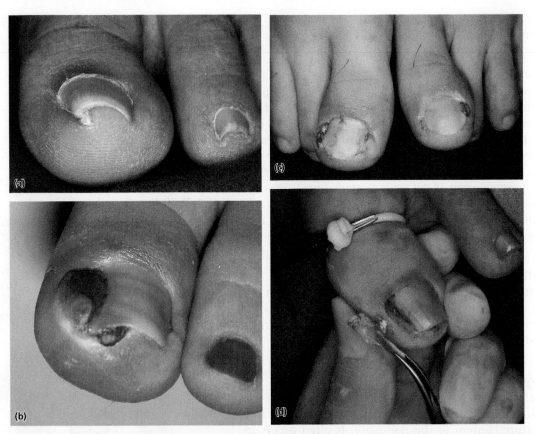

Fig. 19.23 Ingrown nail. a: On the great toe. The sides of the nail grow into the nail fold, causing sharp pain. b,c: Reactive formation of granulation. d: Part of the nail, including the nail matrix, was removed.

CHAPTER 20

Nevi and neurocutaneous syndromes

"Nevus" is Latin for "maternal impression" or "birthmark." It denotes a circumscribed, non-neoplastic skin or mucosal lesion. The term is qualified according to the cell or tissue of origin. Nevi may be caused by hereditary or embryological factors and may appear at any time in life. They progress extremely slowly. The concept of nevi includes what are generally called moles and birthmarks. Nevi are thought to be deformities in the skin made up of aggregated cells at various stages of differentiation, caused by hereditary mosaicism. In understanding nevi, it is helpful to classify them into several types depending on the type of cells that make up the lesion (nevus cells). The classifications are melanocytic nevi (e.g., nevus cell nevus) (Fig. 20.1), epidermal nevi (e.g., verrucous epidermal nevus), mesenchymal cell nevi (e.g., connective tissue nevus), and vascular nevi (e.g., angioma and vascular malformation).

Neurocutaneous syndrome includes nevi formed in the skin and nevoid lesions produced in the systemic organs that cause central nervous symptoms.

Neurocutaneous syndrome is often categorized as a phacomatosis; however, that term has fallen out of use internationally in recent years. This chapter introduces the most common nevi. Angiomas are described in Chapter 21.

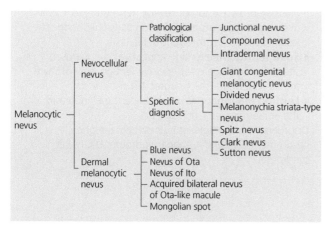

Fig. 20.1 Classification of melanocytic nevi.

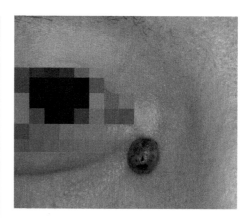

Fig. 20.2-1 Nevus cell nevus.

Shimizu's Dermatology, Second Edition. Hiroshi Shimizu.
© 2017 John Wiley & Sons, Ltd. Published 2017 by John Wiley & Sons, Ltd.

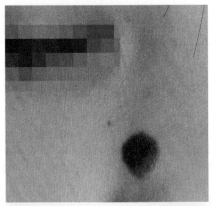

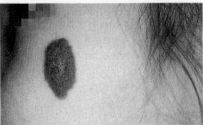

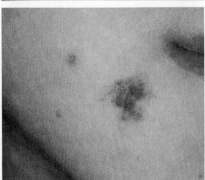

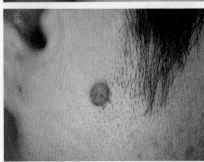

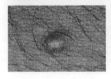 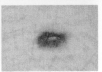

Fig. 20.2-2 Nevus cell nevus.

Nevus

Melanocytic nevi

Nevus cell nevus (synonyms: nevus pigmentosus, pigmented nevus, nevocellular nevus, nevomelanocytic nevus)

- A proliferation of nevus cells (i.e., anaplastic melanocytic cells) causes nevus cell nevus. A small nevus cell nevus is commonly called a mole.
- A hairy, giant, pigmented nevus cell nevus of 20 cm or more in diameter is called a giant congenital melanocytic nevus. It tends to progress to malignant melanoma.

MEMO 20–1 Lentigo

Most cases of the pigmentation that is commonly called lentigo are small nevus cell nevus (mole). When "lentigo" is used to refer to a dermatological disorder, it means a flat, dark brown lesion with localized proliferation of melanocytes as seen under UV radiation; no increase of nevus cells is found in the lesion.
- **Lentigo simplex:** a partly irregularly shaped flat blackish-brown lesion of several millimeters to 15 mm in diameter appears at birth or in early childhood. The lesion remains flat throughout life.
- **Solar lentigo:** the lentigo appears at sun-exposed sites in middle age or after. Solar lentigo is a synonym for senile lentigo (see Chapter 16).
- **Lentigo maligna:** this is a malignant melanoma in the epidermis (see Chapter 22).

Disorders with multiple lentigines: Peutz–Jeghers syndrome, Cronkhite–Canada syndrome, LEOPARD syndrome.

MEMO 20–2 Birthmark

Various cutaneous disorders are included in what is commonly called a birthmark. Middle-sized nevus cell nevus, Mongolian macule, café au lait spot, subcutaneous bleeding and capillary malformation (salmon patch) are included.

- Nevus cell nevus is histopathologically classified into junctional nevus, compound nevus, and intradermal nevus.
- Dermoscopic findings are important for diagnosis.
- "Pigmented nevus" may be used as a synonym; however, non-pigmented lesions are often seen.

Clinical features

A nevus cell nevus is a flat-surfaced or verrucous macule or tumor that is brown, black or sometimes normal skin color (Fig. 20.2). It may be accompanied by terminal hair. Nevus cell nevi are clinically classified by size into three types. A nevus cell nevus is commonly called a mole or lentigo, and it varies in size from several millimeters to 1.5 cm in diameter. Most nevus cell nevi are acquired. They are not present at birth but first appear between the ages of 3 and 4 and gradually increase in number and size to peak in one's 20s to 30s. The average number of nevus cell nevi in an individual is about 10–50. The color of the nevus fades after it has reached the peak and the cells of the nevus are replaced by fat tissue or fibrous tissue. A nevus cell nevus of 1.5–20 cm diameter is called a "black birthmark" and it often occurs in the scalp and neck region. Many of these are congenital and present at birth; they enlarge and become distinct with age. When the diameter exceeds 20 cm, the nevus is called a giant congenital melanocytic nevus. Some types of nevi have specific clinical features.

Pathogenesis

Nevus cells are derived from neural crests and proliferate abnormally, resulting in blackish-brown pigmented macules. Melanocytes and Schwann cells are derived from neural crests; however, nevus cells do not differentiate into either of these (Fig. 20.3).

Pathology

Nevus cell nevi are classified by location of proliferation into junctional nevus, compound nevus, and intradermal nevus (see Fig. 20.3). The clinical features of each type are distinctive.

Diagnosis and differential diagnosis

Nevus cell nevus should be differentiated from early malignant melanoma (see Chapter 22). In differentiation, dermoscopic findings are useful (see Chapter 3).

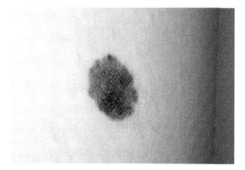
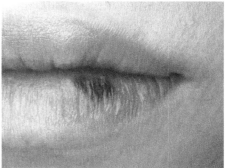
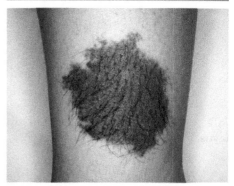
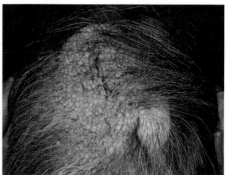

Fig. 20.2-3 Nevus cell nevus.

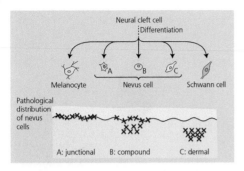

Fig. 20.3 Origin of nevus cells and histological classification of nevus cell nevi.

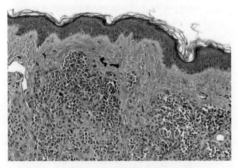

Fig. 20.4 Histopathology of nevus cell nevus.

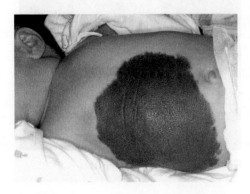

Fig. 20.5 Giant congenital melanocytic nevus.

Treatment

Even when the dermoscopic findings are benign, follow-up is necessary. Surgical removal is the basic treatment for cases with lesions in the palms and soles whose major axis exceeds 6 mm, which tend to have a high likelihood of malignancy, and in cases with a relatively large nevus cell nevus. Surgical removal and skin grafting are generally done for giant congenital melanocytic nevus. When it is too large for removal, long-term follow-up may be chosen to observe for any signs of malignant melanoma.

Common types of nevus cell nevi
Junctional nevus

Nevus cells are localized in the dermo-epidermal junction. Junctional nevus is a compound of large cubical cells that have slightly eosinophilic cytoplasm, function similarly to melanocytes (i.e., the cells produce melanin in great quantities) and resemble keratinocytes morphologically.

Compound nevus

This is a combination of junctional nevus and intradermal nevus. Many compound nevi tend to be small nevus cell nevi.

Intradermal nevus

Most of the nevus cells are localized in the dermis (Fig. 20.4). Melanin production is markedly low in cells in the deeper areas. The cells are small and appear cubic or spindled, resembling Schwann cells. Pedunculated and papillary compound nevus that occurs in the trunk is called Unna nevus. Dome-shaped nevus with vellus hair, which often occurs in the face, is called Miesher's nevus.

Specific types of nevus cell nevi
Giant congenital melanocytic nevus

Giant congenital melanocytic nevi generally exceed 20 cm in diameter. They are seen at birth, sometimes accompanied by black bristles (giant hairy pigmented nevus; Fig. 20.5). Malignant melanoma may develop, and central nervous symptoms (neurocutaneous melanosis) sometimes accompany this condition.

Divided nevus

Divided medium-sized nevus cell nevi distribute predominantly on the upper and lower eyelids. With the eye closed, they appear to be a single lesion. The color is blackish-brown. They are found at birth in most cases (Fig. 20.6).

Melanonychia striata-type nevus

Black lines appear longitudinally on the nail plate from nevus cells in the nail bed (Fig. 20.7) (see Chapter 19). Most cases are benign nevus cell nevus in the nail matrix but there is a high possibility of malignant melanoma when the pigmentation is found in the proximal nail fold (Hutchinson's sign).

Spitz nevus (synonyms: juvenile melanoma, spindle and epithelioid cell nevus)

- This specific subtype of nevus cell nevus frequently occurs in children and young adults.
- It appears suddenly on the scalp or neck region in most cases and enlarges quickly to about 1 cm in diameter. The periphery may become reddish.
- The clinical and histopathological features may resemble those of malignant melanoma; nevertheless, Spitz nevus is benign and may resolve spontaneously.

Clinical features

It occurs most commonly in children but also in adult men and women. It is a small, dome-shaped nodule, usually solitary, ranging in color from light pink to reddish-brown or black and ranging in size from several millimeters to 2 cm (Fig. 20.8). It appears suddenly on the scalp and neck in most cases and enlarges. Because it may be accompanied by dark brown pigmentation (Reed nevus), Spitz nevus is sometimes difficult to differentiate from malignant melanoma. Spitz nevus is benign and does not enlarge beyond a certain size, nor does infiltration occur.

Pathology and diagnosis

Spitz nevus is a compound nevus containing various cells, including spindle cells, epithelioid-like cells, atypical cells, and multinucleated giant cells. Dermal edema, telangiectasia, and inflammatory cell infiltration may occur. These findings resemble those of malignant melanoma; differentiation between Spitz nevus and malignant melanoma is often difficult. The

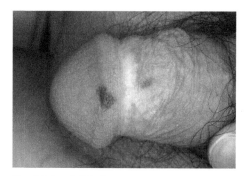

Fig. 20.6　**Divided nevus.**

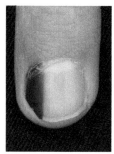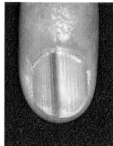

Fig. 20.7　**Melanonychia striata-type nevus.**

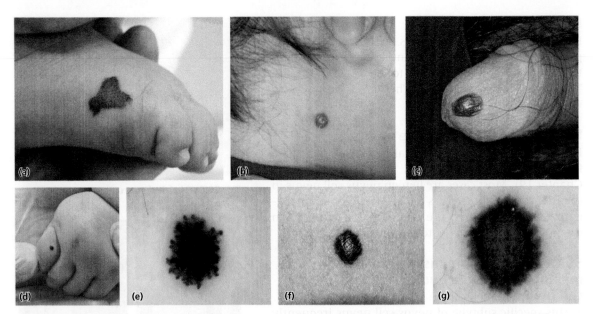

Fig. 20.8 Spitz nevus. a–d,f: Clinical features. e: Dermoscopic image of (d). g: Dermoscopic image of (f).

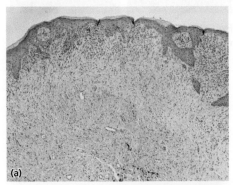

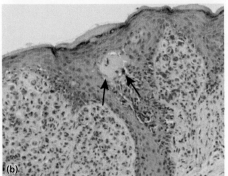

Fig. 20.9 Histopathology of Spitz nevus. a: Spitz nevus at low magnification. b: Spitz nevus at high magnification. Kamino bodies (arrows) are stained by eosin.

basic structural pattern of nevus cell nevus is preserved in Spitz nevus: Its shape is an inverted cone, with a symmetrical structure, and the deeper cells are smaller.

Homogenous non-structural eosinophilic substances called Kamino bodies, which stain well in eosin and stain positive in PAS, are found in the nevus cell nest in 70% of cases (Fig. 20.9). Dermoscopy shows sharply circumscribed pigmented lesions with a characteristic starburst pattern at the periphery (see Chapter 3).

Treatment
Excision is conducted. Spitz nevus does not aggravate but careful differentiation from malignant melanoma is necessary.

Clark nevus (synonyms: dysplastic nevus, atypical nevus)
Clark nevus occurs around puberty. It is a slightly elevated, flat-topped patch or a pigmented nevus cell nevus larger than 5 mm in diameter that has at least two features among the following: irregular shape, vague margin, and irregular pigmentation. Clark nevus is basically benign and disappears with age. Histopathologically, many cases show the findings of compound nevus or junctional nevus. Dermoscopic differentiation from superficial spreading melanoma is necessary. Multiple Clark nevi occur and when the

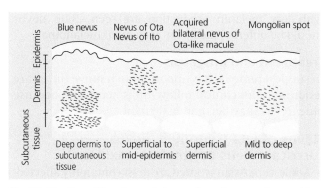

Fig. 20.10 Classification of dermal melanocytic nevi by the distribution of melanocytes.

patient has a family history of similar clinical findings, superficial spreading melanoma is highly possible. The condition is called dysplastic nevus syndrome, which is autosomal dominantly inherited.

See Chapter 16 for Sutton nevus.

Dermal melanocytic nevi

Dermal melanocytes are produced in blue nevus, Mongolian spot, and nevus of Ota (see Fig. 20.1). The clinical features, including the distribution of cells, vary according to the disease (Fig. 20.10).

Blue nevus

- A flat or slightly elevated blue nodule results from proliferation of melanocytes in the dermis (dermal melanocytes).
- It appears between the time of birth and infancy in most cases. The head, extremities, and buttocks are most commonly involved.

Clinical features

A small, firm blue or blackish nodule of 1 cm or less in diameter appears. It may be flat or tumorous (Fig. 20.11). Blue nevi tend to appear singly and to progress gradually. The extremities, head, face, back, and buttocks are most commonly affected. An irregularly shaped, highly elevated lesion that exceeds 1 cm in diameter, called cellular blue nevus, may sometimes form.

Pathology and diagnosis

There is tumorous proliferation of dermal melanocytes, which produce melanin in large quantities, mainly in the middle dermal layer (Fig. 20.12). In cellular blue nevus, spindle-shaped dermal cells resembling Schwann cells

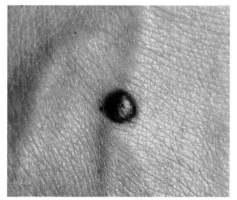

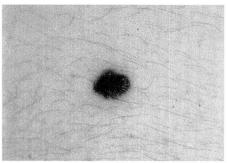

Fig. 20.11 Blue nevus.

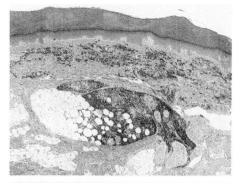

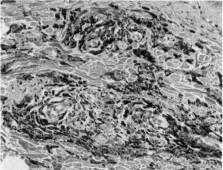

Fig. 20.12 Histopathology of blue nevus.

with low melanin production are seen. Blue nevus should be differentiated from malignant melanoma.

Treatment and prognosis

In surgical removal it is important to remove the entire lesion. Careful clinical follow-up is necessary, because blue nevus may become malignant.

Nevus of Ota (synonym: nevus fuscocaeruleus ophthalmomaxillaris)

* Adolescent Asian women are most commonly affected. A light blue macule appears unilaterally on the skin at the first and second divisions of the trigeminal nerve. Melanosis of the bulbar conjunctiva occurs.
* This nevus is caused by the proliferation of dermal melanocytes and deposition of melanin pigments in the dermal basal cell layer.
* It is not malignant, nor does it heal spontaneously. Laser therapy is effective.

Clinical features

A light blue nevus occurs unilaterally on the skin over the first and second divisions of the trigeminal nerve (eyelids, zygomatic region, lateral forehead, cheek). The nevus is light blue and punctatedly dispersed with various other colors, including brown, red, and dark blue (Fig. 20.13). Nevus of Ota with pigmentation in the sclera, iris, and fundus is called ocular melanosis and is found in about half of cases. Pigmentation may also occur in the tympanic membranes, nasal membranes, pharynx, and palate. A nevus with the same pigmentation as nevus of Ota but in the acrominon and deltoid region is called nevus of Ito or nevus fuscocaeruleus acromiodeltoideus Ito (see Fig. 20.10).

Pathology

Melanocytes are dispersed in the upper to middle dermal layers (see Fig. 20.10). Pigmentation is present in the epidermal basal cell layer.

Treatment

Laser therapy (e.g., alexandrite or Q-switch ruby lasers) is effective.

Acquired bilateral nevus of Ota-like macule (synonym: acquired dermal melanocytosis)

Acquired bilateral nevus of Ota-like macule used to be classified as a subtype of bilateral nevus of

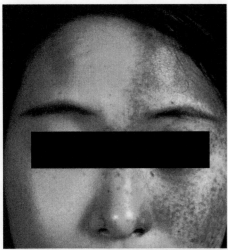
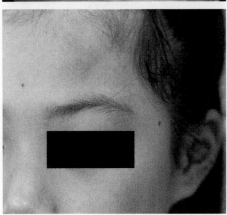

Fig. 20.13-1 Nevus of Ota.

Ota; however, the two are now regarded as distinct diseases. Multiple, punctate, grayish-brown pigmentation of 1–3 mm in diameter occurs on both sides of the forehead and in the zygomatic region and ala nasi (Fig. 20.14). Women between adolescence and middle age, particularly those of Japanese and Chinese descent, are most commonly affected. Histologically, there are proliferated melanocytes in the upper dermal layer. Ocular melanosis is not seen. Laser therapies are effective. Care should be taken in differentiating it from chloasma and in addressing the complication of chloasma (see Chapter 16).

Mongolian spot (synonym: congenital dermal melanocytosis)
Clinical features and pathology
Mongolian spot occurs in the lumbosacral regions and buttocks of newborns. Nearly 100% of Asians, 80–90% of Africans (in whom the blue color tends to be invisible), and 5% of Caucasians are affected. The blue hue intensifies until the age of two and then gradually fades, generally disappearing between 4 and 10 years of age. Mongolian spot is differentiated from nevus of Ota by its lack of brownish tone. Mongolian spot on sites other than the lumbosacral regions and buttocks (e.g., on the face or extremities) is called aberrant or ectopic Mongolian spot (Fig. 20.15). Histopathologically, increases in melanocytes in the middle to lower dermal layers are seen (see Fig. 20.10).

Treatment
Mongolian spots generally disappear spontaneously. The risk of malignancy does not increase even if the spot remains. Clearly marginated, large or ectopic Mongolian spots tend not to disappear spontaneously. Early laser therapy should be considered for cosmetic reasons (Fig. 20.16).

Epidermal nevi

Verrucous epidermal nevus (synonyms: linear epidermal nevus, epidermal nevus)
Definition and pathogenesis
Hyperplasia of epidermal keratinocytes results in localized or systematized verrucous nevus that enlarges gradually and becomes distinct. Internationally, epidermal

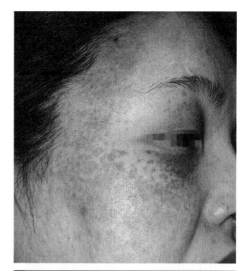

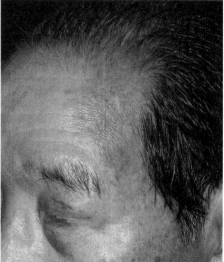

Fig. 20.13-2 Nevus of Ota.

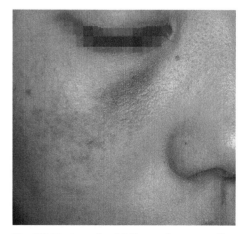

Fig. 20.14 Acquired bilateral nevus of Ota-like macule.

nevi is a generic term for nevi that originate from epidermal cells, including for nevus sebaceous (see next section).

Clinical features

Rough-surfaced verrucous papules or nodules are present at birth or in early childhood. They spread gradually, aggregate and form plaques of various sizes (Fig. 20.17). Although they may be localized, in most cases they are unilateral and arranged systematically along the Blaschko lines (see Fig. 1.4). A generalized type spreads over the whole body.

Although epidermal nevus tends to be asymptomatic, it may be accompanied by itching and eczematous changes. In inflammatory linear verrucous epidermal nevus (ILVEN), multiple intensely itchy light pink verrucous papules occur, most commonly on the lower legs of girls. They coalesce, lichenify and arrange in a linear pattern (Fig. 20.18).

Central nervous symptoms and skeletal abnormality are seen in rare cases; this is called epidermal nevus syndrome.

Pathology

Papilloma-like proliferation occurs in the epidermis. Lymphocytic infiltration or parakeratosis occurs in ILVEN. Granular degeneration also occurs in some cases, and mutation in the keratin 1 or 10 gene is found. This type of case can be considered as mosaic epidermolytic ichthyosis (see Chapter 15).

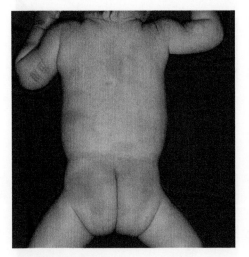

Fig. 20.15-1 Aberrant or ectopic Mongolian spot.

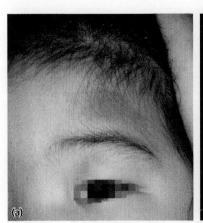
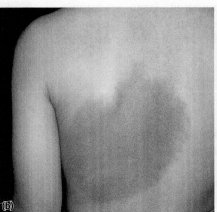
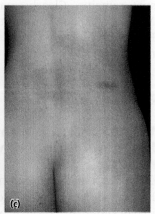

Fig. 20.15-2 Aberrant or ectopic Mongolian spot. a: Forehead. b: Back. c: Lumbar region.

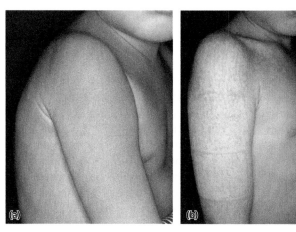

Fig. 20.16 Laser treatment of aberrant Mongolian spot.
a: Mongolian spot on the shoulder and the right arm
(pretreatment). b: Mongolian spot after one session of
alexandrite laser therapy.

Treatment

Epidermal nevi do not disappear or become malignant. Surgical removal, cryotherapy or carbon dioxide laser therapy is used. When itching is intense (e.g., in the case of ILVEN), topical steroids are used.

Sebaceous nevus (synonym: organoid nevus)

- This is caused by abnormal proliferation of various cells that originate in the epidermis, dermal appendages, and connective tissue.
- It is present at birth. The scalp and face are most commonly affected. Sebaceous nevus on the scalp leads to alopecia.
- Removal is considered, because tumors such as trichoblastoma and basal cell carcinoma may develop.

Clinical features

Sebaceous nevus occurs most frequently on the head and face. It is seen on 0.3% of newborns (Fig. 20.19). Sebaceous nevus, which tends to appear singly, forms a round or linear lesion along the Blaschko lines. The lesion is usually a 1–10 cm long, hairless, slightly elevated yellowish plaque. The lesion increases in elevation and gradually becomes verrucous and brownish in puberty. At middle age and after, or sometimes at puberty, the lesion worsens and additional epithelial tumors appear. Epithelial tumors such as dermal appendage tumors (e.g.,

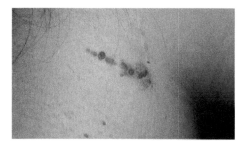

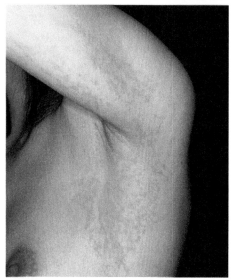

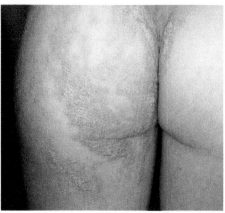

Fig. 20.17-1 Verrucous epidermal nevus.

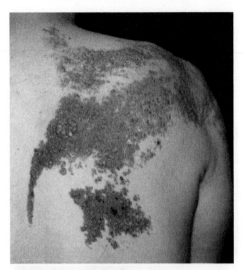

Fig. 20.17-2 Verrucous epidermal nevus.

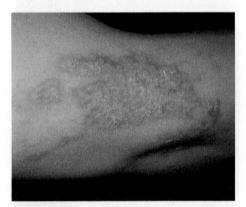

Fig. 20.18 Inflammatory linear verrucous epidermal nevus.

syringocystadenoma papilliferum, trichoblastoma, outer root sheath tumor (see Chapter 21)) and basal cell carcinomas may occur secondarily.

Pathology
In the early stage, mild acanthosis and proliferation of premature pilosebaceous tissues are seen. As the elevation increases, maturation of the pilosebaceous tissues, papilloma-like proliferation of the epidermis, ectopic proliferation of the apocrine glands and abnormality of dermal connective tissue occur. In the late stage, additional epithelial tumorous proliferation in the follicular and sweat gland tissues occurs (Fig. 20.20).

Treatment and prognosis
Surgical excision is conducted when secondary tumor is suspected or there are cosmetic concerns. The occurrence rate of malignant tumors in life is thought to be 5% or lower.

Supernumerary nipple, accessory mammary tissue
Supernumerary nipple is a condition in which more than one pair of primordia remains. The primordia of the mammary glands, which exist along the milk line from the axillary fossae, normally disappear except for one pair on the chest. A brown patch or a palpable nodule about 30% of the size of the primary mammary papilla appears on the axillary fossae or directly under the breast in most cases. Supernumerary nipples are seen in about 2% of men and women, and the chances of finding them in women are high. Swelling, pain, and galactopoiesis may occur during pregnancy. Breast cancer may occur in rare cases.

Nevus comedonicus
Dilated hair follicles with a black keratin plug aggregate or form a cord-like pattern (Fig. 20.21). They often occur between the time of birth and age 10. The face, neck, precordial region, abdomen, and scalp are frequently affected.

Eccrine nevus
Congenital localized hamartoma occurs in the eccrine sweat glands. A hyperhidrotic nodule and a plaque form. When accompanied by angioma, it is called eccrine angiomatous hamartoma, and it most frequently occurs on the extremities.

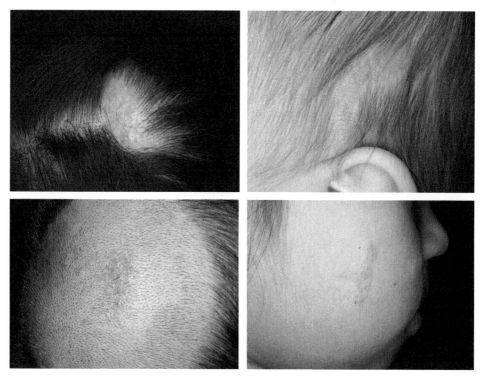

Fig. 20.19 Nevus sebaceous. Nevus sebaceous and hair loss on the scalp.

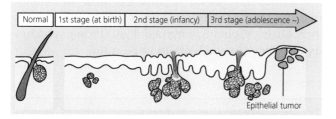

Fig. 20.20 Histopathology of nevus sebaceous classified into three stages. The pathological and clinical features of the sebaceous glands gradually change with age. Normal first stage (at birth), second stage (infancy), third stage (adolescence onward) epithelial tumor (trichoblastoma, basal cell carcinoma and the like).

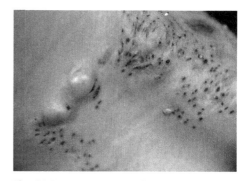

Fig. 20.21 Nevus comedonicus.

Apocrine nevus

A proliferation of apocrine glands often accompanies sebaceous nevus; however, there is a hamartoma called apocrine nevus, in which only the proliferation of apocrine sweat glands is seen. Papules and small nodules occur in the scalp or axillary fossae.

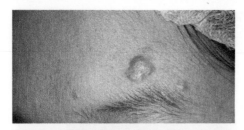

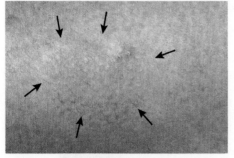

Fig. 20.22 Connective tissue nevus.

Mesenchymal cell nevi

Connective tissue nevus

Proliferation of collagen fibers, elastic fibers or muco-polysaccharides results in slightly elevated plaques or nodules of normal skin color mainly on the trunk (Fig. 20.22). Connective tissue nevus often occurs secondarily to various underlying primary disorders (Table 20.1).

Nevus lipomatosus cutaneous superficialis

Ectopic proliferation of fat cells in the dermis results in soft yellow nodules of several centimeters in diameter (Fig. 20.23). They are present at birth in some cases; other cases occur later in life.

Cartilage nevus

Dome-shaped, cartilage-containing papules of normal skin color appear. Cartilage nevus in the ear region, called accessory ear or ear tag, accompanies embryonic developmental failure of the branchial arch.

Smooth muscle hamartoma (synonym: nevus leiomyomatosus)

This is a hamartoma in the arrector pili (Fig. 20.24). The lumbar and sacral regions are most commonly involved. The onset in most cases is within 6 months after birth. Vaguely margined light brown patches appear. They may be hairy in some cases.

Table 20.1 Underlying diseases of connective tissue nevus.

Increase in...	Disorder	Most common site	Feature
Collagen fibers	Tuberous sclerosis	Lumbar region, buttocks and back sacral region	Shagreen patch
	Multiple endocrine neoplasia type 1	Neck, upper back	This disease is suspected when multiple lesions are present.
	Proteus syndrome	Palm	Hands and feet are larger than normal. Body growth is unbalanced and abnormal
	Familial cutaneous collagenoma	Back	Very rare. Increases in adolescence and later
Elastic fibers	Buschke–Ollendorf syndrome	Abdominal area	Multiple firm flat nodules appear and coalesce.
Mucopolysaccharides	Hunter syndrome	Extremities, chest	Multiple slightly firm papules occur.

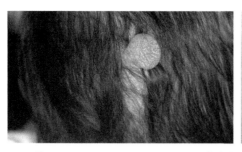
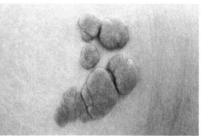

Fig. 20.23 Nevus lipomatosus cutaneous superficialis.

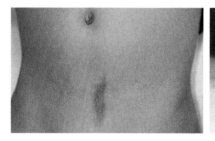
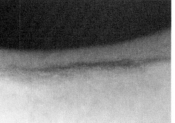
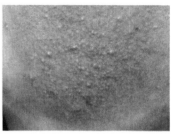

Fig. 20.24 Smooth muscle hamartoma.

Other nevi accompanied by skin pigmentation

Café au lait spot (macule)

Café au lait spots are clearly marginated macules of 0.5–10 cm in diameter; changes other than color are not seen (Fig. 20.25). Café au lait spots are present at birth and become distinct by the age of 2–3 years. Single lesions are seen in about 10% of men and women. Histopathologically, proliferation of melanocytic nevus cells is not present, but there is an increase in melanin granules in the basal layer. When multiple café au lait spots are found, neurofibromatosis type 1 or McCune–Albright syndrome is suspected. Concealing cosmetics and laser therapy are useful.

Nevus spilus

In Asia, particularly in Japan, the term is often used for café au lait spots without underlying disorder (see Fig. 20.25). Dispersed small nevus cell nevi in light brown macules are called nevus spilus or specked lentiginous nevus (Fig. 20.26).

Becker's nevus (synonym: nevus spilus tardivus)

Irregularly shaped, patchy light brown pigmentation first appears. It coalesces with newly produced macules at the periphery and enlarges to a diameter of several

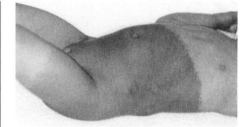
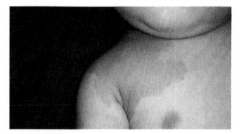

Fig. 20.25 Café au lait spot.

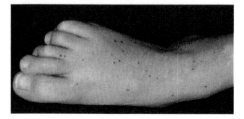

Fig. 20.26 Nevus spilus, speckled lentiginous nevus.

MEMO 20–3 McCune–Albright syndrome

McCune-Albright syndrome is thought to be caused by mosaicism in cells that have *GNAS1* gene mutations. It is characterized by café au lait spots, precocious puberty and fibrous dysplasia of the bones. The café au lait spots found in this disorder have irregular shapes and are described as "coast of Maine spots."

Table 20.2 Comparison of café au lait spot and Becker's nevus.

	Café au lait spot	Becker's nevus
Onset	At birth	Around adolescence
Most common site	Whole body	Shoulders, lumbar region
Complications	Neurofibromatosis may occur.	Very rare (Becker's nevus syndrome)
Hypertrichosis	None	Uncommon
Color	Pale brown to dark brown	Darker
Size of eruption	Large and small mixed	Many are large.
Pathological findings	Increase in melanin pigments in the epidermal basal cell layer	Increase in melanin in the basal cell layer and changes in the dermis and increase of arrector pili muscle

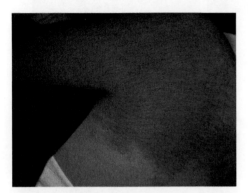

Fig. 20.27 Becker's nevus.

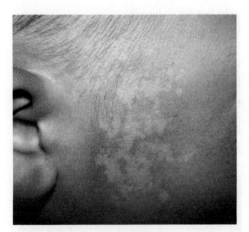

Fig. 20.28 Nevus anemicus.

centimeters to 20 cm (Fig. 20.27). Hypertrichosis often occurs several months to several years after onset. Histopathologically, Becker's nevus resembles café au lait spot; however, some regard it as a subtype of smooth muscle hamartoma, because of the proliferation of smooth muscle fibers in the dermis and the bristles in the lesion. Laser therapy is more effective than for café au lait spots (Table 20.2).

Nevus anemicus

A sharply circumscribed white patch occurs, often on the upper chest, when the skin is flushed by bathing or rubbing (Fig. 20.28). Known to be capillary dysfunction (catecholamine sensitivity), it may accompany neurofibromatosis type 1 (NF1) or nodular sclerosis.

See Chapter 16 for nevus depigmentosus.

Neurocutaneous syndromes

Neurofibromatosis type 1 (NF1) (synonym: von Recklinghausen's disease)

- Cells that originate from neural crests proliferate. Café au lait spot, neurofibroma, nervous tumor, and abnormal formation of bones are the main symptoms.

- It is caused by a mutation in the gene that produces neurofibromin. It is autosomal dominantly inherited.
- Characteristic skin lesions are multiple pigmentation (café au lait spots) at birth, and soft tumors (neurofibromas) and nevus anemicus after infancy.
- Surgical removal and laser therapy are conducted. Care should be taken in observing for any signs of malignant changes in neurofibromas.

Clinical features

Café au lait spot

Café au lait spots of various sizes are seen on 95% of newborns. The spots enlarge with age (Fig. 20.29). A café au lait spot with a diameter of 1 cm or less is called an ephelides-like pigmented patch (small Recklinghausen spot), which appears in infancy and aggregates in the axillary fossae and groin (freckling).

Café au lait spot is clearly defined, with a smooth margin. Diffuse plexiform neurofibroma or pachydermatocele may develop from a large lesion.

Neurofibroma

A neurofibroma is a soft tumor of normal skin color or light brownish-pink that can occur on any site of the skin (Fig. 20.30). Neurofibromas vary in shape and texture: some are pedunculated or elevated in a dome shape, others are palpable and soft, resembling a hernia. Neurofibromas first appear between childhood and puberty, after which they gradually increase in size and number. They may increase rapidly during pregnancy and after delivery.

Valvular or hanging neurofibroma is called diffuse plexiform neurofibroma or pachydermatocele (Fig. 20.31). Restricted body movement and bleeding in the tumor tend to occur and may be life-threatening.

Nodular plexiform neurofibroma, a neurofibroma in the peripheral nerves, is a slightly palpable, spindle-shaped or string-of-beads-shaped tumor that appears on the skin over the subcutaneous nerves and is accompanied by tenderness or radiating pain. Surgical removal of the neutofibroma results in the abscission of nerves.

Other skin lesions caused by NF1

Nevus anemicus or glomus tumor (see Chapter 21) may occur in some cases of NF1. Xanthoendothelioma (see Chapter 21) may appear on the face and scalp of

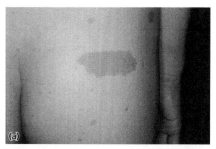

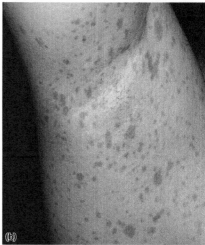

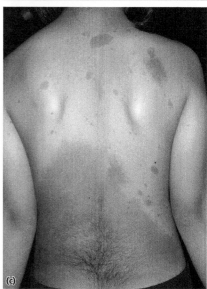

Fig. 20.29 Café au lait spot caused by NF1. a: Large café au lait spot. b: Multiple ephelides-like pigmented patches.
c: Multiple café au lait spots. A large macule may have terminal hair.

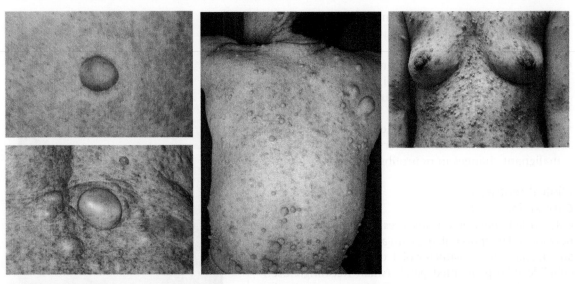

Fig. 20.30 Neurofibroma caused by NF1.

infants. Diffuse plexiform neurofibroma and neuro-fibroma in the peripheral nerves may worsen and develop into malignant peripheral nerve sheath tumor.

Other symptoms of NF1

Neurofibroma in the brain and spiral nerves, glioma, convulsive seizure, and mental retardation may occur. Abnormal formation of bones is characteristically seen in patients with NF1. Spinal deformity (e.g., scoliosis in many cases), thoracic deformity or deformity in the bones of the extremities (e.g., congenital pseudoarthrosis) and defect in the cranial bones are found. An ocular symptom of NF1 is iridic nodules, called Lisch nodules (Fig. 20.32); optic nerve glioma may occur. Pheochromocytoma and gastrointestinal tumors may occur.

Classification

Neurofibromatosis is pathologically classified into eight types: NF1 through NF8. NF1 is the most common, occurring in 1 in 3000 births. It is autosomal dominantly inherited, and half of all NF1 cases are sporadic and caused by genetic mutation. NF2 has been identified as an independent disorder. It is discussed in the next section. A small proportion of cases are thought to be caused by mosaicism, because the symptoms manifest in a segmental manner (e.g., NF5).

Pathogenesis

The causative gene is the gene that codes for neurofibromin, in chromosome 17 (17qll.2). Mutation in the gene that contains 17qll.2, which controls RAS functions, is thought to result in the cell proliferation of NF1. The rate of occurrence of NF1 in carriers of the mutant gene is complete (i.e., the penetration rate is 100%); however, the clinical manifestations vary greatly by case.

Pathology

See the section on neurofibroma (Chapter 21).

Laboratory findings and diagnosis (Table 20.3)

The likelihood of this disorder is extremely high if six or more café au lait spots exceeding 5 mm in diameter are found before puberty or if six or more café au lait spots exceeding 15 mm in diameter are found after puberty (the six-spot criterion). MRI may show unidentified bright objects, mainly in the cerebellum.

Treatment

Café au lait spots are treated by laser therapy and dermabrasion. Cosmetic concealers are also used. Neurofibromas are surgically removed in cases with cosmetic problems. When a diffuse plexiform neurofibroma is excised, there is a risk of massive perioperative hemorrhage.

Prognosis

The prognosis tends to be good. Regular follow-up for any signs of spinal disorders, malignant changes in neurofibromas, and high blood pressure should be done.

Neurofibromatosis type 2 (NF2)

A firm, elastic, sharply margined subcutaneous neurilemmoma (see Chapter 21) is the main cutaneous symptom. Café au lait spots may be found, but freckling (six or more spots) is not found. A few neurofibromas are sometimes found. Neurilemmoma on the auditory nerve (schwannoma of the vestibule nerve) and multiple tumors on the central nerve (e.g., meningioma and neurilemmoma in the spinal nerve) are the main symptoms of neurofibromatosis type 2.

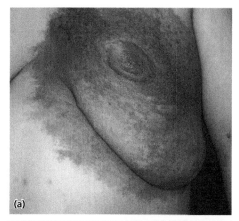

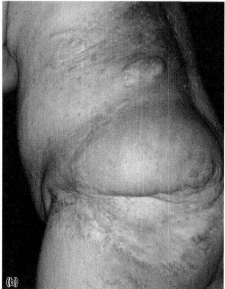

Fig. 20.31 Diffuse plexiform neurofibroma, pachydermatocele. a: Affected breast. **b:** Side of the body. The lesion has been partially removed by excision and suturing.

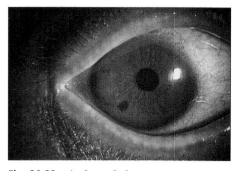

Fig. 20.32 Lisch nodule.

Table 20.3 Diagnostic criteria of neurofibromatosis type 1.

1 Major symptoms
1) Café au lait spot Macules are flat and in various colors, from the pale brown of milky coffee to dark brown. Each macule is of a single color. The macules are often oval. The edge of the macule is roundish and smooth. 2) Neurofibroma Multiple neurofibromas occur on the whole body around adolescence. Nodular plexiform neurofibroma in the peripheral nerves and diffuse plexiform neurofibroma may occur.
2 Other symptoms
a) Bone changes: deformities in the spine, thorax and extremities, defects in the cranial and facial bones b) Ocular symptoms: Lisch nodule, optic nerve glioma c) Cutaneous symptoms: ephelides-like pigmented patches, hairy brown-blue macules, nevus anemicus, juvenile xanthogranuloma d) Brain and spinal tumors: neurofibroma of the brain and spinal nerves, meningioma, nerve glioma e) Abnormal electroencephalogram f) Chromaffinoma g) Malignant neurilemmoma
3 Diagnostic points
Diagnosis is correct if café au lait spots and neurofibroma are found. A child (pretumorous stage) with six or more café au lait spots each 1.5 cm or greater in diameter is suspected of this disorder. Diagnosis is done based on other symptoms and the family history. However, a child may often have normal parents. Adult cases often have unclear café au lait spots. The diagnosis is done mainly based on the neurofibroma.

Partly adapted from the website of the Japan Intractable Diseases Information Center: www.nanbyou.or.jp/.

The first signs of this disorder are hearing loss or disequilibrium in puberty. Quadriplegia is induced by enlargement of the tumor. Ocular symptoms include juvenile cataract.

Pathogenesis and epidemiology

Neurofibromatosis 2 is autosomal dominantly inherited. It occurs in 1 in 40,000 persons. About half of the cases are sporadic. The causative gene is the NF2 gene on chromosome 22 (22q12), which codes for a protein called merlin (moesin-ezrin-radxin-like protein), whose structure is similar to that of cytoskeletal proteins. The normal form of the gene is thought to inhibit tumor formation; however, the mechanism is unknown.

Treatment and prognosis

Total resection of the neurotumor is the basic treatment. Removal may impair hearing. Because tumors enlarge unexpectedly, it is difficult to determine the policy of treatment considering the prognosis for cases with NF2. NF2 has a worse prognosis than NF1.

Tuberous sclerosis complex (synonyms: Bourneville disease, Bourneville–Pringle disease)

- The main symptoms are multiple facial angiofibromas, mental retardation, and epilepsy.
- It is autosomal dominantly inherited. The causative genes are *TSC1* and *TSC2*.
- It is characterized by white leaf-shaped macules in infancy and multiple papules (angiofibroma) that occur around the nose in and after early childhood. Shagreen patch and Koenen's tumor are also important findings.
- Care should be taken for any signs of lymphangioleiomyomatosis of the lung, angiomyolipoma of the kidney, and rhabdomyoma of the heart.

Clinical features

Facial angiofibroma

Multiple firm papules of normal skin color or light pink and 10 cm or less in diameter appear around age 2 in about 90% of cases. The papules appear symmetrically on the nasolabial sulcus, the cheeks and the area around the nose (Fig. 20.33). In puberty, the eruptions rapidly increase and coalesce to take on a tumorous or plaque-like appearance. The eruptions stop increasing in adulthood. The eruptions are of high specificity, although similar eruptions may occur in multiple endocrine neoplasia type 1.

Shagreen patch

Shagreen refers to leather with dimples like sharkskin. Shagreen patch is a connective tissue nevus caused by increases in collagen fibers (see Table 20.1). Firm, flatly elevated lesions of about 1–10 cm in diameter occur, mainly on the lumbar region and buttocks, coalescing in an arabesque pattern. These are found in about 50% of the cases, and they often become marked after puberty.

White leaf-shaped macules, hypomelanotic macules

White leaf-shaped macules are oblong nevus depigmentosus (see Chapter 16) of less than 3 cm in diameter caused by reduced production of melanin, appearing most frequently on the trunk and lower legs. They are seen in about half of all cases with tuberous sclerosis. The onset is usually infancy, and

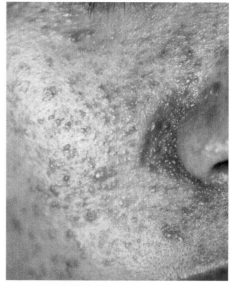

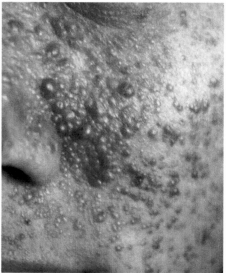

Fig. 20.33 Tuberous sclerosis.
Angiofibroma on the face.

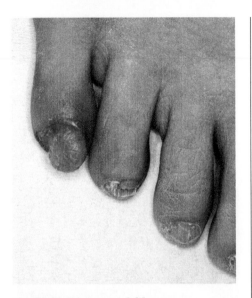

Fig. 20.34 Periungual fibroma, Koenen's tumor.

prompt discovery is important. Wood's lamp is helpful for observation. The lesions tend to disappear with age.

Periungual fibroma, Koenen's tumor

Fibrokeratoma (see Chapter 21) appears at the edge of the nail plate. It rarely appears under the nail plate (Fig. 20.34). Small spindle-shaped hyperkeratotic nodules of 2–10 mm in diameter and of light pink to brown appear. Periungual fibroma occurs on the toes of 90% of adult tuberous sclerosis patients.

Central nervous symptoms

Epilepsy and mental retardation are the main central nervous symptoms. Central nervous symptoms are seen in about 80% of patients with tuberous sclerosis within 1 year after birth.

Other symptoms of tuberous sclerosis

Translucent tumor (astrocytic hamartoma) in the retina accompanied by visual field defect may occur. Lymphangioleiomyomatosis (LAM) of the lung may be caused in rare cases. Rhabdomyoma occurs in the heart of about half of all infant patients. Angiomyolipoma (AML), renal failure from hydronephrosis, and renal cyst occur.

Pathogenesis

The genes responsible for tuberous sclerosis are *TSC1* (tuberous sclerosis complex 1) on chromosome 9 (9q34) and *TSC2* on chromosome 16 (16p13.3). Both are thought to play a role in tumor suppression. Although tuberous sclerosis is autosomal dominantly inherited, about two-thirds of all cases are sporadic.

Laboratory findings

Nodule-like calcium deposition on the lateral ventricular walls and basal nuclei (subependymal giant cell astrocytoma) and enlargement of the lateral ventricle are found by head CT scan. A nodule-like tumor is observed by MRI in the cerebral cortex.

Treatment and prognosis

Dermabrasion, excision, cryotherapy, and laser therapy are conducted on the cutaneous lesions for cosmetic reasons, which nevertheless tend to recur. Antiepileptic drugs are useful for convulsive seizures. The prognosis depends on the severity of the cerebral tumorous, heart, and renal lesions.

Peutz–Jeghers syndrome

- Mutation in the *LKB1* gene is responsible for Peutz–Jeghers syndrome. It is autosomal dominantly inherited.
- It is characterized by pigmentation on the lips, oral mucosa, and distal extremities, and by gastrointestinal polyposis.
- Intussusception may develop as a result of gastrointestinal polyps. Careful observation is required, because gastrointestinal cancer may occur.

Clinical features
Skin pigmentation
Flat, sharply margined, blackish-brown macules of 2–10 mm diameter occur symmetrically on the lips, oral mucosa, palms, and soles (distal extremities in particular) (Fig. 20.35). The disorder is asymptomatic. The longitudinal axis of the macule runs parallel to the dermatoglyphic lines. Dermoscopic findings show that pigmentation is darkest in the crista cutis (parallel ridge pattern). The pigmentation appears between birth and infancy and tends to exacerbate with age.

The lesions in the fingers and toes tend to fade in adulthood.

Gastrointestinal polyposis
Gastrointestinal polyposis may occur in any part of the gastrointestinal tract other than the esophagus, especially in the jejunum. A single lesion or more than ten lesions may be produced. They tend to cause intussusception leading to intense abdominal pain and melena. Most cases of gastrointestinal polyposis are histopathologically hamartomas; the tissue structure of the lesion is normal and the rate of occurrence of malignant tumors is lower than those for other types of gastrointestinal polyposis (Table 20.4).

Pathogenesis
Peutz–Jeghers syndrome is autosomal dominantly inherited; however, about half of all cases occur

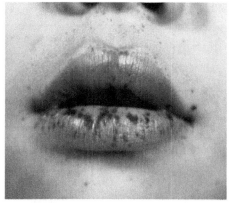
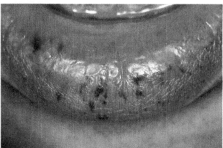
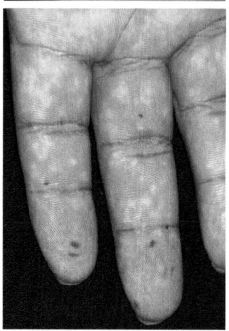

Fig. 20.35 Peutz–Jeghers syndrome.
Pigmentation occurred on the lips and hand.

Table 20.4 Major cutaneous symptoms accompanying gastrointestinal polyposis.

Disease	Inheritance pattern	Sites of polyp formation	Skin symptoms
Peutz–Jeghers syndrome	Autosomal dominant	The entire digestive tract (excluding the esophagus)	Pigmented macules on the lips, oral mucosa and palms
Cronkhite–Canada syndrome	Not inherited	Mainly the stomach and large intestine	Alopecia, nail plate abnormality, pigmented macules on the dorsum of the hands
Gardner syndrome	Autosomal dominant	Large intestine in most cases	Multiple epidermal cysts, fibromas, osteomas, dental dysplasia
Turcot syndrome	Autosomal recessive	Large intestine	Café au lait spot, multiple lipomas
Cowden syndrome	Autosomal dominant	The entire digestive tract (including the esophagus)	Hyperkeratotic papules on the face and extremities, papilloma in the oral mucosa

MEMO 20-4 Laugier–Hunziker–Barans syndrome

Pigmentation resembling that in Peutz–Jeghers syndrome appears on the distal extremities and lips; however, gastrointestinal polyposis is not found.

sporadically. It is caused by mutation in the LKB1 gene on chromosome 19 (19p13.3). The LKB1 gene codes for serine-threonine kinase 11 and is thought to be a tumor suppressor gene.

Pathology

Melanocytes and melanin pigment increase in the epidermal basal layer. There is hyperpigmentation in the crista profunda intermedia, which is the thick portion of the epidermis. The cutaneous lesions do not show malignancy.

Differential diagnosis

As with Peutz–Jeghers syndrome, Cronkhite–Canada syndrome is characterized by gastrointestinal polyposis and pigmentation. However, the onset of Cronkhite–Canada syndrome is middle age or later. Alopecia, hypopigmented patches, and abnormality of the nail plate also occur in Cronkhite–Canada syndrome. The macules are vaguely marginated; histopathologically, proliferation of melanocytes is not found in Cronkhite–Canada syndrome.

Treatment and prognosis

Laser therapy, dermabrasion, and cryotherapy are effective in reducing pigmentation. Endoscopic or surgical excision is conducted on gastrointestinal polyps.

Incontinentia pigmenti (synonym: Bloch–Sulzberger syndrome)

- The skin lesions take a characteristic course, starting with blistering and erythema at birth, progressing to papules and pigmentation, and then disappearing (Figs. 20.36–20.38).
- Mutation in the *NEMO* gene causes incontinentia pigmenti. It is X-chromosome dominantly inherited; female patients greatly outnumber male patients.
- The prognosis is good. Ocular symptoms and deformity are treated.

Clinical features

Cutaneous symptoms

Incontinentia pigmenti is classified by the clinical features. The cutaneous lesions occur along the Blaschko lines (see Fig. 1.4) at any stage.

- **First stage (vesicular stage):** vesicles accompanied by erythema appear, most commonly on the trunk and extremities. The onset is at birth or within 2 weeks after birth. They become pustular or erosive, persisting for several days to several months before healing gradually. Eruptions may recur (see Fig. 20.36).
- **Second stage (verrucous stage):** multiple hyperkeratotic verrucous papules occur, mainly on the distal extremities. The symptoms of the second stage occur after the blisters of the first stage subside, or right after the first stage. Some lesions on the dorsal hands may be found at birth. Most cases resolve in several months, but some persist until adulthood (see Fig. 20.37).
- **Third stage (hyperpigmented stage):** grayish-brown or purplish-brown pigmentation occurs at sites where the first- and second-stage eruptions were. The hyperpigmentation may be the only cutaneous symptom. The lesions become distinct about 6 months after birth. The pigmentation often appears as a whorl or a marbled pattern (see Fig. 20.38).
- **Fourth stage (regression stage):** the pigmentation begins to disappear at age 4 or 5, disappearing completely at puberty in most cases. Pigmentation may persist in adulthood in some cases. About half of all cases heal with mild depigmented scarring.
- **Other symptoms:** eruptions result in alopecia cicatricans on the scalp in about 25% of cases (see Fig. 20.37a). Deformity of the nails, including the ridges, and frizzled hair may occur.

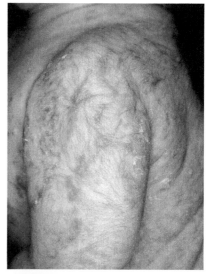

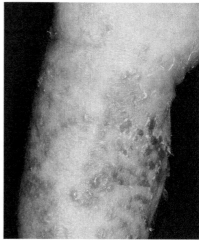

Fig. 20.36-1 Incontinentia pigmenti at the vesicular stage.

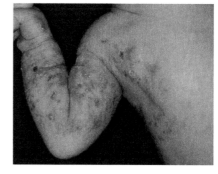

Fig. 20.36-2 Incontinentia pigmenti at the vesicular stage.

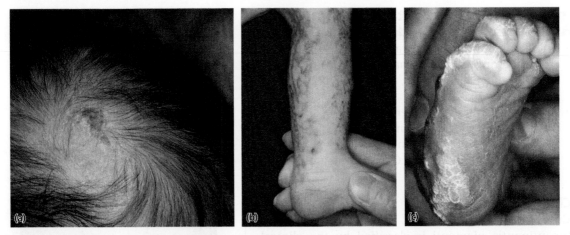

Fig. 20.37 Incontinentia pigmenti at the verrucous stage. a: Eruptions on the scalp. Alopecia also occurred. b: Reticular pigmentation. c: Verrucous eruptions accompanied by severe hyperkeratosis, which resembles verrucous epidermal nevus.

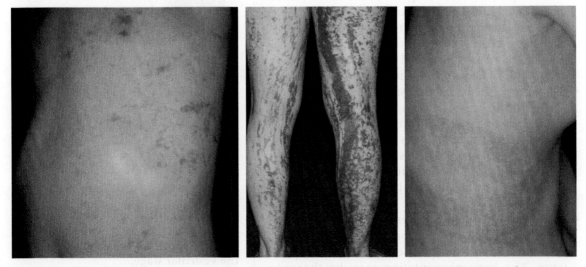

Fig. 20.38 Incontinentia pigmenti at the pigmented stage. Pigmentation appears in various degrees.

MEMO 20–5 Hypomelanosis of Ito

Partially hypopigmented macules (nevus depigmentosus; see Chapter 16) appear on the trunk around 2 years after birth. The lesions distribute along the Blaschko lines. They generally appear asymmetrically and in two or more parts of the body. Systemic symptoms resembling those found in incontinentia pigmenti occur, such as epilepsy, mental retardation and abnormality in dental formation; however, hypomelanosis of Ito is an independent disease with unknown causative genes.

Systemic symptoms

Ocular symptoms occur unilaterally in about 30% of the cases. Strabismus, cataract, optic nerve atrophy, retinal detachment, and blindness may occur. Central nervous symptoms, including epilepsy, mental retardation, microcephaly, and hydrocephalia, may be caused. Odontogenesis imperfecta and abnormal formation of bones (e.g., hyperdactylia) may occur.

Pathogenesis and epidemiology

Incontinentia pigmenti is caused by a mutation in *NEMO* (NF-κB essential modulator). NF-κB is a protein that is involved in inflammatory reactions and apoptosis. Many aspects of the onset mechanism of incontinentia pigmenti are unknown. It is X-linked dominantly inherited. More than 95% of all patients are females. Most male fetuses with the genetic abnormality are not carried to term; however, some may be born with Klinefelter syndrome (XXY) or mosaicism.

Pathology and laboratory findings

There is marked eosinophilic infiltration in the intraepidermal blisters in the first stage (Fig. 20.39). Elevated levels of eosinophils are seen in the peripheral blood. Verrucous papules in the second stage are histopathologically similar to epidermal nevus. Melanophages are observed in large numbers in the upper dermal layer of pigmentation at the third stage (histological pigmentary incontinence). In the fourth stage, melanophages decrease.

Diagnosis and treatment

The condition is sometimes misdiagnosed as epidermolysis bullosa because of the blistering at birth. As the skin lesion heals spontaneously in many cases, symptomatic therapy may be performed if necessary. Early detection is important for the ocular and central nervous symptoms and for the abnormal bone formation. About half of all girls whose mothers have incontinentia pigmenti also have the disease.

Sturge–Weber syndrome

- Sturge–Weber syndrome is a non-hereditary disorder in which capillary malformation in the facial skin, choroid or leptomeninges (i.e., the arachnoid and leptomeninx) occurs.

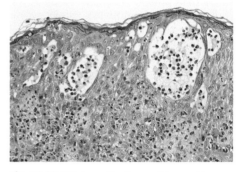

Fig. 20.39 Histopathology of incontinentia pigmenti. First (vesicular) stage. Eosinophilic infiltration in the epidermis is characteristically seen.

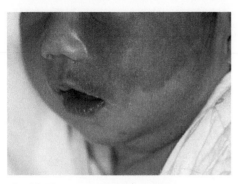

Fig. 20.40 Sturge–Weber syndrome.

MEMO 20–6 Toxic erythema of the newborn, erythema toxicum neonatorum

Toxic erythema of the newborn occurs in about half of all healthy newborns. Dispersed or multiple erythematous lesions or pustules of 1–2 mm in diameter occur. Histopathologically, there is marked eosinophilic infiltration in the epidermis and the upper dermal layer. The lesions spontaneously disappear in several days to several weeks.

- Malformation of capillary blood vessels (hemangioma simplex) occurs in the areas of the face over the first and second divisions of the trigeminal nerve.
- Glaucoma is caused by hemangioma, leading to buphthalmia.

Clinical features

Sturge–Weber syndrome is characterized by capillary malformation in the face, ocular lesions and cerebral nervous symptoms; however, most cases are incomplete, with only facial and cerebral nervous symptoms.

- **Cutaneous symptoms:** capillary malformation (hemangioma simplex, port-wine stain (see Chapter 21)) is seen as erythema at birth. The lesions distribute over the trigeminal nerve of the face. In most cases, the lesions are found over the first or second division of the nerve (Fig. 20.40). The symptoms are unilateral or bilateral. Cutaneous symptoms are seen in 95% or more of cases.
- **Central nervous symptoms:** ictus epilepticus appears in infancy in about 80% of cases. Leptomeningeal angiomatosis occurs on the side with semi-facial angioma, especially on the occipital lobe. Contralateral hemiplegia, atrophy of the cerebral hemisphere, and mental retardation may occur in some cases.
- **Ocular symptoms:** capillary malformation in the choroid occurs on the side with semi-facial angioma, especially in cases with angioma on the eyelid. High fluid pressure is present in the eyes (glaucoma) and the corneal diameter enlarges accordingly, leading to a condition called buphthalmia. The result is blindness in some cases.

The onset of Sturge–Weber syndrome is often in infancy; however, it is sometimes found at birth or in adulthood.

Pathogenesis

Abnormal formation of blood vessels caused by embryonic impairment of the sympathetic nerve is thought to cause Sturge–Weber syndrome; however, the details are unknown. It is congenital; nevertheless, it is known to be non-hereditary in general. It occurs in about 1 in 50,000 people.

Laboratory findings

The double-contoured calcification observed along the cerebral convolution by skull X-ray is called tramline calcification. Head CT scan and MRI are useful for early diagnosis.

Treatment

Laser therapy is performed on cutaneous lesions. When drug therapy is ineffective on convulsive seizures, resection of the brain hemangioma is conducted. For ocular symptoms, early diagnosis and adjustment of ocular pressure are important.

Klippel–Trenaunay–Weber syndrome (synonyms: Klippel–Trenaunay syndrome, Klippel–Weber syndrome)

- Malformation of blood vessels in the extremities and enlargement and extension of the affected limb are observed.
- Spinal curvature is caused by the different length of the extremities, and there is the risk of ulceration and heart failure caused by arteriovenous fistula.
- Symptomatic therapy is the main treatment.

Clinical features and pathogenesis

The cause of Klippel–Trenaunay–Weber syndrome is unknown; however, angiogenesis factor AGGF1 may be involved. Capillary malformation in the skin is present at birth in many cases. Usually only one arm or leg is involved, but sometimes both are involved. It may spread beyond the extremities (Fig. 20.41). Malformation of lymphatic vessels and veins (cavernous angioma, phlebeurysm) also occurs, and edemas and ulceration secondarily occur. The symptoms of Klippel–Trenaunay–Weber syndrome are found at birth or during infancy, and they become distinct with age. Congenital arteriovenous fistula may accompany this disorder (Parkes–Weber syndrome). In Klippel–Trenaunay–Weber syndrome, enlargement and overgrowth of the bone and soft tissue occur, and the extremities may become different in length, with that difference increasing with age. The bone abnormality usually occurs in the leg on the same side of the body as the skin lesion or, rarely, on the opposing side. The different length of the legs results in claudication and compensatory scoliosis. Angioma in internal

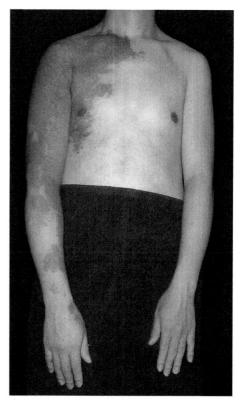

Fig. 20.41 Klippel–Trenaunay–Weber syndrome. The right arm, which is affected by hemangioma, is longer than the left arm.

organs, syndactylism or other dysplasia of fingers and toes, and heart failure may occur.

Severe clotting abnormality (Kasabach–Merritt syndrome; see Chapter 21) may occur in some cases.

Diagnosis and treatment

Diagnosis can be confirmed by the characteristic clinical features, bone radiography, and systemic CT scan. Arteriovenous fistula is examined by thermography, blood gas analysis, and angiography. Symptomatic therapy is the main treatment. Laser therapy is considered for the cutaneous lesions. Ligation or other surgical therapies are performed on arteriovenous fistulae, because they may cause heart failure. To prevent arthropathy and curvature caused by the different lengths of the extremities, orthopedic shoes and osteotomy are helpful.

Neurocutaneous melanosis
Clinical features

Neurocutaneous melanosis is non-familial and occurs in both men and women. Large congenital melanocytic nevus is present on nearly half the trunk (Fig. 20.42) or multiple congenital small- to medium-sized nevus cell nevi disperse over the whole body. These nevi can be a serious cosmetic burden.

Cerebral nervous symptoms such as increased intracranial pressure and secondary hydrocephalia occur. These tend to be accompanied by headache, vomiting, epileptic seizure, and mental retardation. Malignant melanoma often develops on the site of the body with congenital giant melanocytic nevus and leptomeninx.

Pathogenesis

Neurocutaneous melanosis is caused by proliferation of melanoblasts that originate from neural crests in the skin and central nervous system (e.g., leptomeninx).

Treatment

Giant pigmented nevus is removed as completely as possible. The sooner curettage is performed after birth, the better is the result cosmetically. Symptomatic therapies, such as shunting for hydrocephalia and antiepilepsy drugs, are useful for the central nervous symptoms.

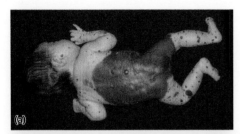
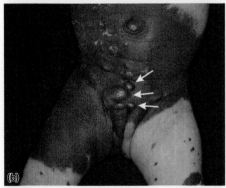

Fig. 20.42-1 Neurocutaneous melanosis. a: On the whole body. b: It is often accompanied by nodules (arrows).

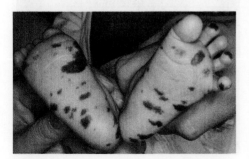

Fig. 20.42-2 Neurocutaneous melanosis. Multiple nevus cell nevi of small to medium sizes occur.

LEOPARD syndrome (synonym: lentiginosis profusa syndrome)

Multiple lentigines appear on the whole body, and abnormal electrocardiogram (e.g., bundle branch block), ocular hypertelorism, maldevelopment of reproductive organs (e.g., cryptorchidism, monorchid, absence of one ovary), short stature, perceptive deafness, and mental retardation occur (MEMO, see Chapter 20). LEOPARD syndrome is caused by mutations in the PTPN11 gene. Relatively small lentigines of 15 mm or less in diameter are distributed all over the body and on the oral mucosa and bulbar conjunctiva at birth (Fig. 20.43). Café au lait spots, leukodermas, and nail malformation also occur. Heart lesion (hypertrophic cardiomyopathy) affects the prognosis most severely.

Nevoid basal cell carcinoma syndrome (synonym: basal cell nevus syndrome)

Nevoid basal cell carcinoma syndrome (NBCCS) is autosomal dominantly inherited, caused by mutations in the *PTCH* gene, a tumor suppressor gene. Small depressions in the palms and soles (corneum-deficient patches of 2–3 mm) occur at infancy and gradually increase, accompanied by multiple basal cell carcinoma (Fig. 20.44). Basal cell carcinoma may occur systemically as dark brown macules and nodules in puberty. Various epithelial cysts, such as epidermal cysts and milia, occur. Multiple cysts of the jaw (odontogenic keratocysts), ocular hypertelorism and central nervous symptoms (e.g., calcification of cerebral falx, medulloblastoma) occur as complications. When basal cell carcinoma is seen in young patients, NBCCS is suspected.

Phacomatosis pigmentovascularis

This is a comorbid disease of capillary malformation in the skin and epidermal/melanocytic nevus (Fig. 20.45). It is known to be non-hereditary. Phacomatosis

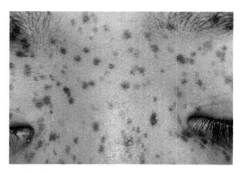

Fig. 20.43 **LEOPARD syndrome.**

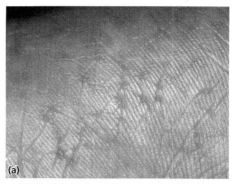

(a)

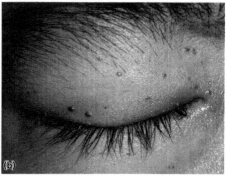

(b)

Fig. 20.44 **Nevoid basal cell carcinoma syndrome.** a: Small concavities (pitting) in the palm. b: Multiple basal cell carcinomas on the eyelid.

MEMO 20–7 LEOPARD syndrome: origin of the term

LEOPARD is an acronym for the following systemic symptoms: L (multiple lentigines), E (electrocardiographic conduction defects), O (ocular hypertelorism), P (pulmonary stenosis), A (abnormalities of genitalia), R (retardation of growth), D (sensorineural deafness).

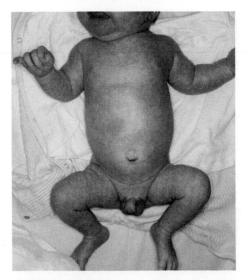

Fig. 20.45 Phacomatosis pigmentovascularis.

pigmentovascularis is classified into four types, depending on the accompanying nevus, and subclassified into type a, which only has cutaneous symptoms, and type b, which has musculoskeletal and ocular symptoms. The four types of accompanying nevi are verrucous epidermal nevus or verrucous nevus cell nevus (type I), dermal melanocytosis (type II), nevus spilus (speckled lentiginous nevus; type III), and dermal melanocytosis and nevus spilus (type IV). Type IIb phacomatosis pigmentovascularis accounts for about 50% of all cases. Sturge–Weber syndrome and Klippel–Trenaunay–Weber syndrome may accompany some cases of phacomatosis pigmentovascularis.

Hereditary hemorrhagic telangiectasia (synonyms: Osler–Rendu–Weber syndrome, Osler's disease)

Osler–Rendu–Weber syndrome is an autosomal dominant inherited disorder in which telangiectasia in the arteriovenous anastomotic region occurs. This disorder is caused by mutations in the TGF-β receptor gene (*ENG, ACVRL1*), which is involved in angiogenesis. Multiple rose pink papules and telangiectasia occur, mainly on the upper part of the

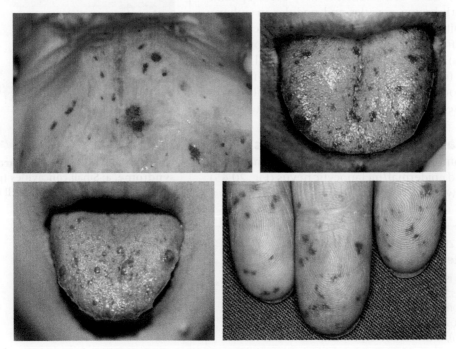

Fig. 20.46 Hereditary hemorrhagic telangiectasia.

body, including the face, lips and tongue, from infancy to after puberty (Fig. 20.46 and Fig. 20.47). The most common first symptom is epitaxis, which recurs; this has diagnostic value. Broken pulmonary arteriovenous fistula may result in hemoptysis, hematothorax, gastrointestinal hemorrhage, and hepatic cirrhosis.

Blue rubber bleb nevus syndrome

In blue rubber bleb nevus syndrome, which is a rare autosomal dominantly inherited disease, malformation of veins (cavernous angioma) occurs in various organs (especially in the skin and digestive tract). The cutaneous symptoms are vaguely marginated blue macules and rubber ball-like dark blue tumors that occur anywhere on the body (Fig. 20.48). The lesions vary in size from several millimeters to 10 cm in diameter. They appear from soon after birth to early childhood, increasing in size with age. Bone deformity may occur secondarily. Malformation of blood vessels in the digestive tract may occur at any site of the organs, including the oral cavity and tongue. The small intestine tends to be most commonly affected, with bleeding that leads to iron-deficiency anemia, intussusception or death from blood loss. Blood vessel malformation may be found in the liver, brain, skeletal muscles or kidneys.

Maffucci syndrome

Malformation of the vascular system of the skin and internal organs and enchondromas occur because the disorder is a congenital mesodermal hypoplasia. Most of the cutaneous lesions are from venous malformation (cavernous angioma), but some are from capillary and lymphatic malformation. Enchondromas are often

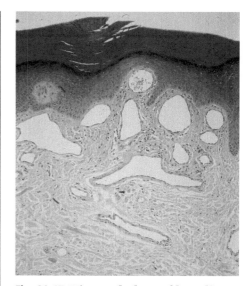

Fig. 20.47 Histopathology of hereditary hemorrhagic telangiectasia.

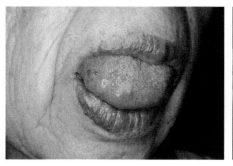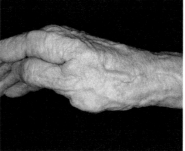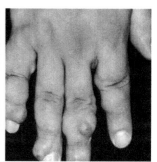

Fig. 20.48 Blue rubber bleb nevus syndrome.

found in the extremities, particularly in the legs, and the lesions are found as subcutaneous nodules. Broken bones in the legs may result in differences in the length of the legs. The disease stops progressing after adolescence; however, chondorosarcomas are found in 30% of cases.

Dyskeratosis congenita (synonym: Zinsser–Cole–Engman syndrome)

The main symptoms are cutaneous reticulated pigmentation, deformity of the nail plates, and oral leukoplakia-like changes. Inheritance of dyskeratosis congenita can be autosomal dominant, autosomal recessive or X-linked. The onset is from early childhood to puberty. Reticular pigmentation on the neck region occurs first. The lesion then spreads to the trunk and extremities, resulting in poikiloderma. Atrophy in the nail plate also occurs. Oral leukoplakia-like change appears most frequently on the tongue, buccal mucosa and genitalia, sometimes becoming malignant. Abnormality in other organs, such as aplastic anemia and pulmonary fibrosis, may occur.

Cutis marmorata telangiectasia congenita

Livedo (Fig. 20.49) appears at birth or shortly thereafter. It often occurs in the legs and may accompany capillary and other venous malformation. The typical skin pigmentation disappears with age, and most cases resolve within 2 years after birth. Although it usually occurs sporadically, there are rare familial cases. Careful examination is necessary, because deformity occurs in the central nervous system, heart, blood vessels, muscles, skeleton, and eyes.

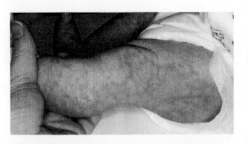

Fig. 20.49 Cutis marmorata telangiectatica congenita.

CHAPTER 21

Benign skin tumors

Skin tumors are examined to determine not only malignancy or benignancy but also the skin component from which the tumor derives. A tumor may originate from keratinocytes, from cells of appendages such as those in sweat glands, or from neural crest cells or mesenchymal cells, including fibroblasts. The pathology, epidemiology, and course of tumors vary depending on the origin of the cells. This chapter classifies benign skin tumors into the subtypes below.

- Epidermal tumors
- Follicular tumors
- Sebaceous tumors
- Sweat gland tumors
- Cysts
- Neural tumors
- Hemangiomas/vascular malformations
- Fibrous tumors
- Histiocytic tumors
- Adipocellular tumors
- Myogenic tumors
- Osteogenic tumors
- Hematopoietic tumors

Tumors originating from epidermal components

Seborrheic keratosis (SK) (synonyms: verruca senilis, senile warts)

- A benign verrucous tumor voccurs most frequently on the face, head or trunk in middle age and beyond. It derives from keratinocytes in the epidermis or infundibular hair follicle.
- Elevated, sharply demarcated, grayish-brown to blackish-brown nodules 1–2 cm in diameter occur.
- Cryotherapy, laser therapy, and excision are the main treatments.
- SK that occurs rapidly in multiple, itchy lesions on the whole body is called Leser–Trélat syndrome. It may be accompanied by internal malignancy.

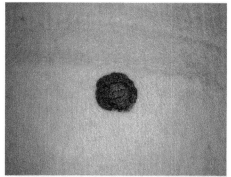
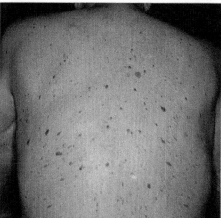

Fig. 21.1-1 Seborrheic keratosis (SK).
Multiple, flatly elevated brown or blackish-brown keratotic papules 1–2 cm in diameter on the back of an elderly man.

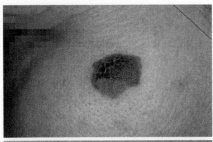

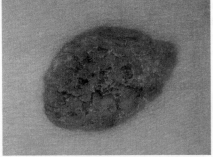

Fig. 21.1-2 Seborrheic keratosis (SK).
The skin lesion resembles clay adhered to
the skin. The surface of the lesion is
keratotic and papillary.

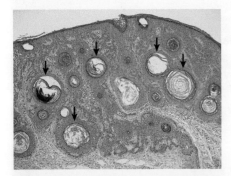

**Fig. 21.2 Histopathology of seborrheic
keratosis (SK).** Pseudo-horn cysts form
(arrows).

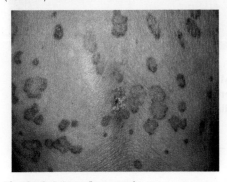

Fig. 21.3-1 Porokeratosis.

Clinical features

Seborrheic keratosis appears in people in their 20s and
is seen in nearly everyone in their 80s and older. As
the synonym "senile warts" suggests, SK is warts
caused by skin aging. Senile freckles (senile lentigo in
Chapter 16) often elevate to form SK. Flat-topped
papules 1–2 cm in diameter, varying in color from
brown to blackish-brown, occur on the face, head, and
trunk (Fig. 21.1). The palms and soles are unaffected.
The surface of the papules is keratotic and often papillary or granular, resembling clay adhered to the skin.
Itching and pain are not usually present.

Pathology

There is upward intraepidermal proliferation of basal
cells and suprabasal cells (exophytic lesion). The ratio of
proliferative cells to normal cells varies. Dysplasia is not
present, but melanin pigmentation occurs in each proliferative cell to a varying degree. Pseudo-horn cyst
formation presents as milia-like cysts on dermoscopy
(Fig. 21.2). Lichenoid inflammatory cell infiltration
called lichen planus-like keratosis is sometimes present.

Diagnosis and differential diagnosis

There are characteristic pathological and dermoscopic
findings (see Chapter 3). The disease should be differentiated from actinic keratosis, Bowen's disease, basal
cell carcinoma, squamous cell carcinoma, malignant
melanoma, keratoacanthoma, verruca plana, and
verruca vulgaris.

Treatment

Treatment is necessary only when there are cosmetic
concerns or suspected malignancy. The lesions do not
disappear spontaneously but increase in number with
age. If necessary, cryotherapy, carbon dioxide gas laser
therapy or surgical removal is conducted.

MEMO 21–1 Leser–Trélat sign

Multiple seborrheic keratoses occur, often
accompanied by itching; they spread to cover
the whole body within a few months. This sign implies
the presence of internal malignancy (stomach cancer, in
particular). Therefore, systemic investigation must be
made for such malignancies when dermatologists see
this phenomenon.

Clear cell acanthoma

A clear cell acanthoma is usually a small, solitary, elastic, firm, dome-shaped or flatly elevated tumor up to 2 cm in diameter. It generally occurs on the lower legs. It may be pedunculated, fungiform or papillomatous. The surface is smooth or granular. The color is usually rose pink, but it may be brown to blackish-brown in some cases. The pathogenesis is unknown. There is a debate over whether clear cell acanthoma is a genuine tumorous lesion or a reactive lesion that accompanies inflammation. Histopathologically, the proliferation of keratinocytes (clear cells) rich in glycogen is observed.

Warty dyskeratoma

In warty dyskeratoma, there are verrucous or flatly elevated small nodules 1–2 cm in diameter that tend to keratinize at the center. The face and head are frequently involved. The condition is largely asymptomatic. Basaloid cells proliferate histopathologically toward the dermis, directly above which cleavage or dyskeratosis appears. Warty dyskeratoma clinically resembles Darier's disease (see Chapter 15). It is surgically removed.

Porokeratosis

- Round, scattered, brown keratotic lesions with elevated rims occur on the extremities, trunk, and face.
- The disorder is asymptomatic and it progresses slowly. In rare cases, there is transformation to squamous cell carcinoma.
- Characteristic pathological features called cornoid lamellae (columns of parakeratotic cells) are observed.
- Excision and administration of oral retinoids are the main treatments.

Clinical features

An elevated keratotic eruption, round or oval in shape, occurs on the extensor surfaces of the extremities and on the trunk and face (Fig. 21.3). Atrophy occurs at the center of the lesion, which becomes slightly concave. Porokeratosis begins as a blackish-brown papule that gradually enlarges centrifugally. It is asymptomatic and progresses slowly for several years without subsiding. Large lesions may aggravate and progress to Bowen's disease or squamous cell carcinoma. Despite the disease name, the eruptions are not associated with the sweat pores. Porokeratosis is clinically divided

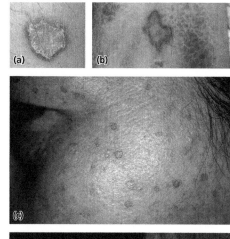
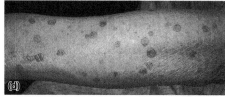
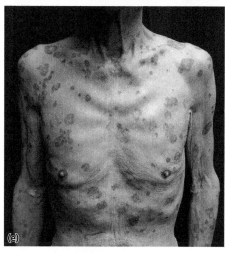

Fig. 21.3-2 Porokeratosis. a,b: Porokeratosis of Mibelli. The eruption is keratotic, with an elevated rim and a diameter of about 2 cm. c,d: Disseminated superficial actinic porokeratosis. The eruptions are slightly elevated at the edge. e: Disseminated superficial porokeratosis.

into the subtypes below. The most frequently seen type is disseminated superficial porokeratosis, which occurs on sun-exposed areas of the body.

Porokeratosis of Mibelli

The eruptions, which appear in infants, are symmetrically dispersed on the distal extremities or face. An individual eruption is typically 1–2 cm in diameter.

Disseminated superficial actinic porokeratosis (DSAP)

Multiple eruptions occur on sun-exposed areas of the body, particularly the extensor surfaces of the extremities in adult women. The multiple eruptions, which are about 1 cm in diameter, may coalesce.

Disseminated superficial porokeratosis

The symptoms resemble those of DSAP; however, eruptions occur at sites other than sun-exposed ones.

Linear porokeratosis

The onset is between birth and early infancy. The eruptions are arranged in a band-like or linear pattern.

Porokeratosis palmaris et plantaris disseminata

Small keratotic papules occur multiply on the palms and soles, spreading to the rest of the body.

Pathogenesis

Porokeratosis is induced by epidermal clones that cause localized dyskeratosis. It may be triggered by UV exposure, external injury or aging. Some cases are autosomal dominant.

Pathology

Acanthosis and hyperkeratosis are found at the periphery of porokeratosis. The rim of the lesion is elevated and there is a cornoid lamella, a column of incompletely keratinized cells. Underneath the cornoid lamella, the granular cell layer is absent (Fig. 21.4). Thinning of the epidermis is present in the concave center of the lesion.

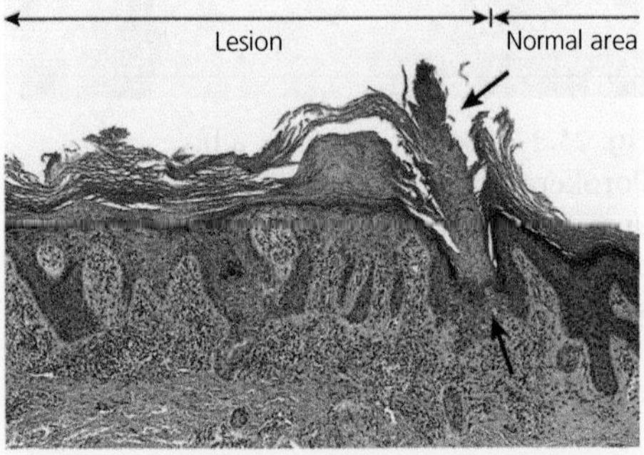

Treatment

Topical keratolytic drugs, excision, electrical coagulation, cryotherapy, dermabrasion, and retinoids are the main treatments. Porokeratosis is chronic and intractable.

Lesion   Normal area

Fig. 21.4 Histopathology of porokeratosis. The cornoid lamella (arrow) around the lesions can be observed by the naked eye as an elevated rim around the skin lesion.

Follicular tumors

Trichofolliculoma

Small, smooth-surfaced, dome-shaped nodules or papules 5–10 mm in diameter occur, most commonly in the nasal region and its peripheries (Fig. 21.5). Trichofolliculoma is characterized by small keratotic cavities with several immature woolly hairs (vellus hairs) at the center. The pathogenesis is unknown. Trichofolliculoma is considered a benign tumor in which the entire follicle – including the inner root sheath, outer root sheath, and dermal hair papilla – differentiates.

Trichoadenoma

A firm, solitary, elastic nodule 1.5 cm or less in diameter appears, most frequently on the face. It is thought to be a tumor whose morphological differentiation falls between that of trichofolliculoma and that of trichoepithelioma. The border between the normal dermis and the trichoadenoma is clear. There are multiple keratin-containing cysts and solid masses of cells in the dermis.

Trichoepithelioma

This benign tumor consists mainly of basal cell-like cells, derived from hair germs that differentiate into various hair components, such as hair papilla. Small papules 2–10 mm in diameter with normal skin color occur around the nose, eyebrows, upper lip, chin, and cheeks. The papules are firm and glossy on the surface. Trichoepithelioma is subdivided into solitary, multiple familial, and desmoplastic subtypes, the last of which shows intense fibrosis histopathologically.

Solitary trichoepithelioma

Solitary trichoepithelioma is the subtype that occurs most frequently. It is non-hereditary. Histopathologically, solitary trichoepithelioma consists of small keratin-containing cysts and basaloid cells, and there is proliferation of dermal stroma. It may be difficult to distinguish from basal cell carcinoma; however, in most cases of solitary trichoepithelioma, there are well-differentiated keratinous cysts and the formation, although incomplete, of hair follicles. In solitary trichoepithelioma, cleavage does not form between the tumor mass and dermal stroma. Foreign body granuloma and calcium deposition may be present.

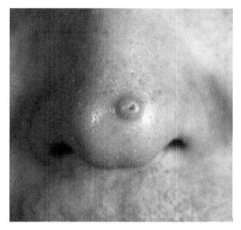

Fig. 21.5 Trichofolliculoma. There is a small keratotic concavity at the center of the lesion. Many fragile young hairs are present.

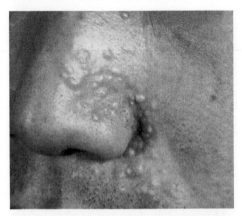

Fig. 21.6 Multiple familial trichoepithelioma. Multiple dome-shaped firm papules 2–10 mm in diameter and normal skin color occur on the face.

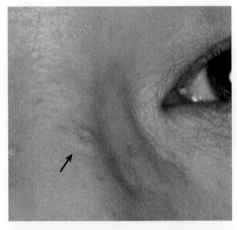

Fig. 21.7 Desmoplastic trichoepithelioma. The skin lesion is 5 mm in diameter, with an elevated rim and small surrounding circular nodules.

Multiple familial trichoepithelioma (synonym: trichoepithelioma papulosum multiplex)

Women are slightly more likely to be affected than men. This condition is autosomal dominant. Abnormality in the cylindromatosis (*CYLD1*) gene has been identified as the cause. The onset is at puberty. Multiple papules of normal skin color occur on the face, mainly around the nose (Fig. 21.6). The papules are similar to the facial angiofibroma seen in tuberous sclerosis (see Chapter 20); however, differentiation from tuberous sclerosis, in which other symptoms such as leukoderma and shagreen patch are present, is possible. Excision or laser therapy is conducted if cosmetically necessary. The tumorous lesions ted to recur.

Desmoplastic trichoepithelioma

Circular nodules or plaques several millimeters to 1 cm in diameter with normal skin color or light yellow color occur, most frequently on the cheeks, forehead, and nasal region of relatively young adult women. The lesions are characterized by elevated edges and concave centers (Fig. 21.7). Histopathologically, the cord-like proliferation of basaloid tumor cells, multiple keratinous cysts, and hyalinized collagen fibrils are present. Differentiation from basal cell carcinoma may be difficult.

Trichoblastoma

A dome-shaped nodule occurs, most frequently on the face or scalp. It consists of fibrous interstitium and tumor cells that resemble follicular germinative cells. It may arise on sebaceous nevi. Differentiation from basal cell carcinoma may be difficult. Distinction from trichoepithelioma remains controversial.

Pilomatricoma (synonyms: calcifiying epithelioma, pilomatrixoma)
Clinical features

A firm, intradermal or subcutaneous tumor 1–2 cm in diameter occurs on the face, neck or upper arm of infants, usually solitarily. The tumor surface is rough and the color is of normal skin or translucent bluish-white. It has the firmness of bone (Fig. 21.8). It may present a blistered appearance. Although it is usually asymptomatic, mild tenderness may be present. Secondary infection may make it difficult to distinguish from inflammatory epidermoid cyst.

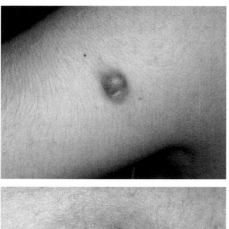

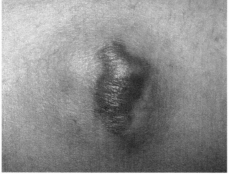

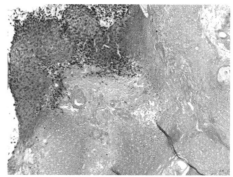

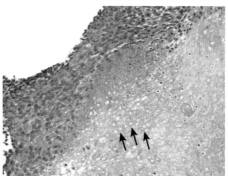

Fig. 21.8 Pilomatricoma. A subcutaneous nodule of 1–2 cm diameter with mild tenderness. Blistering and light pink eruptions may occur.

Fig. 21.9 Histopathology of pilomatricoma. Arrows indicate the shadow cells.

Myotonic dystrophy may induce pilomatricoma. Malignant formation (pilomatrix carcinoma) rarely occurs.

Pathogenesis
Pilomatricoma is a teratoma that originates from the hair follicle bulge. Some cases are caused by genetic abnormality in β-catenin.

Pathology
A sharply margined, irregularly shaped tumor mass appears in the lower dermal layer or subcutaneous tissue. The mass is not covered by a distinct membrane but is surrounded by fibrous connective tissue (Fig. 21.9). The tumor contains basaloid cells (originating from the hair matrix) and shadow cells. Shadow cells, which correspond to hair cortex cells, are enucleated cells that stain eosinophilic. Foreign body granuloma and calcification are seen.

Treatment
The treatment is surgical removal.

MEMO 21–2 Hyperplasia, adenoma, epithelioma

Benign tumors in skin appendages are classified by the degree of cellular differentiation. In order of least abnormal (most differentiated) to most abnormal (least differentiated), they are hyperplasia, adenoma, and epithelioma. When the degree of cellular differentiation is lower than that of epithelioma, the tumor is a blastoma or malignant tumor. A tumor that has components of all three germ layers (ectoderm, mesoblast, endoblast) is called a teratoma.

Trichilemmoma

A verrucous papule 3–8 mm in diameter with normal skin color to light brown color occurs, usually solitarily and most commonly on the face. When multiple papules occur, the possibility of Cowen syndrome (MEMO, see Chapter 21) should be considered. Histopathologically, there are columnar cells arranged in a palisading pattern and a mass of clear cells that resemble outer root sheath cells. Trichilemmal carcinoma occurs in rare cases.

Proliferating trichilemmal cyst

A subcutaneous nodule or tumor 1–10 cm in diameter occurs, most frequently on the scalp. It is pathologically similar to an epidermal cyst or a trichilemmal cyst (described later in this chapter). Erosions and ulcerations may be present on the surface. Trichilemmal keratinization is observed histopathologically. Overproliferation of cell components is also seen. It is thought to originate from the hair follicle isthmus. Malignant proliferating trichilemmal tumor accompanied by atypism is pathologically differentiated from proliferating trichilemmal cyst.

Sebaceous tumors

Sebaceous hyperplasia (synonym: senile sebaceous hyperplasia)

In sebaceous hyperplasia, mature sebaceous glands enlarge to form elevated lesions, most frequently on the face (forehead, cheek, and nose) of elderly people. The lesions are yellowish-white papules or flat nodules 3–8 mm in diameter (Fig. 21.10). Several eruptions occur in most cases. They are centrally umbilicated and may discharge sebum from the center.

Sebaceous adenoma

A yellowish nodule or tumor occurs, most frequently on the face or scalp in middle age. It is a benign tumor that differentiates into sebaceous glands.

Sebaceoma

This is a dome-shaped or pedunculated nodule that occurs on the face or scalp (Fig. 21.11). It may be yellowish. Histopathologically, there is proliferation of tumor cells that resemble basal cells. Some of the tumor cells are anaplastic, and some differentiate to sebaceous cells and ducts.

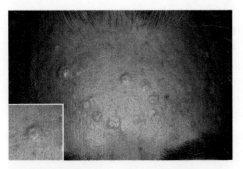

Fig. 21.10 Sebaceous hyperplasia.

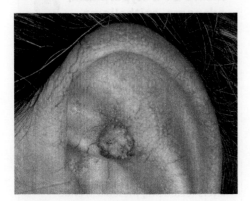

Fig. 21.11 Sebaceoma. A dome-shaped yellowish nodule is seen.

Sweat gland tumors

Eccrine hidrocystoma

A papule of normal skin color or translucent-bluish, 2–3 mm in diameter, occurs on the face, usually solitarily but sometimes more numerously (Fig. 21.12). When there are multiple papules, the number tends to increase in summer and decrease in winter. The skin lesion is thought to be a cystic intradermal channel enlarged by sweat deposition (Fig. 21.13). Decapitation secretion is not seen. Sweat deposition can be identified by needle puncture.

Syringoma
Clinical features

Small, multiple, flatly elevated papules with a diameter of 1–3 mm and normal skin color result from localized proliferation of intradermal sweat ducts. The eyelids are the most commonly affected. The papules may disseminate on the trunk and coalesce (Fig. 21.14). The incidence is higher among women than men, and the disease is seen most often in puberty, when sweat secretion increases. It is asymptomatic and rarely heals spontaneously. (MEMO, see Chapter 17.)

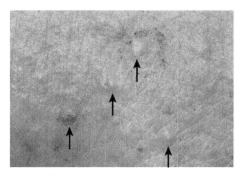

Fig. 21.12 Eccrine hidrocystoma.

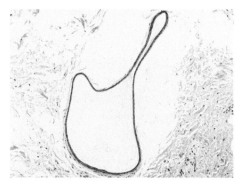

Fig. 21.13 Histopathology of eccrine hidrocystoma.

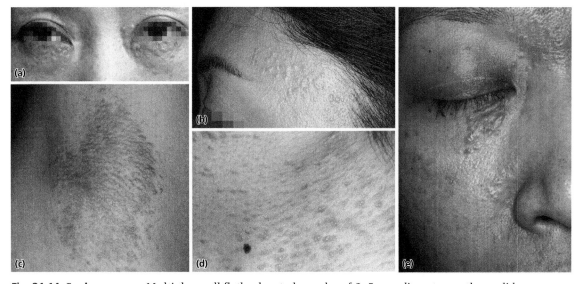

Fig. 21.14 Syringoma. a: Multiple small flatly elevated papules of 2–5 mm diameter on the eyelids. b: Forehead. c: Multiple eruptions of syringoma on the axillary fossa. They coalesce into large plaques. d: The upper chest region. e: Multiple eruptions on the face, with partly coalesced lesions.

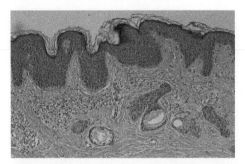

Fig. 21.15 Histopathology of syringoma.
The eruptions contain the tadpole-like or comma-like tumor cells that characterize syringoma.

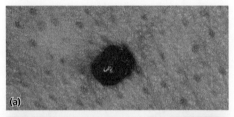

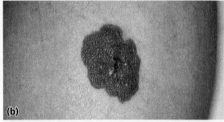

Fig. 21.16 Eccrine poroma. Dark red nodules. a: Pedunculated nodule. b: Dome-shaped nodule.

Pathology

Strands of epithelia form luminal structures of various sizes, with a tadpole-like or comma shape, in the upper and middle dermal layers. The lumen is composed of double-layered mural cells with peripheral proliferation of connective tissue (Fig. 21.15).

Differential diagnosis

Clinically, it is necessary to differentiate syringoma from lupus miliaris disseminatus faciei, milium, angiofibroma, and eccrine hidrocystoma.

Treatment

Treatment is usually unnecessary, as syringoma is asymptomatic and there is no malignant transformation. Carbon dioxide gas laser therapy, cryotherapy, and chemical peeling may be conducted for cosmetic purposes.

Eccrine poroma
Definition and clinical features

Outer cells of eccrine sweat ducts proliferate in eccrine sweat glands. Some of the cells differentiate into sweat duct luminal cells and further into sweat duct excretion cells. A small, dome-shaped or pedunculated nodule occurs on any site of the body, particularly on the soles and palms. The nodules are characterized by dark red color and easy bleeding (Fig. 21.16).

MEMO 21–4 Classification of sweat gland adenomas

Benign tumors that originate from sweat glands in the skin or that differentiate into sweat glands are collectively called hidradenomas. An apocrine hidradenoma divides in the direction of the apocrine glands. An eccrine hidradenoma divides in the direction of the eccrine glands. Hidradenomas are subclassified by the location of the main proliferation into poromas (proliferation is mainly in the epidermal portion of the sweat glands), syringomas (in the dermal sweat duct), and spiradenomas (in the secretory portion). Clear cell hidradenomas, mixed tumors of the skin, cylindromas, hidradenoma papilliferum, and cystadenomas are distinguished by the histopathological findings of the proliferative cells.

Pathology

There is a proliferating nest of poroid cells in the epidermis and the dermis. Eosinophilic cells form small lumens in the focus (cuticular cells; Fig. 21.17). The tumor cells contain large quantities of glycogen.

Treatment

Eccrine poroma may become malignant in rare cases (eccrine porocarcinoma; see Chapter 22). The skin lesion should be surgically removed.

Eccrine spiradenoma

Eccrine spiradenoma is a benign tumor in which there is differentiation of eccrine sweat glands and their intradermal channels. A firm, solitary, sharply margined, intradermal or subcutaneous nodule 1–2 cm in diameter occurs on the face, neck, trunk or upper extremities. The surface of the lesion is normal skin color or bluish, and the spiradenoma is often accompanied by spontaneous pain and tenderness (Fig. 21.18). Histopathologically, large light cells and small dark cells are observed to proliferate in a palisading pattern or in clusters, forming a tubular structure.

Papillary eccrine adenoma

Small solitary nodules of 1–3 cm diameter occur on the extremities. Histopathologically, cystic structures of several sizes and papillary proliferation of the epithelial cells in the lumen are found. Decapitation secretion is not seen. Papillary eccrine adenoma is thought to be a benign tumor that differentiates into the eccrine sweat ducts; however, there has been controversy over whether papillary eccrine adenoma and tubular apocrine adenoma (described later) are different diseases.

Nodular hidradenoma

This is a solitary intradermal nodule that frequently occurs on the face and head. The tumor cells are spindle-shaped dark cells containing long, thin nuclei and round clear cells containing round nuclei. The proportion of the two types of cells varies. When the proportion of the latter cells is high, the condition is called clear cell hidradenoma. It is thought to be a benign tumor that shows differentiation in eccrine or apocrine glands. There may be malignant formation (malignant nodular hidradenoma) in some cases.

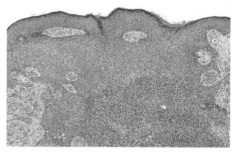

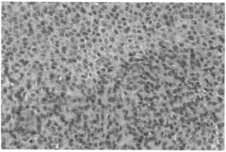

Fig. 21.17　Histopathology of eccrine poroma.

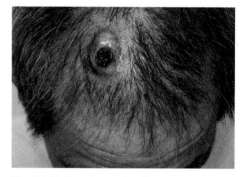

Fig. 21.18　Eccrine spiradenoma.

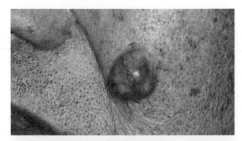

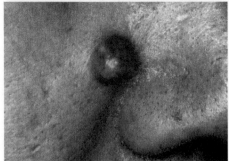

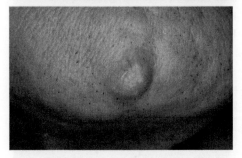

Fig. 21.19 Mixed tumor of the skin.

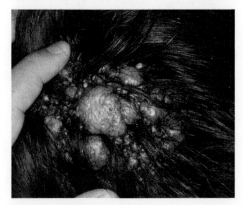

Fig. 21.20 Cylindroma.

Mixed tumor of the skin (synonym: chondroid syringoma)

Relatively firm intradermal or subcutaneous nodules occur, most frequently on the face (upper lip, nose), head, and scalp of young to middle-aged people (Fig. 21.19). Mobility is present at the bottom of the nodule on the skin surface. Characteristically, epithelial tissue that forms luminal structures surrounded by single- or double-layered cell walls is interspersed with mucus-like or cartilage-like mesenchymal tissue. Decapitation secretion and differentiation into follicular cells and sebocytes may be observed. This is thought to be a benign tumor originating from eccrine and apocrine sweat glands. It may be cancerous in rare cases.

Apocrine hidrocystoma

This is a tumor of the apocrine organs. A small, solitary, dome-shaped nodule with a diameter of 2–20 mm occurs around the eye or elsewhere on the face, or on the ear or scalp, of people in middle age or older. The nodule is transparent or bluish. A large cystic structure is found in the dermis. The nodule is composed of single-layered pillar cells that show apocrine secretion and myoepithelial cells that are located on the outer side of the pillar cells. It is usually asymptomatic. Excision may be conducted at the patient's request.

Cylindroma

Cylindroma seldom occurs in ethnic Japanese. Multiple dome-shaped or slightly pedunculated tumors of 1–10 cm diameter and normal to brown skin color occur, most commonly on the scalp of adolescent boys and girls (Fig. 21.20). When the entire scalp is affected, the head has the appearance of being wrapped by a turban (turban tumor). Cylindroma may occur solitarily in rare cases. Multiple cylindroma is an autosomal dominant disorder in which abnormality of the cylindromatosis gene (*CYLD1*) has been identified, as in multiple familial trichoepithelioma. Clusters of tumor cells that show differentiation into sweat glands form a jigsaw puzzle-like pattern. There may be malignant formation in rare cases (malignant cylindroma).

Hidradenoma papilliferum

A small, dome-shaped nodule occurs, often accompanied by erosion and bleeding. It most frequently appears on the female genitalia. The tumor resembles granulation tissue. Histopathologically, there is dense papillary proliferation of glandular epithelial cells with apocrine-type decapitation secretion. Hidradenoma papilliferum is a typical type of apocrine neoplasm.

Syringocystadenoma papilliferum

A verrucous nodule with a rose-pink surface occurs, most commonly on the scalp or face of children. Erosions may sometimes occur (Fig. 21.21). It is an apocrine organic hamartoma and often occurs secondarily to sebaceous nevus. Histopathologically, there is a double-layered luminal structure with long, cylindrical cells on the inner side, cubical cells on the outer side, and marked plasmacytic infiltration in the nodule (Fig. 21.22).

Tubular apocrine adenoma

Tubular apocrine adenoma usually occurs on the scalp and may arise from a sebaceous nevus. The lesion is a nodule of 1–2 cm diameter and of normal skin color or brown. Histopathologically, multiple small cysts and papillary epithelial proliferation are seen, as in papillary eccrine adenoma; however, decapitation secretion is present.

Adenoma of the nipple (synonym: erosive adenomatosis of the nipple)

A benign tumor occurs in the nipple, often accompanied by erosion and exudation. Differentiation from mammary Paget's disease and breast cancer is necessary. Dense papillary proliferation with a luminal structure and decapitation secretion is histopathologically observed. This is a benign tumor derived from the mammary duct in the nipple. The treatment is total excision; unless it is complete, there is recurrence.

Cysts

Epidermoid cyst (synonym: epidermal cyst)
Clinical features
A dome-shaped, intradermal or subcutaneous tumor, usually 1–2 cm in diameter, occurs, most frequently on the head, neck, upper trunk or lumbar region (Fig. 21.23). The tumor adheres to the skin surface; however, the sides and bottom of the tumor mass do not firmly adhere to the peripheral tissue. It tends to occur on sites with hair.

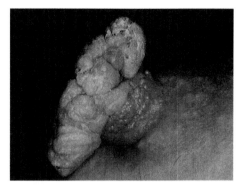

Fig. 21.21 **Syringocystadenoma papilliferum.**

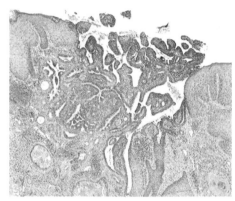

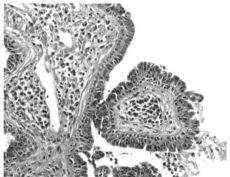

Fig. 21.22 **Histopathology of syringocystadenoma papilliferum.**

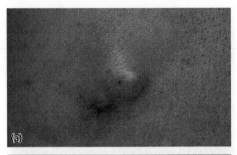

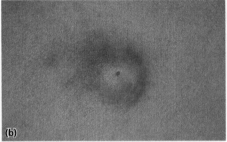

Fig. 21.23 Epidermal cyst. a: There is a black opening at the center of the eruption. b: Secondary infection resulted in reddening and swelling at the periphery.

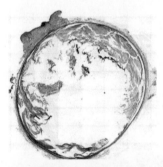

Fig. 21.24 Histopathology of an epidermal cyst.

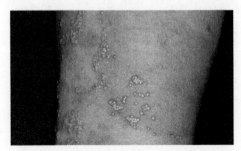

Fig. 21.25 Milium. Lesions on the forearm of a patient with epidermolysis bullosa acquisita (EBA).

Epidermoid cysts are elastic but firm, with a surface color of normal skin or light blue and a black punctate opening at the center. They are asymptomatic. When pressed after excision, the cyst exudes a putrid-smelling, white, gruel-like discharge. Reddening, swelling, and tenderness may be caused by secondary infection and rupture of the cyst walls (inflammatory epidermoid cyst).

Pathogenesis
The epidermis or infundibulum-derived epithelial components invaginate into the dermis and proliferate to form a cyst that contains a keratinous mass. Invagination of the epidermis or of the epithelial components into dermis that is caused by injury or by infection of HPV-57 or HPV-60 is thought to be associated with epidermoid cysts in some cases, in which cases the cysts occur in the palms and soles (see Table 23.1).

Pathology
The wall of the cyst has the same structure as normal epidermis: basal layer, suprabasal cell layer, and granular cell layer (Fig. 21.24). However, in place of the stratum corneum, there are gruel-like, layered keratinous contents. When the keratinous substance is released into the dermis by rupture of the cystic wall, a foreign body granuloma containing multiple polynucleated giant cells may be produced.

Treatment
The cyst is excised.

Milium
Clinical features
A small, firm, white to yellowish-white papule 1–2 mm in diameter occurs immediately below the epidermis (Fig. 21.25). White keratinous contents are discharged by incision. Primary milium occurs most frequently on the eyelids, followed by the cheeks, penis, and labia. Plaques may form. The histological findings are almost the same as those of epidermoid cyst.

Definition and pathogenesis
The pathogenesis of primary milium is thought to be keratotic cyst formation resulting from abnormality of embryonic epithelial buds. Secondary milium occurs after a blistering disease (e.g., dystrophic epidermolysis bullosa, epidermolysis bullosa acquisita), burn

scarring or radiodermatitis. The skin appendages and epidermal cells are damaged by these diseases and proliferate in cyst-like shape under the epidermis.

Treatment

A small incision using a scalpel or a puncture with a hypodermic needle is conducted to remove the spherical white substance.

Dermoid cyst

A dome-shaped subcutaneous nodule with a diameter of 1–4 cm appears, most frequently on the head. It is present at birth. It is often misdiagnosed as an epidermoid cyst. Histopathologically, sebaceous glands and sweat glands are found, as well as cyst walls consisting of epithelial cells.

Trichilemmal cyst (synonym: pilar cyst)

The head is affected in about 90% of cases. Pathologically, a trichilemmal cyst resembles an epidermoid cyst. It is thought to originate from the hair follicle isthmus. Histopathologically, there are cyst walls consisting of epithelial cells, and these cyst walls keratinize without forming a granular cell layer (trichilemmal keratinization). Residual nuclei may be observed in some keratinocytes (Fig. 21.26).

Steatocystoma multiplex

A firm, dome-shaped tumor occurs with a diameter of 3–30 mm in most cases and a color ranging from that of normal skin to light yellow or light blue, frequently on the axillary fossae, upper chest or upper arm (Fig. 21.27). Some cases are associated with follicles. This condition may occur in patients with pachyonychia congenita (see Chapter 19), and mutations in the keratin 17 gene have been reported in patients with this condition. Histopathologically, there are flattened sebaceous glands near or directly attached to the tumor. The cyst wall is composed of intricately multilayered epithelial components.

Eruptive vellus hair cyst

Vellus hair is fuzzy hair. An eruptive vellus hair cyst is derived from a vellus hair follicle. It is an asymptomatic follicular papule of several millimeters in diameter. It occurs most frequently on the chest. The cyst may resemble keratosis pilaris or it may be umbilicated. It may be accompanied by steatocystoma

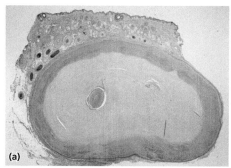

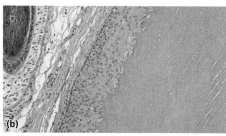

Fig. 21.26 Histopathology of a trichilemmal cyst. a: A cyst in the lower dermal layer. b: Trichilemmal keratinization is observed; tumor cells keratinize without the formation of a granular cell layer.

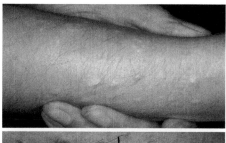

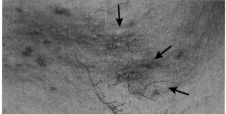

Fig. 21.27 Steatocystoma multiplex. Multiple subcutaneous cysts ranging in diameter from 5 to 10 mm occurred on the forearm and axillary fossa.

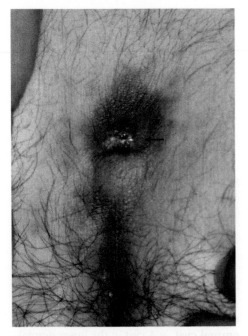

Fig. 21.28 The opening of a fistula caused by a pilonidal sinus on the sacral region.

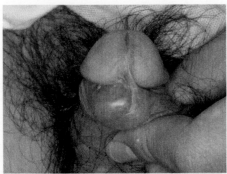

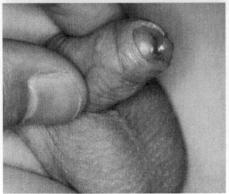

Fig. 21.29 Median raphe cyst of the penis.

multiplex (see the previous section). The cyst wall may contain a sebaceous structure.

Pilonidal sinus (synonyms: pilonidal cyst, pilonidal disease)

Ingrowth of hair leads to the formation of a fistula. The fistula is surrounded by granulomatous tissue or squamous epithelia. It tends to enlarge with recurrence of infection. Young men whose buttocks, particularly the sacral division, are hairy are most frequently affected. Pilonidal sinus may also occur on the occipital region of the head, eyelids, genitalia, axillary fossae, umbilical fossae or interdigital areas. Most cases with interdigital involvement occur occupationally, such as in barbers. The affected site, including the scar tissue, should be completely excised (Fig. 21.28).

Branchial cyst

A branchial cyst is a subcutaneous epidermoid cyst-like nodule that occurs on the preauricular region and neck. As it is caused by branchial debris, mobility is not fully present at the bottom of the cyst. There is a palpable cord-like substance in the cyst. Excision should not be decided quickly. Consultation with a head and neck surgeon is required. Branchial cysts caused by thyrolingual debris are called thyroglossal duct cysts or median cervical cysts.

Median raphe cyst

A tumor of several millimeters in diameter occurs in the penile raphe of young men (Fig. 21.29). It occurs solitarily at the urethral opening in most cases. The cyst may reach several centimeters in diameter. It may occur in the scrotum or perineum. Histopathologically, its wall is composed of single- or several-layered cylindrical epithelia or cubical epithelia that resemble urethral transitional epithelia.

Pseudo-cyst of the auricle

An intense, pulsating cyst occurs unilaterally in the cartilage of the upper part of the auricle. In rare cases, inflammatory symptoms including reddening and sharp pain are present. It most frequently occurs in persons who receive chronic irritation of the auricle, including wrestlers and atopic dermatitis patients. Fluid accumulation (pseudo-cyst) without epithelial components occurs in the auricle cartilage. The treatment is pressure immobilization after puncture or local injection of steroids, although the condition is intractable.

Neural tumors

Neurofibroma

The tumor is dome-shaped, soft and of normal skin color or light pink. It slowly enlarges (Figs 21.30 and 21.31). There are almost no symptoms; however, subcutaneous neurofibroma (nodular plexiform neurofibroma) is often accompanied by tenderness. In neurofibromatosis type 1 (NF1), neurofibromas occur multiply on the whole body. Localized areas, such as the trunk, may be affected by mosaicism (see Chapter 20). Solitary neurofibroma may occur in patients without NF1.

A neurofibroma is thought to be a benign tumor that derives from Schwann cells or from perineural or endoneural cells. Histopathologically, a clearly marginated tumorous lesion that lacks a covering membrane is seen in the region from the dermis to the subcutaneous tissues. Proliferation of spindle-shaped tumor cells and tangled thin collagen fibers woven among the cells are observed. Myxoid stroma and various levels of mast cell infiltration are seen. The tumor cells are S-100 positive.

Neurilemmoma

Clinical features

A neurilemmoma is a benign tumor derived from Schwann cells that forms an axonal myelin sheath. It usually occurs singly but in neurofibromatosis type 2, the neurolemmomas are multiple (see Chapter 20). The tumor is palpable, elastic, firm, spherical, and intradermal or subcutaneous. It may appear in a beaded pattern. It is accompanied by tenderness, and pain may radiate from the pressured site to the periphery. Malignant transformation occurs in rare cases (malignant neurilemmoma).

Pathology

Neurilemmomas are characterized by a biphasic pattern of Antoni A areas and Antoni B areas that is visible by microscopy. Antoni A areas form the cellular component of the lesion and are composed of fairly closely packed spindle cells with tapering, elongated, wavy nuclei and eosinophilic areas with fewer nuclei (verocay bodies). Nuclear palisading is a prominent feature. Antoni B areas are characterized by irregularly scattered spindle or stellate cells set in abundant loose myxoid stroma (Fig. 21.32).

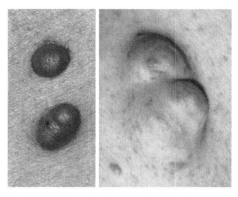

Fig. 21.30 A soft, elevated skin tumor caused by neurofibroma.

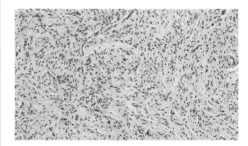

Fig. 21.31 Histopathology of a neurofibroma.

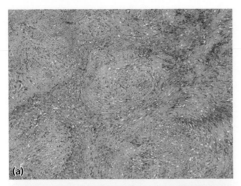

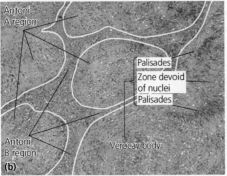

Antoni
A region

Palisades
Zone devoid
of nuclei
Palisades

Antoni
B region

Verocay body

(b)

Fig. 21.32 a: Histopathology of a neurilemmoma (schwannoma). b: Details of the image.

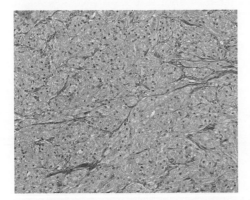

Fig. 21.33 Histopathology of a granular cell tumor.

Treatment

Excision should be conducted carefully, to avoid damaging the displaced nerves.

Traumatic neuroma

A traumatic neuroma, also called an amputation neuroma, is a tumor that occurs in the peripheral nerve stump. Intense spontaneous pain and tenderness are present. Histopathologically, nerve fibers proliferate in all directions and are surrounded by Schwann cells and proliferative fibrotic tissue. Excision may be necessary, depending on the severity of the pain, and neuroanastomosis is performed when possible.

Rudimentary polydactyly

A small nodule 1–2 cm in diameter is present on a digit, often the thumb, at birth. Histopathologically, natural amputation of embryonic polydactylism is thought to cause the outgrowth of nerve fiber bundles and nerve end corpuscles, such as Meissner and Pacinian corpuscles.

Granular cell tumor

A small tumor 3 cm or less in diameter occurs on the skin and in the genital mucosa, tongue, lung, esophagus, stomach, intestine, bladder or uterus. Histopathologically, the tumor is composed of large polygonal cells that contain eosinophilic granules (Fig. 21.33). It is accompanied by acanthosis and is easily misdiagnosed as squamous cell carcinoma. It is thought to originate from Schwann cells. The cytoplasm contains numerous eosinophilic granules. It is resistant to diastase and is PAS positive and S-100 positive. There is malignant transformation in some cases.

Vascular tumors

The vascular anomalies described in this textbook are categorized based on conventional, descriptive terms or histopathological terms. However, the classification is confusing, because "hemangioma" simplex is not tumorous but is a malformation of normal capillaries. The cutaneous vascular anomalies described in this textbook are classified as shown in Table 21.1, according to the classification proposed by the International Society for the Study of Vascular Anomalies (ISSVA).

Table 21.1 Classification of hemangiomas and vascular malformation.

Type of vascular abnormality		Disease	Indirect reference
Hemangioma	Congenital	Infantile hemangioma, GLUT-1 positive	Chapter 21
		Congenital hemangioma	
		Rapidly involuting congenital hemangioma (RICH)	Chapter 21
		Non-involuting congenital hemangioma (NICH)	Chapter 21
		Kaposiform hemangioepithelioma	Chapter 21
		Tufted angioma	Chapter 21
	Acquired	Cherry angioma	Chapter 21
		Glomeruloid hemangioma	Chapter 21
		POEMS syndrome	Chapter 21
		Spindle cell hemangioendothelioma	Chapter 21
		Hemangiopericytoma	Chapter 21
		Pyogenic granuloma	Chapter 21
		Intravascular papillary endothelial hyperplasia	Chapter 21
		Angiolymphoid hyperplasia with eosinophilia (ALHE)	Chapter 21
		Kaposi's sarcoma	Chapter 22
		Angiosarcoma	Chapter 22
Vascular malformation	Capillary	Capillary malformation	Chapter 21
		Sturge–Weber syndrome	Chapter 20
		Phakomatosis pigmentovascularis	Chapter 20
		Telangiectasia	
		Hereditary hemorrhagic telangiectasia	Chapter 20
		Ataxia telangiectasia (AT)	Chapter 11
		Cutis marmorata telangiectatica congenita	Chapter 20
		Spider telangiectasia	Chapter 21
	Venous	Venous malformation	Chapter 21
		Blue rubber bleb nevus syndrome	Chapter 20
		Maffucci syndrome	Chapter 20
		Venous lake	Chapter 21
		Glomuvenous malformation	Chapter 21
	Lymphatic	Lymphatic malformation	Chapter 21
	Arterial	Cutaneous arteriovenous malformation	Chapter 21
	Combined	Capillary lymphatic malformation	Chapter 21
		Other combined	
		Klippel–Trenaunay–Weber syndrome	Chapter 20

Hemangiomas

Infantile hemangioma (synonyms: strawberry mark, strawberry nevus)

- A bright red elevated lesion results from the proliferation of premature capillaries. It appears 3–4 weeks after birth, enlarging until the age of 6 or 7 months.
- The face and arms are often involved. It heals spontaneously with soft scarring in several years.
- Dye laser irradiation is the main treatment. Follow-up without treatment may be chosen.

Clinical features

Shortly after birth, telangiectatic erythema occurs on the face or arms, expanding gradually to form an elevated red tumor by the age of 3–6 months.

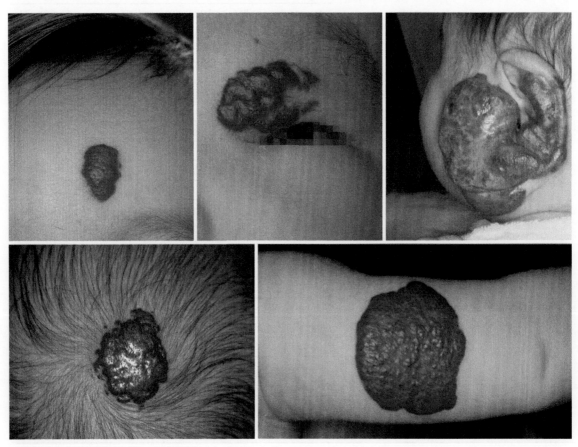

Fig. 21.34 Infantile hemangioma.

This condition is found in about 1% of infants. The lesion resembles a halved strawberry stuck on the skin (Fig. 21.34). The color disappears in diascopy. Ulceration may develop on the lesion. After its peak, the strawberry mark subsides at the stationary phase, in most cases disappearing with light scarring by later childhood.

Pathogenesis and pathology

The primary lesion is a proliferation of vascular endothelial cells. The tumor is bright red and is composed of proliferating premature vessels. Strawberry mark is caused by an angioblast mass; it does not differentiate into normal capillary tissue (Fig. 21.35). GLUT-1 is positive.

Treatment

The conventional policy has been "wait and see." However, in recent years, laser therapy has been performed for cosmetic purposes even in infancy, because scarring may remain after spontaneous healing. The earlier the laser therapy begins, the more effective it is. Systemic administration of steroids or sclerotherapy may be necessary in cases in which the lesion continues to enlarge 6 months after birth, or when the

MEMO 21–5 RICH, NICH

In some cases, the formation of a hemangioma is almost complete at birth, and the lesion disappears rapidly and spontaneously within 6–12 months after birth. In other cases, the lesion does not spontaneously disappear, but slowly enlarges. The former is called rapidly involuting congenital hemangioma (RICH); the latter is called non-involuting congenital hemangioma (NICH).

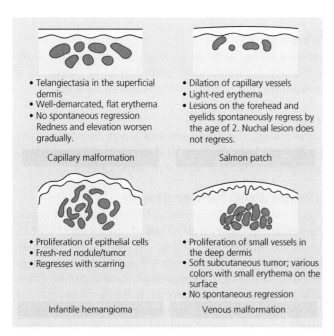

- Telangiectasia in the superficial dermis
- Well-demarcated, flat erythema
- No spontaneous regression Redness and elevation worsen gradually.

Capillary malformation

- Dilation of capillary vessels
- Light-red erythema
- Lesions on the forehead and eyelids spontaneously regress by the age of 2. Nuchal lesion does not regress.

Salmon patch

- Proliferation of epithelial cells
- Fresh-red nodule/tumor
- Regresses with scarring

Infantile hemangioma

- Proliferation of small vessels in the deep dermis
- Soft subcutaneous tumor; various colors with small erythema on the surface
- No spontaneous regression

Venous malformation

Fig. 21.35 Classification of hemangiomas.

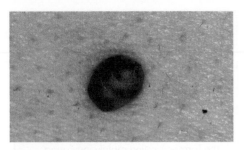

Fig. 21.36 Senile angioma.

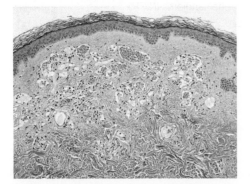

Fig. 21.37 Histopathology of senile angioma.

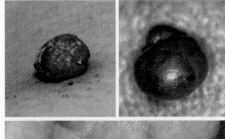

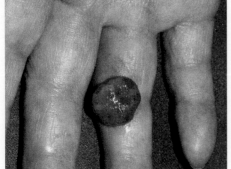

Fig. 21.38-1 Pyogenic granuloma. Soft, pedunculated tumors which are light pink to dark red in color.

lesion is on the lips or when eyelid involvement is causing visual disturbance.

Senile angioma, cherry angioma

Multiple, punctate, glossy, bright red papules occur on the trunk. The onset is after the second decade of life, and the papules become more numerous with age. The pathogenesis is thought to be reactive vascular proliferation. Localized capillary proliferation is histopathologically found in the lower papillary dermis (Fig. 21.36 and Fig. 21.37).

Pyogenic granuloma (synonym: telangiectatic granuloma)
Clinical features

An angioma whose main symptoms are proliferation of capillaries and dilation of vascular lumens is induced by injury. The tumor is soft and pedunculated, ranging in color from bright red to dark red. It is elevated in a dome shape, with a diameter of 5–20 mm (Fig. 21.38). Bleeding is easily caused by injury, leading to ulceration. Pyogenic granuloma in a newborn is often found in the umbilical region (umbilical granuloma). The face of children and the trunk and extremities of adults are most commonly involved. The skin lesion appears suddenly, erodes, and bleeds. Pyogenic granuloma should be differentiated from amelanotic melanoma.

Pathology

Pathologically, there is an angioma accompanied by secondary inflammatory granuloma, or there is a granuloma that is non-angiomatous in structure.

Treatment

Cryotherapy, the application of silver nitrate, carbon dioxide gas laser therapy, and excision are conducted. Topical steroids are effective in some cases.

Glomeruloid hemangioma

This is vascular proliferation. A hemangioma of 1 cm or less in diameter occurs in about half of patients with POEMS syndrome (MEMO, see Chapter 21) (Fig. 21.39). Vascular proliferation factors are secreted and blood estrogen is elevated. Although glomeruloid hemangioma clinically resembles senile angioma, it appears suddenly on the trunk, extremities, and head and neck region of people in their second and third decades. The dome-shaped nodules are too firm to be displaced by digital pressure, and their color is a lighter pink than those in senile angioma.

Kasabach–Merritt syndrome
Clinical features
Large angiomas, platelet decreases, and systemic purpura are present in this syndrome. Subcutaneous induration appears in the first 3 months of life in many cases (Fig. 21.40). The lesions enlarge rapidly and bleed. They form giant tumors that are dark red to purple. Large amounts of platelets are consumed, which leads to edema, minor hemorrhaging, systemic purpura, and ready bleeding. Persistent coagulopathy and thrombocytopenia result in disseminated intravascular coagulation (DIC).

Pathogenesis
Intratumor bleeding is caused by the rapid enlargement of a large angioma in newborns, many of which are kaposiform hemangioepitheliomas and tufted angiomas, leading to platelet consumption. Cutaneous angiomas resemble infantile hemangiomas. Premature cutaneous angiomas are thought to result in hemostasis, platelet consumption, and coagulation factor consumption.

Treatment
Disseminated intravascular coagulation is treated symptomatically. Steroids and anticancer agents are administered, and vascular embolization is conducted.

Tufted angioma (synonym: angioblastoma of Nakagawa)
This begins as an erythema that gradually enlarges to form a flatly elevated, infiltrating plaque (Fig. 21.41). Tufted angioma is a vascular tumor in which immature endothelial cells and pericytes proliferate. The color ranges from light pink to dark purplish-red. The pathogenesis is unknown.

Spindle cell hemangioendothelioma
A bluish subcutaneous tumor occurs, most frequently in the distal areas of the extremities in young persons. Histopathologically, it is composed of dilated vascular lumens and portions of proliferated spindle cells. Multiple tumors occur in localized areas; however, they are benign and non-metastatic.

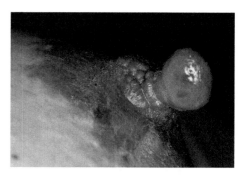

Fig. 21.38-2 Pyogenic granuloma.

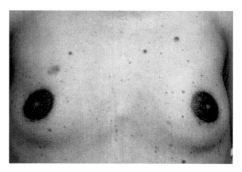

Fig. 21.39 Glomeruloid hemangioma.

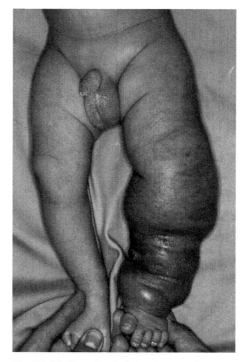

Fig. 21.40 Kasabach–Merritt syndrome.
Large hemangioma in the left leg.

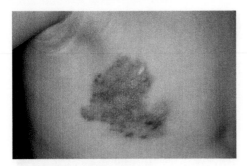

Fig. 21.41 Tufted angioma.

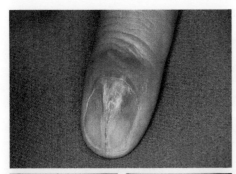
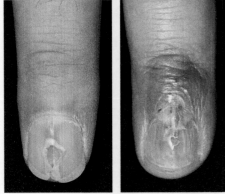

Fig. 21.42-1 Glomus tumor under the nail. Deformity of the nail and severe tenderness occur.

Hemangiopericytoma

A firm, elastic, relatively sharply margined nodule occurs in the lower extremities, the thigh in particular. Histopathologically, round or spindle cells that resemble pericytes proliferate around the capillary lumens, which are covered by a single-layered endothelium.

Intravascular papillary endothelial hyperplasia

The blood vessels proliferate as a result of thrombotic recanalization in the dilated venules. This is a reactive change of thrombotic vessels often seen in adults. A purplish-red nodule occurs, most frequently in the veins of the finger pads. Thrombus formation may cause pain.

Glomus tumor (synonym: glomuvenous malformation)

- This tumor occurs frequently under the nail plate. It is a benign tumor that derives from glomus cells in the neuromyoarterial glomus.
- A firm, dark red to bluish-brown tumor forms in the finger or toe, often under the nail plate. The pain and tenderness are intense.
- Pulsating pain intensifies at night or with exposure to extreme cold.

Clinical features

Glomus tumors can be solitary or multiple, most of them being solitary. A solitary glomus tumor occurs most frequently under the nail plate of individuals age 20 and older. A firm, painful nodule 1 cm or less in diameter occurs, ranging in color from dark red to purplish-red (Fig. 21.42). Glomus tumors are characterized by extreme pain from pressure or exposure to cold water. Multiple glomus tumors can occur in persons of any age. Generally asymptomatic soft tumors of normal skin color to blue and about 1 cm in diameter appear on the whole body. They may appear in a linear pattern in rare cases. Some cases are autosomal dominant.

Pathogenesis

Proliferation of glomus cells (see Chapter 1) leads to hamartoma formation. A hereditary multiple type is thought to be caused by glomuvenous malformation.

Pathology

Glomus cells with eosinophilic cytoplasm and round nuclei proliferate around dilated vascular vessels (Fig. 21.43). Glomus cells stain in desmin and myosin. A solitary glomus tumor is covered by a richly enervated membrane. In multiple glomus tumors, vascular lumens extend in a spongiform pattern.

Differential diagnosis

Multiple glomus tumors are differentiated from blue rubber bleb nevus syndrome (see Chapter 20). Glomus tumors underneath the nail plate should be differentiated from subungual exostosis.

Vascular malformations

Capillary malformation (synonyms: hemangioma simplex, port wine stain, nevus flammeus)

Clinical features

A flat, sharply margined red patch results from capillary telangiectasia in the shallow dermal layer. It is present at birth (Fig. 21.44). The skin lesion remains through life, deepening in color slightly with age. When the face is involved, it may thicken after puberty and multiple nodular elevations may occur (hypertrophic port wine stain). Capillary malformation may occur as a symptom of Sturge–Weber syndrome or Klippel–Trenaunay–Weber syndrome (see Chapter 20).

A light pink, vaguely marginated patch, which is found in the midline region of the face of 20–30% of newborns with a specific type of capillary malformation, is called medial nevus or salmon patch. These lesions on the forehead or eyelids tend to disappear spontaneously by age 2; however, these lesions on the neck, called Unna nevi, do not disappear spontaneously.

Pathogenesis and pathology

Dilation and increase of mature capillaries are found in the upper dermal layer (Fig. 21.45; see also Fig. 21.35).

Treatment

Dye laser therapy is the first-line treatment. Early treatment is desirable. Follow-up without treatment may be chosen for salmon patches. Concealing cosmetics are useful.

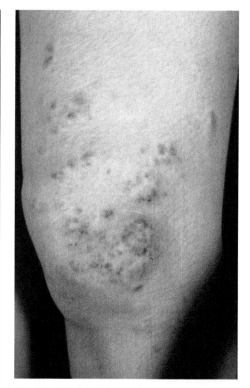

Fig. 21.42-2 Multiple glomus tumors.

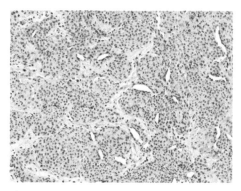

Fig. 21.43 Histopathology of a glomus tumor.

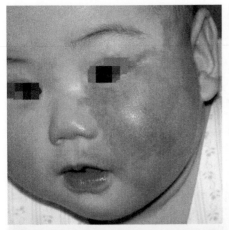

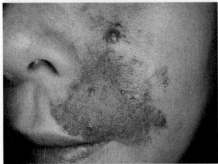

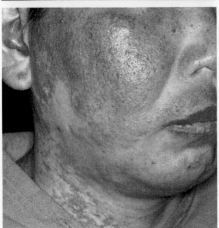

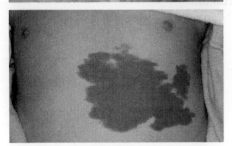

Fig. 21.44-1 Capillary malformation.

Venous malformation (synonym: cavernous hemangioma)

- Malformed veins proliferate in the deep dermal layer.
- A soft, subcutaneous tumor occurs in early childhood. The lesions are normal skin color or light purplish-pink.

Clinical features

Small, mature, malformed vessels (mainly veins) occur in the deep dermal layer (Fig. 21.46; see also Fig. 21.35). The malformed vessels are present at birth; however, many cases are clinically found during infancy. The lesions appear as soft subcutaneous tumors. The color is in the range of normal skin color to light blue or reddish purple. Small erythemas are dispersed on the surface of the tumor. Tenderness is not present. Venous malformation does not heal spontaneously. The condition is usually solitary; however, when it occurs multiply, blue rubber bleb nevus syndrome and neurocutaneous syndromes such as Maffucci syndrome are suspected (see Chapter 20).

Treatment

Excision is conducted for small lesions. Intratumor coagulation (sclerotherapy) is performed. Radiation therapy is ineffective.

Venous lake

A small, slightly elevated, dark blue nodule occurs mainly on the face, lips or auricle of elderly people (Fig. 21.47). Histopathologically, the underlying disease is telangiectasia.

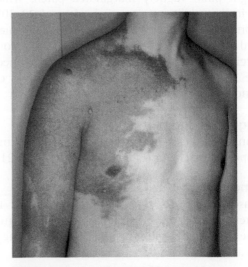

Fig. 21.44-2 Capillary malformation.

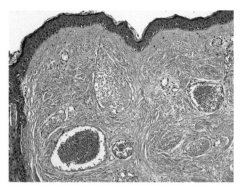

Fig. 21.45 Histopathology of capillary malformation. Dilated capillaries filled with erythrocytes are seen in the dermis, and these have a reddish skin color.

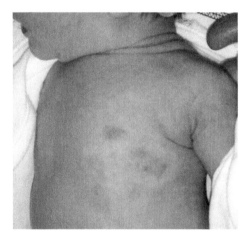

Fig. 21.46 Venous malformation. A tumor with infiltration is seen on the right side of the chest. Abnormality is found in the blood vessels at the center.

Spider telangiectasia (synonyms: vascular spider, spider nevus, spider angioma)

Capillaries extending radially from a red papule of several millimeters diameter give the appearance of a spider spreading its legs (Fig. 21.48; see also Fig. 3.27). The face, neck, shoulders, chest, and upper arms are frequently involved. It is most common in pregnancy or hepatopathy, when estrogen levels are elevated. It may be found in about 15% of healthy individuals. The lesion fades under diascopy. Dye laser therapy is effective. Spider telangiectasia in pregnant women or children disappears spontaneously.

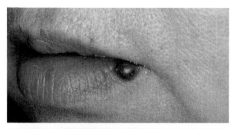

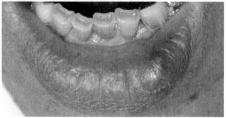

Fig. 21.47 Venous lake.

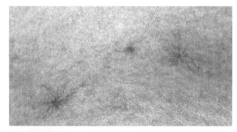

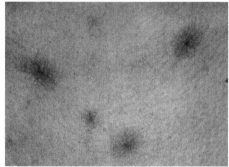

Fig. 21.48 Spider telangiectasia. The dilated capillaries form a web-like pattern.

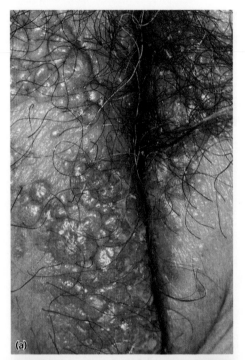
(a)

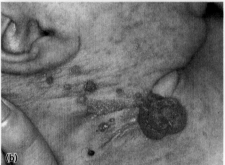
(b)

Fig. 21.49 Lymphatic malformation.
a: Localized lymphangioma. b: Macrocystic lymphatic malformation.

MEMO 21–6 POEMS syndrome (synonyms: Crow–Fukase syndrome, Takatsuki syndrome)

POEMS is an acronym for polyneuropathy, organomegaly of the liver, spleen or lymph nodes, endocrinopathy, monoclonal gammopathy, and skin changes. Various skin lesions, such as glomeruloid hemangiomas, pigmentations, trichosis, scleroderma-like diffuse sclerosis, livedo reticularis, and Raynaud's disease, and clubbed fingers are caused by POEMS syndrome.

Lymphatic malformation (synonym: lymphangioma)

- This is a benign lesion caused by lymphangial hyperplasia and dilation resulting from dysplasia of lymph vessels.
- Vesicles of 1–2 mm diameter aggregate. Bleeding in the vesicles may result in papules whose color ranges from red to black.
- It is surgically removed.
- Postoperative lymphangioma in the axillary fossae or groin after breast cancer or uterus cancer is called lymphangiectasis (acquired lymphangioma).

Classification, clinical features, and pathology

Lymphatic malformations are classified into three subtypes.

- **Lymphangioma circumscriptum:** transparent vesicles several millimeters in diameter aggregate to form irregularly shaped plaques. The vesicles appear reddish from internal bleeding. The thickened epidermis may appear verrucous (Fig. 21.49a). Histopathologically, lymphangiectasia is found in the dermal papillary layer.
- **Macrocystic lymphatic malformation:** this is a large, deep-seated, subcutaneous tumor (Fig. 21.49b). The color ranges from normal to light pink or bluish-purple. The tumor pulsates. Lymph fluid is discharged from the tumor by puncture. The tongue, face, and genitalia are frequently involved. Histopathologically, irregular lymphangiectasia occurs in the subcutaneous and deep dermal layers.
- **Lymphangiectasia (acquired lymphangioma):** lymphangioma occurs postoperatively in the axillary fossae or groin after breast cancer or uterus cancer.

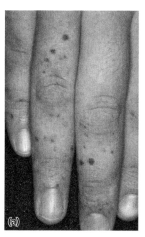 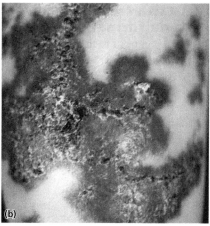 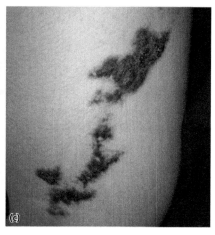

Fig. 21.50 Angiokeratoma. a: Angiokeratoma of Mibelli. b,c: Angiokeratoma circumscriptum naeviforme.

Treatment

Surgical removal and sclerotherapy are the main treatments.

Angiokeratoma

Proliferation of capillaries in the dermal papillae is found, and the hyperkeratinized epidermis surrounding the capillaries appears verrucous (Fig. 21.50 and Fig. 21.51). This is not a type of hemangioma. It is thought to be vasodilation of capillaries or lymphatic malformation in the dermal papillae. Angiokeratoma is classified into five subtypes. Various factors are associated with the occurrence of angiokeratomas.

- **Solitary angiokeratoma:** this is induced reactively by injury, and often occurring on the lower extremities.
- **Angiokeratoma of Mibelli:** chilblains present as a prodrome. The hands and feet are frequently affected (see Fig. 21.50a). It is autosomal dominant.
- **Angiokeratoma scroti (Fordyce):** this is an angioma that occurs in large numbers, mainly in the scrotum of the elderly.
- **Angiokeratoma circumscriptum naeviforme:** verrucous vascular papules arrange themselves linearly on the unilateral extremities and trunk at birth. Crusting is present (see Fig. 21.50b).
- **Angiokeratoma corporis diffusum:** small, multiple papules occur on the trunk of patients with lysosomal storage diseases such as Fabry's disease and Kanzaki's disease (see Chapter 17).

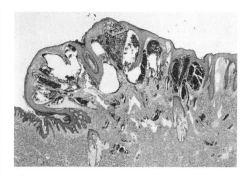

Fig. 21.51 Histopathology of an angiokeratoma. Marked dilation of capillaries in the papillary layer directly under the epidermis.

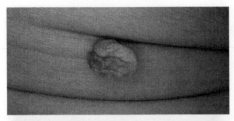
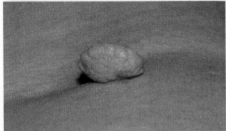
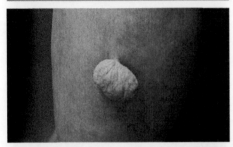
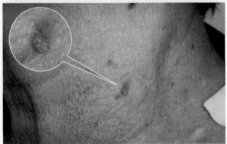

Fig. 21.52 Soft fibroma.

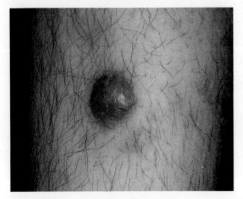

Fig. 21.53-1 Dermatofibroma.

Cutaneous arteriovenous malformation

Congenital vascular malformation and plural embryonic arteriovenous fistulae are the underlying conditions. The skin lesion may resemble a capillary malformation or may be indistinct. It begins to enlarge at a certain point, and swelling occurs accompanied by heat sensation on the surface of the lesion. Pulsation and tremor are present. When the extremities are involved, the lesion enlarges and may cause Klippel–Trenaunay–Weber syndrome (see Chapter 20).

Fibrous tumors

Soft fibroma (synonyms: acrochordon, skin tag, fibroma pendulum)
Clinical features

A soft, dome-shaped or pedunculated tumor with wrinkles on the surface and a color of normal skin or light brown occurs on the neck, axillary fossae or groin (Fig. 21.52). Small, multiple, thread-like tumors 2–3 mm long on the neck and axillary fossae are called acrochorda or skin tags. A solitary, relatively large tumor of about 1 cm on the trunk is called a soft fibroma. An enlarged soft fibroma hanging from the skin is called a soft fibroma pendulum. Soft fibromas tend to occur in obese persons and are more common women; they are thought to relate to skin aging.

Pathology

The primary condition of soft fibroma is the proliferation of collagen bundles with few fibroblasts. In soft fibroma or fibroma pendulum, fat cells are contained in tumors in many cases.

Treatment

The peduncle of the soft fibroma may be excised and the site treated by cryotherapy.

Dermatofibroma (synonym: fibrous histiocytoma)

- This is a firm benign tumor in which fibroblasts or macrophages proliferate in the dermis. It may be caused by external injury, such as insect bites and stings.
- Elevated brown nodules of several millimeters to 2 cm diameter are produced, most commonly on the extremities of adults.

Clinical features and pathogenesis

A dermatofibroma is an intradermal nodule often described as "a button buried shallowly in the skin." The skin of the lesion is brownish (Fig. 21.53). The lesion develops slowly and usually stops changing when it reaches a certain size. In rare cases, a giant dermatofibroma (benign) with a diameter of 5 cm or larger occurs on the lower legs. It is solitary in most cases, but may occur multiply. Tenderness may be present. Connective tissue factors are thought to proliferate reactively against a minor injury and cause dermatofibroma; some dermatologists do not consider it a tumor in the strict sense.

Pathology

Dermal and subcutaneous proliferation of collagen fibers, fibroblasts, and histiocytes occurs (Fig. 21.54). The tumorous cells are blood coagulation factor XIIIa positive and CD34 negative, which differentiates dermatofibroma from dermatofibrosarcoma protuberans (see Chapter 22). Elevated levels of melanin pigment are present in the epidermal basal cell layer. When the main finding is histiocytic proliferation, it is called cellular dermatofibroma, and the tumor is slightly reddish and soft. Dermatofibromas in which fibroblasts and collagen fibers proliferate are called fibrous dermatofibromas. Fibroblasts are scattered among collagen fibers.

Differential diagnosis

When the lesion is firm and blackish or relatively rapidly growing, differentiation from malignant melanoma is necessary. Dermatofibrosarcoma protuberans, tuberous xanthoma, nevus cell nevus, and blue nevus are also differentiated from dermatofibroma.

Treatment

Excision is conducted. It can be left untreated if it has been differentiated from malignant tumors.

Hypertrophic scar and keloid

- A flat, sharply margined, red or brown elevation is caused by proliferation of connective tissue.
- It usually occurs secondary to external injury or operation, but it may occur spontaneously in some cases.

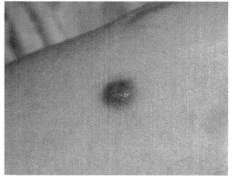
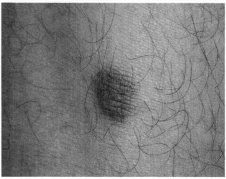

Fig. 21.53-2 Dermatofibroma.

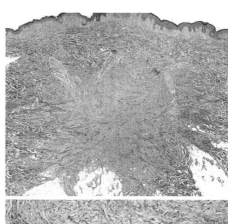
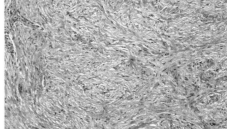

Fig. 21.54 Histopathology of a dermatofibroma.

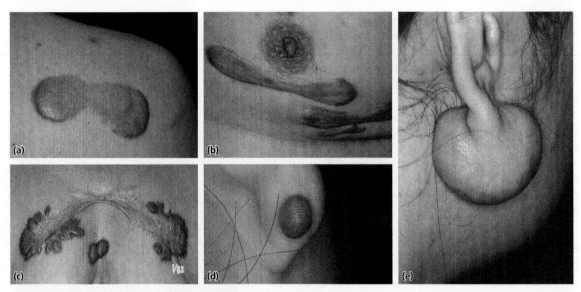

Fig. 21.55 Hypertrophic scar and keloid. a–c: Hypertrophic scar and keloid on the trunk. d,e: Hypertrophic scar and keloid at the site of a former granuloma in the pierced earlobe.

- There is itching and tenderness in the keloid.
- Local injection and steroids are the main treatments. The condition is intractable.

Classification

An elevated reddish-brown lesion occurs on preexisting scarring, caused by excessive production of collagen fibers in fibroblasts. A lesion that atrophies spontaneously within a few years after onset is called a hypertrophic scar. However, a lesion with excessive growth of collagen fibers in which the hyperplastic scar does not disappear is called a keloid. Keloids from ear piercing have been increasing in recent years (Fig. 21.55).

Clinical features

It is triggered by external injury or operation. It usually occurs within 1 month after injury or operation, mostly on the ear, shoulder, and upper part of the trunk. Hypertrophic scars and keloids are flat or dome shaped and sharply demarcated. They range in color from bright red to brown (see Fig. 21.55). True keloids are characterized by gradual enlargement as they progress. When pinched firmly from the side, they are painful (lateral tenderness). Hypertrophic scars do not enlarge beyond the scar width. Lateral tenderness is not present in hypertrophic scars.

Treatment

Hypertrophic scars and keloids are intractable, although pressure dressing, topical steroids, local injection of steroids, and oral tranilast are useful in the early stages. For severe cases and when dysfunction is present, these treatments and radiation therapy are performed after surgical removal.

Palmoplantar fibromatosis

A firm, cord-like substance occurs in the aponeuroses of the palms and soles. It is a deep-seated fibromatosis in which outgrowths of the aponeuroses of the palms and soles are present. The five fingers flex and contract in palmar fibromatosis (Dupuytren's contracture) (Fig. 21.56). Palmoplantar fibromatosis may accompany diabetes mellitus (see Chapter 17).

Pearly penile papule

Multiple, systematized, dome-shaped, whitish papules 1–3 mm in diameter occur on the coronary sulcus of the penis. Pearly penile papules are angiofibromas; they are considered a normal variant and require no therapy. It is necessary to differentiate this condition from condyloma acuminatum (see Chapter 23).

Fibrous papule of the nose

A solitary, firm, dome-shaped papule ranging in color from normal skin color to brown or red and with a diameter of 10 mm or less occurs on the face and neck (Fig. 21.57). Histopathologically, angiofibroma is present.

Acquired digital fibrokeratoma

A small, dome-shaped or cylindrical, protruding, elastic, firm nodule with a hyperkeratotic surface and normal skin color occurs (Fig. 21.58), frequently on the fingers and toes but sometimes on the palms and soles. Nodular sclerosis (see Chapter 20) that occurs around the nail plate is called Koenen tumor. Histopathologically, hyperkeratosis, the proliferation of collagen fibers and fibroblasts, and numerous small vessels are present.

Elastofibroma

A dome-shaped or flat, discoidal tumor occurs bilaterally, usually on the side of the subscapular region. There is proliferation of collagen and elastic fibers (Fig. 21.59).

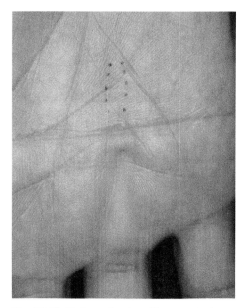

Fig. 21.56 Palmoplantar fibromatosis.
A case of Dupuytren's contracture with flexed and contracted fingers.

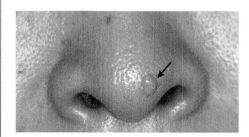

Fig. 21.57 Fibrous papule of the nose.

MEMO 21–8 Infantile digital fibromatosis

This is a fibrous tumor that occurs in the fingers and toes of infants. Histopathologically, it is characterized by the proliferation of myofibroblasts that accompany inclusion bodies. It tends to heal spontaneously. Unless it causes difficulty in walking, only clinical follow-up is recommended.

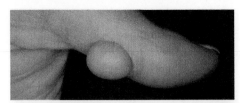

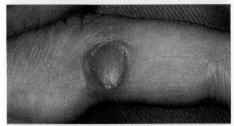

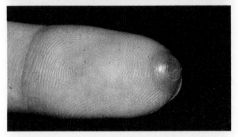

Fig. 21.58 Acquired digital fibrokeratoma.

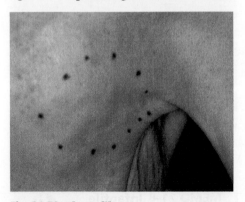

Fig. 21.59 Elastofibroma.

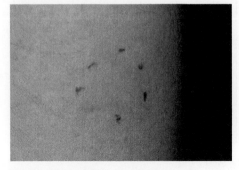

Fig. 21.60 Nodular fasciitis.

Sclerotic fibroma

A dome-shaped nodule of up to 2 cm diameter occurs. Histopathologically, firm collagen fibers are packed densely in a storiform pattern. Because cellular components are largely absent, sclerotic fibroma appears as a well-defined tumor in the dermis. Multiple sclerotic fibromas may be found in patients with Cowden syndrome (MEMO, see Chapter 21).

Nodular fasciitis

Nodular fasciitis occurs frequently in the forearm of men and women in their 30s. External injury may induce it. A subcutaneous nodule 2–3 cm in diameter forms rapidly 1–2 weeks after injury (Fig. 21.60). Tenderness and spontaneous pain often accompany the condition. Histopathologically, premature fibroblast-like cells proliferate in irregular patterns, such as bundles or spirals, seen in the fascia region. Mucin deposition and nuclear division are seen. Differentiation from sarcoma (fibrosarcoma, malignant fibrous histiocytoma, leiomyosarcoma, myxoid liposarcoma, dermatofibrosarcoma protuberans) is necessary. Nodular fasciitis tends to heal spontaneously.

Giant cell tumor of the tendon sheath

A painless intradermal or subcutaneous firm, multilobular nodule of several millimeters to 4 cm diameter occurs, most commonly on the proximal joints of the fingers. The lesion is solitary and of normal skin color. It is thought to be a tendon-derived or synovial membrane-derived tumor that is characterized by the proliferation of histiocyte-like cells and giant cells. It should be completely removed surgically.

Desmoid tumor

This is a firm, deep-seated tumor of several centimeters to 10 cm in diameter and normal skin color. The muscles of the shoulders, chest wall, thighs, and aponeurosis are most frequently involved. It is a benign tumor that histopathologically consists of differentiated fibroblasts and collagen fibers. It slowly enlarges and infiltrates, and has a high probability of recurring after it resolves.

Cutaneous myxoma

This is a soft, asymptomatic, nodular benign tumor up to several centimeters in diameter. Histopathologically, star-shaped or spindled tumor cells appear to float in mucous membrane-like tissue. Cutaneous myxoma is not a mucinosis (see Chapter 17), but an independent disease.

Digital mucous cyst, ganglion

A false cystic lesion containing mucin occurs on the dorsal surface of a finger or toe (Fig. 21.61). It may present a blistered or verrucous appearance. Digital mucous cysts are divided into myxomatous and ganglionic. A myxomatous digital mucous cyst is caused by overproduction of hyaluronic acid by fibroblasts and is essentially focal mucinosis. A ganglionic digital mucous cyst is a joint capsule or tendovaginal hernia. Incomplete removal of the lesion leads to recurrence. Needle aspiration of accumulated mucin, cryotherapy, and local injection of steroids are carried out.

Mucous cyst of the oral mucosa

A soft, dome-shaped tumor of 2–10 mm diameter occurs, predominantly on the lower lip, or on the buccal mucosa and tongue in rare cases (Fig. 21.62). When incised, the tumor discharges transparent yellowish mucin. The pathogenesis is thought to be rupturing of the salivary excretory duct by a bite, leading to salivary flow in the surrounding tissue and the formation of a granuloma.

Histiocytic tumors

Xanthogranuloma (synonym: juvenile xanthogranuloma)

A flat-topped, yellowish or dark-reddish papule or nodule several millimeters to 1 cm in diameter occurs, most frequently on the face, extremities, and trunk (Fig. 21.63). The onset of single or multiple lesions most often occurs at birth or several months thereafter. It disappears spontaneously by the age of 5 or 6 years. Similar eruptions are sometimes seen in adults. Serum lipid is not elevated. The condition should be differentiated from Langerhans cell histiocytosis (see Chapter 22), which may cause similar eruptions.

Histopathologically, juvenile xanthogranuloma is a reactive granuloma composed of histiocytes, xanthoma cells, and Touton giant cells (Fig. 21.64). When complicated with neurofibromatosis type 1 (see Chapter 20), leukemia may be suspected.

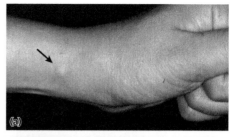
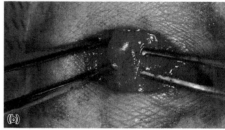
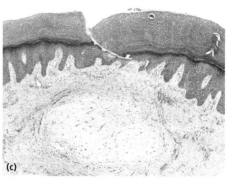

Fig. 21.61 Digital mucous cyst (ganglion). a: Clinical features. b: Surgical excision. c: Histopathology.

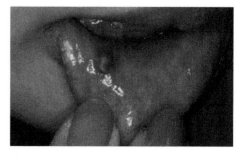

Fig. 21.62 Mucous cyst of the oral mucosa.

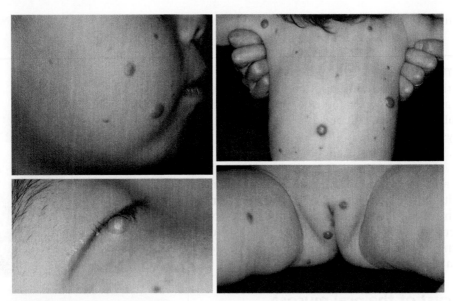

Fig. 21.63 Xanthogranuloma.

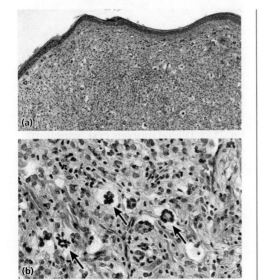

Fig. 21.64 Histopathology of a xantho-granuloma. a: Marked growth of tumor cells. b: Touton giant cells that have phagocytosed fat (arrows).

Verruciform xanthoma

This is a granular-surfaced, pedunculated tumor ranging in color from normal skin color to red and resembling a mulberry, frequently occurring in the genitalia. Serum lipid is not elevated. Histopathologically, there is infiltration of multiple fat-rich foam cells to the dermal papillary and subpapillary layers.

Multicentric reticulohistiocytosis

Firm brown or yellowish papules or nodules occur on the dorsa of the hands and fingers, around the nail plates, and in the elbow regions (Fig. 21.65). They may coalesce and form plaques. Symmetrical and destructive arthritis also occurs. The pathogenesis is thought to be reactive proliferation of phagocytic and activated monocytes or macrophage-derived histiocytes. Infiltration of histiocyte-like cells containing opaque eosinophilic cellular cytoplasm is observed histopathologically.

Benign cephalic histiocytosis

Dispersed reddish-brown patches, papules, and nodules of 3–10 mm in diameter occur, most commonly on the face, earlobes, and neck of infants (Fig. 21.66). Intradermal infiltration of mononuclear histiocyte-like cells is found histopathologically. Differentiation from Langerhans cell histiocytosis (see Chapter 22) is necessary. The tumor cells are CD68 positive, S-100 protein negative, and CD1a negative. The skin lesion usually disappears spontaneously; benign cephalic histiocytosis is thought to be a juvenile xanthogranuloma.

Fat cell tumors

Lipoma
Lipoma may appear on any site of the body surface, singly or multiply (Fig. 21.67). It usually occurs subcutaneously and is soft and highly mobile. The skin lesion is soft and palpable. Lipoma tends to be asymptomatic but pressure on nerves may produce pain.

Proliferation of mature fat tissue is seen. The tumor cells are characterized by a thin covering of connective tissue. Depending on the mesenchymal tissue elements in the skin lesion, lipoma may be called fibrolipoma, angiolipoma or myolipoma. Angiolipoma tends to occur multiply and is often accompanied by tenderness. Lipoblastic cells may also be seen. All these are benign mesenchymal cell tumors. Malignant transformation is rarely seen. Lipomas extend gradually, and excision may be conducted if necessary.

Muscular tissue tumors

Leiomyoma
Leiomyoma derived from the arrector pili muscle is cutaneous leiomyoma, that from the vascular smooth muscle is angioleiomyoma, and that from the dartos fascia is genital leiomyoma. A solitary or sometimes multiple tumor of up to about 1 cm in diameter occurs, often accompanied by pain and tenderness (Fig. 21.68). Angioleiomyoma, which most commonly occurs in the lower extremities of adult women, is accompanied by intense paroxysmal pain caused by exposure to cold. Scrotal leiomyoma is painless. Leiomyosarcoma may occur in rare cases.

Osteosis tumors

Osteoma cutis
Osteoma cutis is ectopic bone formation on the head and on the skin of the extremities. It is divided into primary osteoma cutis, which occurs in newborns and

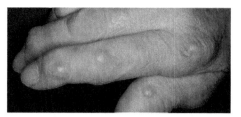
Fig. 21.65 Multicentric reticulohistiocytosis. Multiple firm yellowish nodules and papules occur on the dorsum of the hand and fingers.

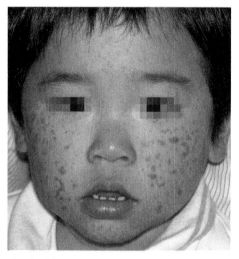
Fig. 21.66 Benign cephalic histiocytosis.

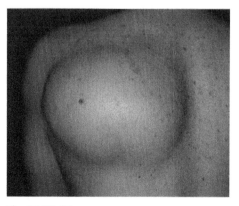
Fig. 21.67 Lipoma.

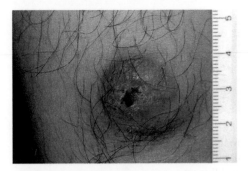

Fig. 21.68 Leiomyoma.

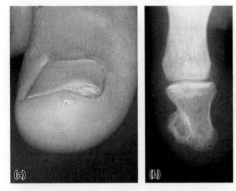

Fig. 21.69 Subungual exostosis. a: Clinical features. b: X-ray image.

infants, and secondary osteoma cutis. Secondary osteoma cutis is caused by inflammation from acne vulgaris. Single or multiple very firm papules, nodules or plaques occur. The lesions may adhere to the bone tissue underneath. In cases with multiple lesions, the possibility of McCune–Albright syndrome (MEMO, see Chapter 20) should be considered.

Subungual exostosis

Bone tissue derived from the distal end of a finger or toe proliferates, pushes the skin up, and appears under the nail plate (Fig. 21.69a). It occurs in people between the ages of 10 and 30. The big toe is most frequently involved. Intense pain and deformity in the nail plate are present. Subungual exostosis should be differentiated from glomus tumor. X-ray is useful (Fig. 21.69b). Excision is the main treatment.

Hematopoietic tumors

Lymphocytoma cutis (synonyms: lymphadenosis benigna cutis, pseudo-lymphoma)

Lymphocytoma cutis may occur as the result of an insect sting or bite, external injury, sunlight or Lyme disease; however, most cases are idiopathic. A dark red, dome-shaped tumor of 1–2 cm diameter occurs, usually on the face (Fig. 21.70). The lesion is elastic and smooth-surfaced. Ulceration does not occur. The lesion appears solitarily in most cases and disappears spontaneously several months after onset. Histopathologically, a lymphoid follicle structure with little atypism forms. Infiltration of various cells, including plasma cells, hystiocytes, and eosinophils, is observed. Differentiation from cutaneous B cell lymphoma is important; follicle formation is the main characteristic of lymphocytoma cutis, various types of cell infiltration are seen, and atypism is not found in lymphocytes. Lymphocytoma cutis has a good prognosis, although it progresses to lymphoma in rare cases.

Kimura's disease

Kimura's disease, whose cause is unknown, occurs commonly on the face of pubertal men. Solitary or multiple, flat or dome-shaped, soft, elastic, partially nodular and subcutaneous or intradermal tumors 5–10 cm in diameter appear. The surface of the lesion is brownish, and itching may be present (Fig. 21.71).

Subcutaneous lymphatic follicle formation and marked eosinophilic infiltration are observed histopathologically. Kimura's disease is characterized by the increase of eosinophils in the peripheral blood and bone marrow, and elevated IgE level.

It may be accompanied by atopic dermatitis and pruritus. Local steroid injection is effective. This condition is chronic. Differentiation between Kimura's disease and angiolymphoid hyperplasia with eosinophilia (ALHE, see the next section) has been controversial.

Angiolymphoid hyperplasia with eosinophilia (ALHE)

A firm, bright or dark red nodule several centimeters in diameter occurs, frequently on the peripheral auriculae, forehead or temporal area (Fig. 21.72). The skin lesion is a vascular proliferation of epithelial cells that contain abundant cytoplasm. Dense infiltration of eosinophils and lymphocytes is often found in the peripheral blood vessels. Although ALHE resembles Kimura's disease when a subcutaneous lesion is present, it can be differentiated from Kimura's disease because it lacks the proliferation of abnormal vessels.

The main treatment for ALHE is local injection of steroids; nevertheless, the disease is intractable. Dye laser therapy is effective in some cases.

Mastocytosis (synonyms: urticaria pigmentosa, mastocytoma)

- Mast cells proliferate and become tumorous.
- Urticaria is caused by rubbing (Darier's sign).

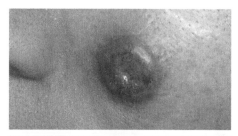
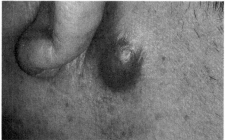
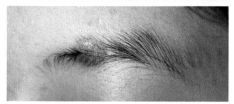
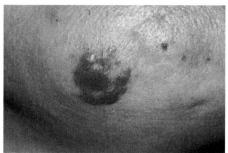

Fig. 21.70 Lymphocytoma cutis.

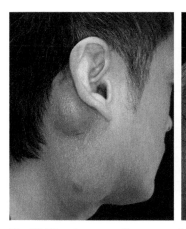
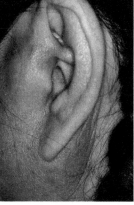

Fig. 21.71 Kimura's disease. Subcutaneous nodule and tumor on the peripheral auriculae.

MEMO 21–9 Lymphocytic infiltration of the skin (Jessner)

An asymptomatic, infiltrative plaque ranging in color from light pink to reddish-brown occurs, most frequently on the face. Although it disappears spontaneously, it may recur. Dense lymphocytic infiltration is found in the dermis, especially in the peripheral appendages. Differentiation from discoid lupus erythematosus (DLE) or malignant lymphoma is important.

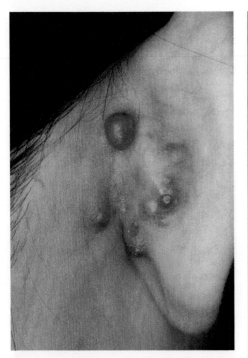

Fig. 21.72 Angiolymphoid hyperplasia with eosinophilia (ALHE). Multiple firm, itching, dark red nodules 3–10 mm in diameter appear.

- It occurs most frequently in infants, healing spontaneously by adulthood. When the onset is in adulthood, the disease is intractable.
- Urticarial attacks may recur in some cases.

Clinical features

The onset of mastocytosis is in the first year after birth, in most cases. The adult type has an onset at puberty or thereafter. In infant mastocytosis, multiple round or spindled brown patches or small nodules of up to 1 cm diameter occur after recurrent urticaria on the face and trunk. A solitary nodule several centimeters in diameter may occur in rare cases (Table 21.2). When mechanical stimulation is applied to sites with eruptions, histamine is released from mast cells, leading to the formation of urticaria (Darier's sign; Fig. 21.73). Urticaria may be caused all over the body by bathing or rubbing with a towel, leading to systemic symptoms such as flushing, nausea, vomiting, diarrhea, stomach ache, fever, cardiac palpitation, breathing difficulty, and shock (urticarial attacks).

In adult mastocytosis, these symptoms first appear at puberty or thereafter, and the eruptions and systemic symptoms tend to be moderate. Darier's sign is not significantly noticeable. In some cases, extremely itchy diffuse eruptions may occur and progress to systemic mastocytosis. Systemic mastocytosis is accompanied by lymph node enlargement, splenohepatomegaly, osteoporosis, and osteosclerosis. Thrombocytopenic bleeding tendency is present. Most cases are indolent systemic mastocytosis; however, the condition may progress to leukemia (mast cell leukemia).

Table 21.2 Classification of cutaneous mastocytosis.

Disease	Typical age of onset	Clinical features
Urticaria pigmentosa	Child > adult	Several to thousands of brown macules and nodules occur. Blisters may form.
Mastocytoma of skin	Child	A brownish nodule occurs singly.
Diffuse cutaneous mastocytosis	Child	The skin on the entire body thickens diffusely and presents an orange peel-like appearance.
Telangiectasia macularis eruptiva perstans	Adult	Multiple vaguely demarcated, dark red macules with capillary dilation occur. Darier's sign is often negative.

Classification and pathogenesis

Mast cells that become tumorous and proliferate in the skin or in the whole body are stimulated, leading to the release of histamine and heparin, which results in urticaria. Mastocytosis in which localized cutaneous lesions occur is called cutaneous mastocytoma. When a solitary lesion occurs, it is called mastocytoma. When tumorous lesions spread to the bone marrow, gastro-intestinal tract or spleen, it is called systemic mastocytosis. The pathogenesis is unknown.

Pathology

In the upper dermal layer, there is abnormal proliferation of polygonal mast cells of various sizes that stain metachromatically in toluidine blue (Fig. 21.74). It is classified by the proliferative pattern into Unna mastocytosis and Róna mastocytosis. In the former, multiple proliferative foci form map-like shapes resembling islands. In the latter, a few dispersed perivascular foci form. Róna mastocytosis with little cell infiltration is often seen in adult mastocytosis. Darier's sign is not clearly observed in many cases. Increases in melanin granules are observed in the epidermal suprabasal cell layer and basal layer in pigmented areas of the skin lesion.

Treatment and prognosis

Any stimulation that may induce the release of histamine, such as bathing or rubbing of the skin, should be avoided. Treatment for urticarial attacks is the same as for general urticaria (administration of antihistamine).

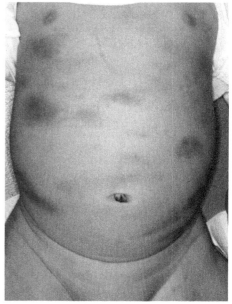
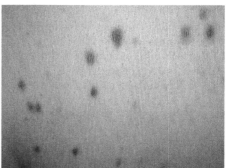

Fig. 21.73-1 Mastocytosis.

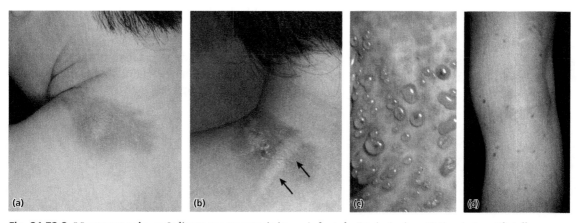

(a)   (b)   (c)   ((d))

Fig. 21.73-2 Mastocytosis. a: Solitary mastocytosis in an infant. b: Darier's sign: Urticaria is artificially caused by mechanical pressure. c: Mastocytosis with blistering. d: Mastocytosis in an adult (lower extremity).

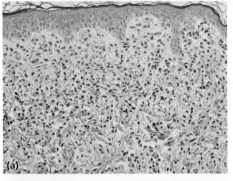

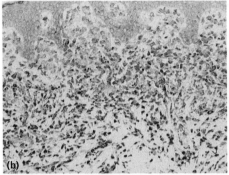

Fig. 21.74 Histopathology of mastocytosis (Unna mastocytosis). a: Mast cells of mastocytosis in HE staining. b: The mast cells stain metachromatically purple, not blue, with toluidine blue (metachromasia).

A solitary mastocytoma may be excised. Infant mastocytosis heals spontaneously in several years, possibly over a dozen years. It does not need treatment, as long as there are few eruptions and no severe attacks. Adult mastocytosis does not heal spontaneously and is intractable.

Plasmacytosis

Multiple brown plaques with palpable infiltration occur, mainly on the trunk (Fig. 21.75). Histopathologically, plasmacytic infiltration is found in many locations. Plasmacytosis is reported from Japan more often than in other areas of the world. Hypergammaglobulinemia and lymph node swelling are present.

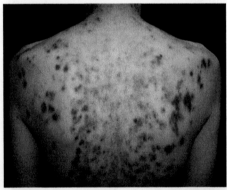

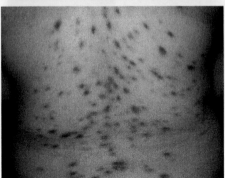

Fig. 21.75 Plasmacytosis.

CHAPTER 22

Malignant skin tumors, lymphomas, and melanomas

Tumors, whether malignant or benign, should be examined to determine the skin component from which they originate. The clinical features, course of progression, and prognosis differ according to the cells from which the tumor derives. Malignant skin tumors may derive from (1) epidermal or follicular keratinocytes, (2) skin appendages such as sebaceous and other sweat glands or (3) intradermal mesenchymal cells. The benign tumors described in Chapter 21 may become malignant, in which case they are given malignant diagnostic names. This chapter introduces malignant tumors, including lymphomas of the skin and melanomas, that have relatively high incidences.

Malignant skin tumors

Epidermal and follicular tumors

Basal cell carcinoma (synonym: basal cell epithelioma)

- This is a malignant skin tumor with a high incidence.
- It is induced by UV light and occurs most commonly in the elderly, particularly on the midline of the face.
- Small grayish-black nodules appear at the edge of the tumor. The center of the tumor may be ulcerated.
- Localized intense infiltration may be present. Metastasis rarely occurs. The prognosis is good.
- Excision is the basic treatment.

Clinical features

Basal cell carcinoma (BCC) occurs most frequently in men and women aged 40 and older. There are small, firm, waxy, glossy, blackish-brown (pearly) nodules at the periphery of the skin lesion (Fig. 22.1). Telangiectasia often occurs in and at the periphery of the lesion. The face, especially its midline, is affected in 80% of cases. The lesion appears blackish-brown in most cases in Asians; however, it is usually normal skin color in Caucasians. BCC is subclassified according to the clinical features.

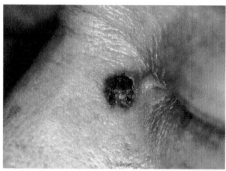
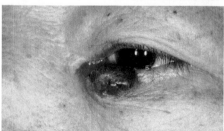
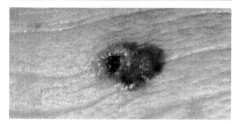

Fig. 22.1-1 Basal cell carcinoma.

Shimizu's Dermatology, Second Edition. Hiroshi Shimizu.
© 2017 John Wiley & Sons, Ltd. Published 2017 by John Wiley & Sons, Ltd.

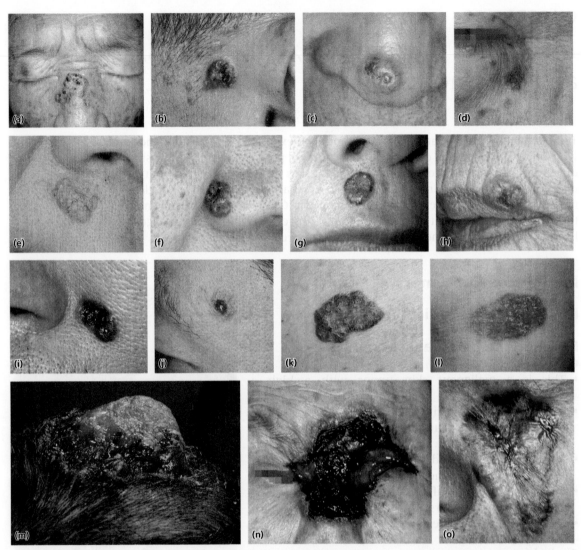

Fig. 22.1-2 Basal cell carcinoma (BCC). Various clinical features are seen. a–j: Nodular BCC. k,l: Superficial BCC. m: BCC. Because the BCC was left untreated, it damaged the bone and infiltrated into the brain. n: BCC that infiltrated into the eyeball. o: Morpheaform BCC.

- **Nodular (ulcerative) BCC:** more than 80% of BCCs are of this type. Small, firm, black nodules coalesce, accompanied by epidermal telangiectasia. The center of the lesion often ulcerates (rodent ulcer).
- **Superficial BCC:** a flatly elevated, infiltrative plaque ranging in color from red to blackish-brown gradually expands. This type often affects the trunk.
- **Morpheaform BCC:** this is an oval, infiltrative plaque with an atrophic, slightly concave center. It resembles morphea (see Chapter 12).

- **Pinkus type (fibroepithelial basal cell carcinoma of Pinkus):** small single or multiple pedunculated tumors occur, often in the midline of the lumbar and back sacral region.

Pathogenesis

Basal cell carcinoma results from the proliferation of the embryonic epithelium (primary epithelial germ cells), which differentiates into various organs. The occurrence of BCC is thought to be associated with abnormality in the *PTCH* and SMO genes. Sunlight, traumatic injury, radiation, and scarring are also associated with the occurrence of BCC.

It may occur secondary to an underlying disease, such as xeroderma pigmentosum, basal cell nevus carcinoma syndrome, chronic radiodermatitis, chronic arsenic poisoning or sebaceous nevus. In such cases, the young may also be affected, and the skin lesions are multiple (Fig. 22.2).

Pathology

Basal cell carcinoma is the proliferation of tumor cells that resemble epidermal basal cells (Fig. 22.3). The cells have a large oval nucleus, a small amount of cytoplasm, and low atypicality. The tumor cells occur in a palisading pattern (palisading arrangement) at the periphery. Connective tissue proliferates around the tumor. BCC is characterized by the presence of spaces between the tumor and the surrounding stroma that result from sectioning (separation artifact). Epidermis-derived and follicle-derived melanocytes are found mingled. The abundance of melanophages in the stroma results in the clinical blackish color. BCCs are histopathologically divided into nodular, adenoid, keratotic, cystic, and other types (Fig. 22.4).

> ### MEMO 22–1 Mohs micrographic surgery
>
> In this technique, a tumor is removed layer by layer while the completeness of tumor removal is determined histopathologically. The removed tissue is flash-frozen as samples to determine whether the tumor has been completely removed. The procedure is mainly used in treating basal cell carcinoma and squamous cell carcinoma. The advantages are the minimal invasiveness from minimal removal and the low recurrence rate.

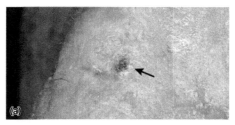
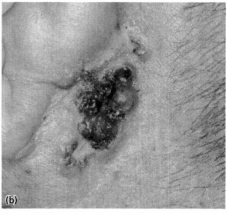

Fig. 22.2 Basal cell carcinoma (BCC) from underlying disease. a: BCC in a patient with xeroderma pigmentosum (group D) (arrow shows the lesion). b: BCC on a sebaceous nevus.

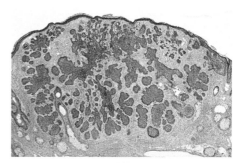
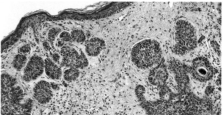

Fig. 22.3 Histopathology of basal cell carcinoma.

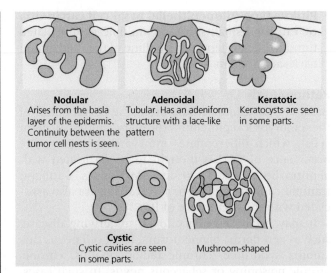

Nodular
Arises from the basla layer of the epidermis. Continuity between the tumor cell nests is seen.

Adenoidal
Tubular. Has an adeniform structure with a lace-like pattern

Keratotic
Keratocysts are seen in some parts.

Cystic
Cystic cavities are seen in some parts.

Mushroom-shaped

Fig. 22.4 Histopathology of basal cell carcinoma.

Differential diagnosis

Basal cell carcinoma should be differentiated from nevus cell nevus, blue nevus, Spitz nevus, seborrheic keratosis, melanoma, acne vulgaris, and pyoderma gangrenosum. Dermoscopy is useful in diagnosing BCC (see Chapter 3). Superficial BCC should be differentiated from psoriasis and Bowen's disease, and morpheaform BCC should be differentiated from morphea, discoid lupus erythematosus, granuloma annulare, and keloid.

Treatment

Surgical removal of the lesion with 3–10 mm of surrounding healthy skin is the basic treatment. As the face is frequently affected, the surgery often involves local skin flap or skin graft. Irradiation therapy, topical chemotherapy, cryotherapy, and photodynamic therapy may be chosen.

Prognosis

Basal cell carcinoma tends not to metastasize. The prognosis is good. Unless excised, however, it continues to proliferate, destroying normal tissue.

Squamous cell carcinoma

- This cancer is caused by the malignant proliferation of keratinocytes.
- In situ lesions, including those of solar keratosis and Bowen's disease, and scarring lesions are sometimes accompanied by squamous cell carcinoma (SCC).

- A firm nodule occurs, frequently on a sun-exposed area of the body. It often necrotizes and ulcerates, giving off a foul odor.
- The less keratinous are the cells, the more undifferentiated and malignant is the cancer.
- Surgical removal, lymph node dissection, radiation therapy, and chemotherapy are the main treatments.

Clinical features

Squamous cell carcinoma occurs in elderly people solitarily on sun-exposed areas of the body, such as the face and the dorsum of the hands. Small papules and nodules appear on preexisting lesions and gradually extend to form tumors or intractable ulcers (Fig. 22.5). They proliferate, taking on a cauliflower-like appearance. The skin lesion is often accompanied by keratinous substances and crusts. When the surface of the lesion ulcerates, secondary bacterial

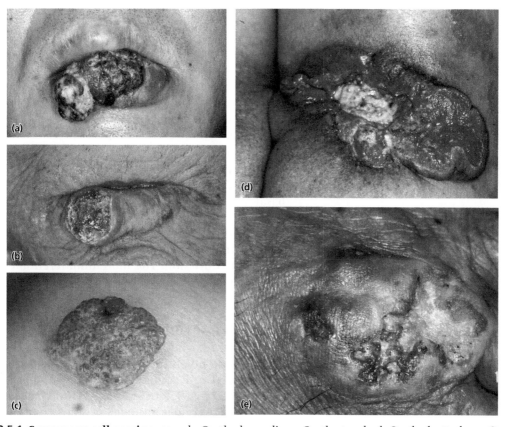

Fig. 22.5-1 Squamous cell carcinoma. a,b: On the lower lip. c: On the trunk. d: On the buttocks. e: On the dorsum of the hand.

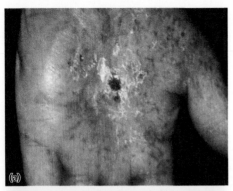

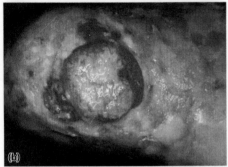

Fig. 22.5-2 Squamous cell carcinoma. a: On the palm, where chronic radiodermatitis occurred. b: In a patient with recessive dystrophic epidermolysis bullosa.

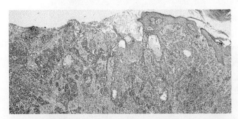

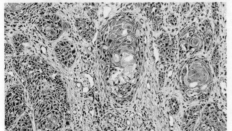

Fig. 22.6 Histopathology of squamous cell carcinoma.

Table 22.1 Preexisting lesions of squamous cell carcinoma.

Type of disease	Disease or condition
Scarring	Burn, chronic radiodermatitis, lupus vulgaris, chronic pyoderma, chronic discoid lupus erythematosus
Precancerous	Bowen's disease, actinic keratosis, actinic cheilitis, leukoplakia, xeroderma pigmentosum, porokeratosis, lichen sclerosis et atrophicus (external genitalia)
Other	Phimosis, congenital premature aging syndromes (Rothmund–Thomson syndrome and the like), dystrophic epidermolysis bullosa, condyloma acuminatum, lichen planus

infection accompanied by distinct odor occurs. SCC tends to spread to the regional lymph nodes, which then feel firm when palpated.

Pathogenesis

Squamous cell carcinoma frequently occurs on a preexisting chronic scarring lesion. In addition to the preceding lesions shown in Table 22.1, carcinogenic factors such as exposure to sunlight (UV), arsenic, tar, and irradiation are associated with onset.

Pathology

Abnormal keratinocytes that destroy the epidermal basal layer are found within the infiltrative and thickened epidermis (Fig. 22.6). SCC is characterized by individual cell keratinization, disturbance in cellular arrangement, nuclear atypicality, cancer pearls, and cellular division. The more undifferentiated and malignant are the cells, the less keratinization may occur.

Diagnosis and differential diagnosis

Differential diagnosis is made by histopathology. Lymph node involvement and distant metastases are determined by ultrasound and computed tomography (CT) to identify the disease stage (TNM classification; Table 22.2). Keratoacanthoma, actinic keratosis, basal cell carcinoma, and deep mycoses are differentiated from SCC.

Table 22.2 TNM classification and stage grouping of SCC (UICC,2002).

T classification (primary lesion)	
T0	Primary lesion is not found.
Tis	Carcinoma in situ
T1	Lesions of 2 cm or less in diameter
T2	Lesions of 2 cm to 5 cm in diameter
T3	Lesions of 5 cm or more in diameter
T4	Lesions that invade tissues deeper than skin (e.g., cartilage, muscle, bone)

N classification (regional lymph nodes)	
N0	Lesions without metastasis in regional lymph node
N1	Lesions with metastasis in regional lymph node

M classification (distant metastasis)	
M0	Lesions without distant metastasis
M1	Lesions with distant metastasis

Staging			
Stage 0	Tis	N0	M0
Stage I	T1	N0	M0
Stage II	T2,3	M0	N0
Stage III	T4	N0	M0
	anyT	N1	M0
Stage IV	anyT	anyN	M1

Treatment

Surgical removal is the first-line treatment. Lesions are excised with 4–10 mm of adjoining normal skin. Radical lymph node dissection is conducted in cases with lymph node involvement. Combined modality therapies, such as irradiation therapy and chemotherapy (Fig. 22.7), are used in progressive cases.

Actinic keratosis (AK) (synonyms: senile keratosis, solar keratosis)

- This is a subtype of squamous cell carcinoma in situ.
- UV exposure induces keratinocytic atypia, particularly in the basal cell layer. The atypical keratinocytes proliferate in the epidermis (dyskeratosis).
- Vaguely marginated erythema or keratotic lesions accompanied by scaling and crusting occur in elderly people, on sun-exposed sites of the body. The disorder is asymptomatic.

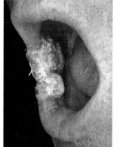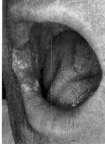

Fig. 22.7 Chemotherapeutic example of squamous cell carcinoma. The lesion markedly reduced in size after intraarterial injection of cisplatin.

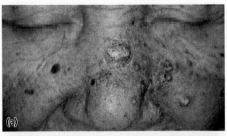

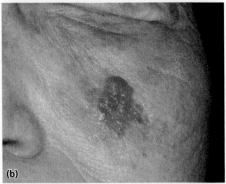

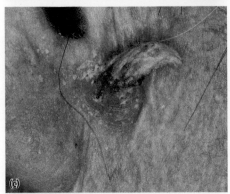

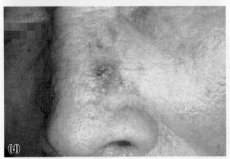

Fig. 22.8 Actinic keratosis. a: Multiple actinic keratosis on the face.
b: Erythematous lesions are present.
c: A cutaneous horn formed on the preauricular area. d: Erythema with keratinization on the nasal dorsum.

- Horn-like protrusions (cutaneous horns) form in cases with marked keratinization.
- Cryotherapy, excision, and topical anticancer agents are the main treatments.

Clinical features

A light-pink erythematous plaque several millimeters to 1 cm in diameter occurs on a sun-exposed area of the body, such as the face or dorsal hand. The plaque is covered with scales and crusts. The margin of the plaque is often vague. Keratinization is usually intense. Grayish-white keratotic nodules or horn-like protrusions (cutaneous horns) may form (Fig. 22.8). The skin lesion occurs singly or multiply, most frequently in people over age 60. Nearly all elderly Caucasians are affected. Actinic keratosis occurs in infancy in patients with xeroderma pigmentosum.

Pathogenesis

Epidermal keratinocytes that are damaged by chronic UV exposure proliferate abnormally in the dermis. This is a type of squamous cell carcinoma in situ.

Pathology

There are six histological types of actinic keratosis (Fig. 22.9, Table 22.3). Malignant changes are localized in the epidermis, and follicular and sweat pore regions remain normal. Atypism is found in the lower epidermal basal layer. Solar elastosis is present in the dermis.

Diagnosis and differential diagnosis

Skin biopsy is conducted when it is difficult to differentiate actinic keratosis from seborrheic keratosis and senile lentigo.

Treatment and prognosis

The tumor is excised. Other treatment options include cryotherapy and topical application of anticancer agents such as 5-FU and imiquimod. Some cases progress to squamous cell carcinoma, often indicated by aggravation and enlargement of the peripheral erythema and rapid enlargement of ulcers.

Bowen's disease

- This is a type of squamous cell carcinoma in situ.
- It presents as a sharply marginated plaque, ranging from reddish-brown to blackish-brown, with a diameter of 1–10 cm.

Table 22.3 Histopathological findings of actinic keratosis.

Type	Findings
Commonly found in all types	Parakeratosis, atypical suprabasal cells, hyperkeratosis, solar elastosis
Hypertrophic	Mainly acanthosis and hyperkeratosis
Atrophic	Atrophy of the epidermal basal cell layer, loss of the epidermal rete ridges
Bowenoid	Findings resembling those of Bowen's disease.
Acantholytic	Acantholysis immediately above the epidermal basal cell layer
Pigmented	Increase in melanin granules
Lichenoid	Marked lichenoid reaction

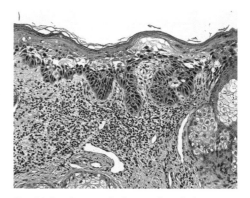

Fig. 22.9 Histopathology of actinic keratosis. Marked atypism is observed, especially in the lower epidermal layer.

MEMO 22–2 Verrucous carcinoma

This is a subtype of squamous cell carcinoma with low-grade malignancy in which elevated keratotic nodules form (See figures).

Although localized proliferation of the tumor cells in the nodules is marked, the nodules rarely metastasize to other organs. Human papillomavirus is associated in some cases. Verrucous carcinoma is classified by the affected site into oral mucous verrucous carcinoma (oral florid papillomatosis; MEMO, see Chapter 22), genital verrucous carcinoma, and plantar verrucous carcinoma. Surgical removal is the most reliable treatment.

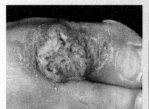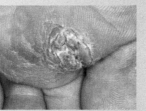

MEMO 22–3 Oral florid papillomatosis

A keratotic or infiltrative plaque varying in shape from papillary to cauliflower-like occurs on the lip or oral mucosa of the elderly. It is a type of verrucous carcinoma. There are cases that are associated with human papillomavirus, smoking, and leukoplakia. Severe thickening and keratinization of the epidermis are pathologically observed; however, infiltrative proliferation is not present.

MEMO 22–4 Actinic cheilitis

Dryness, cracking, and erosion on the lips occur in association with UV exposure. The condition is chronic and intractable, persisting for many years. It is an actinic keratosis on the lips and is understood as a carcinoma precursor.

MEMO 22–5 Arsenical keratosis

This skin disease is caused by chronic arsenic poisoning. Multiple hyperkeratotic papules resembling clavi appear on the palms and soles, and the lesions coalesce and form verrucous plaques. Erythemas with scaling may occur on the trunk. Arsenical keratosis may progress to squamous cell carcinoma, an infiltrative cancer. Basal cell carcinoma may occur as a complication. Other skin diseases associated with chronic arsenic poisoning include multiple Bowen's disease and arsenic melanosis, in which raindrop pigmentation and depigmentation are present. Machine oil keratosis and tar keratosis are examples of other chemical-induced precancers.

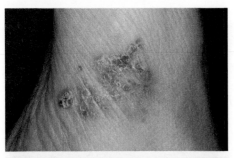

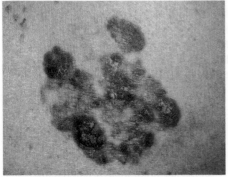

Fig. 22.10-1 Bowen's disease.

- Multiple lesions may be induced by chronic arsenic poisoning.
- Histopathologically, atypical cells are seen in all layers of the epidermis. It is characterized by individual cell keratinization and cell clumping.
- Surgical removal and cryotherapy are the main treatments.

Clinical features

Bowen's disease occurs solitarily, in elderly people. A round or oval, flatly elevated, relatively sharply edged infiltrative plaque of several centimeters in diameter forms, ranging from brown to reddish-brown. Underneath the scales and crusts that cover the plaque, red erosion is present (Fig. 22.10). Small nodules may be present.

Pathology

The pathological findings are those of squamous cell carcinoma in situ. Hyperkeratosis, parakeratosis, dyskeratosis (keratinization of individual cells), and multinucleated dyskeratotic cells (clumping cells) are found in the epidermis. These atypical cells proliferate in all the epidermal layers (Fig. 22.11).

Pathogenesis

The cause of solitary Bowen's disease is unknown in many cases. UV exposure and human papillomavirus may induce the disease. Multiple Bowen's disease is highly associated with arsenic intake. Therefore, history taking on predisposing factors is important, such as the location of birth and the possibility of chronic agricultural chemical poisoning (e.g., from arsenic).

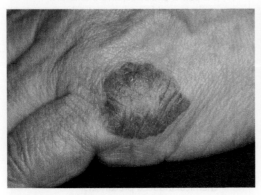

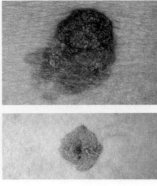

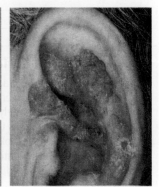

Fig. 22.10-2 Bowen's disease.

MEMO 22–6 Erythroplasia of Queyrat

Erythroplasia of Queyrat is a Bowen's disease that occurs in the penis (left figure). The lesion is red and presents as a velvet plaque. Similar lesions occur in the female external genitalia or in the oral cavity (right figure). Erythroplasia of Queyrat tends to progress to squamous cell carcinoma.

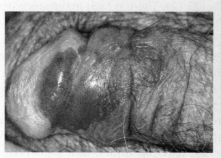
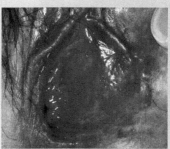

It is differentiated from chronic eczema, psoriasis, actinic keratosis, extramammary Paget's disease, and the superficial type of basal cell carcinoma. Differential diagnosis is made by skin biopsy.

Treatment
Surgical removal is the first-line treatment. Topical anticancer agents (5-FU, imiquimod, bleomycin) and cryotherapy are also useful.

Prognosis
Unless treated, the lesion destroys the epidermal basement membrane and progresses to squamous cell carcinoma.

Leukoplakia
Definition
A white patch or plaque occurs in the mucous membranes and at the mucocutaneous junction. The WHO defines oral leukoplakia as a white patch or plaque that cannot be characterized clinically or pathologically as any other disease, such as lichen planus candidiasis. However, in dermatology, a condition with patches of white plaques, including those caused by various diseases, is often clinically called leukoplakia. It is important to recognize that some cases of leukoplakia are precancerous and can progress to squamous cell carcinoma.

Clinical features
Men over age 50, especially smokers, are most commonly affected. The oral cavity and lips are most frequently

MEMO 22–7 (Oral) Hairy leukoplakia

White plaques with a hairy appearance occur in the oral cavity, particularly on the sides of the tongue. An opportunistic infection of the EB virus, it is strongly associated with HIV infection.

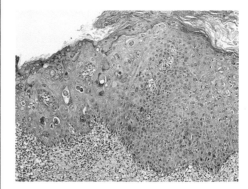

Fig. 22.11 Histopathology of Bowen's disease. Dyskeratotic cells and clumping cells are present in all epidermal layers.

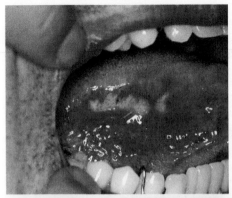

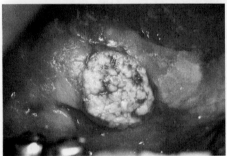

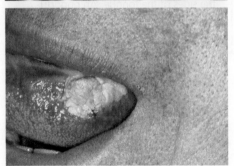

Fig. 22.12 Leukoplakia.

involved. The tongue, nipples, and genital membranes (glans penis, vagina, perianal region) are affected. The lesion is often a slightly infiltrative, clearly marginated plaque with various morphological findings (smooth-surfaced, keratinous, verrucous, papillary, and/or erosive) (Fig. 22.12). There is high malignancy when an erythroplasia-like lesion is produced (erythroleukoplakia).

Pathogenesis, diagnosis, and differential diagnosis

It is thought that smoking may induce cellular atypism, leading to leukoplakia of the mucosa. Disorders that produce white plaques include lichen planus, discoid lupus erythematosus, syphilis, candidiasis, white sponge nevus, external injury, and graft-versus-host disease. Skin biopsy is necessary for differential diagnosis.

Pathology

The epidermis thickens, caused by hyperkeratosis. Varying degrees of atypism and dyskeratosis are found in the keratinized cells.

Treatment

If there is malignancy, treatment by surgical excision, the administration of topical anticancer agents, laser therapy or cryotherapy should be carried out. Complete smoking cessation is necessary.

Keratoacanthoma

- This appears suddenly and solitarily on the face or dorsal hand, grows rapidly, and forms a dome-shaped, cratered nodule.
- Most cases heal spontaneously in several months.
- It is important to differentiate it from squamous cell carcinoma, which it closely resembles histopathologically. Generally, excision is recommended.

Clinical features

More than 90% of cases involve the face. Middle-aged and older men are most frequently affected. Keratoacanthoma is solitary in most cases. In young people with xeroderma pigmentosum, the lesions tend to occur multiply.

A small papule occurs and rapidly enlarges in several weeks to a diameter of 1–2 cm, resulting in the formation of a dome-shaped or hemispheric nodule (Fig. 22.13). The nodule is clearly marginated and elastically soft or firm, and ranges from normal skin color to light pink or dark red. After it rapidly enlarges to a certain size, keratinization occurs at the center of the nodule, to form a large keratin plug and a crater-like appearance (keratin-filled crater). Many cases heal spontaneously in several months, with scarring.

Pathogenesis

Many years of exposure to sun (UV) or tar, as well as human papillomavirus infection, smoking and external injury, are associated with the occurrence of keratoacanthoma.

Pathology

Hyperkeratosis is found at the center of the tumor, whose periphery is surrounded by proliferating supra-basal cells (Fig. 22.14). The suprabasal cells are charac-terized by clear eosinophilic cytoplasm and atypia, which resembles squamous cell carcinoma. Tumor cells appear to infiltrate the dermis, and lymphocytes and neutrophils infiltrate below the tumor. Keratoacanthoma is thought to be well-differentiated squamous cell carci-noma or pseudo-carcinoma.

Differential diagnosis

It is necessary to differentiate keratoacanthoma from squamous cell carcinoma (Table 22.4). In SCC, the border between the edge of the tumor and normal tissue is unclear, and there is asymmetrical mor-phology and a high tendency to infiltration. Squamous cell carcinoma enlarges far more slowly than keratoac-anthoma. Keratoacanthoma is also differentiated from basal cell carcinoma and molluscum contagiosum.

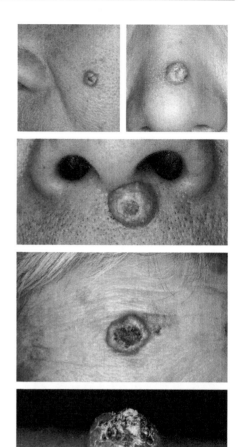

Fig. 22.13-1 Keratoacanthoma.
Keratoacanthoma is characterized by dome-shaped nodules with a volcano-like center.

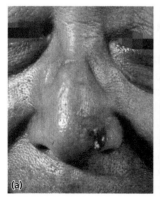 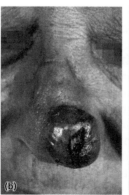 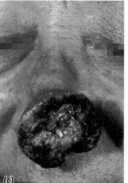 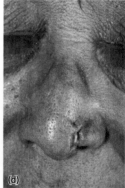

Fig. 22.13-2 Natural history of keratoacanthoma (from onset to spontaneous resolution). a: Onset. The lesion begins as a dome-shaped tumor 1 cm in diameter. b: The tumor gradually grows. c: It grows further. The center ruptures spontaneously. d: The lesion heals without treatment, with slight scarring.

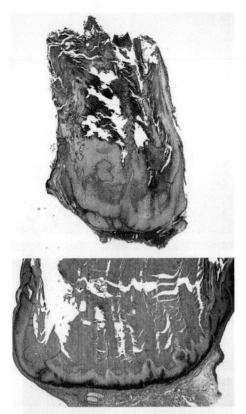

Fig. 22.14 Histopathology of keratoac-anthoma. There is marked hyperkeratosis at the center of the tumor. Suprabasal cells proliferate to envelop the tumor.

Table 22.4 Clinical differences between keratoacanthoma and squamous cell carcinoma (SCC).

	Keratoacanthoma	SCC
Site of onset	Most frequently the face (in 90% or more of cases)	Sites of preexisting lesions
Shape of eruption	Volcano-like	Erosive, cauliflower-like appearance
Eruption size change	1–2 cm in diameter at the peak	Slowly enlarges
Multiple, or solitary?	Solitary in many cases, multiple in some cases	Solitary in most cases
Growth	Proliferates by the week	Proliferates by the month to the year
Spontaneous regression?	Yes	No
Lymph node invasion?	No	Yes

Treatment

For diagnosis, it is necessary to examine the overall structure of the skin lesion. Total resection of the skin lesion, which is simultaneously a treatment, is recommended. If a pathological diagnosis is made, follow-up may be offered instead of treatment until the condition resolves. Irradiation, topical application or local injection of steroids or bleomycin, and administration of oral etretinate and cryotherapy are useful.

Sebaceous gland tumors

Sebaceous carcinoma

Sebaceous carcinoma is a skin cancer derived from sebaceous glands. Many cases of sebaceous carcinoma are of the ocular type, derived from meibomian gland tissue. Extraocular types derived from the sebaceous glands of the skin are rare. An orange-colored nodule occurs (Fig. 22.15). Histopathologically, the tumor cell nest contains atypical clear sebaceous cells. In the autosomal dominantly inherited Muir–Torre syndrome, multiple benign or malignant sebaceous tumors occur, often accompanied by visceral malignancies.

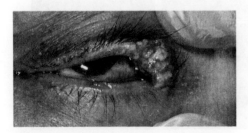

Fig. 22.15 Sebaceous carcinoma in the meibomian gland.

Follicular tumors

Trichilemmal carcinoma, malignant proliferating trichilemmal cyst, and malignant pilomatricoma are included in the rare types of malignant tumors derived from various cells of the hair follicles.

Sweat gland tumors

Mammary Paget's disease

- Infiltrative eczema-like erythema or erosion occurs on and around the nipples.
- The condition occurs most commonly in the opening of the lactiferous ducts of middle-aged women. It is a carcinoma in situ that derives from the lactiferous duct epithelia. It corresponds to breast cancer.
- A nodule does not form in most cases.
- It is not itchy, nor does it respond to topical steroids. Mammary Paget's disease can be distinguished from eczema by these characteristics.
- The treatments are the same as those for breast cancer.

Clinical features

A plaque with clearly circumscribed erythema, erosion, infiltration, and crusts appears, mainly on the nipple. The lesion gradually enlarges to the areola mammae and the surrounding area (Fig. 22.16). The lesion is slightly firm, palpable, and usually unilateral. Middle-aged women are most frequently affected. Bilateral mammary Paget's disease and mammary Paget's disease in men are extremely rare. Mammary Paget's disease accounts for 1–4% of all breast cancer cases. As the disease progresses, a palpable tumor forms in the breast and metastasizes to the regional lymph node (mainly the axillary lymph node).

Pathogenesis and pathology

Mammary Paget's disease is regarded as an intraductal carcinoma. Large, clear Paget cells are found in the epidermis, lactiferous ducts, and mammary glands. Although the skin lesion does not clinically appear to be severe, Paget cells often infiltrate lactiferous ducts and mammary glands more extensively than is clinically obvious. Immunostaining is positive for CK7 and CEA.

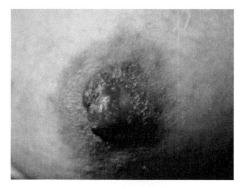

Fig. 22.16 Mammary Paget's disease. Infiltrative erythema is present on the nipple. The treatment for this disease is generally the same as for breast cancer.

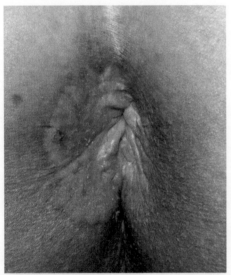

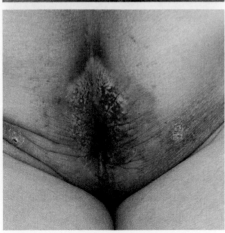

Fig. 22.17-1 Extramammary Paget's disease in the perianal region.

Differential diagnosis

Chronic eczema, tinea corporis, and basal cell carcinoma should be distinguished from mammary Paget's disease. Intractable eczematous lesions on the breast that do not respond to topical agents should be suspected of being mammary Paget's disease.

Treatment

The treatments are the same as those for breast cancer.

Extramammary Paget's disease

- Elderly people account for the majority of cases. Eczematous erythema and erosions resembling those found in mammary Paget's disease occur.
- It is thought to be an intraepidermal cancer that originates from the apocrine glands. The genitalia, anal region, and axillary fossae are most frequently involved.
- It occasionally destroys the basement membranes and progresses to invasive carcinoma.

Clinical features

Extramammary Paget's disease occurs most commonly in the elderly. A bright red infiltrative plaque resembling mammary Paget's disease appears (Fig. 22.17), most frequently on the genitalia, and less frequently on the perianal region, perineum, axillary fossa or umbilical region. Eczema, dermatitis or candidiasis may occur secondarily, and vaguely marginated lesions accompanied by itchiness may form. The lesion gradually spreads, with melanin deposition at the periphery in some cases. Extramammary Paget's disease occasionally destroys the basement membranes and develops a palpable small tumor in the lesion (Fig. 22.18). Regional lymph node metastasis occurs in advanced cases, in which case the prognosis is poor.

Pathogenesis

Extramammary Paget's disease is thought to originate from apocrine sweat gland cells.

Pathology

Large, bright, scattered or aggregated Paget cells are found in the epidermis, sweat ducts, and follicles (Fig. 22.19). The cells are positive for PAS, Alcian blue, CEA, and GCDFP-15, and negative for CK20.

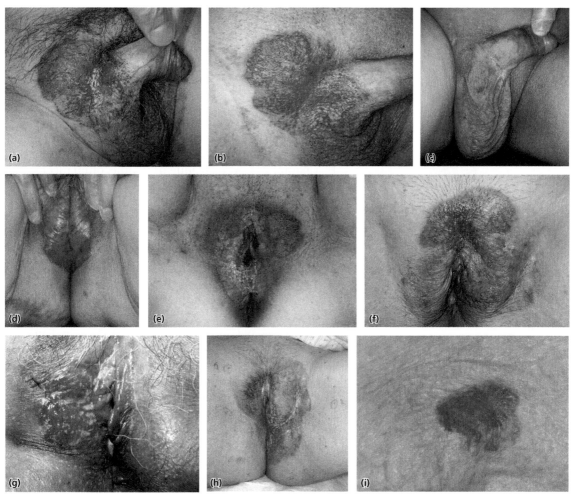

Fig. 22.17-2 Extramammary Paget's disease. a,b: Sharply demarcated erythematous plaques. c: A mix of hypopigmented macules and erythematous plaques. d–h: Extramammary Paget's disease on the labia majora of an elderly woman. i: Extramammary Paget's disease on the axillary fossa.

Differential diagnosis

Eczema, dermatitis, candidiasis, tinea cruris, Bowen's disease, Hailey–Hailey disease, and pemphigus vegetans are distinguished from extramammary Paget's disease. Tumor cells that resemble Paget cells may be seen in patients with dermal infiltration from rectal cancer or urinary tract cancer (Paget phenomenon). GCDFP-15 and CK20 staining are useful for differentiation. In the case of Paget phenomenon, GCDFP-15 is negative and CK20 is positive.

Treatment

To determine the area of the lesion, mapping biopsy is done (i.e., the locations of cancer cells are determined

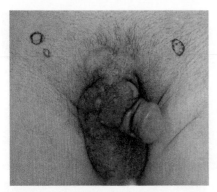

Fig. 22.18 Invasive extramammary Paget's disease that had been left untreated for a long time. A flat lesion elevated gradually, forming infiltrative nodules. The lesion destroyed the basal membrane and infiltrated the deep portions of the dermis. Metastasis to the regional lymph node was observed.

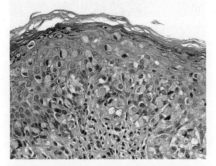

Fig. 22.19 Histopathology of extramammary Paget's disease. There are scattered Paget cells with large, clear cytoplasm.

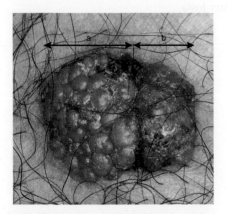

Fig. 22.20 Eccrine porocarcinoma arising from eccrine poroma. a: Eccrine porocarcinoma (malignant). b: Eccrine poroma (benign).

by collecting specimens in punch biopsies around the clinically determined lesion) and photodynamic diagnosis (PDD) is undertaken (see Chapter 5). The basic treatment is extensive surgical removal with a 1–3 cm margin including the peripheral normal skin. Irradiation and photodynamic therapies may be used in some cases.

Eccrine porocarcinoma

This is a malignant form of eccrine poroma (see Chapter 21). A red plaque or nodule, often ulcerative, occurs, most frequently on the lower legs of elderly people (Fig. 22.20). In most cases, eccrine porocarcinoma is clinically observed as a tumor that is a mix of eccrine poroma and eccrine porocarcinoma.

Microcystic adnexal carcinoma (MAC) (synonyms: syringoid eccrine carcinoma, sclerosing sweat duct carcinoma)

A firm, discoid, intradermal nodule 1–3 cm in diameter occurs, most commonly around the mouth of persons of middle age or older. The pathological findings resemble those of syringoma (see Chapter 21). Intense infiltration deep into the subcutaneous areas and slight atypism are found. Distant metastasis occurs rarely. After extensive resection, the site should be examined histopathologically for any remaining original lesions, because of the high frequency of local recurrence. For this reason, Mohs microsurgery is also effective.

Mucinous carcinoma of the skin

A nodule 2–3 cm in diameter occurs, frequently on the face or scalp (Fig. 22.21). The tumor is covered by abundant mucin. Mucinous carcinoma of the skin is thought to originate from eccrine sweat glands or apocrine sweat glands. The nuclei of tumor cells show slight atypism. Metastatic carcinoma of the skin with extreme mucus production from internal malignancies should be distinguished from mucinous carcinoma of the skin.

Nervous system tumors

Merkel cell carcinoma

- This skin cancer originates from Merkel cells of the epidermis. These cells are thought to be tactile receptor cells.

- A highly malignant, domed red tumor forms on the head, neck or extremities of elderly people.
- Extensive resection, irradiation, and chemotherapy are the main treatments.

Clinical features
A firm, domed nodule varying in color from light pink to purplish-red and with a diameter of 1–3 cm occurs, most frequently on the head and neck of elderly women (Fig. 22.22). The condition is usually asymptomatic.

Pathology
Small cells that lack cytoplasm and have round nuclei are found in a dense palisading pattern (Fig. 22.23). Dense-core granules that resemble Merkel cells are found on electron microscopy (Fig. 22.24). Immuno-histochemically, neuron-specific enolase (NSE) and chromogranin A are positive, and on CK20 staining the cytoplasm stains in a dot-like pattern.

Diagnosis and differential diagnosis
Merkel cell carcinoma is diagnosed by clinical features and histopathological tests. Adnexal malignant tumors, amelanotic malignant melanoma, and lymphoma are differentiated from it. Metastasis of small cell lung cancer to the skin presents the same pathology as Merkel cell carcinoma. If this carcinoma is suspected, examination for lung cancer should be performed. In small cell lung cancer, CK20 is generally negative.

Treatment and prognosis
Because of its metastatic and recurrent tendency, extensive excision and lymph node dissection are carried out. Radiation therapy and chemotherapy are also useful. Rare cases with spontaneous healing have been reported.

Malignant peripheral nerve sheath tumor (MPNST)
Malignant peripheral nerve sheath tumor is a malignant tumor that originates from Schwann cells. MPNST may occur in patients with neurofibromatosis type 1 (see Chapter 20). Extensive excision, amputation of the extremities, and chemotherapy are carried out. The prognosis is poor.

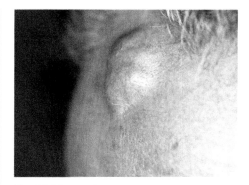

Fig. 22.21 Mucinous carcinoma of the skin.

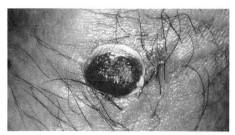

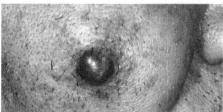

Fig. 22.22 Merkel cell carcinoma.

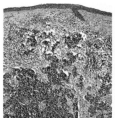 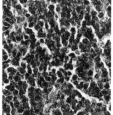

Fig. 22.23 Histopathology of Merkel cell carcinoma.

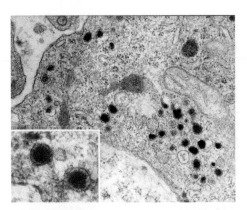

Fig. 22.24 Electron microscopic image of Merkel cell carcinoma, enlarged image of dense-core granules.

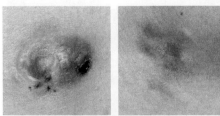

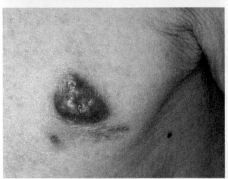

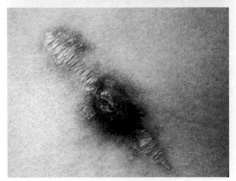

Fig. 22.25 Dermatofibrosarcoma protuberans.

Mesenchymal tumors

Fibrous tissue tumors
Dermatofibrosarcoma protuberans

Dermatofibrosarcoma protuberans (DFSP) is a malignant tumor that is thought to derive from fibroblasts, myofibroblasts or histiocytes. The trunk of adult men is most commonly involved. It begins as an intradermal or subcutaneous nodule that slowly forms a dome-shaped or fungiform tumor at the local site (Fig. 22.25). The tumor is firm and dark reddish-brown, often accompanied by erosion or crusts. A characteristic swirl arrangement of tumor cells and fibers called a storiform pattern is observed on histopathology (Fig. 22.26). Nuclear division and atypism are absent. The tumor cells are usually negative for blood coagulation factor XIIIa and positive for CD34. DFSP rarely metastasizes (fewer than 10% of cases); however, extensive resection is necessary because of its high tendency to recur locally.

Atypical fibroxanthoma

A firm nodule occurs, most frequently on a sun-exposed area in an elderly person. Spindle-shaped or histiocyte-like cells with low malignancy are found from the dermis to the subcutaneous layers. Some consider this identical to superficial malignant fibrous histiocytoma (MFH).

Epithelioid sarcoma

This is a rare malignant tumor. It occurs most commonly at the ends of the extremities and progresses relatively slowly. It begins as intradermal or subcutaneous nodules that gradually increase in number and size (Fig. 22.27). Epithelial cells with abundant eosinophilic components as observed histopathologically proliferate in a sheet-like formation or a palisading pattern. The center of the nodule is necrotic in many cases.

Epithelioid sarcoma should be differentiated from granuloma annulare and rheumatoid nodules. Epithelioid sarcoma cells are immunohistochemically keratin positive. Extensive resection is the basic treatment. When epithelioid sarcoma metastasizes, lymph nodes are often involved and the prognosis is poor.

Synovial sarcoma

A soft, painful tumor occurs, frequently in the large joint of an extremity, particularly in the knee of young adults. In rare cases, it occurs subcutaneously or subfascially. Chromosomal translocation t(X; 18) (p11.2;

Table 22.5 Classification of malignant fibrous histiocytoma (MFH).

Former classification	Disease name by WHO classification (2002)
Storiform-pleomorphic MFH	Undifferentiated high-grade pleomorphic sarcoma
Myxoid MFH	Myxofibrosarcoma
Giant cell MFH	Undifferentiated pleomorphic sarcoma with giant cells
Inflammatory MFH	Undifferentiated pleomorphic sarcoma with prominent inflammation
Angiomatoid MFH	Angiomatoid fibrous histiocytoma

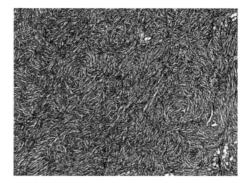

Fig. 22.26 Histopathology of dermatofibrosarcoma protuberans. Storiform pattern.

q11.2) is characteristically found in the cells of the sarcoma. The tumor grows slowly and metastasizes. The prognosis is poor. Extensive resection, chemotherapy, and long-term follow-up are essential.

Malignant fibrous histiocytoma

The proximal limb muscles and retroperitoneum of adults are most commonly involved. A painless, lobulated, multinodular subcutaneous tumor occurs in most cases (Fig. 22.28). Malignant fibrous histiocytoma (MFH) is composed of highly atypical fibroblast-like cells and histiocyte-like cells. It displays various pathological features, including giant cells and inflammatory cellular infiltration. This is the most frequently occurring soft tissue sarcoma; however, there is controversy over whether MFH is an independent entity. The WHO has proposed the classification shown in Table 22.5. The prognosis tends to be poor.

Tumors of fat cells
Liposarcoma

A liposarcoma is a malignant mesenchymal tumor that originates from fat cells. It is deep-seated, clearly defined, large, and nearly asymptomatic. According to the WHO classification, the malignant tumors are the well-differentiated, dedifferentiated, myxoid, round cell, and pleomorphic types. Well-differentiated liposarcoma, also called atypical lipomatous tumor, has a good prognosis. Extensive resection and chemotherapy are the main treatments.

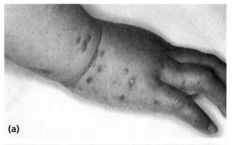

(a)

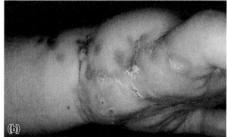

(b)

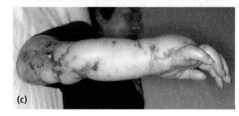

(c)

Fig. 22.27 The course of epithelioid sarcoma. a: It begins as nodules 1 cm in diameter. b,c: The nodules gradually increase in number. The tumors become infiltrative and enlarged.

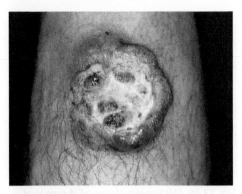

Fig. 22.28 Malignant fibrous histiocytoma.

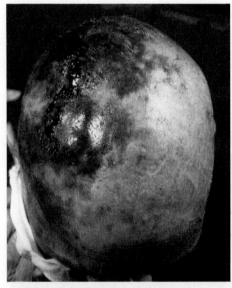

Fig. 22.29-1 Angiosarcoma. Partly ulcerative lesions.

Tumors of muscular cells

Leiomyosarcoma and rhabdomyosarcoma are rare malignant tumors of muscular cells. Their prognosis is poor. Leiomyosarcoma occurs on the extremities of elderly people. Spindle-shaped cells with strong atypism and differentiation to smooth muscles are seen. Rhabdomyosarcoma occurs as three types: in the head and neck of infants (embryonic), in the extremities of young adults (alveolar), and in elderly people (pleomorphic).

Vascular tumors
Angiosarcoma (synonym: malignant angioendothelioma)

- Vaguely marginated, dark reddish-violet erythema, bloody blisters, and easily bleeding elevated plaques form, most frequently on the head and face of elderly people.
- This is a malignant tumor caused by proliferation of endothelial cells in the blood vessels and lymph vessels.
- It tends to metastasize hematogenously to the lungs. The prognosis is poor.

Clinical features

Angiosarcoma is induced in some cases by minor external injury. A small purpura first appears and progressively enlarges to present an edematous dark red plaque (Fig. 22.29). The plaque easily bleeds and forms erosion and crusts, resulting in exudative ulceration. As it progresses, nodules appear, metastasizing to the lungs, pleural membranes, liver, and lymph nodes, leading to hemopneumothorax and death in many cases.

Angiosarcoma that occurs at sites with prolonged postoperative lymphedema is called Stewart–Treves syndrome. Angiosarcoma often accompanies lymphedema in the upper extremities after mastectomy (axillary lymph node dissection). Angiosarcoma occurs after irradiation therapy in rare cases.

Pathology

Markedly atypical tumor cells proliferate, forming a luminal structure (Fig. 22.30). Immunostaining is positive for UEA-I, CD31, CD34, and blood coagulation factor VIII-related antigen (von Willebrand factor) in many cases.

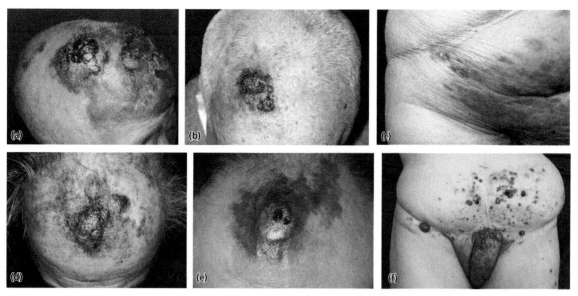

Fig. 22.29-2 Angiosarcoma. a,b,d,e: Dark red erythema and an elevated plaque form. c,f: Angiosarcoma on lymphedema.

Diagnosis and differential diagnosis

Angiosarcoma should be differentiated from subcutaneous hematoma, melanoma, and malignant lymphoma. When angiosarcoma is suspected, biopsy is carried out for diagnosis. As most cases have already progressed at the time of diagnosis, various tests are performed to examine the systemic condition. Because metastasis to other organs, the lungs in particular, influences the prognosis, chest X-ray, abdominal computed tomography (CT) and magnetic resonance imaging (MRI), and nuclear medicine imaging are conducted.

Treatment and prognosis

In cases at the early stages with good systemic condition and no metastasis, combination therapy of extensive resection and irradiation or chemotherapy is conducted. Local recurrence often occurs in angiosarcoma. IV drip or local or arterial injection of genetically altered IL-2 may also be given. The 5-year survival rate is 12–33%.

Kaposi's sarcoma

- The lower legs and feet of elderly people and patients with immunodeficiency are most frequently affected.

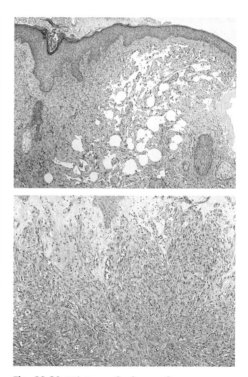

Fig. 22.30 Histopathology of angiosarcoma.

- This cancer is characterized by endothelial and vascular proliferation. Edema first appears, forming a firm nodule that is accompanied by intense pain and easy bleeding.
- The lymph nodes and internal organs are involved. Patients may die from the bleeding of internal organs.
- HHV-8 is associated with onset.
- Irradiation therapy and chemotherapy are the main treatments.

Clinical features

Kaposi's sarcoma occurs on the extremities, particularly on the feet, gradually spreading to the proximal areas. The progression begins with a patch stage, followed by a plaque stage and then a nodule stage. Multiple, purplish-brown patches or angioma-like papules appear in the skin and mucosa (Fig. 22.31), rapidly spreading and forming elevated plaques that become firm nodules.

The eruptions themselves are largely painless but secondary lymphedema causes sharp pain. In progressive cases, infiltration occurs in the lymph nodes, gastrointestinal tract, liver, lungs, and bones, causing various symptoms.

Classification and pathogenesis

Kaposi's sarcoma occurs when human herpes virus type 8 (HHV-8) infection causes malignant transformation in endocapillary cells. Kaposi's sarcoma is classified into four types based on the underlying primary disorder, the country of residence, and various other factors. The types are classic (often occuring among elderly Jewish or Eastern Europeans), African endemic (often occurring among young Africans), immunosuppressive treatment related (caused by the use of immunosuppressants after organ transplant), and HIV associated (epidemic). The HIV-associated type progresses rapidly, whereas the other types progress slowly.

Pathology

Non-specific proliferation of capillary vessels is the only pathological finding in the early stage. In the patch stage, irregularly shaped vascular lumens proliferate, and bleeding and mild atypism in cells are present. In the plaque stage, marked proliferation of

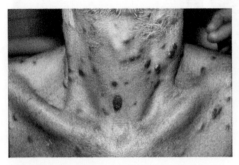

Fig. 22.31 Multiple Kaposi's sarcomas in a patient with AIDS.

spindle cells around the blood vessels is found and the pathological findings resemble those of angiosarcoma. In the nodular stage, the tumor cells proliferate in bundles and multiple spaces filled with erythrocytes form between the cells (Fig. 22.32).

Treatment

Irradiation therapy and combination chemotherapy are the main treatments. Surgical removal may be conducted on localized lesions. For the HIV-related type, highly active antiretroviral therapy (HAART) (see Chapter 23) is effective. For the immunosuppressive treatment-related type, reduction or cessation of immunosuppressants improves the condition.

Histiocytic tumors
Langerhans cell histiocytosis (synonym: histiocytosis X)

Malignant Langerhans cells proliferate in systemic organs such as the skin, liver, spleen, lymph nodes, and lungs, and in the bone marrow. Langerhans cell histiocytosis (LCH) was classified by age of onset and clinical features into Letterer–Siwe disease, Hand–Schüller–Christian disease, and eosinophilic granuloma. In recent years, these types have come to be unified under the name of LCH. Cutaneous symptoms are found in 60–80% of patients with LCH. Reddish plaques resembling eczema, and hemorrhagic papules, crusts, and purpura occur, mainly in the seborrheic areas (Fig. 22.33). Eruptions resembling xanthogranuloma (see Chapter 21) may occur in some cases. Histologically, epidermotropic large histiocyte-like cells proliferate in the dermis, and the tumor cells are positive for CD1a (Fig. 22.34) and S-100 proteins.

- **Letterer–Siwe disease:** this occurs suddenly in infancy. Hemorrhagic papules appear over the whole body, accompanied by fever, splenohepatomegaly, pulmonary lesion, and pancytopenia. Seborrheic dermatitis-like lesions occur on the scalp. Chemotherapy and hematopoietic stem cell transplantation are carried out. The prognosis is poor.
- **Hand–Schüller–Christian disease:** this occurs most frequently in early childhood. The three main symptoms are osteolytic lesions in the skull, ocular proptosis, and diabetes insipidus. Granulomatous and xanthomatous eruptions appear. LCH may subside spontaneously in some cases.

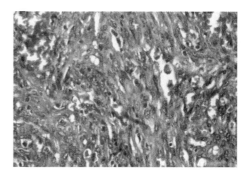

Fig. 22.32 Histopathology of Kaposi's sarcoma.

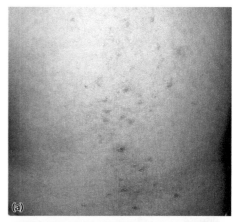

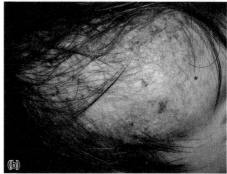

Fig. 22.33 Langerhans cell histiocytosis.
a: Multiple keratotic, erythematous plaques on the trunk. b: Eczema-like plaques on the scalp. Alopecia, pustules, and crusts are present.

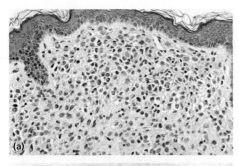

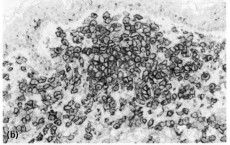

Fig. 22.34 Histopathology of Langerhans cell histiocytosis. a: H&E staining image of Langerhans cells. There is marked infiltrative proliferation of Langerhans cells in the upper dermal layer. b: CD1a chromatic staining of Langerhans cells. There are CD1a-positive infiltrative cells.

MEMO 22–8 Congenital self-healing histiocytosis

This is also called Hashimoto–Pitzker disease.

Within several weeks after birth, red to brownish papules or nodules of 2–20 mm in diameter disseminate over the whole body. There is proliferation of Langerhans cells. Langerhans cell histiocytosis may be difficult to differentiate from congenital self-healing histiocytosis but in the latter, the eruptions disappear spontaneously in several weeks to a year.

• **Granuloma:** this occurs in late childhood and adulthood. Single or dispersed osteolytic lesions are found in the skull and vertebral column. Histopathologically, marked infiltration of histiocyte-like cells and eosinophils is observed. The prognosis is good.

Metastatic carcinoma of the skin

This is a visceral cancer that metastasizes to the skin transcoelomically, hematogenously or lymphogenously. The primary cancer in many cases is in the mammary glands, lungs, colon, uterus or ovaries. Metastatic carcinoma of the skin is a terminal symptom of a primary cancer. Multiple, asymptomatic, intradermal or subcutaneous nodules occur in most cases (Fig. 22.35). The clinical types are as follows.

• **Carcinoma erysipelatodes:** reddening and palpable infiltration suddenly appear, resembling erysipelatodes. It is accompanied by lymphangitis carcinomatosa.

• **Alopecia neoplastica:** tumor cells metastasize to the scalp. Localized alopecia occurs.

• **Sister Mary Joseph nodule:** a nodule occurs in the umbilical region from metastasis of digestive organ cancers, including colon and pancreatic cancer. The primary cancer in most cases is at the terminal stages; the prognosis is poor, with most patients dying within months.

Malignant lymphomas and other hematopoietic tumors

Lymphoma is a malignant tumor of the lymphoid lineage cells. It can be a Hodgkin or a non-Hodgkin lymphoma. Cutaneous lymphoma, a non-Hodgkin lymphoma, is classified into primary, in which tumor cells are found only in the skin at the time of diagnosis, and secondary, in which primary cancerous lesions are found in other parts of the body and the skin symptoms are the result of metastasis. This section focuses on primary cutaneous lymphoma.

Classification

Cutaneous lymphoma is the second most common extranodal lymphoma after those that occur in the gastrointestinal tract or nasopharyngeal region. There were several classifications of primary cutaneous lymphoma in use when the WHO/EORTC proposed a new classification in 2005 (Table 22.6). The new classification has been gaining ground. It is based on the proliferative cells (T cells, NK cells, B cells, blood progenitor cells), the clinical findings, the surface marker, and the degree of cellular differentiation. In Japan, 90% of primary cutaneous lymphomas are T cell-derived (cutaneous T cell lymphoma).

Diagnosis

Histopathological examination is essential in determining the type. H&E staining and the expression of various surface markers, T cell receptors (TCR), and immuno-globulin (Ig) are immunohistochemically examined. The origin of the tumor cells and their monoclonality are investigated by identifying the gene rearrangement of the TCR or the immunoglobulins. To identify the disease stage, the following should be considered: various image analyses (CT, positron emission tomography [PET], ultra-sound, digestive tract imaging), peripheral blood tests (flow cytometry, lactate dehydrogenase [LDH], soluble IL-2 receptor (MEMO, see Chapter 22), HTLV-1, Epstein–Barr virus [EBV] antibody, *Borrelia* antibody) and biopsies (bone marrow puncture, lymph node biopsy).

Major disorders are discussed below.

Cutaneous T cell lymphoma

Mycosis fungoides

- This is the most frequently occurring T cell lymphoma.
- It progresses slowly, over a period of a few years to several dozen years. The three stages are classified morphologically as patch, plaque, and tumor.

MEMO 22–9 Soluble IL-2 receptor (sIL-2R)

The IL-2 receptor has α, β, and γ subunits. The α chain is expressed in activated T cells only, and it flows into the peripheral blood. The α ells ov is called sIL-2R. sIL-2R increases under the condition where T cells are activated and proliferate. sIL-2R also increases when malignant lymphoma (ATLL, in particular), viral infection or collagen disease is present. The sIL-2R level is said to reflect the progression of malignant lymphoma. When patients with lymphoma catch a cold, the level temporarily increases.

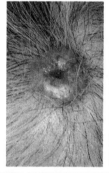
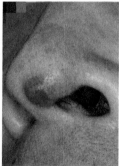

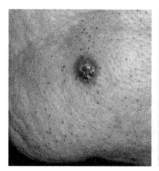
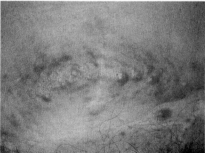
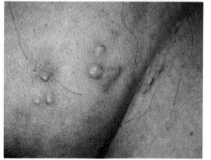

Fig. 22.35 Metastatic carcinoma of the skin.

Table 22.6 Types of primary cutaneous lymphoma.

Cutaneous T cell lymphoma (CTCL)/NK cell lymphoma
Mycosis fungoides (MF)   Sézary syndrome (SS)   Adult T cell leukemia/lymphoma (ATLL)   Primary cutaneous CD30⁺ T cell lymphoproliferative disorders   • Primary cutaneous anaplastic large cell lymphoma   • Lymphomatoid papulosis   Subcutaneous panniculitis-like T cell lymphoma   Extranodal NK/T cell lymphoma, nasal type   Hydroa vacciniforme-like lymphoma   Primary cutaneous g/d T cell lymphoma   Primary cutaneous CD8⁺ aggressive epidermotropic cytotoxic T cell lymphoma   Primary cutaneous CD4⁺ small/medium T cell lymphoma   Peripheral T cell lymphphoma, not otherwise specified
Cutaneous B cell lymphoma (CBCL)
Primary cutaneous marginal zone B cell lymphoma   Primary cutaneous follicle center lymphoma (PCFCL)   Primary cutaneous diffuse large B cell lymphoma, leg type   Primary cutaneous diffuse large B cell lymphoma, other   Intravascular large B cell lymphoma
Precursor hematological neoplasm
CD4⁺/CD56⁺ hematodermic neoplasm, blastic NK cell lymphoma

Adapted from Kim YH., et al., *Blood* 2007; 110: 497.

MEMO 22–10 Subtypes and other diseases related to mycosis fungoides Folliculotropic MF

In folliculotropic MF, tumor cell infiltration in the follicular epithelium exceeds that in the epidermis. Multiple follicular papules occur and coalesce. The progression tends to be rapid.

MEMO 22–11 Pagetoid reticulosis (Woringer–Kolopp)

Pagetoid reticulosis is a subtype of MF in which tumor infiltration shows marked epidermotropism. The name comes from the pathological findings, which resemble those of Paget's disease. A single red plaque with keratinization appears on a lower extremity.

MEMO 22–12 Follicular mucinosis

Decalvant plaques occur, and histopathological changes in hair follicles and mucin deposition are found. Cases as a complication of MF have been reported (see Chapter 17).

- It does not spread to other organs until the final stage.
- Atypical lymphocytic infiltration (Pautrier's micro-abscess) in the epidermis is a characteristic histo-pathological finding.
- The first-line treatments are topical steroids and UV irradiation therapy. Combination chemotherapy is given at the final stage.

Clinical features

Mycosis fungoides (MF) follows a course that is divided into three stages, according to the skin clinical features of the eruptions (Fig. 22.36). In the early stage, eczema, dermatitis or psoriasis-like eruptions occur, persisting for up to 10 years (patch stage). The skin lesion becomes infiltrative and flatly elevated (plaque stage). Several years later, tumors form, metastasize to lymph nodes, and infiltrate other organs (tumor stage).

MEMO 22–13 Gene rearrangement analysis

Rearrangement of the T cell receptor (TCR) and immunoglobulin (Ig) genes occurs during lymphocyte differentiation for recognition of non-self, which leads to various antigenic recognitions. In
lymphoma, lymphocytes proliferate monoclonally and there is often one rearrangement pattern to the
TCR/Ig gene. Thus, Southern blotting from skin lesion tissue is useful for differentiating between lymphoma
and benign diseases. When the gene encoding TCR/Ig is excised by a restriction enzyme and the tissue is
lymphoma (monoclonal), a single band is observed in electrophoresis; in the case of a benign reactive
disease (polyclonal), there is no specific band in electrophoresis. These findings are helpful for diagnosing
the malignancy of tissues and blood (gene rearrangement analysis, GRA).

In T cell lymphoma, the β chain (Cβ region) of the TCR gene is mainly detected, because the majority of
the tumor cells derive from α and β lymphocytes. Rearrangement of the Jγ region is positive in most T cell
lymphomas, because the γ chain is rearranged first in the process of T cell differentiation. In B cell lymphoma, rearrangement of the heavy-chain J region (IgH-JH) is mainly detected. Detection using PCR is also
used, because comparatively large amounts of tissue samples (>0.25 to 0.5 g) are necessary in the
Southern blotting detection of gene rearrangement.

It should be noted that rearrangement may be positive in lichen planus or pseudo-lymphoma, because a
portion of the monoclonal proliferation is detected.

Patch stage (erythematous stage)

Multiple erythemas of various shapes and sizes,
accompanied by moderate scaling, occur on the trunk
and extremities. MF at this stage is sometimes clinically indistinguishable from seborrheic dermatitis,
psoriasis, pityriasis rosea (Gibert), and parapsoriasis. It
may respond to topical steroids; however, eruptions
spread with repeated exacerbation and remission for
up to a few dozen years. As the eruptions progress,
they are often accompanied by skin atrophy and pigmentation (poikiloderma). Many cases of parapsoriasis en plaque (see Chapter 15) progress to MF.
Parapsoriasis en plaque itself is considered to be a type
of MF at the patch stage.

Plaque stage (infiltrative stage)

Circular or horseshoe-shaped, flatly elevated, red or
reddish-brown eruptions with palpable infiltration
appear. Scaling is often present. The eruptions progress
to the tumor stage with repeated exacerbation and
remission.

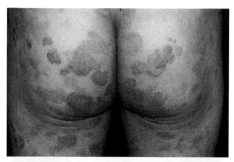
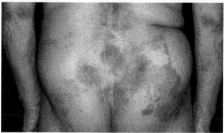

**Fig. 22.36-1 Mycosis fungoides at the
erythematous stage.**

Tumor stage

Dome-shaped, elevated, elastic, dark red tumors occur.
The surface is smooth at first but may later become
partly erosive and ulcerate. In the tumor stage, the
lesions progress rapidly and infiltrate the lymph nodes
and internal organs (stage of visceral dissemination).
They rarely become leukemic. Immunodeficiency and

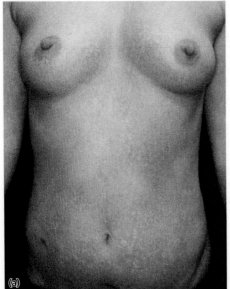

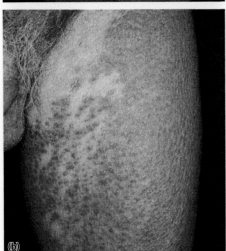

Fig. 22.36-2 Mycosis fungoides (MF). a: Mycosis fungoides at the erythematous stage. b: Folliculotropic lesions of MF.

resulting infections, and lesions of internal organs lead to death in 1–2 years in many cases.

Pathology
Patch stage
Lymphocytic infiltration occurs in the superficial dermis. Lymphocytic infiltration without spongiosis occurs in the epidermis (epidermotropism). Atypical lymphocytes are observed in some cases.

Plaque stage
Markedly dense, band-like cellular infiltration occurs in the upper dermal layer. Large atypical cells containing deeply constricted nuclei are found among the infiltrative lymphocytes. Epidermotropism becomes distinct. Multiple honeycomb epidermal lymphocytic infiltration, called Pautrier's microabscess (Fig. 22.37), is observed.

Tumor stage
Epidermotropism is lost. Atypical lymphocytes infiltrate all dermal layers and subcutaneous tissue.

Infiltrative tumor cells have CD4$^+$ T cell surface markers (CD3$^+$, CD4$^+$, CD5$^-$, and CD20$^-$). CE7 and CD26, which appear in normal T cells, are often negative.

Diagnosis and differential diagnosis
Until MF progresses to the final stages, there are few abnormal findings in blood and biochemical tests. MF is diagnosed by the clinical features and histopathological findings. As characteristic findings of MF are difficult to obtain in the early stages, skin biopsies may be conducted repeatedly at certain intervals in suspected cases. Gene rearrangement analysis of the tissue is useful. Disorders that should be differentiated from MF include eczema, dermatitis (atopic dermatitis, in particular), psoriasis, parapsoriasis, and adult T cell leukemia/lymphoma.

Treatment
Determine the TNMB classification (Table 22.7), and consider the treatments. Phototherapies such as PUVA and narrow-band UVB inhibit the progression of lesions in the patch and plaque stages, to some extent. Topical steroids and interferon are also useful. Progressive cases, such as MF in the tumor stage, are treated with electron beam irradiation and

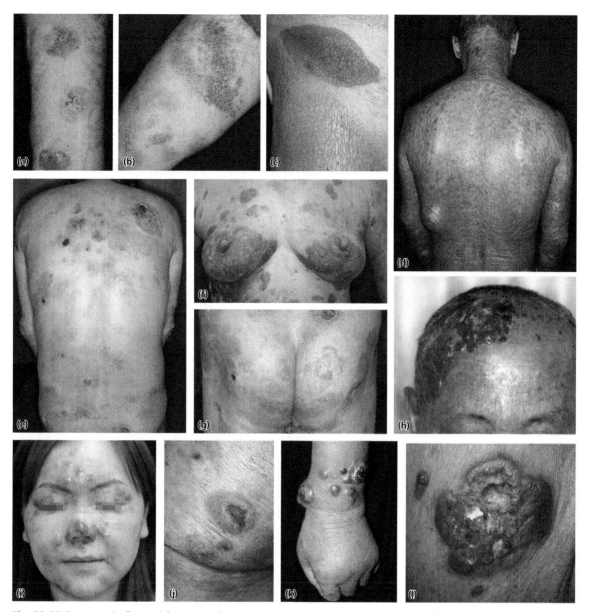

Fig. 22.36-3 Mycosis fungoides. a–c: Plaque stage. d–l: Tumor stage. Severely infiltrative ulcers form.

chemotherapy (e.g., CHOP therapy; the treatment is the same as for non-Hodgkin lymphoma) (Table 22.8).

Sézary syndrome

- Sézary syndrome (SS) is a primary cutaneous T cell lymphoma.
- Intense itching is present. The main symptoms are erythroderma, swelling of superficial lymph nodes,

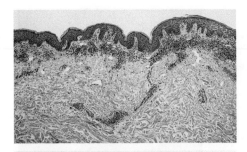

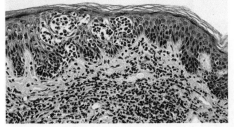

Fig. 22.37 Histopathology of mycosis fungoides. Histological image of mycosis fungoides somewhere between the erythematous and plaque stages. Atypical lymphocytes invade the epidermis and form a microabscess (Pautrier's microabscess).

Table 22.7 Stage grouping of mycosis fungoides and Sézary syndrome (ISCL/EORTC, 2007).

T: Skin lesion characteristics and ranges
T1: Less than 10% of the skin surface
T1a (Patch only), T1b (plaque and patch)
T2: 10% or more of the skin surface
T2a (Patch only), T2b (plaque and patch)
T3: One or more tumors (1 cm or greater in diameter)
T4: Erythroderma (80% or more of the skin surface)

NCI classification of lymph node
NCI LN0: No atypical lymphocytes*
NCI LN1: Solitary atypical lymphocytes are seen, but they are not clustered.
NCI LN2: Numerous atypical lymphocytes are seen, or clusters of 3–6 cells are found.
NCI LN3: Lymphocytes form large clusters, but the basic structure of the lymph node is maintained.
NCI LN4: The structure of the lymph node is partially or entirely lost by the proliferation of atypical lymphocytes or tumor cells.

M: Visceral
M0: No visceral organ involvement is found
M1: Visceral involvement is found (confirmed pathologically)

B: Peripheral blood
B0: 5% or less atypical lymphocytes in peripheral blood lymphocytes
B0a: (No clone expansion), B0b: (Clone expansion is found.)
B1: The number of atypical lymphocytes exceeds 5%, but the criterion of B2 is not met.
B1a: (No clone expansion), B1b: (Clone expansion is found.)
B2: 1000/mL or higher Sézary cells (with clone expansion)

* Abnormal lymph node: firm, irregular, clustered, and immovable, with a diameter of 1.5 cm or more.
Adapted from Olsen E., et al. *Blood* 2007; 110: 1713.

Table 22.8 Therapeutic examples of CHOP used in the tumor stage of mycosis fungoides.

Drug	Dose	Administration example	day				
			1	2	3	4	5
Cyclophosphamide	750 mg/m²	Instillation for 3 hours	↓				
Doxorubicin	50 mg/m²	Instillation for 1 hour	↓				
Vincristine	1.4 mg/m²	Instillation for 1 hour	↓				
Prednisolone	100 mg/body	Oral administration	↓	↓	↓	↓	↓

and the appearance of atypical lymphocytes in the peripheral blood.

- The laboratory findings and treatments are largely the same as those for mycosis fungoides.

Definition

Sézary syndrome is a primary cutaneous T cell lymphoma with the three main symptoms of erythroderma, swelling of superficial lymph nodes, and the appearance of atypical lymphocytes in the peripheral blood. Cases that satisfy the conditions described in T4 and B2 of the TNMB classification in Table 22.7 are diagnosed as Sézary syndrome.

Clinical features

Men over age 50 are most frequently affected. Erythema accompanied by scaling over the whole body surface occurs diffusely, presenting as erythroderma that covers 80% or more of the body surface (Fig. 22.38). Intense itching is often present. Swelling of the superficial lymph nodes, exceeding 1.5 cm in the clinical image, and splenohepatomegaly are present. The systemic symptoms tend to be mild, and fever is not present. As SS progresses, nodular eruptions occur and may infiltrate into the internal organs.

Pathology and laboratory findings

Leukocytosis and lymphocyte atypicality are found in the peripheral blood. These atypical lymphocytes, called Sézary cells, have nuclei with deep invaginations as seen in the cells found in epidermis affected by mycosis fungoides, and they contain superficial markers of CD4+ T cells. Band-like or perivascular lymphocytic infiltration including Sézary cells is found in the upper dermal layer of the areas with erythroderma. Pautrier's microabscess may occur in the epidermis (see Fig. 22.37).

Adult T cell leukemia/lymphoma

- This is a hematopoietic malignancy caused by human T cell leukemia virus type 1 (HTLV-1).
- Multiple, firm, reddish-brown skin tumors with dome-shaped elevation appear. Various skin symptoms, including erythroderma and elevated, scaling plaques, are present.
- Serum anti-HTLV-1 antibodies are positive. Characteristic "flower cells" are found in the peripheral blood.

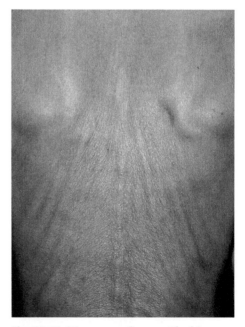

Fig. 22.38 Sézary syndrome. Flushing accompanied by intense itching occurs on the whole body.

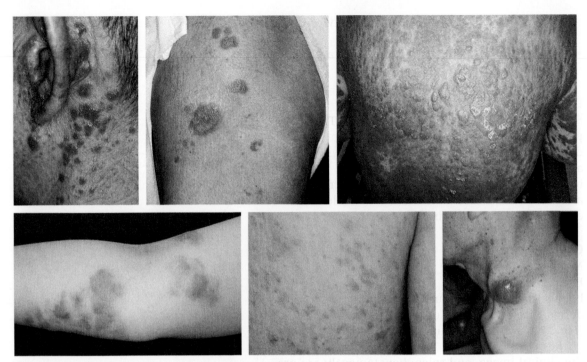

Fig. 22.39-1 Adult T cell leukemia/lymphoma.

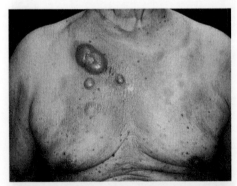

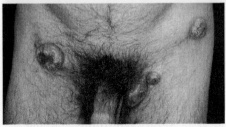

**Fig. 22.39-2 Adult T cell leukemia/
lymphoma.**

Clinical features

Adult T cell leukemia/lymphoma (ATLL) is classified by the course of progression into several types, including the smoldering, chronic, acute, acute transformative, and lymphoma types. Cutaneous lesions are seen in about 60% of ATLL patients and in all variants. Multiple, firm, dome-shaped, reddish-brown tumors occur, ranging in size from several millimeters to 10 cm. They may be accompanied by scaling, infiltrative elevated reddish-brown plaques, and erythroderma (Fig. 22.39). Besides the characteristic eruptions (specific eruptions) with tumor cell infiltration, non-specific eruptions caused by immunodeficiency, various infections such as candidiasis and herpes zoster, and urticaria, acquired ichthyosis, palmoplantar keratosis, and eczema-like eruptions also appear. As ATLL progresses, opportunistic infection is caused by fungi or viruses resulting from cellular immunodeficiency. There are systemic symptoms such as lymph node enlargement, splenohepatomegaly, fever, and fatigue. The patient tends to develop hypercalcemia.

Epidemiology

The incidence varies by region. The incubation period between transmission and development of ATLL is usually more than 40 years. In Japan, about 1.2 million people have tested positive for the anti-HTLV-1 antibody, and it is estimated that 1 out of 1000 of these develops ATLL every year (the lifetime incidence rate is said to be 3–5%). Worldwide, many patients are from the Caribbean and Africa.

The routes of infection may be through mother-to-child contact, sexual activity or blood. Most cases are mother-to-child transmission through breast milk. In the cases transmitted through sexual activity in adult life, ATLL seldom develops. Most patients are over age 40 but rare cases in young people have been reported.

Pathogenesis

Human T cell leukemia virus type 1, a retrovirus (RNA virus), infects CD4$^+$ T cells and produces proviral DNA by means of enzyme reverse transcriptase. The provirus DNA is integrated in the host DNA. It is thought that monoclonal proliferation of T cells is induced by various factors, including the portions of DNA in which the proviral DNA is integrated. Generally, HTLV-1 is not detected as a viral particle. Infection occurs from the invasion of infected T cells in blood, breast milk or semen.

Laboratory findings and diagnosis

Serum anti-HTLV-1 antibodies are positive. Southern blot is performed using peripheral blood or skin tissue to identify monoclonal integration of HTLV-1 proviral DNA into tumor cells. In some subtypes, there is a marked increase of leukocytes (100,000 to several hundred thousand/mL) and atypical lymphocytes called flower cells in the peripheral blood (Fig. 22.40), increased LDH in the blood, increased serum calcium and soluble IL-2 receptor. ATLL is classified into subtypes according to the severity of these changes (Table 22.9).

Treatment and prognosis

Patients with the chronic or smoldering type of ATLL are followed up to check for signs of acute transformation. The acute, lymphoma, and acute transformative types are treated with conventional chemotherapy (e.g., LSG15). The prognosis is poor, and the 3-year

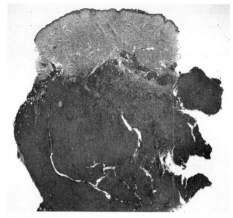
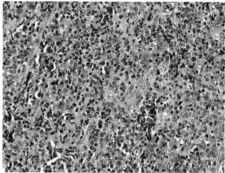

Fig. 22.40　Histopathology of adult T cell leukemia/lymphoma.

Table 22.9 Clinical characteristics and types of adult T cell leukemia/lymphoma.

		Smoldering	Chronic	Lymphoma	Acute
Anti-HTLV-1 antibody		+	+	+	+
Number of lymphocytes (× 10⁹/L)		<4	≥4a	<4	*
Atypical T-cells		≥5%	+	≤1%	+
Flower cells		Often	Often	None	+
LDH		≤1.5N	≤2N	*	*
Ca concentration (mg/dL)		<11	<11	*	*
Lymph node infiltration		None	*	+	*
Tumor lesion	Skin	**	*	*	*
	Lungs	**	*	*	*
	Liver	None	*	*	*
	Spleen	None	*	*	*
	Central nervous system	None	None	*	*
	Bones	None	None	*	*
	Ascites	None	None	*	*
	Pleural effusion	None	None	*	*
	Digestive tract	None	None	*	*

N: Uppermost normal value,
*: Unnecessary for diagnosis,
**: Necessary for diagnosis of cases in which peripheral atypical T cells account for 5% or less of total leukocytes.
a: T lymphocyte density is 3.5 × 10⁹/L or more.
b: When atypical T lymphocytes account for 5% or less of total leukocytes, histological diagnosis is necessary.
(Adapted from Shimoyama M. Diagnostic criteria and classificat ion of clinical subtypes of adult T cell leukaemia-lymphoma. A report from the Lymphoma Study Group (1984–87). *Br J Haematol* 1991; 79: 428–37).

survival rate is 20–30%. Hematopoietic stem cell transplantation may be carried out. Intravenous fluid and calcitonin are administered for hypercalcemia.

Primary cutaneous anaplastic large cell lymphoma

Primary cutaneous anaplastic large cell lymphoma is a CD30⁺ lymphoinfiltrative cutaneous T cell lymphoma. In many cases, a single nodule or papule occurs, often accompanied by erosion (Fig. 22.41). On histopathology, infiltration of large atypical cells is found, which resembles that of Hodgkin disease. CD30 antigen (Ki-1 antigen) is positive in 75% or more of the tumor cells. The final diagnosis should be carefully made, because CD30⁺ infiltration is also seen in mycosis fungoides and other types of lymphoma. Irradiation therapy and surgical removal are carried. The prognosis is generally good.

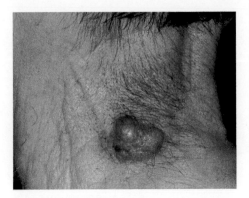

Fig. 22.41 Primary cutaneous anaplastic large cell lymphoma.

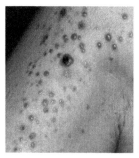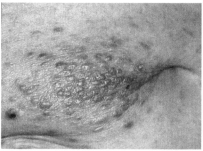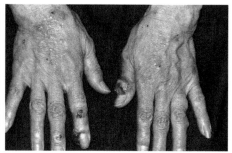

Fig. 22.42-1 **Lymphomatoid papulosis.**

Lymphomatoid papulosis

Lymphomatoid papulosis begins as reddish-brown papules of several millimeters to 1 cm in diameter on the trunk and extremities, which are accompanied by scaling and bloody crusts or necrotic spots in the center. The eruptions heal spontaneously in 2–3 weeks with moderate scarring and pigmentation. The eruptions often recur for many years, and new eruptions are present together with older ones (Fig. 22.42). Histopathologically, CD30+ large atypical cells are found together with the leakage of erythrocytes and eosinophilic infiltration. This disorder is thought to be on the spectrum of anaplastic large cell lymphomas. Clinically, it shows benign characteristics. When it does not spontaneously disappear, topical steroids and PUVA therapy are administered.

Extranodal NK/T cell lymphoma, nasal type

Extranodal NK/T cell lymphoma is a malignant disorder with proliferation mainly of natural killer (NK) cells. The majority of NK/T cell lymphomas occur in the

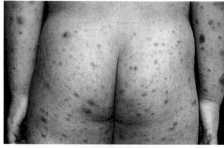

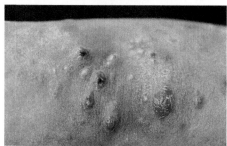

Fig. 22.42-2 **Lymphomatoid papulosis.**

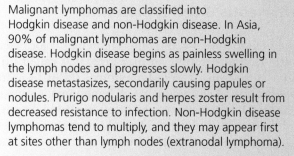

MEMO 22–14 Hodgkin disease and non-Hodgkin disease

Malignant lymphomas are classified into Hodgkin disease and non-Hodgkin disease. In Asia, 90% of malignant lymphomas are non-Hodgkin disease. Hodgkin disease begins as painless swelling in the lymph nodes and progresses slowly. Hodgkin disease metastasizes, secondarily causing papules or nodules. Prurigo nodularis and herpes zoster result from decreased resistance to infection. Non-Hodgkin disease lymphomas tend to multiply, and they may appear first at sites other than lymph nodes (extranodal lymphoma).

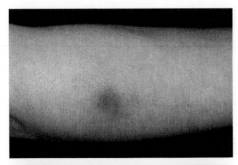

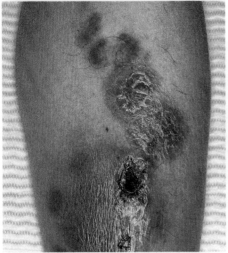

Fig. 22.43 Extranodal natural killer/T cell lymphoma.

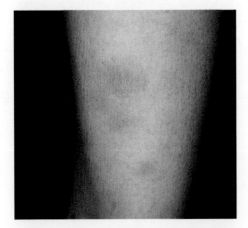

Fig. 22.44 Subcutaneous panniculitis-like T cell lymphoma. Erythema nodosum-like erythema is accompanied by tenderness and panniculitis. Histopathological observation revealed the infiltration of lymphoma cells.

nasopharyngeal region and form skin lesions as a result of metastasis (secondary cutaneous lymphoma). Primary cutaneous lymphoma without the involvement of other organs is also present. An association between the EB virus and extranodal nasal T/NK cell lymphomas has been suggested. Plaques easily become erosive and subcutaneous nodules occur in the trunk and extremities (Fig. 22.43). Swelling of the face, eyelids, and lips, aphtha in the lips, and chilblain-like eruptions may be present. Cases with multiple lesions or infiltration in multiple organs have a poor prognosis.

Hydroa vacciniforme-like lymphoma

Hydroa vacciniforme used to be attributed to photosensitivity with unknown cause (see Chapter 13). The cause is now thought to be proliferation of NK/T cells from EB viral infection, and the disorder is classified as a type of cutaneous lymphoma. Papules or blisters accompanied by central umbilication and necrosis occur on sun-exposed areas such as the dorsal hands and cheeks. Edema appears on the eyelids, lips, and face.

Subcutaneous panniculitis-like T cell lymphoma (SPTCL)

Panniculitis-like clinical features resemble those of erythema nodosum (Fig. 22.44). It is very likely that certain disorders with poor prognosis that used to be diagnosed as Weber–Christian disease or cytophagic histiocytic panniculitis are included in this disorder. The tumor cells derive from CD8+ cytotoxic T cells and infiltrate the surrounding individual subcutaneous fat cells (rimming). Macrophages that have phagocytosed the nuclear debris are seen. The prognosis is often poor if hemophagocytic syndrome occurs.

Cutaneous B cell lymphoma

When cutaneous B cell lymphoma remains localized to the skin at the time of diagnosis, it is called primary cutaneous B cell lymphoma (PCBCL). The classification of cutaneous B cell lymphoma is shown in Table 22.6. A localized red or purplish-red plaque, nodule or tumor occurs. Multiple papules, nodules or infiltrating erythema occur in some cases. The

Table 22.10 Differentiation of B cells and cellular surface traits.

Mature phase	Tumor	TdT	Cellular surface trait	clg
Lymphatic stem cell	B-ALL	+		$H^{O/R}L^O$
	B-ALL	+	CD19	$H^R L^O$
	B-ALL	+	CD19, CD10	$H^R L^{R/O}$
	B-ALL	+	CD19, CD10, CD20	$H^R L^{R/O}$
Pro B cell	B-ALL	+	CD19, CD10, CD20	$H^R L^{R/O}$
Pre B cell	B-ALL, CLL	+	CD19, CD20, CD21, IgM	$\mu\ H^R L^R$
Immature B cell	CLL		CD19, CD20, CD21, CD35, IgM, IgD, Fc, (CD5)	Ig $H^R L^R$
Mature B cell	ML, PL, HCL		CD19, CD20, (CD21), Fc, (CD10), CD35, IgG, IgA, IgM	Ig $H^R L^R$
Plasma cell-like B cell	ML, MG, HCL		CD19, CD20, CD35, CD38, IgM, Fc, PCA-1, (PC-1)	Ig $H^R L^R$
Plasma cell	MM		CD38, PC-1, PCA-1	Ig $H^R L^R$

TdT: terminal deoxynucleotidyl transferase, clg: Immunoglobulin class, H: Immunoglobulin heavy chain,
L: Immunoglobulin light chain,
O: No rearrangement, R: gene rearrangement, Fc: Fc receptor of IgG, B-ALL: B-cell acute lymphocytic leukemia,
CLL: Chronic lymphocytic leukemia, PL: Prolymphocytic leukemia, ML: Malignant lymphoma, HCL: Hairy-cell leukemia,
MG: Macroglobulinemia, MM: Multiple myeloma.
(Hase T, et al. B-cell lymphomas. In: Hori Y, et al., editors. *Cutaneous Lymphoma Atlas*. Bunkodo; 1996: 82–5).

eruption rarely ulcerates. The skin surface is normal, and a layer that lacks lymphocyte infiltration (Grenz zone) is seen directly under the dermis. Erosive lymphocytic infiltration occurs in the dermis; the deeper the infiltration, the more severe it tends to be (bottom-heavy appearance). B cell-specific antigens are expressed, but T cell surface antigens are not detected (Table 22.10). The monoclonality of the immunoglobulin gene becomes apparent; gene rearrangement analysis is useful for differential diagnosis. The main treatment is radiation therapy and surgical removal. Chemotherapy and administration of rituximab are carried out in cases with multiple lesions.

Primary cutaneous marginal zone B cell lymphoma

Primary cutaneous marginal zone B cell lymphoma often occurs in the trunk and extremities (Fig. 22.45). The tumor includes mature B cells that form the marginal zone and plasma cell-like cells. The tumor cells are CD5⁻ and CD10⁻. The 5-year survival rate is nearly 100%. Surgical removal and irradiation therapy are often carried out. In the 2008 WHO classification, primary cutaneous marginal zone B cell lymphoma

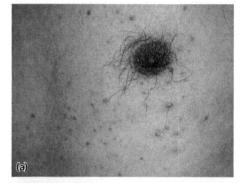
(a)

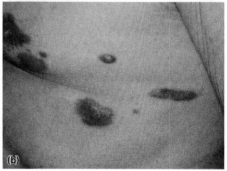
(b)

Fig. 22.45-1 Primary cutaneous marginal zone B cell lymphoma.

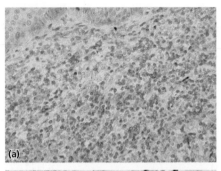

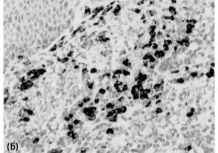

Fig. 22.45-2 Primary cutaneous marginal zone B cell lymphoma. a: Negative IgGl chain staining of case b in Fig. 22.45-1. b: Positive IgGk chain staining of case b in Fig. 22.45-1.

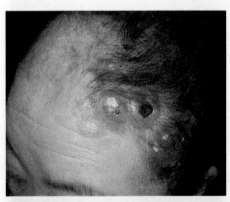

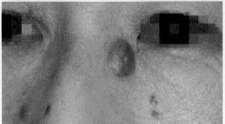

Fig. 22.46 Primary cutaneous follicle center lymphoma.

was reclassified as an extranodal marginal zone lymphoma of mucosa-associated lymphoid tissue (MALT lymphoma).

Primary cutaneous follicle center lymphoma

Primary cutaneous follicle center lymphoma often occurs in the head and neck region and trunk. Mid-sized to large cells that resemble follicular center cells proliferate (Fig. 22.46). The tumor cells are CD10⁺ and bcl-2⁻. A follicular structure is not always present. The prognosis is good, with a 5-year survival rate of 95%. The main treatments are surgical removal and irradiation therapy.

Primary cutaneous diffuse large B cell lymphoma

Primary cutaneous diffuse large B cell lymphoma is classified into the leg type and other. In the leg type, the lesions are mainly found in the lower extremities of elderly people. Large, very atypical follicular center cells or immunoblast-like cells proliferate diffusely (Fig. 22.47). The prognosis is rather poor, with a 5-year survival rate of about 50%.

Other hematopoietic tumors

Leukemia cutis

This specific eruption is caused by infiltration of leukemic tumor cells from blood into the skin. Papules, nodules, tumors, and erythroderma are the main cutaneous symptoms (Fig. 22.48). It occurs frequently in adult T cell leukemia, acute monocytic leukemia, and acute transformation of chronic myelogenous leukemia. Skin lesions that accompany leukemia but are not caused by the direct infiltration of tumor cells are called non-specific eruptions, and they may appear as urticaria, erythema multiforme, erythema nodosum, pruritus or pigmentation.

Multiple myeloma

Atypical plasma cells proliferate in the bone marrow. The bone lesions spread to the skin, where they form the cutaneous symptom of firm nodules. Multiple nodules may occur through hematogenous metastasis in rare cases. Purpura may be caused by cryoglobulinemia

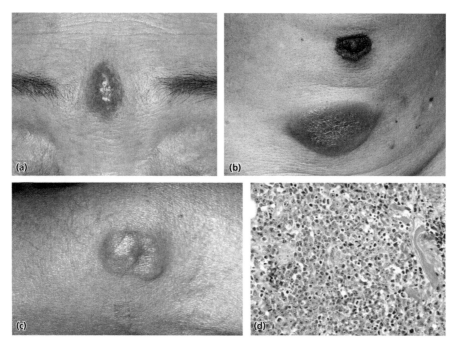

Fig. 22.47 Primary cutaneous diffuse large B cell lymphoma. a: A small nodule on the glabella. b: A tumor on the chest. c: A small, light pink nodule. d: Pathological findings of case c. The proliferation of large atypical lymphocytes with nuclei of characteristic shape is seen. Nuclear division is also seen.

(see Chapter 11) and amyloidosis (see Chapter 17) as a cutaneous symptom in some cases.

(Malignant) melanoma

- A malignant tumor of the melanocytes, this is classified into the following melanomas: nodular, superficial spreading, acral lentiginous, and lentigo maligna. Lesions of all types are blackish and vaguely marginated.
- It tends to metastasize lymphogenously or hematogenously, to infiltrate the lungs and bones, and to be highly malignant.
- Early detection and surgical removal are essential. Other treatments are largely ineffective.

Classification

Melanoma is classified by clinical features and pathology into nodular, superficial spreading, acral lentiginous, and lentigo maligna (Fig. 22.49, Table 22.11). There are many other types that do not fit these categories, such as an intermediate type and an unclassifiable type.

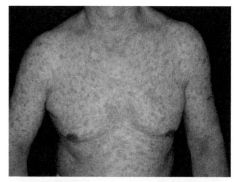

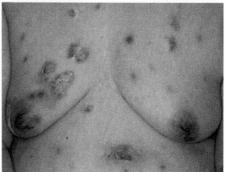

Fig. 22.48 Leukemia cutis.

Table 22.11 Clinical and pathological findings of the four major types of melanoma.

1 Nodular melanoma (NM)
A dome-shaped nodular lesion occurs, often accompanied by ulceration. The lesion progresses to the vertical growth phase without undergoing the radial growth phase in most cases. Therefore, rapid metastasis may occur. The prognosis is poor. It may occur on any site of the body. Atypical tumor cells proliferate in the vertical direction. Proliferation of tumor cells is almost never seen around the nodules.
2 Superficial spreading melanoma (SSM)
Pigmented spots appear. They enlarge over the course of several months to several years. Some of the spots elevate and progress to the vertical growth phase. The epidermis thickens slightly. There are large, clear melanoma cells that resemble Paget cells in all epidermal layers.
3 Acral lentiginous melanoma (ALM)
The ends of extremities, fingernails, and toenails are most frequently involved. ALM begins with light brown macules that continue to enlarge over the course of up to a dozen years. Nodules appear on the macules. When a nail is affected, a black macule may spread beyond the nail fold (Hutchinson's sign). There is acanthosis and extension of the epidermal rete ridges. Atypical melanocytes proliferate in the lower epidermal layer.
4 Lentigo maligna melanoma (LMM)
A blackish-brown spot first appears. It gradually enlarges over the course of decades. Because of the mild progression over a long period of time, the primary black spot is often misdiagnosed as lentigo. The precursor pigmented macule of LMM is called lentigo maligna. Sun-exposed areas of the body such as the face are most frequently involved. The epidermal rete ridges disappear. Atypical melanocytes are scattered in the basement of the atrophied epidermis. Solar elastosis is caused in the upper dermal layer.

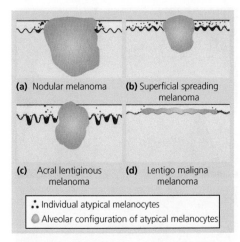

(a) Nodular melanoma **(b)** Superficial spreading melanoma

(c) Acral lentiginous melanoma **(d)** Lentigo maligna melanoma

⁖ Individual atypical melanocytes
◉ Alveolar configuration of atypical melanocytes

Fig. 22.49 Classification of melanoma (Clark's level).

Clinical features

The distinguishing clinical features of the four types are listed in Table 22.11. All types of melanoma begin as a horizontal proliferation of tumor cells in the epidermis (radial growth phase). In this phase, a dark brown or black patch is observed clinically. After the patch enlarges to a certain size, the tumor cells begin to proliferate vertically (vertical growth phase). The patch partially elevates and forms a black nodule, erosion, and ulcer (Fig. 22.50). When the patch progresses to the vertical growth phase, the risk of metastasis increases sharply. Metastasis is lymphatic in most cases; satellite lesions form around the primary location and metastasize to the regional lymph nodes, resulting in distant metastases in organs such as the lungs, liver, and brain.

Melanocytes continue to produce melanin after they become malignant; the skin lesion in most cases becomes blackish-brown. The five characteristic clinical features of melanoma are initialed as ABCDE (Table 22.12). In rare cases, the melanoma cells lack melanin production. This is called amelanotic melanoma, and it has an even worse prognosis.

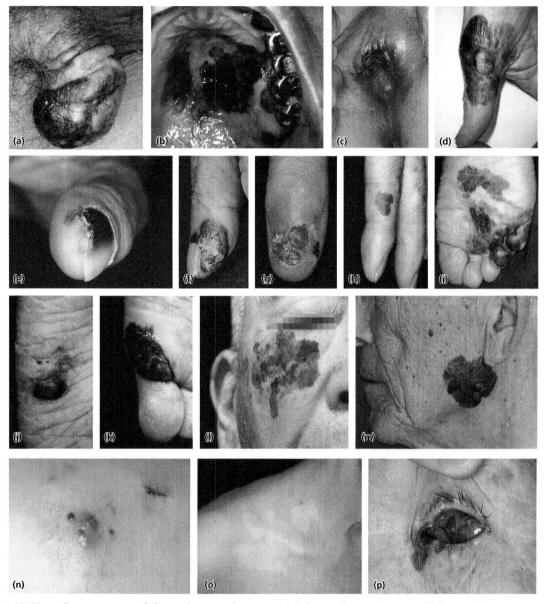

Fig. 22.50 Melanoma. a: Nodular melanoma. b,c: Superficial spreading melanoma. d–k: Acral lentiginous melanoma. l,m: Lentigo maligna melanoma. n: Metastatic melanoma of the skin. o: Leukoderma in a patient with progressive melanoma. p: Conjunctival melanoma.

Pathogenesis and epidemiology

Melanoma is caused by malignant melanocytes in normal skin, or it may originate from a nevus cell nevus (e.g., Clark nevus and large congenital melanocytic nevus), blue nevus or xeroderma pigmentosum. External injury, UV radiation, blisters caused by footwear, clavus

Table 22.12 Clinical characteristics of melanoma (ABCDE).

Finding	Feature
A	Asymmetry
B	Borderline irregularity
C	Color variegation
D	Diameter enlargement (over 6 mm)
E	Elevation of surface

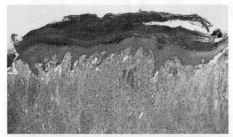
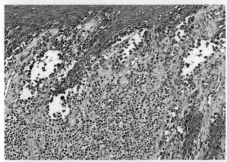
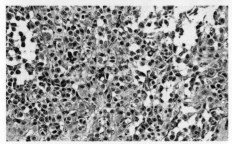

Fig. 22.51 Histopathology of melanoma. Atypical melanocytes proliferate in the epidermis and dermis. When the melanomas are clinically blackish, the tumor cells contain large quantities of melanin pigment.

removal, chilblains, and burn scarring may also induce melanoma. Melanomas occur not only in the skin, but also in other organs that have melanocytes, such as the eye socket, oral cavity, and nasal mucosa. Melanomas may occur multiply in the skin as a result of metastasis from the primary lesion in another organ.

The incidence and the site of origin depend greatly on environmental factors and on intrinsic factors, including race and genetic background. Sun exposure is the most notable environmental factor. The disorder occurs frequently in Caucasians, from a lack of natural protection against UV (i.e., little melanin pigment in the skin), particularly on sun-exposed areas. It rarely occurs in persons of African descent, whose protective capacity is high, and when it does occur, it is most frequent at the ends of the extremities. Asians fall between these two extremes. For example, in Japan about two people in 100,000 have this disorder, and in Australia more than 20 people in 100,000 have malignant melanoma annually. In recent years, the incidence of melanoma has been increasing worldwide. This is attributed to demographic aging, lifestyle changes such as clothing, and depletion of the ozone layer.

Pathology

In all types of melanoma, atypical melanocytes of various sizes proliferate in the epidermis and dermis. The cells often coalesce to form vaguely defined tumor nests of various sizes (Fig. 22.51).

Each type of melanoma presents a characteristic infiltration pattern of atypical cells (see Table 22.11). The depth of tumor cell infiltration is the important factor in determining prognosis, as judged by the distance from the upper part of the granular cell layer to the deepest part of the lesion (Breslow's tumor thickness). The Clark classification uses levels I–V, according to the depth of the infiltrating cell invasion.

Diagnosis

The clinical findings of the tumor are the most important factor in diagnosis. Whenever a blackish-brown lesion is found, melanoma should be suspected. Dermoscopic findings such as parallel ridge pattern and atypical pigment network are useful for diagnosis (see Chapter 3). Biopsy used to be avoided, because it was thought that partial removal promotes dissemination of the tumor; however, biopsy is basically safe if it is done at the early stage and the surrounding tissue is excised with the lesion. Immunopathologically,

MEMO 22–15 Sentinel lymph node biopsy

When a radioactive isotope or a pigment such as indigo carmine is injected locally into a malignant tumor, the substance flows in the lymph vessels and temporarily accumulates in the regional lymph node. A lymph node that takes in pigment or radioactive isotope is called a sentinel lymph node (SLN), and it is thought to be the first lymph node that the lymphogenously metastasizing tumor cells reach. Early detection of lymph node metastasis for a malignant tumor is possible if the sentinel lymph node is selectively biopsied. When the biopsy is negative, it is possible to avoid highly invasive lymph node dissection, leading to quality of life improvement. This biopsy is called sentinel lymph node biopsy, and it may be conducted for melanomas.

the tumor cells are positive for S-100, HMB-45, and MART-1 (Melan A).

The TNM classification and the disease stage are determined after diagnosis (Table 22.13 and Table 22.14). Lymph node involvement and distant metastasis are examined by ultrasound, CT, and PET. Sentinel lymph node biopsy (MEMO, see Chapter 22) is useful. 5-s-Cysteinyl dosa in the blood is measured as a marker for tumor metastasis in the progressive stage (see Chapter 1).

Differential diagnosis

Melanoma should be differentiated from nevus cell nevus, Spitz nevus, basal cell carcinoma, senile lentigo, pyogenic granuloma, squamous cell carcinoma, verruca vulgaris, angiosarcoma, and subungual hemorrhage. Dermoscopy is useful in many cases.

Treatment

Treatments are chosen according to the stage of melanoma. If the tumor is shallower than 2 mm, it should be removed with a 1 cm margin of healthy skin. If the tumor is deeper than 2 mm, the lesion should be removed with a 2 cm margin of healthy skin. Skin grafting, skin flap, lymph node dissection, and amputation of fingers, toes, and other extremities may be considered. When the disease progresses beyond stage IB, then DAV-feron therapy (local injection of dacarbazine, nimustine hydrochloride, vincristine, and IFN-β) and feron maintenance therapy (once a month local injection of IFN-β) should be considered as postoperative adjunctive treatments. Careful

Table 22.13 TNM classification of melanoma.

T classification Tumor thickness	
Tis: NA	
T1 ≤1 mm	a: Ulceration is not found, and the number of cell divisions <1/mm². b: Ulceration is found, and the number of cell divisions >1/mm².
T2 1.01~ 2.0 mm	a: Without ulceration. b: With ulceration
T3 2.01~ 4.0 mm	a: Without ulceration. b: With ulceration
pT4 > 4.0 mm	a: Without ulceration. b: With ulceration
N classification Number of metastatic lymph nodes	Degree of metastasis in lymph nodes
N0: No metastasis is found in the regional lymph nodes.	
N1: 1 lymph node is involved.	a: Micrometastasis b: Macrometastasis
N2: 2–3 lymph nodes are involved.	a: Micrometastasis b: Macrometastais c: Without lymphatic metastasis, in-transit metastasis or with satellite lesions
N3: 4 or more metastatic lymph nodes, metastatic lymph nodes coalesce, in-transit metastasis with lymphatic metastasis, or formation of satellite lesions	
M classification Location of distant metastasis	Serum lactate dehydrogenase (LDH)
M0: No distant metastases	N/A
M1a: Metastases in the distant skin, subcutaneous or lymph nodes	Normal
M1b: Metastases in the lungs	Normal
M1c: Metastases in other internal organs	Normal Elevated
Any distant metastasis	

Micrometastasis is a condition that is diagnosed by sentinel lymph node biopsy.
Macrometastasis is clinically found lymphatic metastasis that is confirmed histopathologically.

clinical follow-up is necessary for early detection of recurrence or metastasis.

In cases of stage IV with distant metastasis, surgery is rarely performed; instead, chemotherapy using mainly dacarbazine, irradiation therapy, and immunotherapy is administered. The patient responds to chemotherapy in fewer than 30% of cases. There is no effective treatment. It is necessary to choose therapies in consideration of the patient's quality of life.

Prognosis

The depth of tumor cell infiltration and metastasis are important factors in determining prognosis. Five-year survival rates for stages 0–IV are approximately 100%, 95%, 70%, 50%, and 10%.

Table 22.14 Classification of anatomical stage of melanoma (AJCC/UICC, 2010).

	Clinical staging*				Histopathological staging†		
	T classification	N classification	M classification		T classification	N classification	M classification
Stage 0	Tis	N0	M0	Stage 0	Tis	N0	M0
Stage IA	T1a	N0	M0	Stage IA	T1a	N0	M0
Stage IB	T1b	N0	M0	Stage IB	T1b	N0	M0
	T2a	N0	M0		T2a	N0	M0
Stage IIA	T2b	N0	M0	Stage IIA	T2b	N0	M0
	T3a	N0	M0		T3a	N0	M0
Stage IIB	T3b	N0	M0	Stage IIB	T3b	N0	M0
	T4a	N0	M0		T4a	N0	M0
Stage IIC	T4b	N0	M0	Stage IIC	T4b	N0	M0
				Stage IIIA	T1a-4a	N1a	M0
					T1a-4a	N2a	M0
Stage III	any T	N>N0	M0	Stage IIIB	T1b-4b	N1a	M0
					T1b-4b	N2a	M0
					T1a-4a	N1b	M0
					T1a-4a	N2b	M0
					T1a-4a	N2c	M0
				Stage IIIC	T1b-4b	N1b	M0
					T1b-4b	N2b	M0
					T1b-4b	N2c	M0
					any T	N3	M0
Stage IV	any T	any N	M1	Stage IV	any T	any N	M1

* In clinical staging, assessment is done based on the pathological findings of the primary lesion, findings from physical examination, and examination using imaging. Generally, total excision of the primary lesion is done, and staging is done after assessing the metastasis of local lymph nodes and distant metastases.
† In pathological staging, assessment is done based on the pathological assessment of the primary lesion and the lymph nodes. Information is collected by sentinel lymph node biopsy or lymph node dissection. However, cases with pathological staging of 0 or IA are treated as exceptions. Pathological assessment of lymph nodes is not required.
Source: Japan Association of Dermatologic Surgery. *Dermatologic Surgery*. Tokyo: Gakken Medical Shujunsha Co. Ltd., 2010, p. 414.

CHAPTER 23

Viral infections

A virus is a particle of DNA or RNA enclosed by structural proteins. Viruses infect cells and proliferate to cause viral infections. Viral skin diseases are classified according to three groups of clinical features: (1) degeneration of keratinocytes and blistering (e.g., in herpes simplex and herpes zoster), (2) tumorous changes in keratinocytes (e.g., in verruca vulgaris), and (3) generalized skin lesions on the whole body (e.g., in measles and rubella). The first two groups are caused by viral infection in epidermal keratinocytes; the last group is caused by systemic viral infection (viremia). This chapter introduces various viral skin diseases, including HIV infection.

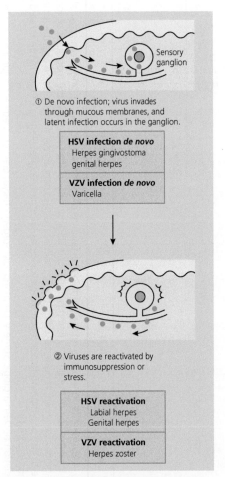

① De novo infection; virus invades through mucous membranes, and latent infection occurs in the ganglion.

| HSV infection *de novo* |
| Herpes gingivostoma |
| genital herpes |

| VZV infection *de novo* |
| Varicella |

② Viruses are reactivated by immunosuppression or stress.

| HSV reactivation |
| Labial herpes |
| Genital herpes |

| VZV reactivation |
| Herpes zoster |

Fig. 23.1 Mechanism of infection by HSV and VZV. HSV, herpes simplex virus; VZV, varciella zoster virus.

Viral infections whose main symptom is blistering

Herpes simplex viral infection (synonym: herpes simplex)

- This is caused by infection or reactivation of herpes simplex virus type 1 (HSV-1) or type 2 (HSV-2).
- Vesicles (herpes) aggregate, accompanied by pain.
- HSV-1 causes herpes labialis, herpes gingivostomatitis, and Kaposi's varicelliform eruption.
- HSV-2 causes herpes genitalis. In recent years, the number of herpes genitalis cases caused by HSV-1 has been increasing.
- The clinical findings are the most important factors in diagnosis. Detection of the viral antigen and the Tzanck test are useful for diagnosis.
- The main treatment is administration of antiviral drugs (e.g., aciclovir).

Pathogenesis

Herpes simplex is caused by herpes simplex virus type 1 (HSV-1) or type 2 (HSV-2). The oral cavity, eyes, and genitalia are affected by HSV-1, whereas the genitalia are mainly involved in HSV-2. The infection pattern of HSV is shown in Figure 23.1. The virus enters the skin

---

Shimizu's Dermatology, Second Edition. Hiroshi Shimizu.
© 2017 John Wiley & Sons, Ltd. Published 2017 by John Wiley & Sons, Ltd.

through a minor external injury or through the oral mucosa, eyes or genitalia. It travels along the sensory nerve axons to reach the trigeminal ganglia or lumbosacral spinal cord ganglia. In 90% of cases, primary infection does not progress beyond latency; however, symptoms such as herpes gingivostomatitis may be apparent in infants or in people with immunodeficiency. After the symptoms subside, viral DNA remains in the gangliocytes. HSV is characterized by reactivation caused by stress or the common cold. Some viruses may travel along the axons in an anterograde direction to reach the skin and cause recurrence of skin symptoms.

Clinical features

The initial latency is between 2 and 10 days. Localized aggregations of small herpetic blisters occur in primary infection. They may occur on any part of the body, but particularly the lips, genitalia, and fingers (Fig. 23.2). Severely erosive plaques accompanied by fever or lymph node enlargement occur (herpes gingivostomatitis), and vesicles may appear on the whole body (Kaposi's varicelliform eruption). Symptoms caused by reactivation are often milder than those at the initial infection. Cases with repeated recurrence may cause serious mental distress.

Pathology

Repetitive replication of viral DNA leads to ballooning degeneration and reticular degeneration of infected keratinocytes (Fig. 23.3). These degenerated keratinocytes are observed as balloon cells containing intranuclear inclusion bodies evident on smear staining of the blister contents (Tzanck test) (see Fig. 23.3).

Laboratory findings

The Tzanck test and detection of the virus using monoclonal antibodies are carried out using blister contents, and serological diagnosis is conducted. HSV-infected keratinocytes are easily and quickly observed by the Tzanck test. Immunofluorescence (IF) using monoclonal antibody detection is conducted to differentiate between HSV-1, HSV-2, and varicella zoster virus (VZV).

Herpes types and treatments

Antiviral drugs such as aciclovir are given topically, orally or intravenously, depending on the severity of

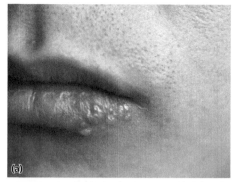
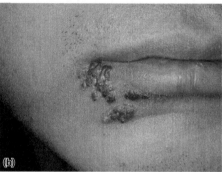
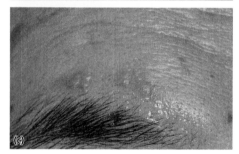

Fig. 23.2 Herpes simplex. a,b: Vesicles aggregated around the lips (herpes labialis) caused by herpes simplex. c: Affected eyebrow. d: Genital herpes.

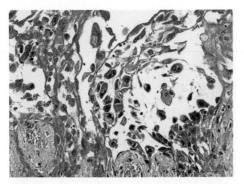

Fig. 23.3 Histopathology of herpes simplex. There is necrotic degeneration in epidermal cells. The giant cells contain inclusion bodies (ballooning cells).

MEMO 23–1 Airborne infection and droplet infection

Airborne infection (droplet nuclei infection): Infectious agents in droplets are dispersed into the air. The moisture in the droplets evaporates to form light droplet nuclei of 5 μm or smaller. The pathogenicity of the infectious agents is maintained after they become nuclei, and the nuclei float in the air for a long time. Infection occurs when the nuclei are inhaled. This type of infectious agent is the same as those of measles, varicella, and tuberculosis.

Droplet infection: Infection occurs when infectious agents from the patient, which are dispersed by coughing or sneezing, adhere to the mucosa of others. The droplet moves less than 1 m because the particle that contains the virus has a diameter of more than 5 μm. This type of infectious agent is the same as those of influenza, rubella, and bacterial pneumonia.

the symptoms. In cases of herpes genitalis with a strong tendency to recur, continuous administration of aciclovir is effective in controlling recurrences.

Herpes labialis (cold sore)

This is the most common clinical form of herpes simplex seen in adults. Most cases are caused by reactivated HSV-1. About 30% of adults are thought to have experienced herpes labialis. Herpes labialis most frequently occurs on the lips and their periphery, including the nostrils, cheeks, and orbital region. Prodromes such as itching, burning sensation, and discomfort appear in about half of all cases. After a day or two, edematous erythema appears and small blisters with central umbilication occur and aggregate, sometimes coalescing to form irregularly shaped blisters. The blisters soon form pustules, erosions, and crusts. They heal in about 1 week.

Herpes gingivostomatitis

This type occurs most frequently in initial infection of HSV-1 in infancy; however, it may also occur in adults. After about 5 days of latency, multiple painful vesicles and erosions occur in the oral mucosa, tongue, and lips. These symptoms are accompanied by discomfort, high fever, and enlargement of the regional lymph node. The fever generally subsides in 3–5 days, and the disorder heals in about 2 weeks.

Kaposi's varicelliform eruption (synonym: eczema herpeticum)

Kaposi's varicelliform eruption occurs most frequently in infants with atopic dermatitis or eczema. Repeated recurrences may be seen in adult patients with atopic dermatitis or in those with immunodeficiency. Primary infection or reactivation of HSV-1 (HSV-2 in some cases) causes Kaposi's varicelliform eruptions. Acute high fever, swelling in systemic lymph nodes, and multiple vesicles on top of eczematous lesions occur. They are surrounded by red haloes, and coalesce into large erosions (Fig. 23.4). Pustules, bleeding, and bacterial infection, particularly of *Streptococcus pyogenes*, often accompany Kaposi's varicelliform eruption. The face and upper body are commonly involved; in breast-fed infants, the lesions often occur over the whole body. The eruptions usually form crusts in 4–5 days; however, eruptions occur successively.

Genital herpes (herpes genitalis)

Genital herpes is typically transmitted through sexual activity. Although men and women in adolescence and older are frequently affected, it may also occur in infants in rare cases. It may be transmitted to an infant by the hands of the mother or a nurse. The causative virus in most cases is HSV-2; however, the number of cases caused by HSV-1 has been increasing in recent years. Severely painful small blisters or erosions form in the glans penis or foreskin of adult men, or in the labia or perineal region of adult women. The inguinal lymph node may become painful and enlarged. The lesions usually disappear spontaneously in 2–4 weeks; however, when the sacral nerve root is involved, it may leave urinary disturbance. The cases caused by HSV-2 infection have a strong tendency to recur. Eruptions repeatedly recur in several weeks in some cases.

Herpetic whitlow

HSV-1 (or HSV-2 in some cases) invades the body from a minor injury in the tip of a finger, leading to the aggregated formation of painful blisters and pustules on the fingers. Blisters on the fingers are not as fragile as those on other sites of the body. Dentists and infants who have a habit of finger sucking may be infected. The condition is recurrent and heals in 2–4 weeks.

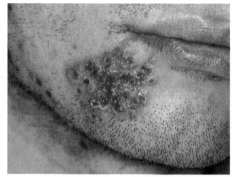
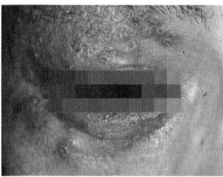
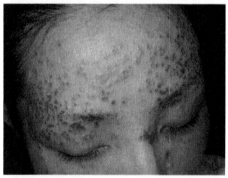
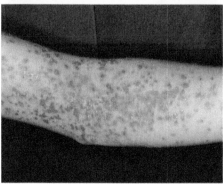

Fig. 23.4-1 Kaposi's varicelliform eruption. The eruptions are rimmed with a vivid red halo. The vesicles coalesce into a large erosion.

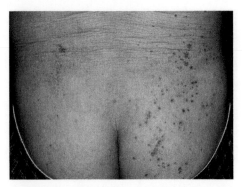

Fig. 23.4-2 Kaposi's varicelliform eruption.

MEMO 23–2 Names of human herpesviruses

Human herpesvirus 1 – herpes simplex virus type 1 (HSV-1)
Human herpesvirus 2 – herpes simplex virus type 2 (HSV-2)
Human herpesvirus 3 – varicella zoster (VZV)
Human herpesvirus 4 – Epstein–Barr virus (EBV)
Human herpesvirus 5 – cytomegalovirus (CMV)
Human herpesvirus 6 – human herpes virus type 6 (HSV-6)
Human herpesvirus 7 – human herpes virus type 7 (HSV-7)
Human herpesvirus 8 – human herpes virus type 8 (HSV-8)

Varicella

- This is commonly known as chickenpox. Infants are most frequently affected.
- Varicella is caused by infection of the varicella zoster virus (VZV), which is extremely infectious.
- A fever occurs concurrently with the emergence of erythematous papules on the whole body. Eruptions progress in the course of vesicles, pustules and crusts, and healing. New eruptions continue to occur such that preexisting eruptions appear together with new eruptions. They heal in 7–10 days.
- The main treatments are antiviral drug administration and symptomatic therapies. Aspirin is contraindicated in infants and children.

Clinical features

After a latency of 2–3 weeks, erythematous papules appear on the whole body, accompanied by fever (37–38°C) and systemic fatigue. Varicella is characterized by small blisters with red haloes that resemble insect bites and by blisters that form on the scalp. Blistering also occurs in the oral mucosa and palpebral conjunctiva. The eruptions are accompanied by itching. They progress in the order of erythema, papules, blisters, pustules, and crusts, over the course of several days. Because the eruptions continue to appear, preexisting eruptions are found together with newly formed ones (Fig. 23.5). Varicella heals in 7–10 days, without scarring (Fig. 23.6). If the eruptions are scratched or secondarily infected, they heal with moderate scarring.

The main complications are secondary bacterial infections (impetigo contagiosa and cellulitis), pneumonia, encephalitis (with meningeal irritation signs such as high fever and headache), unilateral high-frequency deafness (thought to be a symptom of

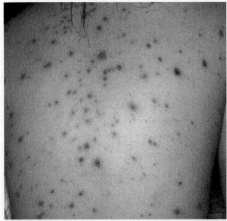

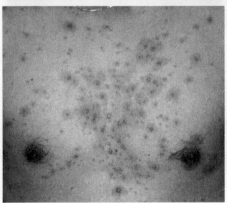

Fig. 23.5-1 Varicella in an adult.

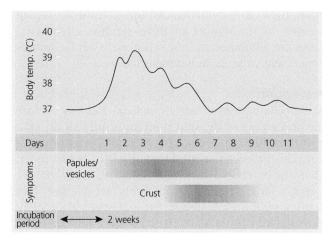

Fig. 23.6 The clinical course of varicella/chickenpox.

Ramsay–Hunt syndrome), and Reye syndrome (cerebritis and fatty liver).

Pathogenesis and epidemiology
Varicella is caused by infection with the VZV. This virus enters the upper respiratory tract by airborne or contact infection and proliferates in the regional lymph nodes, inducing primary viremia. The virus further proliferates in the liver and spleen, leading to secondary viremia, and it reaches the skin, resulting in blistering. The rate of latent infection is reported to be about 5%. Varicella occurs most frequently between weaning and early childhood. Ninety-five percent of children aged nine years have the antibodies. The age of initial infection has risen in recent years; varicella in adults is increasing. In adult cases, varicella is often accompanied by encephalitis and pneumonia, and it can easily become severe.

Laboratory findings and diagnosis
The Tzanck test is useful for early diagnosis. Infected keratinocytes are observed as balloon cells. Immunofluorescence using monoclonal antibodies of blister contents and measurement of the serum antibody titer are carried out.

Treatment
Oral antiviral drugs are often used to stop infection from worsening. Symptomatic therapies such as oral antihistamines against itching and topical petrolatum or antibiotic ointments for eruptions are the main treatments for infants. Phenol and zinc oxide ointments are

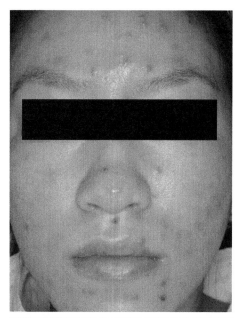

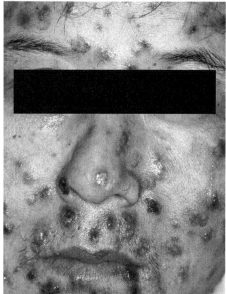

Fig. 23.5-2 Varicella.

often used as treatments. Aspirin is contraindicated because of the danger of Reye syndrome. Antiviral drugs are administered intravenously to adults, immunodeficient patients, and newborns.

Prevention

A varicella patient is infectious from 1–2 days before the occurrence of the skin symptoms until all the skin eruptions have crusted over. Within 72 h after infection, the onset can be inhibited by varicella vaccine in 60–80% of cases. Oral antiviral drugs may reduce symptomatic severity in patients who have had contact with an affected individual, even after 72 h. Varicella can be fatal in patients with immunodeficiency; human immunoglobulin containing high anti-VZV antibody titer is used as a treatment in some cases.

Herpes zoster

- Herpes zoster is caused by reactivation of latent VZV in the ganglia.
- Band-like herpetic aggregations of small blisters form on certain innervated regions. Pain is present in areas over the involved nerves.
- The blisters may disseminate on the whole body in cases with immunodeficiency.
- The pain that persists after healing is called postherpetic neuralgia (PHN). When the ears and peripheral regions are involved, hearing loss and peripheral facial paralysis may occur (Ramsay–Hunt syndrome).

Clinical features

Herpes zoster symptoms are divided into cutaneous and nervous. Prodromes such as neuralgic pain and abnormal paresthesia often occur several days before the eruptions manifest. After a few days, edematous erythema with small blisters appears at sites of pain or paresthesia.

Mucocutaneous symptoms

Edematous erythema appears in band-like patterns over certain innervated regions. The skin over the intercostal nerve is most frequently involved, followed by the trigeminal area of the face (Fig. 23.7). Later, small vesicles occur and transform into aggregated blisters (herpetic blisters). All these blisters progress in the same course, which is different from varicella, in which preexisting blisters are found concurrently with

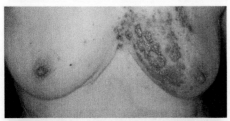
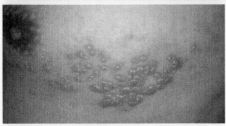

Fig. 23.7-1 Herpes zoster.

MEMO 23–3 Zoster-associated pain (ZAP)

In herpes zoster, acute pain occurs in the early period and as postherpetic neuralgia (PHN), which is a sharp pain caused by irreversible nerve degeneration. NSAIDs are effective only for the former. The two types of pain in combination tend to be called ZAP.

newly formed ones. The blisters soon rupture and become erosions. They heal after crust formation in 2–3 weeks.

Nervous symptoms
Neuralgic pain is often present several days before the onset of eruptions. Sharp pain peaks 7–10 days after the occurrence of skin lesions. The degree of pain varies from that causing slight perceptual dysfunction to severe pain that causes insomnia. Paralysis may occur in some cases. In most cases, the pain subsides with remission of the eruptions.

Herpes zoster subtypes
- **Generalized herpes zoster:** in patients who are immunocompromised as a result of steroid or immunosuppressant intake or a primary disease, small blisters may spread over the whole body several days after manifestation of the typical eruptions of herpes zoster. The infection prevention measures used for varicella are required.
- **Herpes zoster with eye symptoms:** complications involving the eyes, such as conjunctivitis and keratitis, may occur in herpes zoster at the first division of the trigeminal area (ophthalmic nerve). The result is the occurrence of acute retinal necrosis that can lead to blindness in rare cases. Herpes zoster on the nasal dorsum often induces eye complications (Hutchinson's sign).
- **Ramsay–Hunt syndrome:** the external auditory canal and auricle are involved. Peripheral facial palsy and acoustic nerve impairment are present. The pathogenesis is thought to be pressure exerted on the facial nerve by the geniculate ganglia. In some cases, facial palsy is the only symptom and there is no blistering.
- **Postherpetic neuralgia (PHN):** neuralgia may persist after the eruptions disappear. The pathogenesis is thought to be irreversible nerve degeneration. It often occurs after the onset of herpes zoster in elderly people or in those whose eruptions were severe. The degree of pain varies from persistent localized discomfort to severe paroxysmal pain causing insomnia that persists for several years.

Pathogenesis and epidemiology
Herpes zoster is caused by reactivation of latent VZV. During the course of varicella, VZV travels to the

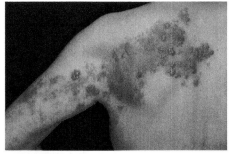
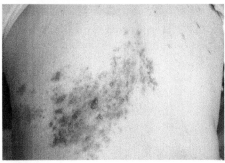
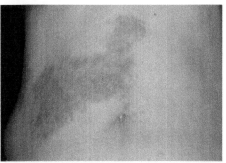
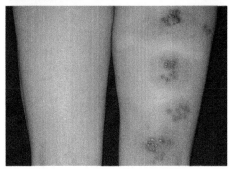

Fig. 23.7-2 Herpes zoster on various sites of the body.

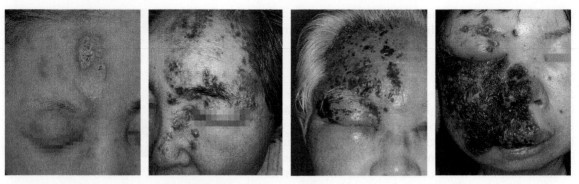

Fig. 23.7-3 Herpes zoster on the first and second divisions of the trigeminal nerve. Eye symptoms such as conjunctivitis and keratitis occur as complications in some cases.

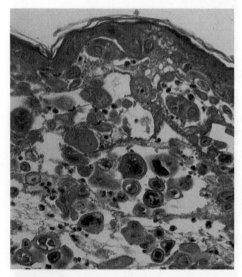

Fig. 23.8 Histopathology of herpes zoster. Many ballooning cells in the blister.

sensory nerves to reach the ganglia, whose dorsal root cells remain latently infected after varicella heals and the anti-VZV antibodies increase. Stress, aging, malignant tumor, and immunodeficiency can trigger reproliferation of VZV (see Fig. 23.1) and cause herpes zoster. Herpes zoster occurs most frequently in people between the ages of 10 and 30, and over 50.

Diagnosis and examinations

The Tzanck test (Fig. 23.8), detection of viral antigens, and serological diagnosis are carried out, as for cases of herpes simplex and varicella. Early ophthalmological examination should be conducted on any lesions involved in the first division of the trigeminal area. When the ears and peripheral regions are involved, particular care should be taken in detecting facial palsy.

Treatment and prognosis

The main purpose of treatment is to alleviate the sharp pain in the acute stages to prevent complications and sequelae. As a basic treatment, antiviral drugs are administered, orally at the early stages and intravenously in severe cases. Non-steroidal antiinflammatory drugs (NSAIDs) and vitamin B12 are used as symptomatic therapy. After the first infection, patients obtain permanent immunity due to reactivated cell-mediated immunity.

As treatments for PHN, oral vitamin B12, pregabalin, and antidepressants are administered; thermotherapy, low-level laser therapy, and other physical therapies are given; and nerve block is instigated. Cases with intense symptoms may be treated at a pain clinic.

Viral infections whose main symptom is verruca

Verruca vulgaris, common wart
- This is caused by human papillomavirus (HPV) infection.
- It occurs most frequently on the fingers, toes, soles, and dorsal surfaces of the hands. It is largely asymptomatic.
- Liquid nitrogen cryotherapy, topical glutaraldehyde application, carbon dioxide gas laser therapy, and electrosurgery are useful. Some cases heal spontaneously.

Pathogenesis
Verruca vulgaris is caused by the human papillomavirus (HPV), a virus in the Papovaviridae family. The most frequent HPV infection is HPV-2 (Table 23.1). The virus invades the skin from a minor external injury and infects the keratinocytes. It replicates simultaneously with differentiation of keratinocytes, leading to the maturation of viral particles in the granular cell layer. The viral particles are released concurrently with exfoliation of the verruca, causing spread to other areas.

Clinical features
Verruca vulgaris occurs most commonly on the hands and feet of infants. After a latency of 1–6 months, it begins with small papules. They enlarge, elevating in verrucous shape and reaching several millimeters to several centimeters in diameter (Fig. 23.9). Usually multiple but sometimes solitary eruptions of verruca

Table 23.1 HPV types and clinical symptoms.

Type	Symptoms
1	Myrmecia
2, 4, 7	Verruca vulgaris
3, 10	Verruca plana
5, 8	Epidermodysplasia verruciformis
57, 60	Epidermoid cyst of the sole
6, 11	Condyloma acuminatum
16, 18, 31, 33–35, 39, 40, 51–59	Cervical dysplasia, endocervical cancer

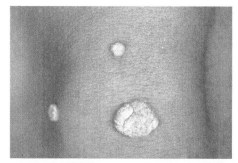
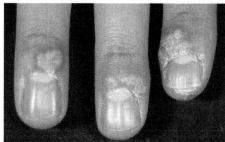
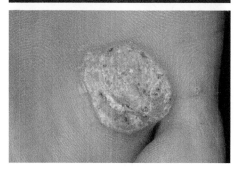

Fig. 23.9-1 Verruca vulgaris.

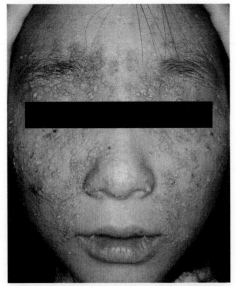

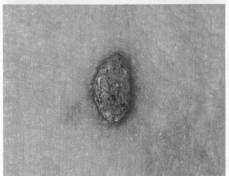

Fig. 23.9-2 Verruca vulgaris.

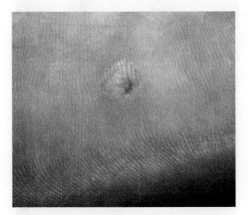

Fig. 23.10 Myrmecia. A dome-shaped nodule occurs, accompanied by tenderness.

vulgaris aggregate, coalesce, and may form plaques. It is largely asymptomatic.

There are some types of verruca vulgaris that are given characteristic clinical diagnostic names according to the clinical features, type of virus, and the affected site.

Plantar wart

This is verruca vulgaris on the soles of the feet. A keratotic lesion forms without distinct elevation. It resembles tylosis and clavus, but can be differentiated from those by scraping. If surface scraping of the keratotic lesion causes petechiae, the diagnosis is plantar wart (see Chapter 15).

Myrmecia

A small, dome-shaped nodule forms on the palms and soles (Fig. 23.10). Also called deep palmoplantar wart, it is caused by HPV-1 infection. It has a red, cratered appearance. Tenderness is often present. It is a type of plantar wart.

Pigmented wart

The main cause is infection by HPV-4, or by HPV-60 in rare cases. It has the clinical features of verruca vulgaris and blackish pigmentation; it is also called a black wart.

Punctate wart

A punctate wart is caused by HPV-63. Multiple punctate, white keratotic lesions occur on the palms and soles.

Filiform wart

A long, thin protrusion of several millimeters in diameter occurs on the face, head or neck (Fig. 23.11). It is a type of verruca vulgaris.

Pathology

There is hyperkeratosis, parakeratosis, and thickening of the granular cell layer with papillary acanthosis of the epidermis. Cells with vacuolar degeneration and large keratohyaline granules are found in the granular cell layer. These cellular changes, called koilocytosis, are characteristic of HPV infection (Fig. 23.12).

Treatment

The main treatment for verruca vulgaris is liquid nitrogen cryotherapy. Surgical removal and cauterization by carbon dioxide gas laser are conducted at sites where cryotherapy is not fully effective, including palms and soles. Topical application of activated vitamin D3, monochloroacetate or glutaraldehyde, and local injection of bleomycin are carried out. The lesion may heal spontaneously after the occurrence of inflammatory reactions.

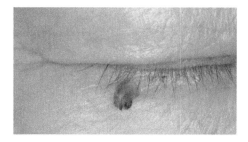

Fig. 23.11 Filiform wart.

Verruca plana, plane wart, flat wart (synonym: verruca plana juvenilis)
Clinical features and pathogenesis
A flat wart is a viral wart that is often caused by HPV-3 or HPV-10. Multiple slightly elevated, flat papules 2–10 mm in diameter occur on the face (forehead and cheeks). These may coalesce or appear in a linear pattern from autoinfection (Köbner phenomenon) (Fig. 23.13). The papules are normal skin color or light pink and nearly asymptomatic. When they disappear spontaneously, inflammatory symptoms such as itching and reddening occur, and the warts heal with scaling. However, flat warts may persist for several years.

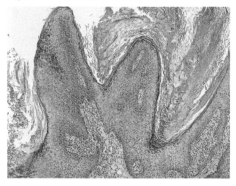

Fig. 23.12 Histopathology of verruca vulgaris.

Treatment
Liquid nitrogen cryotherapy is recommended.

Condyloma acuminatum
- Genital papillary papules are caused by HPV-6 or HPV-11. This is a sexually transmitted infection.
- Latency is 2–3 months.
- Liquid nitrogen cryotherapy, topical imiquimod, and surgical removal are the main treatments.

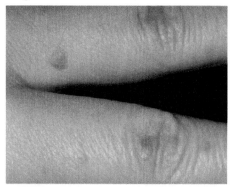

Epidemiology, pathogenesis, and clinical features
Condyloma acuminatum is caused by HPV-6 or HPV-11. Most cases occur in the sexually active years, transmitted through sexual activity. The latency is 2–3 months. Multiple verrucous papules of papillary, cockscomb or cauliflower shape occur in the genitals or perianal region (Fig. 23.14). Keratinization is rarely present. The papules are infiltrative at the surface and may give off a foul odor. Condyloma acuminatum may enlarge, keratinize, and ulcerate. Large condyloma acuminatum on the penis is called a Buschke–Lowenstein tumor, which is considered to be a type of verrucous carcinoma (MEMO; see Chapter 22).

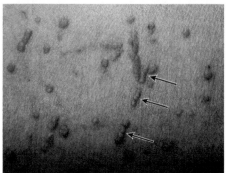

Fig. 23.13 Flat wart. Köbner phenomenon (arrows) is seen (bottom).

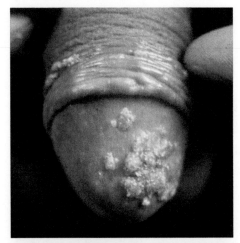

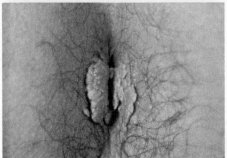

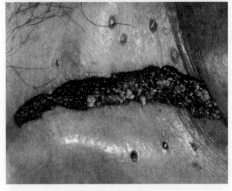

Fig. 23.14 Condyloma acuminatum.

Diagnosis and differential diagnosis

Condyloma acuminatum can be diagnosed by the clinical features; however, biopsy may be needed for differential diagnosis, such as from Bowenoid papulosis (see next section). It is necessary to differentiate condyloma acuminatum from pearly penile papule and vestibular papillae of the vulva, which are physiological changes (see Chapter 21).

Treatment

Treatments including cryotherapy are administered as for cases of verruca vulgaris. Topical application of imiquimods has been used in recent years.

Bowenoid papulosis

Multiple flatly elevated black papules 2–20 mm in diameter occur on the genitalia of young people (Fig. 23.15). The small papules may coalesce and form plaques. It is usually asymptomatic. HPV-16 is detected in the lesion. It is thought to be an atypical type of condyloma acuminatum (see previous section). Bowenoid papulosis is histopathologically indistinguishable from Bowen's disease (see Chapter 22). It rarely becomes malignant, and it may heal spontaneously. The prognosis is good. Cryotherapy and electrical cauterization are the main treatments.

Epidermodysplasia verruciformis

Epidermodysplasia verruciformis is a rare autosomal recessive inherited disease in which verrucous lesions occur in patients with congenital cellular immunodeficiency against HPV. Abnormalities of the *EVER1* and *EVER2* genes have been reported as predisposing factors. The main causative viruses are HPV-5, HPV-8, HPV-17, and HPV-20. Relatively large, flat wart-like, reddish-brown keratotic patches that resemble seborrheic keratosis appear on sunlight-exposed areas, such as the dorsal surfaces of the hands, even from early childhood (Fig. 23.16). The lesions often coalesce to form plaques or reticular arrangements. Pityriasis versicolor-like leukoderma and erythema may occur. Multiple bright and enlarged clear dysplastic cells are observed histopathologically in the upper suprabasal cell layer.

The eruptions gradually spread over the whole body surface. Malignant skin tumor (e.g., squamous cell carcinoma, basal cell carcinoma, Bowen's disease) occurs in about half of adolescent and older patients. Sunscreen is used preventively. Oral retinoid administration is effective.

Molluscum contagiosum

- This is caused by molluscum contagiosum viral infection.
- It occurs most frequently in young children. Multiple molluscum contagiosum may appear on the face of patients with AIDS.
- Small, multiple, dome-shaped nodules 2–10 mm in diameter occur. Autoinfection is caused by the adhesion of wart contents to the epidermis.
- Tweezer excision of the wart using a pair of trachoma forceps is the most effective treatment.

Clinical features

The latency of molluscum contagiosum is between 14 and 50 days. The disorder is most common in children, who tend to be predominantly affected on the trunk, extremities, genitalia, lower abdomen, and medial thigh. Multiple, small, dome-shaped papules 2–10 mm in diameter occur. The eruptions are flat and glossy on the surface and umbilicated in the center (Fig. 23.17). The eruptions contain an opaque white gruel-like substance. Erythema and inflammation occur at the periphery of the eruption. The eruptions are asymptomatic except for mild itching.

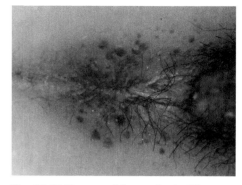

Fig. 23.15 Bowenoid papulosis. The papules caused by Bowenoid papulosis are blackish in most cases, or close to normal skin color in some cases.

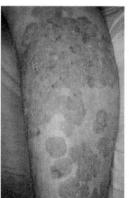 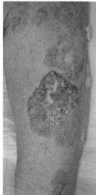 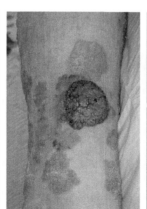 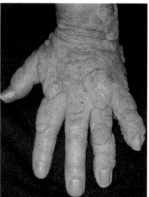

Fig. 23.16 Epidermodysplasia verruciformis. Large, flat, verrucous, reddish-brown keratotic macules occur. The eruptions elevate and form tumors in some cases.

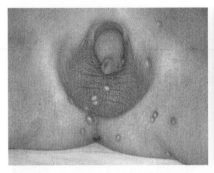 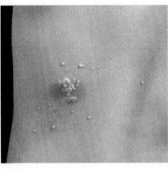 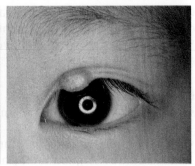

Fig. 23.17 Molluscum contagiosum. The small papules are glossy on the surface and umbilicated at the center.

Pathogenesis and epidemiology

Warts are produced by the *Molluscum contagiosum* virus, in the Poxviridae family. The virus invades the skin from a minor external injury or hair follicle and proliferates in the suprabasal cells of the epidermis. When the lesions are scratched, the contents adhere to the epidermis and cause autoinfection. In recent years, infections in healthy children at swimming schools, in adults from sexually transmitted infections, and in patients with immunodeficiency have been increasing.

Pathology

Molluscum contagiosum is characterized by lobulated, endophytic hyperplasia that produces a circumscribed intracutaneous pseudo-tumor. The keratinocytes contain very large intracytoplasmic inclusions (molluscum bodies) (Fig. 23.18).

Complications

When typical eruptions are found, diagnosing molluscum contagiosum is easy. Young children with atopic dermatitis are frequently affected. When the lesions are scratched, eruptions may not be clearly seen. Sudden occurrence of multiple molluscum contagiosum in adults, on the face in particular, is strongly suggestive of AIDS involvement.

Treatment

The lesions are removed using trachoma forceps. Cryocoagulation therapy and application of 40% silver nitrate are also useful. Molluscum contagiosum spontaneously disappears in several months. When it is asymptomatic, follow-up may be chosen as a treatment option.

Fig. 23.18 Histopathology of molluscum contagiosum.

Viral infections with generalized skin lesions

Measles

- This is an infectious disease caused by the measles virus. Young children are most frequently affected.
- A fever and common cold-like symptoms occur after an incubation period of about 2 weeks. When the fever subsides, white macules called Koplik's spots appear in the oral mucosa. Fever recurs (diphasic fever) with catarrhal symptoms, and eruptions and skin lesions appear over the whole body. The fever subsides rapidly in 3–4 days with exfoliation of the eruptions. Healing occurs with pigmentation.
- Otitis media, pneumonia, encephalitis, and subacute sclerosing panencephalitis (SSPE) may occur as complications.

Clinical features

The clinical features of measles appear after an incubation period of 10–14 days (Fig. 23.19). The clinical course of measles is divided into the catarrh stage (the first 5 days from onset), the eruption stage (the next 5 days), and the recovery stage (Fig. 23.20).

Catarrh (prodrome stage)

A fever of about 38°C and catarrhal symptoms such as nasal discharge, sneezing, eye discharge, and cough persist for 3–4 days. At this stage, the respiratory secretions, lacrimal fluid, and saliva are at their most infectious. On the last 1–2 days of the catarrhal symptoms, punctate white macules called Koplik's spots appear on the buccal mucosa and sometimes on the gums at almost the same time as the fever subsides (Fig. 23.21).

Second stage (eruption)

After the fever subsides, it recurs, accompanied by eruptions and aggravation of the common cold-like symptoms. It persists for 3–4 days (diphasic fever). Dark reddish edematous erythema occurs first at the opisthotic areas and on the cheeks, then spreading to the trunk and extremities. The erythema enlarges and coalesces, forming irregular shapes with a reticular pattern.

Third stage (recovery)

The fever subsides in several days. Healing is with exfoliation of eruptions and pigmentation.

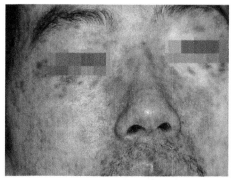
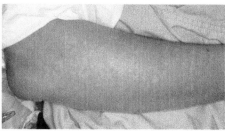

Fig. 23.19 Measles.

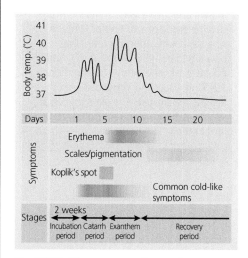

Fig. 23.20 The course of measles.

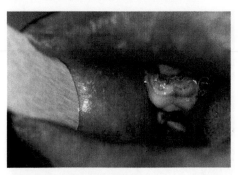

Fig. 23.21 Koplik's spots.

MEMO 23–4 Variola (synonym: smallpox)

Variola is caused by infection of the upper respiratory mucosa by *Orthopoxvirus variola*. Infection is by droplet or contact. This pathogen is so virulent that it used to be fatal in many cases; however, Jenner's cowpox vaccine made prevention possible. A smallpox eradication program was developed in 1958 by the WHO, and no cases of variola have occurred since 1977. In 1980, the WHO declared the disease eradicated. The virus is kept at secure institutions in biosafety level 4 labs in the US and Russia.

Modified measles

When measles infection occurs in a person who has incomplete immunity to measles, mild measles with an atypical clinical course occurs, called modified measles. It may occur in infants younger than 3 months who have antigens of maternal origin, people who have been given γ-globulin prophylactically or those who received vaccination several years before.

Complications

Pneumonia, otitis media, measles encephalitis, and SSPE may occur as complications. The pneumonia and encephalitis may be fatal. Aggravation of tuberculosis may occur in measles patients.

Pathogenesis

The causative virus is in the family Paramyxoviridae, genus *Morbillivirus*. Infants in the first 3 months after birth are not infected by the measles virus, because of the maternal-to-fetal transfer of passive immunity. Infants between the age of 3 months and early childhood are most commonly affected. The measles virus is highly infectious and invades by the airborne route. It proliferates in the epithelial cells of the nasopharynx, resulting in viremia. Subclinical infection rarely occurs; more than 95% of infected patients show apparent infection. Affected individuals gain strong permanent immunity.

Diagnosis and differential diagnosis

Decreases in both neutrophils and lymphocytes (leukocytopenia) and increases in lactate dehydrogenase (LDH) are observed by peripheral blood examination. Serological assay of antibody responses, viral isolation of respiratory secretions, and PCR analysis are useful for diagnosis. It is differentiated from other viral infections, including rubella and exanthema subitum, and from scarlet fever, drug eruptions, erythema multiforme, Kawasaki's disease, and sepsis (Fig. 23.22).

Treatment

There is no effective treatment for measles. Bedrest, keeping the body warm, and oral antipyretics and antitussives are recommended as symptomatic therapies. Bacterial complications are treated with antibiotics. Human immunoglobulin may be used in severe cases.

Prevention

When the route of infection has been defined and no more than 5 days have passed after infection, the onset can be prevented or symptoms mitigated by intramuscular injection of human immunoglobulin. Vaccination is effective only within the first 72 h after infection. A live, highly attenuated vaccine is used for immunization. The rate of immunity obtained is 95% or higher.

Rubella

- Caused by the rubella virus, this is commonly known as German measles or "three-day measles."
- The main symptoms are eruptions, enlarged lymph nodes (the postauricular lymph node, in particular), and fever.
- Eruptions and fever occur concurrently. Papular erythema accompanied by moderate itching on the face spreads to the whole body surface and does not coalesce. Healing is without scaling or pigmentation.
- Rubella infection in early pregnancy may induce congenital rubella syndrome in the fetus. Pregnant women must avoid rubella infection and vaccination.

Clinical features

The clinical course is shown in Figure 23.23. After a latency of 2–3 weeks, the systemic lymph nodes enlarge. Enlargement in the postauricular region and cervical lymph node is particularly noticeable and persists for several weeks. In some cases, it begins with eruptions and fever without lymph node enlargement. Several days later, papular erythema and itching spread over the whole body accompanied by moderate fever (Fig. 23.24). Unlike measles, the eruptions of rubella are solitary and do not usually coalesce. They disappear without scaling or pigmentation in 3–5 days. Petechiae-like enanthema called Forschheimer spots occurs in the palate mucosa in about half of all cases.

Complications

Encephalitis, meningitis, thrombocytopenic purpura in infancy and arthritis in adulthood occur as complications. If a woman is infected in or before her fifth month of pregnancy, the newborn may also be affected (congenital rubella syndrome, CRS).

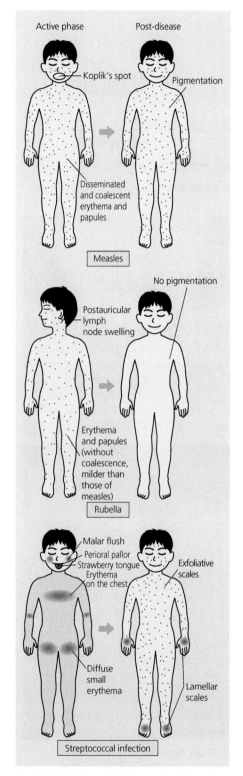

Fig. 23.22 Differential diagnosis of measles.

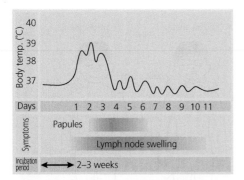

Fig. 23.23 The course of rubella.

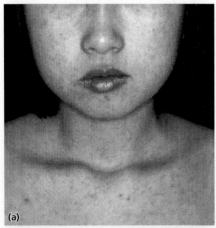

Fig. 23.24 Rubella. a: Erythematous papules on the face and upper chest. b: Erythematous papules on the trunk.

Pathogenesis

The rubella virus, an RNA virus in the family Togaviridae, genus *Rubivirus*, invades the body from the upper respiratory tract by droplet infection or contact infection, proliferates in the regional lymph node, and causes viremia resulting in rubella. Permanent immunity is obtained after the first infection, although reinfection occurs in rare cases. Most patients are between 5 and 15 years old. Rubella tends to occur in spring and summer epidemics at intervals of 3–10 years.

Laboratory findings, diagnosis, and differential diagnosis

Leukocytopenia, thrombocytopenia, and atypical lymphocytes are found by peripheral blood test. Increased antibody titer is observed by serological assay. Cases with moderate symptoms are diagnosed by the clinical course and epidemic circumstances. Other viral infections such as measles, exanthema subitum, and scarlet fever should be differentiated from rubella (see Fig. 23.22).

Treatment and prevention

Symptomatic treatments are helpful.

Exanthema subitum, roseola infantum

* This is caused by human herpesvirus (HHV) types 6 and 7. Breast-fed infants are most commonly affected.
* A high fever occurs suddenly and persists for 3 or 4 days. As the fever subsides, measles-like eruptions appear on the whole body. They do not coalesce, but disappear without pigmentation in 2–3 days.
* Febrile convulsions may occur as a complication.

Clinical features

After a 2-week latency, an acute high fever of 38–39°C occurs and persists for 3–4 days. Infected children in most cases appear normal. Diarrhea and moderate cough often occur. About the time when the fever subsides, light pink macules occur on the face and trunk. They do not coalesce, but disappear without pigmentation in 2–3 days (Fig. 23.25). Seizures may occur during the febrile period in 6–15% of patients. Acute encephalitis or liver dysfunction may occur as a complication in rare cases.

Pathogenesis

The causative viruses are thought to be HHV-6 type B and HHV-7. Although HHV-6 is spread by saliva transfer, newborns are not infected because of maternal passive immunity; infants between the ages of 6 months and 3 years are affected.

Diagnosis and treatment

Exanthema subitum can be diagnosed by the characteristic clinical features. In about two-thirds of cases, enlargement and reddening occur in the lymph follicles at the base of the uvula. These findings are helpful for diagnosis. Symptomatic treatments are helpful. Aspirin is contraindicated because of the danger of Reye syndrome.

Erythema infectiosum (synonym: fifth disease, slapped cheek disease)

- Erythema infectiosum is caused by human parvovirus B19. It is commonly known as slapped cheek disease.
- Flush appears in the cheeks, and papular erythema occurs on the extremities, coalescing to present lacy, reticulated eruptions that predominate in the extremities. These heal without scaling or pigmentation in about 1 week.
- Infection in pregnancy may lead to fetal hydrops. If patients with hemolytic anemia are infected, acute pure red cell aplasia occurs, resulting in marked anemia.

Clinical features

Erythema infectiosum is commonly known as fifth or slapped cheek disease. It tends to occur in spring and summer epidemics. It occurs most frequently in children between 4 and 10 years of age; however, there are also cases in which adults, especially mothers and nurses, are infected by infants and children. Latency is between 4 and 14 days. Erythema infectiosum may begin with mild prodromal symptoms. Influenza-like catarrhal symptoms occur in some cases. Erythema that resembles a hand slap occurs suddenly on both cheeks and disappears in 1–4 days (Fig. 23.26). A day or two after the facial lesion manifests, erythematous lesions of about 1 cm diameter occur on the extensor surfaces of the arms first, and then the legs. These coalesce gradually and begin to heal at the center, leaving the characteristic lacy, reticulated pattern. When the trunk is involved, no lacy pattern is present. The

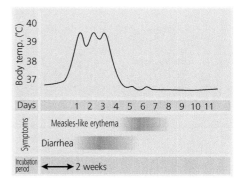

Fig. 23.25 The course of exanthema subitum/roseola infantum.

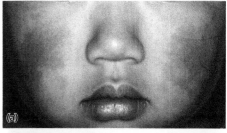

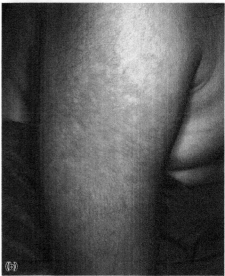

Fig. 23.26 Erythema infectiosum. a: Erythema on the cheeks ("slapped cheek"). b: Erythema on the upper arm.

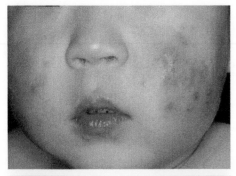

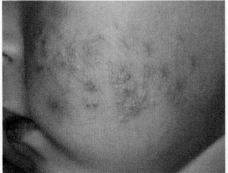

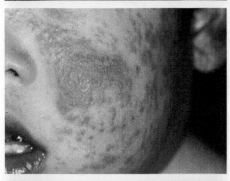

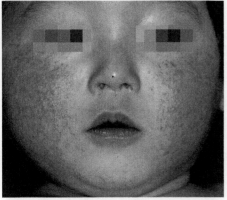

Fig. 23.27-1 Gianotti-Crosti syndrome.
Multiple infiltrative erythematous papules
on the cheeks. Coalesced plaques are seen.

eruptions disappear without scaling or pigmentation in about 1 week.

In adult cases, the slapped cheek erythematous lesions are indistinct, and non-specific erythematous lesions, joint pain, and elevated antinuclear antibody level are observed. Cases of erythema infectiosum in adults should be differentiated from collagen diseases.

Infection before 20 weeks of pregnancy may lead to fetal hydrops or fetal death. Rapid decrease of erythrocytes (aplastic crisis caused by acute pure red cell aplasia) occurs in cases with hemolytic anemia or immunodeficiency as an underlying condition, leading to marked anemia.

Pathogenesis

Erythema infectiosum is caused by droplet infection of human parvovirus B19, which is in the *Parvovirus* genus of DNA viruses. The virus invades the body by respiratory infection and proliferates within erythroblasts of the bone marrow in 4–7 days, resulting in viremia. Manifest infection occurs in 70% of infant cases and 30% of adult cases.

Treatment

No specific antiviral therapy is available. Accessory symptoms are treated symptomatically. Recurrence of cutaneous lesions may be caused by sunlight exposure or exercise for several weeks after healing.

Gianotti–Crosti syndrome (synonym: papular acrodermatitis of childhood)

- Papules appear on the legs, ascending to the arms and face.
- It is caused by infection with hepatitis B virus or Epstein–Barr virus. It occurs most frequently in infants.

Clinical features

Gianotti–Crosti syndrome occurs most frequently in infants between the ages of 6 months and 12 years. Multiple, flat, light pink to dark red papules 3–4 mm in diameter suddenly appear solitarily and symmetrically on the legs and buttocks. The lesions rapidly ascend to the arms and face in 3–4 days. Multiple infiltrative red papules and coalesced plaques on the cheeks and extensor surfaces of the arms are characteristic features of Gianotti–Crosti syndrome (Fig. 23.27). The trunk, palms, and soles are rarely involved. Although it is accompanied by mild itching, cases caused by hepatitis B virus are often asymptomatic. The lesions disappear with mild scaling in about 1 month. Enlargement of the superficial lymph node and liver, elevation of liver enzymes, fever, loss of appetite, diarrhea, and common cold-like symptoms may occur.

Pathogenesis

Gianotti–Crosti syndrome has been reported to be caused by the hepatitis B virus, the Epstein–Barr virus, cytomegaloviruses, coxsackieviruses, RS viruses, and rotaviruses. It is thought that the initial infection by these viruses causes eruptions characteristic of allergic reactions. The frequency of cases caused by the EB virus is high.

Treatment and disease course

Follow-up without treatment may be chosen because the condition generally resolves naturally. When the causative virus is the hepatitis B virus and HB antigens persist after the eruptions disappear, the patient may become an HBV carrier.

Hand, foot, and mouth disease (HFMD)

- These eruptions are caused by coxsackievirus A16 or enterovirus 71. Breast-fed infants are most commonly affected.
- After a latency of several days, erosion, papules, and small vesicles appear in the distal portions of the extremities and oral mucosa. The lesions disappear in 4–7 days.
- When caused by enterovirus 71, HFMD may be accompanied by meningitis.
- The only treatment that is usually necessary is oral hydration.

Clinical features

Hand, foot, and mouth disease occurs after 2–5 days of latency. In about half of all cases, slight fever and common cold-like symptoms are present for 1 or 2 days. Lesions in the oral cavity are present in nearly all cases. Erythematous eruptions of 2–3 mm diameter that number from a few to several dozen occur on the buccal mucosa and tongue. They gradually form blisters, erosions or aphtha-like erosions with red haloes. The sharp pain that accompanies the oral lesions may cause difficulty in drinking that may result in dehydration. Lesions in the extremities are seen in about two-thirds of cases. Dispersed small oval blisters with red

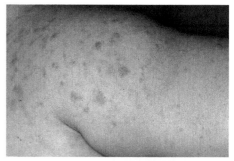
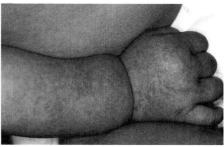

Fig. 23.27-2 Gianotti–Crosti syndrome.
Multiple infiltrative erythematous papules on the extensor surface of the upper extremities. Coalesced plaques are seen.

MEMO 23–5 Gianotti–Crosti syndrome and Gianotti–Crosti disease

The term "Gianotti–Crosti disease" may be used for the condition caused by the hepatitis B virus, and "Gianotti–Crosti syndrome" for conditions caused by other viruses.

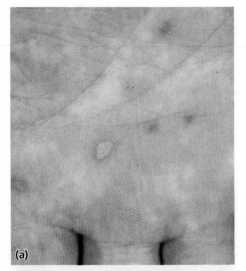

(a)

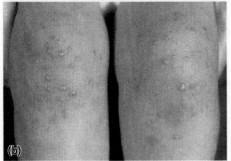

(b)

Fig. 23.28-1 Hand, foot, and mouth disease. a: Vesicles are accompanied by red haloes and slight tenderness. b: Eruptions on the knees.

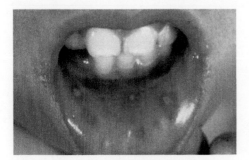

Fig. 23.28-2 Hand, foot, and mouth disease. Vesicles are accompanied by sharp pain and aphtha in the oral mucosa.

haloes appear on the hands, soles, knee joints, and buttocks (Fig. 23.28). The blister's long axis is often parallel to the dermatoglyphic line. Some degree of tenderness, but not itching, may accompany these. The lesions disappear in 7–10 days. When caused by enterovirus 71, HFMD may be accompanied by aseptic meningitis.

Pathogenesis and epidemiology
The main causative viruses are coxsackievirus A16 and enterovirus 71. These proliferate in the intestinal tract and are found in stool and pharyngeal secretions. The viruses are spread by droplet, oral, and contact routes. The infectiousness is so high that widespread outbreaks sometimes occur in hospitals. Infectious virus in stool is found 2–4 weeks after the disappearance of symptoms. It most commonly occurs in children under the age of 10 years and in summer epidemics.

Treatment and prognosis
The only treatment that is usually necessary is oral hydration. When high fever, headache, and vomiting continue, complication with meningitis is suspected. Permanent immunity is obtained from the first infection; however, multiple infections may occur because the causative viruses are multiple.

Infectious mononucleosis
- Infectious mononucleosis is caused by infection with the Epstein–Barr virus (EBV). It occurs most frequently in puberty.
- The main symptoms are high fever, pharyngeal pain, and swelling in the cervical lymph nodes. Rubella-like and measles-like eruptions and erythema multiforme appear.
- Symptomatic therapy is the main treatment. Penicillin-containing drugs and aspirin are contraindicated.

Clinical features
The latency of infectious mononucleosis is 1–2 months. After prodromes such as headache and generalized fatigue persisting for several days, a high fever (higher than 39°C) and intense pharyngeal pain occur. Eruptions appear 4–10 days after the onset in about 20% of cases (Fig. 23.29). Various skin symptoms occur, including rubella-like eruptions, urticarial erythema, and erythema multiforme. The eruptions subside spontaneously in several days.

If the pharyngeal pain is misdiagnosed as bacterial pharyngeal pain and antibacterial drugs are administered, particularly penicillin-containing drugs, then a hypersensitive reaction is induced that aggravates the eruptions. Intense swelling and tenderness occur in the systemic lymph nodes, particularly in the cervical lymph nodes. Splenohepatomegaly accompanied by hepatic dysfunction often occurs.

The fever subsides in 7–10 days, after which the symptoms gradually subside. Thrombocytopenia, hemolytic anemia, meningitis, encephalitis, and Guillain–Barré syndrome occur as complications.

Pathogenesis and epidemiology

Infectious mononucleosis is caused by infection with the EBV. Permanent immunity is obtained from the first infection. EBV is always present in the oral cavity, and it easily spreads orally or through inhalation. The virus invades the body, proliferates in the epithelial cells of the pharyngeal mucosa and travels to the regional lymph node. It immortalizes B cells by latently infecting them through CD21 on their surfaces.

It is thought that the B cells induce cellular immunity (CD8$^+$ T cells and NK cells), which causes infectious mononucleosis. Over 90% of adults are previously infected. Initial infection generally occurs by the age of 3 years, and most cases are latent infections. Conversely, when the first infection occurs in adolescence, apparent infection takes place as infectious mononucleosis in about half of the cases. It occurs most frequently in adolescents between the ages of 14 and 18, regardless of the season. Patients are often infected by the mother in the case of young children, and by the opposite sex in the case of patients in puberty and later; infectious mononucleosis is commonly called "kissing disease."

Laboratory findings

Leukocyte levels are elevated. Numerous large cells called atypical lymphocytes appear. These cells are not B cells infected by EBV but CD8$^+$ T cells activated to exclude infected cells. Increased serum aspartate aminotransferase (AST), alanine aminotransferase (ALT), and alkaline phosphatase (ALP) titers resulting from liver dysfunction and antibodies produced by infected B cells lead to elevated levels of polyclonal human immunoglobulin. Measurement of EBV antibody titer (Fig. 23.30) is useful for diagnosis. The diagnostic criteria for children are listed in Table 23.2.

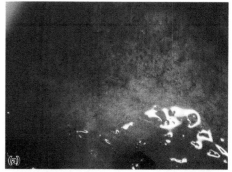
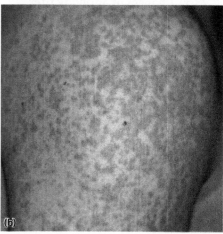
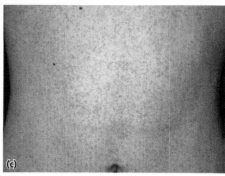

Fig. 23.29 Infectious mononucleosis.
a: Lesion on the soft palate. b: Lesion on the shoulder and upper arm. c: Lesion on the trunk.

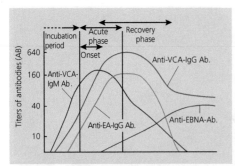

Fig. 23.30 Changes of antibody titer related to EBV, and staging of infectious mononucleosis. Source: Akira I. Infectious mononucleosis. In Ogawa S (ed.) *Standard Textbook of Internal Medicine*, 7th edn. Tokyo: Nakayama Shoten, 2009, p. 99.

Table 23.2 Diagnostic criteria for infectious mononucleosis in infants.

1 Clinical features: at least 3 items positive
a. Fever b. Tonsillitis, pharyngitis c. Swelling of lymph node of the neck region ($\geq$1 cm) d. Hepatomegaly (under 4 years old: $\geq$1.5 cm) e. Palpable splenomegaly
2 Blood findings
a. Lymphocytes $\geq$50% or 5000/mL, and b. Atypical lymphocytes/HLA-DR + cells $\geq$10%, or $\geq$1000/mL
3 EBV antibody test (acute EBV infection): acute-stage EBNA antibody negative and positive in one or more of the following
a. VCA-IgM antibody is initially positive but later turns negative. b. VCA-IgG antibody titer is elevated by a factor of 4 or more. c. EA antibody transitorily increases. d. VCA-IgG antibody is positive from the initial stage, and EBNA antibody turns positive later. e. EBNA-IgM antibody is positive/EBNA-IgG antibody is negative.

Source: Wakiguchi H. Infection (virus infection, herpes virus infection, Epstein-Barr virus infection). In Shiraki K, et al. (eds) *Pediatrics*, 2nd edn. Tokyo: Igaku-Shoin, 2002, p. 539.

Treatment

There are no specific treatments for infectious mononucleosis, other than bedrest and symptomatic therapies. Drugs containing aspirin or penicillin are contraindicated: aspirin may cause Reye syndrome and penicillin may induce a severe hypersensitive reaction. Chronic active EBV infection may occur in rare cases of patients with infectious mononucleosis.

Specific viral infectious diseases

Acquired immunodeficiency syndrome (AIDS)

- Diagnosis is confirmed when the CD4$^+$ T cell count is found to be reduced by HIV and the diagnostic criteria are met.
- The infection routes are sexual activity, blood infection, and mother-to-child transmission.

- Mucocutaneous symptoms such as Kaposi's sarcoma, oral candidiasis, molluscum contagiosum, and seborrheic dermatitis may be helpful for diagnosis. Herpes zoster, *Cryptococcus* infection, tinea, and drug eruptions often occur.

Cutaneous symptoms of AIDS

The symptoms of AIDS (Fig. 23.31) are listed below. A decreased CD4+ T cell count is associated with AIDS.

Kaposi's sarcoma

In Japan, homosexual males are most commonly affected. Multicentric nodules ranging from reddish-purple to blackish-brown occur most frequently. See Chapter 22, for details.

Mucocutaneous infectious disease

Candidiasis occurs in the oral cavity in all cases of AIDS; it has diagnostic value. Herpes simplex and herpes zoster are easily caused and tend to become generalized and severe. Molluscum contagiosum appears multiply on the face. Verruca vulgaris, *Cryptococcus* infection, tinea, and impetigo also occur and become intractable, displaying atypical clinical features in many cases.

Drug-induced skin reactions

Eruptions caused by drug therapies for opportunistic infections (e.g., pneumocystis pneumonia) frequently occur. Eruptions caused by anti-HIV drugs often occur: Stevens–Johnson syndrome from nevirapine, anaphylactic shock from abacavir, and lipodystrophy from reverse transcriptase inhibitors and protease inhibitors should be noted.

Other symptoms

Seborrheic dermatitis, psoriasis vulgaris, and eosinophilic pustular folliculitis often occur.

Systemic symptoms of AIDS

Primary HIV infection progresses to the asymptomatic stage and then to symptomatic HIV infection, resulting in the onset of AIDS (Fig. 23.32).

Primary HIV infection (acute HIV infection)

Three to 6 weeks after infection, fever, fatigue, sore throat, headache, diarrhea, and enlarged lymph nodes, as well as papular eruptions on the whole body, occur and resolve.

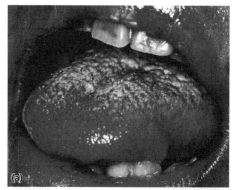
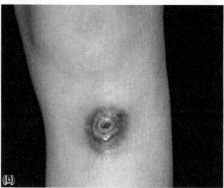
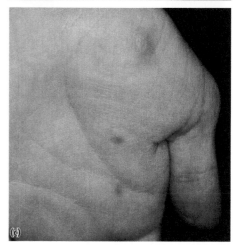

Fig. 23.31-1 Cutaneous lesions in a patient with AIDS. a: Candidiasis of the tongue. b: Ulceration by non-tuberculous mycobacteria on a lower extremity. c: Macular syphilide on the palm.

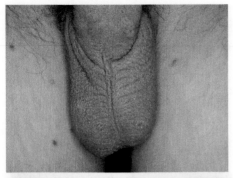

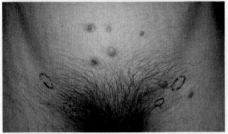

Fig. 23.31-2 Cutaneous lesions in a patient with AIDS. Papular syphilide: Multiple infiltrative, light pink papules 5–10 mm in diameter occur.

Asymptomatic stage (asymptomatic carrier)

This stage of clinical latency lasts for 5–10 years. The CD4+ T cell count gradually decreases. The patient begins to develop herpes zoster, oral candidiasis, and seborrheic dermatitis because of compromised immunity.

Progression from HIV to AIDS

HIV RNA levels begin to rise, and the CD4+ T cell count falls below 200 per microliter. Opportunistic infection and Kaposi's sarcoma occur.

Epidemiology

HIV/AIDS-infected patients numbered 35.3 million worldwide at the end of 2013. The main endemic areas are Africa, Latin America, and Asia. The prevalence has stabilized in Asia.

Pathogenesis and mechanism of infection

AIDS is caused by infection with the human immuno-deficiency virus, which is classified in the *Lentivirus* genus of the Retroviridae family; the virus can be isolated from blood, serum, genital secretions, breast milk, cerebrospinal fluid, urine, saliva, and lacrimal fluid. The main infection routes are sexual activity, blood infection (from blood products, transfusion, the sharing of needles for drugs, needle-stick accidents), and mother-to-child infection.

HIV targets CD4+ T cells and macrophages. The virus invades the cells by binding gp120 on the virus to CD4 on the target cells. In recent years, other coreceptors besides CD4 have been found to be involved.

When HIV invades the cells, proviral DNA is produced by HIV reverse transcriptase and transcribed into lymphocytic DNA by integrase, leading to latent infection. Viral particles synthesized from the implanted DNA mature from the action of protease, and then bud (Fig. 23.33).

Diagnosis and examination

Anti-HIV antibody screening is conducted by enzyme-linked immunosorbent assay (ELISA). Although the test is highly sensitive, it is ineffective for differential diagnosis because there are false positives in patients with autoimmune disease and it takes 6–8 weeks after HIV infection for antibodies to be produced (window period). Screenings that show positive must be

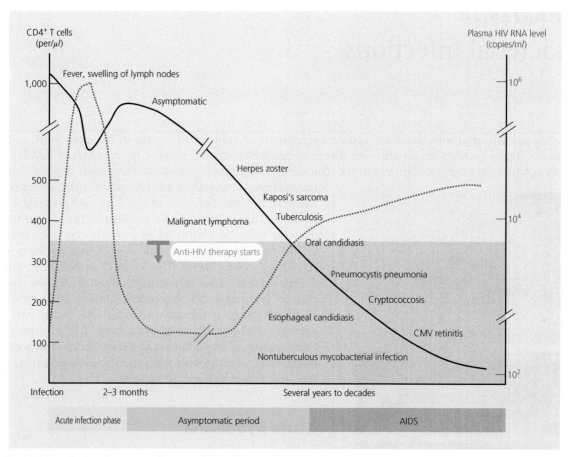

Fig. 23.32 Relation between the number of CD4⁺ T cells in an HIV patient and the course of opportunistic infection.

reexamined by more specific tests, such as Western blot or TaqMan PCR.

The nucleic acid amplification test (NAAT) is used for testing during a short window of about 3 weeks.

Treatment

Reverse transcriptase inhibitors such as azidothymidine (AZT) work effectively as anti-HIV drugs. Highly active antiretroviral therapy (HAART) with reverse transcriptase inhibitors and protease inhibitors such as indinavir (IDV) improves the prognosis significantly. Combination therapy of anti-HIV drugs is helpful. In recent years, coreceptor inhibitors (particularly CCR5) and integrase inhibitors have been developed.

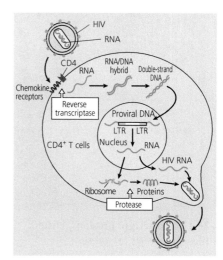

Fig. 23.33 Life cycle of the human immunodeficiency virus (HIV).

CHAPTER 24
Bacterial infections

Cutaneous bacterial infections are caused by resident or transient bacteria in the epidermis and mucosa. These bacteria invade the skin where its barrier function is weaker, such as at hair follicles, sweat glands, and sites of minor trauma. The occurrence of symptoms after infection depends on the balance between the amount and virulence of the bacteria and the defenses of the host. When a cutaneous bacterial infection is suspected, the causative bacteria must be identified by culture and microbial sensitivity test in order for the appropriate antibacterial drugs to be chosen. This chapter introduces four main subtypes of bacterial infections, classified by the clinical features, and the representative diseases of each subtype: acute cutaneous infections (acute pyoderma), chronic cutaneous infections (chronic pyoderma), systemic infections caused by toxins produced by bacteria, and diseases with specific clinical features that are caused by specific bacteria.

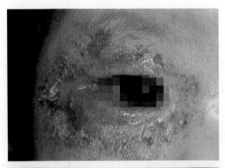

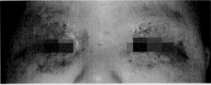

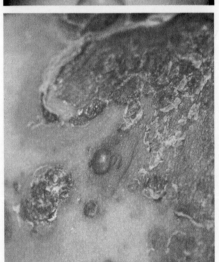

Fig. 24.1-1 Impetigo. Erosions, blisters, pustules, and crusts are present.

Acute pyoderma

Impetigo, impetigo contagiosa
- Bacterial infection occurs under the stratum corneum, producing toxins that cause blisters and crusts. The infection spreads by autoinoculation.
- Infants are most frequently affected. Impetigo is divided into bullous impetigo, with blistering, and non-bullous impetigo, with crusts. The causative bacteria are *Staphylococcus aureus* and group A β-hemolytic *Streptococcus*, respectively.
- Systemic administration of cefem antibiotics is the main treatment.

Bullous impetigo
Clinical features
Bullous impetigo occurs most commonly in infants, during the summer. It often spreads through epidemic outbreaks at daycare centers or nursery schools. It tends

Shimizu's Dermatology, Second Edition. Hiroshi Shimizu.
© 2017 John Wiley & Sons, Ltd. Published 2017 by John Wiley & Sons, Ltd.

to occur at sites of minor trauma, insect bite, eczema or atopic dermatitis when those sites are scratched. Bullous impetigo begins as an itchy, slightly inflammatory vesicle that enlarges to form flaccid blisters. The blisters easily break and become erosive, forming new blisters by peripheral spreading or dispersal to distant locations (Fig. 24.1). Bullous impetigo is transmitted by contact with an infected person. Nikolsky's sign is negative. It heals without scarring. It may progress to staphylococcal scalded skin syndrome (SSSS).

Pathogenesis

Staphylococcus aureus proliferates in the stratum corneum, producing exfoliative toxin (ET), which digests desmoglein 1 in the epidermis and leads to intraepidermal blisters (see Chapter 1 and Chapter 14).

Differential diagnosis

Insect bites in which blisters are severely inflammatory and contain sterile components can be distinguished from bullous impetigo. In staphylococcal scalded skin syndrome (SSSS), the characteristic features are lesions around the eyes and mouth, systemic symptoms including fever, and positive Nikolsky's sign; it should be differentiated from bullous impetigo. Cases with adult onset should be differentiated from pemphigus foliaceus, in which mildly increased serum anti-Dsg1 antibody titers may be observed. The skin should be kept clean. To prevent transmission, patients should not share towels until crusts have formed. Topical application of antibiotic ointments and oral cefem antibiotics are useful.

Non-bullous impetigo
Clinical features and epidemiology

A few blisters form. Non-bullous impetigo begins as small erythema, followed by multiple pustules and the formation of yellowish-brown crusts. The crusts are thick and firmly adherent; they discharge pus when pressured. Pain and swelling occur in the regional lymph node, often accompanied by pharyngeal pain and fever. The onset of non-bullous impetigo is acute and is independent of age and season. The prevalence has been increasing among patients with atopic dermatitis.

Pathogenesis

The condition is caused by subcorneal infection of group A β-hemolytic *Streptococcus* (*Streptococcus pyogenes*)

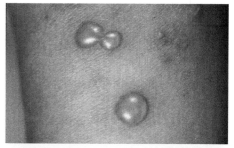
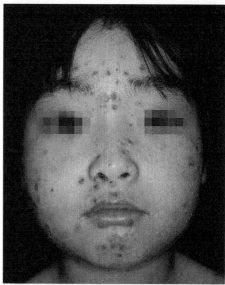
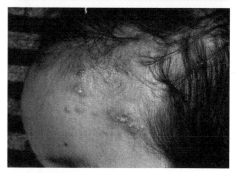

Fig. 24.1-2 Impetigo. Disseminated vesicles and pustules appear on the arms and face.

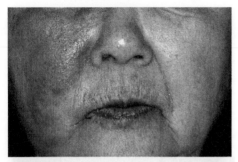

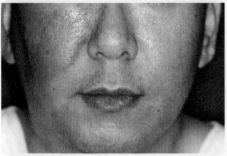

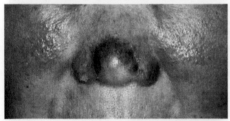

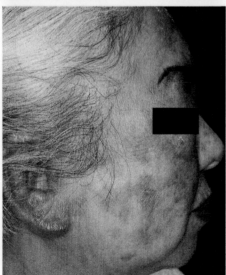

Fig. 24.2 Erysipelas. Sharply demarcated, edematous erythema on the face. It is accompanied by tenderness and flush.

or *Staphylococcus aureus*. Mixed infections of the two types are frequently found.

Differential diagnosis

It is difficult to distinguish non-bullous impetigo from Kaposi's varicelliform eruption, particularly in children with atopic dermatitis. The two conditions may occur at the same time.

Treatment

Oral antibiotics are the first-line treatment. Urine analysis is conducted in cases with streptococcal non-bullous impetigo, because glomerulonephritis may occur as a complication. To prevent nephritis, the administration of oral antibiotics is continued for at least 10 days after remission of the eruptions.

Erysipelas

- This is most often caused by group A β-hemolytic streptococcal infection (*Streptococcus pyogenes*).
- The face is most frequently affected. Sharply demarcated edematous erythemas rapidly spread and sudden fever occurs. Intense tenderness and burning sensation are present.
- Because *Streptococcus pyogenes* is not easily detected by culture, the ASO and ASK values are also measured.
- Systemic administration of penicillin and cefem antibiotics is the first-line treatment.

Clinical features

Sharply demarcated edematous erythemas accompanied by chills and fever occur suddenly, frequently on the face and legs. Fever may occur 1–2 days before the cutaneous symptoms. The erythema surface is tense and glossy. There is intense burning sensation and tenderness. Blistering may occur on the edematous erythema (erysipelas bullosa). The eruptions spread

---

MEMO 24–1 Ecthyma

Ecthyma at the early stage resembles impetigo contagiosa; however, the lesion rapidly spreads to the dermis and gangrene with red halo forms. Group A β-hemolytic streptococci are frequently detected in the test. Multiple lesions similar to those in ecthyma are caused by *Pseudomonas aeruginosa* in patients with immunological deficiency (ecthyma gangrenosum).

rapidly and centrifugally. When the face is involved, first one side is affected and then the other (Fig. 24.2). Swelling of the regional lymph nodes, including in the neck and inguinal regions, generally accompanies the condition. Nausea and vomiting may be present. The eruptions may recur repeatedly on previously affected sites; this is called recurrent erysipelas.

Pathogenesis

Erysipelas is a purulent inflammatory disease that primarily affects the dermis. It can be understood as shallow cellulitis (see next section) localized in the dermis. It is most frequently caused by group A β-hemolytic *Streptococcus*. *Streptococcus pyogenes* of other groups, *Staphylococcus aureus*, and *Streptococcus pneumoniae* may cause symptoms similar to those of erysipelas. Infections may be induced by external injury, including microinjury in the external auditory canal caused by ear picking, and by tonsillitis, chronic venous insufficiency, and tinea pedis. Recurrent erysipelas tends to occur in patients with lymphatic edema.

Laboratory findings

Antistreptolysin O (ASO) and antistreptokinase (ASK) increase as a result of streptococcal infection. Elevated erythrocyte sedimentation rate, leukocytosis (left shift of the nuclei in leukocytes), and C-reactive protein (CRP) positivity are observed. The rate of bacterial detection from tissue fragments is low.

Diagnosis and differential diagnosis

Cellulitis is more deeply seated than erysipelas (see Fig. 24.3), and its erythema edges are less clearly defined. Necrotizing fasciitis can be distinguished from erysipelas by the rapidly progressing necrotic lesions and intense systemic symptoms. Facial erysipelas at an early stage is particularly difficult to distinguish from herpes zoster, contact dermatitis, and insect bites.

When the lesions are present in the legs, thrombophlebitis, deep vein thrombosis, Sweet syndrome, sclerosing panniculitis, and carcinoma erysipelatodes must be differentiated from erysipelas.

Treatment

Erysipelas responds well to oral or intravenous antibiotics such as penicillin drugs and first-generation

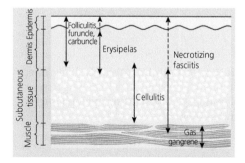

Fig. 24.3 Acute pyoderma classified by the depth of the affected skin.

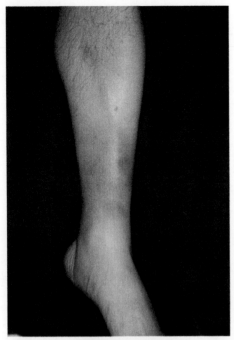

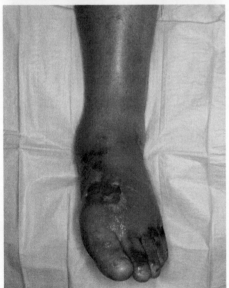

Fig. 24.4-1 Cellulitis. Vaguely demarcated erythema, swelling, localized temperature elevation, localized flush, and tenderness are present.

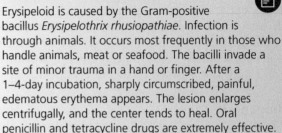

MEMO 24–2 Erysipeloid

Erysipeloid is caused by the Gram-positive bacillus *Erysipelothrix rhusiopathiae*. Infection is through animals. It occurs most frequently in those who handle animals, meat or seafood. The bacilli invade a site of minor trauma in a hand or finger. After a 1–4-day incubation, sharply circumscribed, painful, edematous erythema appears. The lesion enlarges centrifugally, and the center tends to heal. Oral penicillin and tetracycline drugs are extremely effective.

cefem. Administration of oral antibiotics is continued for 10 days after remission to avoid recurrence and prevent the complication of nephritis.

Cellulitis

- This acute purulent inflammation occurs in the deep dermal layer and subcutaneous tissue (Fig. 24.3).
- Vaguely demarcated erythema, swelling, localized heat sensation, and sharp pain occur acutely on the face and extremities.
- It may progress to necrotizing fasciitis or septicemia.
- The main treatments are systemic administration of antibiotics and resting of the affected area.

Clinical features

The face and extremities, particularly the lower legs, are most frequently involved. Cellulitis begins with ill-demarcated erythema, swelling, and localized burning sensation. The lesions spread quickly and are accompanied by tenderness and spontaneous pain (Fig. 24.4). The centers of the lesions may become soft and form blisters and pustules. Systemic symptoms such as fever, headache, chills, and arthralgia are present. Lymphangitis or swelling of the regional lymph node may occur as a complication. Red lines originating from the lesions and leading to proximal areas may be found. Cellulitis may progress to necrotizing fasciitis (see Fig. 24.16) or septicemia.

Pathogenesis

Most cases of cellulitis are caused by *Staphylococcus aureus*. Group A β-hemolytic *Streptococcus* and *Haemophilus influenzae* are among the causative species. Bacteria usually invade the skin through a minor cutaneous ulcer, folliculitis or tinea pedis, causing cellulitis secondarily; however, the entry route may not be identifiable. Chronic venous insufficiency and lymphatic edema may induce cellulitis. Adult cases may occur with underlying disease, including diabetes and AIDS. In infants, immunodeficiency may be found as the underlying condition.

Differential diagnosis

Lesions caused by erysipelas are superficial and sharply circumscribed; however, differentiation from cellulitis is difficult. Necrotizing fasciitis is accompanied by purpura, blisters, bloody blisters, and severe systemic symptoms. Thrombophlebitis, deep vein thrombosis, erythema nodosum, insect bites, eosinophilic cellulitis, and herpes zoster should also be differentiated from cellulitis.

Treatment

Systemic administration of cefem antibiotics is the main treatment. Resting of the affected area and administration of intravenous cefem antibiotics under hospitalization should be done if possible. Necrotizing fasciitis is suspected when non-localized symptoms are present, including high fever, abnormally high leukocyte and CRP levels, and marked systemic symptoms.

Folliculitis

- This is a shallow, localized bacterial infection in a hair follicle. It is a small pustule accompanied by erythema.
- It may progress to furuncle or carbuncle.
- The main treatments are skin care and topical or oral antibiotics.

Clinical features

Erythemas and pustules accompanied by mild pain occur at the hair follicle (Fig. 24.5). Acne vulgaris (see Chapter 19) is a type of folliculitis. It heals in several days without scarring in most cases. When the condition progresses to deep-seated folliculitis, nodules form and inflammation intensifies (furuncle or carbuncle; see next section). Deep-seated folliculitis in the barba areas (moustache, beard, sideburns) is called sycosis vulgaris. Erythematous lesions with crusts may coalesce into plaques.

Pathogenesis

A hair follicle is infected by *Staphylococcus aureus* or *Staphylococcus epidermidis*. A minor trauma, obstruction or scratch around a hair follicle, or the topical

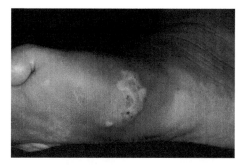

Fig. 24.4-2 Cellulitis.

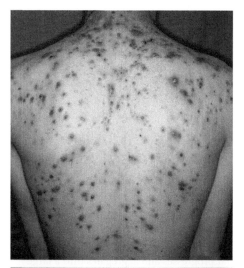

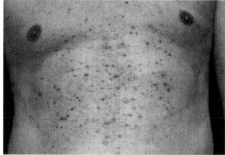

Fig. 24.5 Folliculitis caused by *Malassezia furfur* (see Chapter 25).

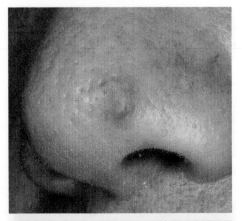

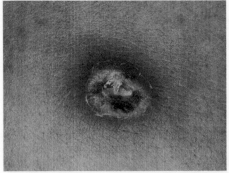

Fig. 24.6 Furuncle (top) from folliculitis that progressed to form an abscess. A carbuncle (bottom) results from a furuncle that progresses and aggregates into a large abscess.

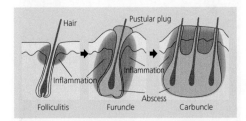

Fig. 24.7 Classification of bacterial infectious diseases of the hair follicles.

application of steroids, may induce the infection. The hair follicle becomes inflamed.

Treatment

When there are only a few eruptions, keeping the affected area clean or using topical retinoids is effective. Topical or oral antibiotics are used in cases with multiple eruptions or for sycosis vulgaris.

Furuncle, carbuncle

- This is advanced folliculitis. A pustular plug forms at the center of the skin lesion. There is purulent swelling.
- It is called a furuncle when a single hair follicle is involved, and a carbuncle when the furuncle spreads to multiple hair follicles.
- The administration of antibiotics, and incision and drainage of pus are the main treatments.

Clinical features

A small red follicular papule or pustule (folliculitis) appears, accompanied by induration (Fig. 24.6). Reddening, necrosis, spontaneous pain, and localized burning sensation become marked. The induration softens and becomes an abscess in several days to a few weeks. The inflammatory symptoms quickly subside when the pus discharges. It heals leaving a small scar. When this type of lesion occurs in a single follicle, it is called furuncle. When a furuncle repeatedly recurs over a long period of time or when multiple furuncles occur, it is called furunculosis. Immunodeficiency from diabetes, internal malignancy or AIDS may underlie some cases of furunculosis.

A carbuncle is an aggravated furuncle whose inflammation spreads to multiple peripheral hair follicles (Fig. 24.7). Carbuncles are dome-shaped, reddish or swelling indurations with several pustular plugs at the top (see Fig. 24.6). They are often accompanied by sharp pain and systemic symptoms such as fever and fatigue. The back, nape of the neck, and thighs are often involved.

Diagnosis

Painful, inflamed swelling occurs in the hair follicle. Diagnosis can be confirmed when a pustular plug is seen at the center of the eruption. It may be difficult to differentiate furuncle or carbuncle from inflammatory epidermal cyst (see Chapter 21).

Differential diagnosis

An inflammatory epidermal cyst is an epidermoid cyst that is infected with bacteria and develops abscesses. White gruel-like contents and the cyst wall discharge from the dome-shaped elevation when a small incision is made. Hidradenitis suppurativa occurs, most frequently at sites with apocrine sweat glands, such as axillary fossae, and it progresses slowly.

Treatment

Antibiotics are administered orally, or intravenously in severe cases. Incision and drainage of pus under local anesthesia is conducted in cases with palpable pulsation.

Bacterial paronychia (synonyms: whitlow, felon)

- This is purulent inflammation around the nail plate of the fingers and toes. An abraded wound or ingrown nail often induces the condition.
- The main symptoms are reddening and swelling, and abscess formation accompanied by pulsating sharp pain.
- Administration of oral antibiotics, and incision and drainage of pus are the main treatments.

Clinical features

Sharp throbbing pain, swelling, reddening, burning sensation, and abscess are caused by bacterial infection in the skin and subcutaneous tissue of the periungual region of the finger (Fig. 24.8). The nail plate may appear green when the infection is caused by *Pseudomonas aeruginosa* (green nail; see Chapter 19). The nail may exfoliate.

Pathogenesis

The main causes of bacterial paronychia are *Staphylococcus aureus*, *Streptococcus pyogenes*, and *Pseudomonas aeruginosa*. Puncture wounds, ingrown nails, and adhesive tape often induce it.

Diagnosis and treatment

Mucous cyst, glomus tumor, Osler's node, herpetic whitlow, and candidal paronychia should be differentiated from bacterial paronychia. Resting and cooling the affected site and administering topical and oral antibiotics are the main treatments. Incision and drainage of pus are considered if necessary.

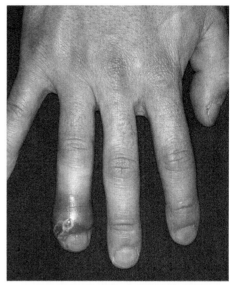
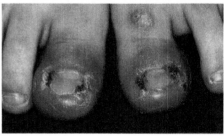

Fig. 24.8 Bacterial paronychia. Purulent inflammation occurs in the fingers, toes, and nails, and their periphery. It is accompanied by severe tenderness.

Multiple sweat gland abscesses in infants (synonym: periporitis staphylogenes)

Multiple painful pustules, subcutaneous indurations, and abscesses occur on the face, scalp, back, and buttocks of newborns and infants, most frequently in summer. The condition may be accompanied by moderate fever. Miliaria (see Chapter 19) appears as a precursor, with *Staphylococcus aureus* infection in the obstructed eccrine glands resulting in multiple sweat gland abscesses. Oral or topical antibiotics are administered. Incision and drainage of pus may be done. Prevention by frequent changes of clothes and proper skin hygiene is important.

Chronic pyodermas

Definition and classification

Chronic pyoderma is a general term for chronic purulent diseases in which multiple obliterative lesions of hair follicles are infected by bacteria, leading to prolonged inflammatory reaction or granulomatous inflammation. It is most frequently caused by *Staphylococcus aureus, Staphylococcus epidermidis*, and coliform bacteria. Multiple abscesses with intricately netted fistulae occur, and the lesions excrete pus. Many diagnostic names for chronic pyoderma exist but they all refer to the same disease. The axillary fossae, scalp, and buttocks are most commonly involved.

Treatment and prognosis

Keeping the affected area clean and using oral or topical antibiotics are effective. It is necessary to use oral tetracycline drugs for long periods of time in many cases. Incision and drainage of pus, and removal and skin graft may be carried out in some cases. Squamous cell carcinoma may originate from these conditions.

Hidradenitis suppurativa

This is hidradenitis in the opening of a hair follicle contained in an apocrine sweat gland. The follicular opening is blocked, leading to deposition of secretion which results in chronic infection (Fig. 24.9). One or several subcutaneous nodules about 5 mm in diameter occur, most frequently on the axillary fossae of women. The nodules soften, rupture, excrete pus, and heal

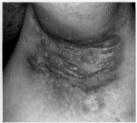

Fig. 24.9 Hidradenitis suppurativa.
Subcutaneous nodules of several millimeters in diameter on the axillary fossae rupture spontaneously. The lesions soften and coalesce, leading to the formation of scarring plaques.

with scarring. Other sites with apocrine sweat glands, such as the genitalia, anus, and breasts, may also be involved.

Keloidal folliculitis
Folliculitis appears multiply and continuously on the occipital and nuchal regions of middle-aged men. Infiltration in the lesion gradually becomes intense, and connective tissue proliferates and forms a keloidal plaque (Fig. 24.10). Abscess formation and secretion of pus may be present in severe cases. Differentiation from kerion (see Chapter 25) is necessary.

Pyoderma chronica glutealis
Middle-aged men are most frequently affected. Acne-like pustules or papules appear on the lumbar region, genitalia, and thighs, gradually coalescing into a large, infiltrative plaque. Abscesses with intricately netted fistulae form, which excrete pus when pressed (Fig. 24.11). There is hidradenitis suppurativa or acne conglobata as an underlying disease in many cases.

Systemic infections

Staphylococcal scalded skin syndrome (synonym: staphylococcal toxic epidermal necrolysis)
- The condition occurs most frequently in infants and children up to age 6. Fever and reddening around the mouth or eyes first appear, followed by painful exfoliation, erosions, and blistering.
- Exfoliative toxin A produced by *Staphylococcus aureus* digests desmoglein 1 in the desmosomes of the epidermis, leading to blisters and erosions.
- Nikolsky's sign is positive.
- Systemic management and care, and administration of antibiotics are the main treatments.

Clinical features
Staphylococcal scalded skin syndrome (SSSS) occurs most frequently in infants and children up to age 6; it is extremely rare in adults. It begins with reddening and blistering around the mouth, nostrils, and periocular area. This is accompanied by systemic symptoms,

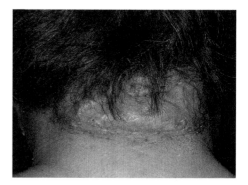

Fig. 24.10 Keloidal folliculitis. Scarring with thick plaques on the back of the head and neck.

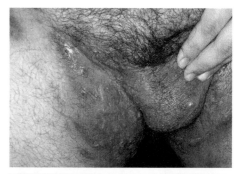

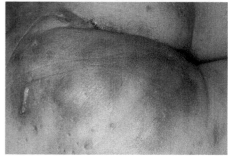

Fig. 24.11 Pyoderma chronica glutealis. Large infiltrative plaques accompanied by pustules, papules, fistulae, and abscesses spread to the crotch.

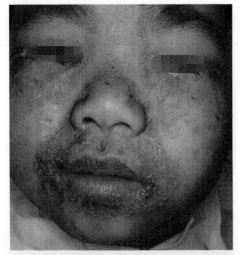

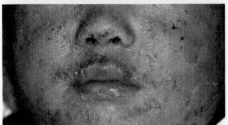

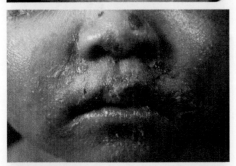

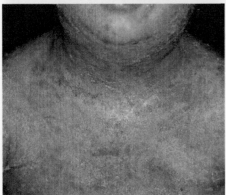

Fig. 24.12-1 Staphylococcal scalded skin syndrome (SSSS). SSSS is characterized by facial features that include fissures around the mouth, eye discharge, and crust formation.

such as a fever, irritability, and poor appetite. Radial fissures around the mouth, eye discharge, and crust formation result in characteristic facial features. Erythema occurs on the neck, axillary fossae, and groin in 2–3 days, and the whole body skin begins to exfoliate as if burned, which leads to erosions (Fig. 24.12). Skin at sites that appear normal is painful when touched, and the skin exfoliates easily by friction. (Nikolsky's sign is positive.) The mucous membranes tend not to be affected. Exfoliation on the scalp can occur in rare cases. Systemic administration of antibiotics accelerates exfoliation, and SSSS begins to heal. The entire course of SSSS is typically 1–2 weeks (Fig. 24.13).

Pathogenesis

Staphylococcal scalded skin syndrome is caused by exfoliative toxin A (ETA) produced by *Staphylococcus aureus*. The nasopharynx, conjunctivae, external ears, and navel are most frequently infected. ETA spreads to the whole body by blood circulation and cleaves desmoglein 1, a desmosomal structural protein. Pemphigus foliaceus-like acantholytic and intraepidermal blisters and erosions form on the upper epidermal layer (see Chapter 1 and Chapter 14).

Diagnosis and differential diagnosis

Staphylococcal scalded skin syndrome can be diagnosed by the characteristic facial features, burn-like erosions, marked Nikolsky's sign, and normality of oral mucosa. *Staphylococcus aureus* is detected in a throat swab culture. Differential diagnosis from toxic epidermal necrolysis (TEN) is done by examining the following:

- any drug history that might be suspected as a cause
- the presence of marked lesions in the oral mucosa
- the presence of erythema multiforme
- histopathological finding of necrosis in all the epidermal layers.

Multiple bullous impetigo is differentiated by features such as the absence of facial features characteristic of SSSS, negative Nikolsky's sign, lack of systemic symptoms, and pus found in the blisters.

Treatment

Treatment involves hospitalization and systemic care, including transfusions and intravenous antibiotics effective against *Staphylococcus aureus*. The affected site is treated with topical ointments that contain antibiotics or petrolatum. SSSS tends to have a good prognosis but it may become severe, with sepsis or pneumonia appearing as a complication in infants and immunodeficient adults.

Toxic shock syndrome (synonym: staphylococcal toxic shock syndrome)

Toxic shock syndrome (TSS) is caused by an exotoxin called toxic shock syndrome toxin (TSS toxin-1 or TSST-1), which is produced by *Staphylococcus aureus* (methicillin-resistant *Staphylococcus aureus* [MRSA] in most cases). It may occur in burn patients and in women who use sanitary tampons. TSS is a systemic toxic disease whose main symptoms are acute fever, decreased blood pressure, scarlet fever-like erythema, and multiple organ dysfunction. Diffuse erythema is accompanied by systemic fatigue, chills, headache, arthralgia, vomiting, and diarrhea (Fig. 24.14). The administration of high-dose antibiotics and antishock therapy should be carried out immediately. The eruptions heal with scaling in 1–2 weeks.

Scarlet fever

- This is an erythematous exanthema and enanthema caused by toxins from group A β-hemolytic streptococci (GAS).
- It begins with pharyngeal pain and high fever. It is characterized by reddening of the tongue (strawberry tongue) and dense erythema over the whole body.
- Eruptions do not appear around the mouth (perioral pallor).
- Penicillin is administered. Nephritis and rheumatic fever may occur.

Clinical features

Scarlet fever most frequently occurs in late childhood. The incubation period is 1–5 days. It begins with a sudden fever and pharyngeal pain, soon followed by strawberry tongue. At the early stage, tongue fur is seen in many cases. However, this resolves in a day or two, leaving the typical strawberry tongue. Cutaneous eruptions appear within 1–2 days. Small vivid red follicular papules appear on the neck region. The lesions spread to the face, trunk, and extremities in a few days. The lesions coalesce and feature mild itching. The surface of the affected areas has a rough, sandpaper-like texture. Diffuse erythema appears on the face, except around the mouth and nasal alae (perioral pallor). Generally, the palms and soles are not involved. Hemorrhagic lesions in the soft palate

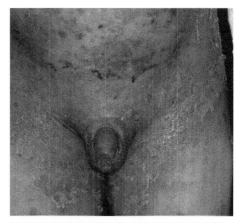
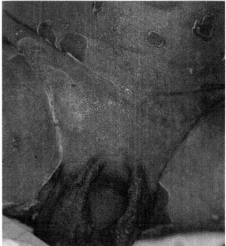
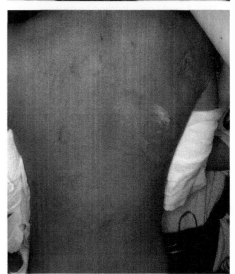

Fig. 24.12-2 Staphylococcal scalded skin syndrome. There is burn-like exfoliation and erosion of the skin on the whole body. Nikolsky phenomenon is positive.

MEMO 24–4 Toxic shock-like syndrome (synonym: severe invasive strepto-coccal infection, streptococcal toxic shock syndrome)

The main cause is superantigens such as streptococcal pyogenic exotoxin (SpeA) or SpeC, produced by strepto-cocci. Swelling in the extremities and fever occur, rapidly progressing to necrotizing fasciitis, multiple organ failure, and shock.

MEMO 24–5 Superantigens

The immunological response between antigen-presenting cells and T cells is usually mediated by a certain antigen. However, recent studies have discovered molecules, called super-antigens, that induce T cell activation whether or not the antigen is specific to the T cell receptor. T cells are activated abnormally by superantigen TSST-1 and SpeC, leading to severe systemic inflammatory reactions.

and systemic lymph node enlargement also occur. The fever resolves on the third or fourth day. The eruptions heal after scaling without pigmentation. Clinical features that characterize scarlet fever are shown in Fig. 24.15.

Pathogenesis

Eruptions are caused on the whole body by an exo-toxin (streptococcal pyogenic exotoxin B) produced by *Streptococcus pyogenes*. This bacterium first infects the

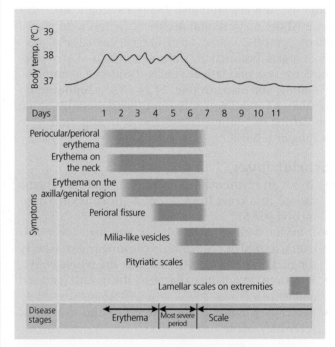

Fig. 24.13 Clinical course of staphylococcal scalded skin syndrome.

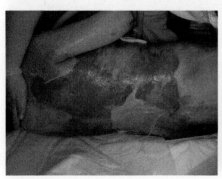
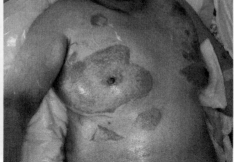
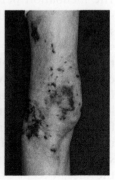

Fig. 24.14 Toxic shock syndrome.

palatal tonsil or skin. Infection by *Staphylococcus aureus*, which produces enterotoxin (staphylococcal entero-toxin B), may cause scarlet fever-like symptoms (staphylococcal scarlet fever).

Laboratory findings and diagnosis

Bacteria are detected from the primary infection site, such as the pharynx. The rapid diagnostic test kit (Strep A) is also useful. Leukocytosis and left shift of the nuclei in leukocytes are found. ASO and ASK levels rise 1–3 weeks after the initial infection.

Differential diagnosis

See Figure 23.22 for the difference between scarlet fever and viral eruptions, including rubella. Differentia-tion from drug eruptions and SSSS may be necessary in some cases. The clinical findings of Kawasaki's disease are very similar to those of scarlet fever but Kawasaki's disease has three distinct features: the period of fever is long, pharyngeal culture is negative, and the palms, toes, and bulbar conjunctivae are involved.

Treatment and prognosis

Oral penicillin G and cefem antibiotics are the first-line treatments. Although the eruptions disappear in 2–3 days, medication should be continued for at least 2 weeks, because if it is stopped early, *Strep-tococcus* may proliferate again in the pharynx, caus-ing complications such as nephritis or rheumatic fever. After cessation of medication, periodic exam-inations such as urine test are necessary to detect bacteria.

Necrotizing fasciitis

- This is an acute bacterial infection in the subcuta-neous tissue and superficial fascia (see Fig. 24.3). The extremities and genitalia of people in middle age and older are most frequently affected.
- The main systemic symptoms are reddening and swelling of the skin, ulceration, and fever accompa-nied by intense pain.
- The administration of large doses of antibiotics at an early stage and debridement are necessary. Multiple organ failure may lead to death.

Clinical features

The extremities (lower legs in particular), genitalia, and abdomen of people over age 40 are most

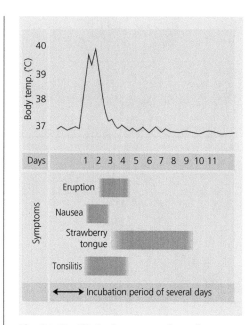

Fig. 24.15 Clinical course of scarlet fever.

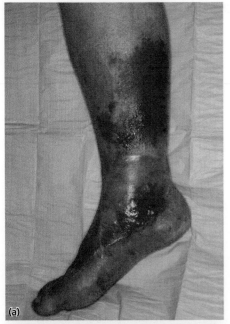

(a)

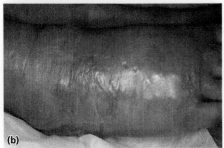

(b)

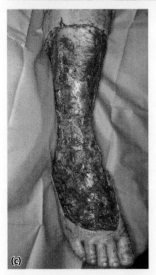

(c)

Fig. 24.16 Necrotizing fasciitis.
a,b: Generalized purpura, blisters, bloody blisters, necrosis, and ulceration progress quickly. c: Surgical debridement was performed on the lesion. The subcutaneous tissues, including the fascia, are affected.

frequently affected. Necrotizing fasciitis begins with localized reddening and swelling. In 1–3 days, purpura, blisters, bloody blisters, and ulcers occur (Fig. 24.16). Sense of touch diminishes with progression of the fasciitis. Even when the periphery of the lesion appears normal to the naked eye, the subcutaneous tissue is affected. Necrotizing fasciitis is accompanied by intense systemic symptoms, such as high fever, severe arthralgia, muscle pain, shock, and multiple organ failure. Necrotizing fasciitis of the male genitalia is called Fournier's gangrene. Necrotizing fasciitis frequently occurs as a complication of toxic shock-like syndrome (MEMO, see Chapter 24).

Pathogenesis

The main causative bacteria are *Streptococcus pyogenes* and anaerobes such as *Bacteroides fragilis* and *Peptostreptococcus anaerobius*. *Streptococcus pyogenes* may infect healthy persons, leading to a sudden onset of necrotizing fasciitis. Anaerobic bacteria tend to infect individuals with an underlying disease, such as diabetes. Subcutaneous gas may be found (non-clostridial gas gangrene; see next section). In some cases, a microinjury or tinea pedis induces necrotizing fasciitis; however, details of the pathogenesis are unclear.

Pathology

Edema is marked throughout the dermis. Necrosis, blockage of the blood vessels, and infiltration of polymorphonuclear leukocytes occur from the lower dermal layer to the underlying fat tissue and fascia.

Laboratory findings

Leukocytosis, left shift of the nuclei in leukocytes, elevated levels of CRP, liver failure, and coagulation abnormality (when disseminated intravascular coagulation [DIC] is caused) are present. Prior to administration of antibiotics, bacteria are detected from the puncture fluid, necrotizing tissue at debridement, and the blood. Gram stain is useful in detecting bacteria in pus and tissue. Magnetic resonance imaging (MRI), computed tomography (CT), and X-ray images are helpful in testing for the depth and size of lesions and for any retention of gas.

Differential diagnosis

Some cases are difficult to differentiate from ordinary cellulitis; however, necrotizing fasciitis is characterized by rapid progression of the skin lesions, purpura and bloody blisters, and intense systemic symptoms. The spread of inflammation and the involvement of fascia can be determined by MRI.

Treatment and prognosis

Large doses of antibiotics (e.g., penicillin, clindamycin) and surgical debridement in the early stages are essential. Unless treated in the early stages, the prognosis is extremely poor.

Gas gangrene

- Most cases are caused by anaerobic bacteria, such as those of the genus *Clostridium*. Mortality is high.
- Intense systemic symptoms, muscular necrosis, and aerogenesis occur. There is crepitation from gas in the tissues.
- Rapid surgical debridement in the early stages, high-dose antibiotics, and hyperbaric oxygen therapy are the main treatments.

Clinical features

Six to 72 h after injury, gas gangrene begins with localized sharp pain. Systemic symptoms such as chills and tachycardia occur. The skin becomes dark purple or blackish and hematoid serous blisters form. Liquefactive necrosis occurs in muscle tissue. The lesion swells from the gas produced by the bacteria (Fig. 24.17a). The affected site releases foul odor. When the site is pressed, the gas moves, causing crepitation. Bubbles are observed by X-ray (Fig. 24.17b). If left untreated, multiple organ failure occurs, resulting in death.

Pathogenesis

Gas gangrene is most frequently caused by *Clostridium perfringens*. This bacterium exists in soil and sometimes in the feces of humans and animals, invading the muscle tissue through severely crushed and contaminated wounds from traffic accidents and the like. Non-clostridial gas gangrene is caused by *Bacteroides fragilis* and other bacteria. These bacteria grow in anaerobic environments and produce exotoxins containing proteolytic enzymes that induce hemolysis and shock.

Diagnosis, treatment, and prevention

Gram staining of the exudative fluid is conducted. If Gram-positive bacilli are observed and neutrophils are not found, the possibility of clostridial gas gangrene is

> **MEMO 24–6 "Killer bugs"**
>
> Infections caused by so-called "killer bugs" result in necrotizing fasciitis and shock in several hours to several days after the onset of the condition. The mortality rate for this infection is very high. The causative bacteria are group A β-hemolytic streptococci in toxic shock-like syndrome (TSLS) (MEMO, see Chapter 24) and *Vibrio vulnificus*.

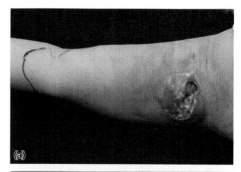

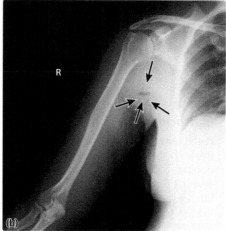

Fig. 24.17 Gas gangrene. a: Clinical features. b: X-ray image (arrows show bubbles).

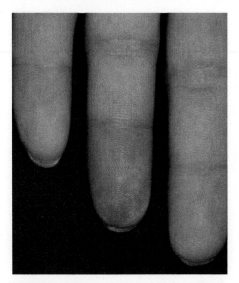

Fig. 24.18 Osler's node. Painful erythema on the fingers.

MEMO 24–7 *Vibrio vulnificus*

Vibrio vulnificus proliferates in the body of people with immunodeficiency or cirrhosis of the liver after consumption of undercooked seafood or contact with contaminated seawater. It causes necrotizing fasciitis. The mortality rate is 50–70%; the prognosis is extremely poor.

MEMO 24–8 *Pasteurella multocida* infection

Pasteurella multocida invade the body through cat or dog scratches or bites. Localized cellulitis occurs several days after infection. Swelling is intense, and subcutaneous abscesses tend to form. Early administration of antibiotics is important.

very high. Surgical debridement is carried out immediately, and large doses of penicillin G or cefem antibacterial drugs are administered. Proliferation of anaerobic bacteria can be prevented by opening the lesion. Hyperbaric oxygen therapy is effective in treating clostridial gas gangrene. Systemic care is performed for shock, kidney failure, and DIC. Amputation of extremities may be necessary in severe cases.

Sepsis

Sepsis occurs when bacteria from a localized cutaneous infection, such as an abscess, cellulitis or erysipelas, becomes aggravated and disseminates to the bloodstream. Thrombosis caused by bacteria in the blood or immunological reaction mediated by various cytokines induces septic vasculitis, resulting in erythemas, purpuras, bloody blisters, and pustules.

Osler's node

Osler's node often accompanies subacute infective endocarditis. Erythema and red papules occur on the finger pads and palm (Fig. 24.18). Sharp pain occurs as a precursor, and a brown patch appears and then disappears in a few days. Osler's node accompanied by painless light pink erythema on the finger pads and palm is called Janeway lesion. These conditions are caused most often by *Staphylococcus aureus*. Osler's node is known to appear in 15% of infectious endocarditis cases.

Other bacterial infections

Trichomycosis palmellina (synonyms: trichomycosis axillaris, trichomycosis pubis)

This disorder occurs most frequently in adolescence. Bacteria in colloidal suspension, ranging from yellowish-brown to white, attach in clusters to axillary or pubic hairs. The hairs appear to be yellowish and swollen. Although it is usually asymptomatic, hyperhidrosis and foul odor may be present. The pathogenesis in most cases is infection caused by *Corynebacterium tenuis*. The affected hairs fluoresce as yellow, white or blue under Wood's lamp. The treatments are hygiene improvement, antisepsis, shaving of hair, and topical antibiotics such as clindamycin gel.

Erythrasma
Clinical features and pathogenesis
Erythrasma is caused by infection of the stratum corneum by the Gram-positive bacillus *Corynebacterium minutissimum*. Moist intertriginous regions such as the genitocrural region, axillary fossae, and interdigital clefts are most commonly involved. Erythrasma presents as sharply margined, red or reddish-brown patches on whose surface thin, fine scales attach. Thick yellowish scales appear in interdigital clefts. Papules or blisters do not occur. The center of the lesion does not heal, which distinguishes erythrasma from tinea. Erythrasma tends to be asymptomatic, and there may be itching and burning in rare cases.

Diagnosis and examinations
It is difficult to differentiate erythrasma in the toe clefts from tinea pedis; however, coral-red fluorescence of erythrasma observed under Wood's lamp, which is caused by coproporphyrin III produced by the bacteria, is diagnostic. Since erythrasma and tinea pedis are present together in many cases, mycological examination of the scales is necessary. Gram-positive short bacilli are observed in the scales of the lesion. Potassium hydroxide slide examination is also performed, because erythrasma in the toe clefts accompanies tinea pedis in many cases.

Treatment
Topical imidazole antifungal agents and oral erythromycin are effective.

Cat scratch disease, cat scratch fever
Cat scratch disease (CSD) is caused by infection with the Gram-negative bacillus *Bartonella henselae*. The infection is caused by cat bites, scratches or licks. Fleas may cause infection. After several days to 2 weeks of incubation, red papules 3–5 mm in diameter and small blisters appear at the site of injury. In 1–3 weeks after the appearance of skin lesions, painful swelling in the regional lymph nodes occurs, and abscesses form. Systemic symptoms including fever and headache may accompany the condition. It spontaneously heals after several weeks to a few months in most cases. If the condition persists, oral antibacterial drugs such as cefem antibiotics, tetracycline or macrolides are administered.

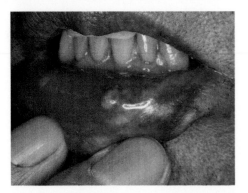

Fig. 24.19 Actinomycosis. A small nodule on the lower lip. *Actinomyces israelii* was detected by excision.

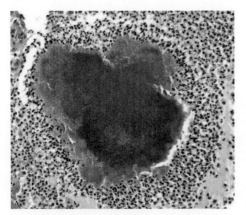

Fig. 24.20 Histopathology of actinomycosis. A cluster of *Actinomyces israelii*, called a granule or drüse, is observed in the microabscess.

Actinomycosis
Clinical features and classification

Actinomycosis is classified by the primary site into cervicofacial, thoracic, and abdominal actinomycosis. Of these three subtypes, cervicofacial actinomycosis, which is often induced by dental caries and accompanied by skin lesions, accounts for about half of all actinomycosis cases. Thoracic actinomycosis and abdominal actinomycosis are accompanied by lesions in the internal organs; unless there is a fistula that affects the skin, these two subtypes are not addressed in dermatology.

Gram-positive bacilli, mainly *Actinomyces israelii*, a microbe resident in the human oral cavity, tonsillar fossae, and dental plaques, invades the body from a minor injury, proliferates and forms a lesion. Reddening, swelling, and induration occur, forming dark red subcutaneous nodules (Fig. 24.19). The nodules form abscesses where fistulae are produced, excreting pus for a long period of time. A chronic suppurative granulomatous lesion is produced. Mild fever and pain are present in most cases. Actinomycosis is nearly asymptomatic; however, there is difficulty opening the mouth when the masticatory muscle is involved.

Pathology

Inflammatory granulomatous lesions accompanied by abscesses and fibrotic tissue occur. Actinomycosis is characterized by bacterial masses in the abscess called sulfur granules (drüsen) (Fig. 24.20).

Diagnosis and treatment

Actinomycosis should be differentiated from nocardiosis, external dental fistula, and inflammatory epidermal cyst. Antibiotics such as penicillin are administered orally.

External dental fistula

As a result of progression of dental caries, alveolar osteitis or infection in a maxillary cyst, pus is excreted at the exit of a fistula formed on the skin right outside the originally affected site (Fig. 24.21). Dental treatment is necessary. It may be misdiagnosed as subcutaneous ulcers, such as epidermal cysts or actinomycosis. When reddening or pus discharge is found on the cheek or lower jaw, this condition is suspected. Examinations using imaging, such as X-ray examination (panoramic radiography), are conducted.

Nocardiosis
Clinical features

Nocardia asteroides is the causative species in most cases. Skin lesions caused by nocardiosis are divided by morphology into three subtypes: nocardia mycetoma, which forms subcutaneous nodules in the foot; localized cutaneous nocardiosis, in which pustules and subcutaneous abscess form; and cutaneous lymphatic nocardiosis, in which the lesion enlarges on skin over the lymph vessels. In the case of pulmonary nocardiosis, the bacteria spread hematogenously to form red nodules over the whole body. These conditions occur as opportunistic infections in immunodeficient patients, such as those with AIDS. See Chapter 25 for mycetoma.

Laboratory findings, diagnosis, and treatment

Granules in pus or sputum smears are examined. Cultures are obtained on Sabouraud glucose agar medium, or *Nocardia* is identified by skin biopsy. Bone is investigated by bone X-ray. The most effective drug for each case is chosen from among a sulfamethoxazole/trimethoprim (ST) mixture, minocycline or penicillin. Treatment is continued for several months. For cases in which all drugs are ineffective or bone is involved, surgical removal is performed.

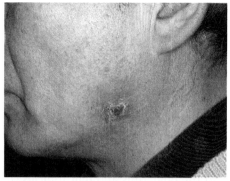
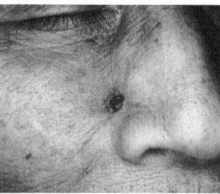

Fig. 24.21 External dental fistula. A fistula in the lower jaw from inflammation of the dental root, which was caused by dental caries.

CHAPTER 25
Fungal diseases

Fungi are eukaryotic microorganisms that have a cell wall and do not photosynthesize. Instead, they parasitize organisms or exist autonomously as spores. Fungal infections are called mycoses. In superficial mycoses (tinea, candidiasis, pityriasis versicolor), fungi parasitize shallow sites no deeper than the epidermis and hair follicles. In subcutaneous mycoses (sporotrichosis, chromoblastomycosis), the fungi tend to parasitize the dermis and deeper layers.

Table 25.1 Classification of dermatophytes (Blue letters indicate the more important ones).

Trichophyton
T. rubrum
T. mentagrophytes
T. verrucosum
T. tonsurans
T. violaceum
T. schoenleinii
T. concentricum
T. equinum
Microsporum
M. canis
M. gypseum
M. audouinii
M. cookie
M. equinum
M. ferrugineum
M. gallinae
M. nanum
Epidermophyton
E. floccosum

Superficial mycoses

Tinea (dermatophytosis)

- Tinea is caused by dermatophytes (fungi of the genus *Trichophyton*) that parasitize the skin, the stratum corneum in particular.
- It goes by various common names, depending on the affected site. The main subtypes are tinea pedis (commonly called athlete's foot), tinea capitis (scald head), tinea corporis (serpigo), and tinea cruris (jock itch).
- Tinea with intense inflammation and loss of scalp hair is called kerion.
- The causative dermatophyte is microscopically identified from scales of the lesion or nail by using a potassium hydroxide solution. The type of dermatophyte is identified by fungal culture.
- The treatments are topical or oral antifungal agents.

Classification
Fungi called dermatophytes parasitize the skin, causing dermatophytosis. Dermatophytes are divided into three genera, each with various species (Table 25.1). The most common dermatophytes are *Trichophyton rubrum* and *Trichophyton mentagrophytes*. Because dermatophytes feed on keratin, they usually infect the stratum corneum, nails, and hair follicles, causing lesions. Inflammation may spread deeper to the dermis and subcutaneous tissue. Inappropriate treatment,

---

Shimizu's Dermatology, Second Edition. Hiroshi Shimizu.
© 2017 John Wiley & Sons, Ltd. Published 2017 by John Wiley & Sons, Ltd.

such as the use of topical steroids, may cause dermatophytes to proliferate in the dermis and subcutaneous
tissue (MEMO, see Chapter 25).

Laboratory findings and diagnosis

The potassium hydroxide test (see Chapter 5) is performed using a specimen taken from a scale, blister covering, nail or hair. The diagnosis of dermatophytosis is
confirmed when dermatophytes containing cross-walls
of 3–4 mm in width or segmental spores are found
(Fig. 25.1 and Fig. 25.2). Dermatophytes are not detected
in the erosive surface, which lacks keratins. When there
is any possibility of tinea being present, this microscopy
test should be done. Other major tests include culture in
Sabouraud glucose agar for color tone and morphological observation of the colonies, morphological
observation of conidia by slide culture, and molecular
examination by PCR or in situ hybridization.

Treatment

The basic treatment for all sites infected with tinea
superficialis, except hairy areas, is the application of a
topical antifungal agent. This is continued for several
weeks, and the affected site is kept clean to prevent
aggravation or recurrence. For tinea superficialis on
hairy areas, intractable tinea and tinea profunda (e.g.,
kerion, hyperkeratotic tinea pedis and tinea manus,
tinea unguium, and granuloma trichophyticum), useful treatments are oral itraconazole and terbinafine
hydrochloride.

Tinea pedis (synonyms: ringworm of the foot, athlete's foot)

This is commonly called athlete's foot. More than half
of all tinea cases are tinea pedis. The most common
causative fungus is *Trichophyton rubrum*, followed by
Trichophyton mentagrophytes. Tinea pedis is classified by
clinical features into three subtypes. In any of the subtypes, when the lesions spread to the dorsa of the feet,
ring-shaped lesions resembling the lesions of tinea
corporis form.

Interdigital erosive

This is the most common of the three subtypes. The
fourth toe cleft is most commonly affected. It begins
with erythema and vesicles on the interdigital region,
leading to scaling. The skin lesion often softens with
sweat, becoming whitish, then exfoliating and becoming

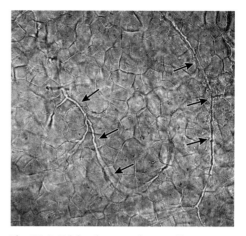

Fig. 25.1 *Trichophyton rubrum.* Filamentous
hyphae (arrows) are observed microscopically
in the horny cell layer with the addition of
KOH solution.

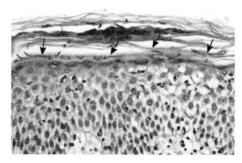

**Fig. 25.2 Histopathology of tinea (PAS
staining).** Filamentous hyphae (arrows)
are observed in the stratum corneum.

**MEMO 25–1 Potassium
hydroxide direct
microscopy for tinea**

Dermatophytes are identified by direct
microscopic examination of scales or
nails in cases with untreated tinea of
the skin or nail. The administration of
oral drugs is contraindicated without
positive confirmation for tinea.

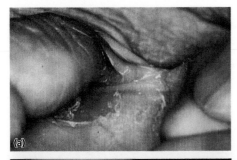

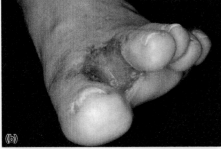

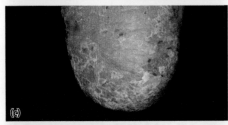

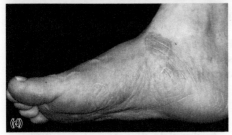

Fig. 25.3 Tinea pedis. a: Interdigital type. b: Interdigital type with secondary infection. c: Chronic hyperkeratotic type. Partially healed erosions are observed at sites where the patient has peeled off the stratum corneum. d: Vesiculo-bullous type. Scales form on the dry lesion.

MEMO 25–2 Fungi and molds

Molds and mushrooms are fungi. Yeasts are also regarded as uninuclear fungi. A fungus consists of a hypha that is long and thin, and a spore that is usually spherical and that proliferates by germination. Spores parasitize humans by becoming airborne and attaching to the body, where they form hyphae and reproduce sexually or asexually. Spores may be elongated, depending on the environment, resembling hyphae (pseudo-hyphae). When cultured, as in slide culture, for example, they form characteristic hyphae and asexual spores that are called conidiophores and conidia. The conidium consists of the macroconidium and the microconidium. Disease-causing fungi may be identified by the features of the hyphae.

erosive (Fig. 25.3). Itching is intense. Secondary infection from erosion may cause sharp pain or cellulitis. Interdigital erosive tinea pedis in patients with diabetes in particular tends to lead to intractable ulcers, cellulitis, lymphangitis or necrotizing fasciitis.

Vesiculo-bullous

The plantar arch, the base of the toes, and the sides of the feet are most frequently involved. Multiple vesicles occur and then dry, leading to scaling. It tends to appear during wet seasons and subside in autumn.

Chronic hyperkeratotic

This type occurs most frequently on the soles and heels. The causative dermatophyte is *Trichophyton rubrum*. Diffused hyperkeratosis and roughness of the skin are present. Itching is rarely present, but sharp pain results from cracking. This type is resistant to topical agents; oral antifungals are effective.

Tinea unguium

Tinea unguium frequently occurs on the first toe, often secondary to tinea pedis. Usually, white nail (leukonychia) first appears at the tip of the toenail and gradually spreads to the nail matrix. The nail becomes fragile and shatters when cut with clippers (MEMO, see Chapter 25; Fig. 25.4). The fungal elements occur mostly in the deeper portions of the nail plate and in the hyperkeratotic nail bed, rather than on the surface of the nail plate. It is often left untreated for a long period because of its asymptomatic nature. Dermatophytes spread

MEMO 25–3 Subtypes of tinea unguium

Tinea unguium is classified into four subtypes.
- **Distal and lateral subungual onychomycosis:** the most common subtype, it progresses from tinea pedis to tinea of the nail bed and the nail matrix.
- **Superficial white onychomycosis:** the surface of the nail becomes whitish.
- **Proximal subungual onychomycosis:** the nail starts to become whitish from the nail matrix.
- **Total dystrophic onychomycosis:** the whole nail is affected by *Trichophyton*. It becomes brittle and thick, resulting in onychogryphosis.

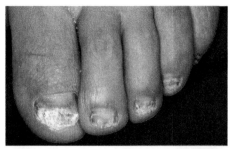
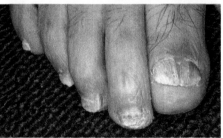
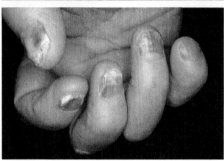

Fig. 25.4 Tinea unguium.

from tinea unguium skin lesions to tinea pedis skin lesions, causing autoinfection and intrafamilial infection. It is sometimes difficult to improve with topical agents. Oral antifungal drugs are more effective.

Tinea manus

The skin lesion may be hyperkeratotic, vesicular or scaling. The majority of patients have tinea pedis as a complication. One hand, rather than both, tends to be involved (Fig. 25.5). Topical antifungal agents are the main treatment.

Tinea corporis

It appears as small erythematous papules on the trunk and extremities, gradually spreading centrifugally. The papules tend to heal centrally, giving the lesions a ring shape (Fig. 25.6). The center of the lesion subsides with mildly abnormal pigmentation, but the periphery is elevated, and papules, vesicles, and scales form there. Itching is present. As in tinea pedis, the causative dermatophyte in most cases of tinea corporis is *Trichophyton rubrum*. Tinea corporis is occasionally caused by *Microsporum canis*, which parasitizes dogs and cats. It often affects the faces of young children (tinea faciei; Fig. 25.7). It is characterized by intense inflammatory symptoms.

Tinea cruris

Commonly called "jock itch," tinea cruris is frequently found in adult men and is accompanied by tinea pedis. Ring-shaped erythematous lesions resembling those of tinea corporis form in the crotch and buttocks. Itching is intense. The lesions often appear symmetrically. The scrotum is rarely involved. For intractable cases that have been left untreated for many years, it may be necessary to use oral antifungal agents.

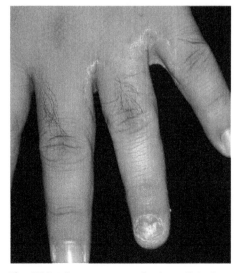

Fig. 25.5 Tinea manus. The interdigital areas, fingers, and fingernails are frequently affected.

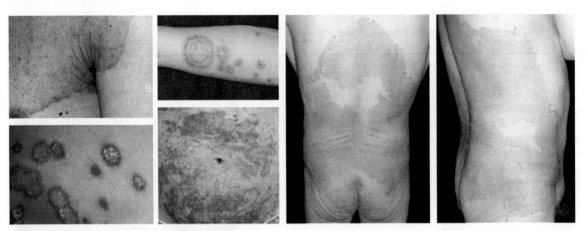

Fig. 25.6 Tinea corporis. Erythematous lesions enlarge centrifugally. The center tends to heal and the rim elevates in a banked shape.

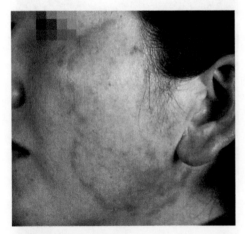

Fig. 25.7 Tinea faciei.

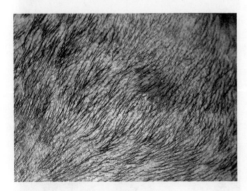

Fig. 25.8 Tinea capitis.

Tinea capitis

Commonly called "scald head," tinea capitis occurs most frequently in children. Fungal infection occurs on the hair. *Trichophyton* infection in hair follicles results in sharply demarcated alopecia of the scalp. There are dry pityroid scales and short, broken hairs in the lesion.

Tinea capitis accompanied by black dot formation at the follicles after the hairs break off is called black dot ringworm. The symptoms, such as itching and sharp pain, are mild, and many cases are not accompanied by inflammation (Fig. 25.8).

MEMO 25–4 Tinea incognito

If tinea is misdiagnosed or self-judged as eczema and topical steroids are misused for treatment, the inflammation subsides and the characteristic central healing or ring-shaped erythema in the lesion is not distinctly observed. This complicates diagnosis, and such clinical manifestation is called tinea incognito. Tinea incognito presents clinically atypical cutaneous symptoms (See Figures).

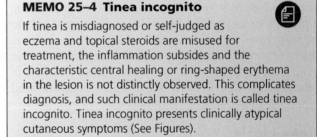
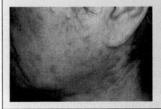
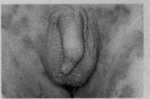

Kerion

Kerion occurs with misuse of topical steroids. Inflammation in the dermis may accompany follicular tinea such as tinea capitis. In kerion erythema, follicular papules, pustules, and flat or dome-shaped abscesses occur (Fig. 25.9). The lesions are accompanied by sharp pain, mild pulsation, and discharge of pus. The hairs in the lesion fall out. Systemic symptoms include swelling of the regional lymph nodes and fever. The most common causative agent of kerion is *Microsporum canis*, which infects humans through their pets. Infants are most frequently affected. The incidence of *Trichophyton tonsurans* infection has been increasing in recent years (MEMO, see Chapter 25). Histopathologically, *Trichophyton* infection is found in hair; inflammatory cellular infiltration occurs in peripheral follicles. However, *Trichophyton* does not proliferate in the dermis.

Sycosis trichophytica

The upper lip and its periphery in middle-aged men are most frequently involved (Fig. 25.10). Reddening and swelling occur in the entire area with facial hair (moustache, beard, sideburns). Pus is discharged from

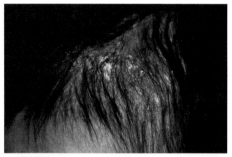
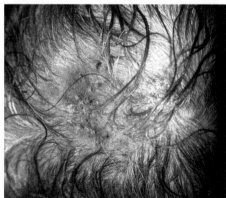

Fig. 25.9 Kerion celsi.

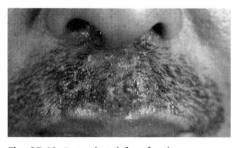

Fig. 25.10 Sycosis trichophytica.

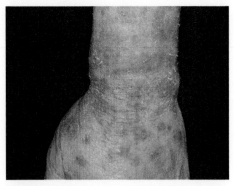

Fig. 25.11 Granuloma trichophyticum. An infiltrative skin lesion from prolonged use of topical steroids to treat tinea corporis. This was misdiagnosed as eczema.

Table 25.2 The *Candida* species most frequently cultured from humans.

C. albicans
C. parapsilosis
C. glabrata
C. tropicalis
C. krusei
C. guilliermondii
C. kefyr

the hair follicles and the hairs come out easily when pulled. Most cases are caused by shaving or misuse of steroids. The treatments are those for kerion (see section above), because the conditions of tinea barbae are similar to those of kerion.

Granuloma trichophyticum (synonym: Majocchi granuloma)

When topical steroids are mistakenly used on tinea corporis on the lower leg, for example, nodules occur intradermally or subcutaneously. Flat infiltrative plaques or large tumorous plaques may form. Clinically, differentiation from erythema induratum (see Chapter 18) is necessary (Fig. 25.11).

Candidiasis

- This is an infection of the skin or mucous membrane caused by yeasts of the genus *Candida*.
- It is described according to the location and clinical features as candida intertrigo, erythema mycoticum infantile, candidal paronychia or thrush.
- It may also occur as an occupational disease in workers whose hands are in frequent contact with water, or as a sexually transmitted infection (STI) or an opportunistic infection.
- The affected site should be kept clean and dry. The antifungal imidazole is applied topically.

Classification, pathogenesis, and clinical features

Fungi of the genus *Candida* are biphasic fungi (yeast-like fungi) that can take the form of yeast or hyphae, depending on the conditions of culture. There are 7–10 virulent *Candida* species (Table 25.2). The main causative species is known to be *Candida albicans*.

Because the fugi normally inhabit the oral cavity, colon and vagina, a positive result from culturing fungi taken from a skin lesion does not necessarily mean that the diagnosis is candidiasis. Proliferation of *Candida* should be confirmed directly by microscopy of scales, leukorrhea or nail fragments.

Candidiasis tends to infect individuals with an underlying disease, such as diabetes, those who have used oral steroids for an extended period or those with immunodeficiency, such as AIDS patients. Internal infection, such as gastrointestinal candidiasis, may occur.

Candidiasis can also be an endogenous mycosis or an opportunistic infection.

Diagnosis

Racemose spores and pseudo-hyphae are observed by direct microscopy with potassium hydroxide solution (Fig. 25.12). Differentiation of candidiasis from tinea is confirmed when spores are found and the bacterial threads have branches but not septa. Test samples are collected from pustules, scales, the stratum corneum of the nail, the tongue fur or leukorrhea using a surgical scalpel or adhesive tape. When cultured in Sabouraud glucose agar at 25°C, white or cream-colored aggregations of *Candida* form in 2–3 days. In cases of candidemia or internal infection, the Cand-Tec R test is positive and the blood β-D-glucan value is elevated.

Treatment

Most cases are improved by bathing, cleansing, applying zinc oxide ointment, and keeping the affected site dry. Topical antifungal agents are used. In oral candidiasis, gargling with amphotericin B syrup or applying miconazole gel is useful. Vaginal suppositories containing miconazole are used to treat genital candidiasis in women. Oral and intravenous antifungal drugs may be necessary in severe cases.

Candidal intertrigo

Sharply marginated erythemas with scales and small pustules at the periphery are induced by sweating or poor hygiene in intertriginous regions, such as the genitocrural region, buttocks, neck, nuchal region, axillary fossae, and inframammary region. When the condition progresses, the lesions become erosive and tend to develop secondary bacterial infection. Mild itching and sharp pain may be present. Candidal intertrigo should be differentiated from tinea corporis, seborrheic dermatitis, irritant contact dermatitis, Hailey–Hailey disease, and extramammary Paget's disease.

Candidal intertrigo occurring in the crotch of infants is called candida diaper dermatitis or erythema mycoticum infantile. The incidence is highest during summer, from increased perspiration. Candidal intertrigo should be differentiated from miliaria and diaper dermatitis (irritant contact dermatitis).

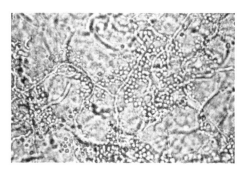

Fig. 25.12 Microscopy of *Candida* in KOH solution. Filamentous pseudo-hyphae and racemose spores are present.

MEMO 25–7
(1→3)-β-D-glucan

(1→3)-β-D-glucan is a component of the fungal cellular wall. Its serum value is high in deep fungal infections with invasive lesions (candidemia, aspergillosis) and in pneumocystis pneumonia. (1→3)-β-D-glucan is useful in early detection of these disorders but it is not species specific.

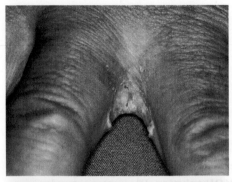

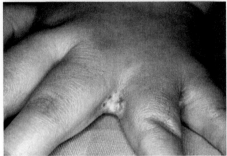

Fig. 25.13 Interdigital candidiasis (erosio interdigitalis blastomycetica). The third interdigital area is most frequently involved.

Erosio interdigitalis blastomycetica (synonym: interdigital candidiasis)

The third interdigital cleft is most frequently involved. Erythemas appear on the interdigital areas and gradually enlarge. The center of the erythema becomes vivid red and erosive, with an infiltrative white rim (Fig. 25.13). It may be accompanied by bacterial infection and mild pain or itching. It frequently occurs in those whose hands are exposed to water for extended periods, such as workers in dining establishments.

Candidal paronychia

As with interdigital candidiasis, this often occurs in those whose hands are in water for extended periods. Reddening and swelling occur in the periungual region of the fingers (Fig. 25.14). Pus may be discharged from the nail by pressure. Deformities may appear at the nail root. It is intractable. Even with the use of an effective antifungal agent, healing takes several months, and the condition tends to recur.

MEMO 25–8 Black hairy tongue

A hairy change varying in color from black to brown is observed on the surface of the tongue (See Figure). There may be blackish pigmentation without hair. It is asymptomatic. The color comes from the production of a pigment (sulfur compound) from abnormal hyperkeratosis of the lingual papillae to which bacteria attach. It may be caused by microbial substitution. Guidance on hygiene is given, and topical antifungal agents are administered.

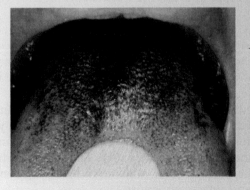

Candidal onychomycosis (synonym: nail candidiasis)

Thickening, deformity, and fragmentation of the nail plate occur (Fig. 25.15). It is not possible to differentiate candidal onychomycosis from tinea unguium clinically; fungal culture is necessary for confirmation of diagnosis.

Oral candidiasis

This is also known as thrush. A white pseudo-membrane or "fur" attaches to the oral mucosa and tongue, accompanied by inflammatory flush. Burning sensation and gustatory anesthesia are present. Erosive plaques form at the site where the pseudo-membrane detaches, causing sharp pain. It often occurs in newborns as a transbirth canal infection and heals spontaneously in 1–2 weeks. Oral candidiasis in adults often occurs in patients with diabetes or immunodeficiency. Oral candidiasis also occurs as an early symptom of AIDS.

Genital candidiasis (candidal vulvovaginitis, candidal balanitis)

Genital candidiasis is experienced at least once in life by 75% of otherwise healthy women. There is erosive reddening, the formation of white "fur," and white vaginal discharge. It tends to aggravate or become chronic in pregnant women and in adult women with diabetes. In male cases, reddening and scaling occur on the corona of the glans penis and the foreskin. Some cases are sexually transmitted.

Chronic mucocutaneous candidiasis

Various types of candidiasis appear in childhood, accompanying underlying disease such as endocrine abnormality and progressing slowly. Some cases are inherited in an autosomal recessive or dominant manner. Multiple skin lesions occur. Chronic mucocutaneous candidiasis (CMC) accompanies hyperkeratosis and tends to form thick crusts. Histopathologically, granulomas may form (candidal granuloma). In adult cases, complications with thymoma or AIDS are seen. CMC is refractory. Oral or intravenous antifungal agents are used, but the condition tends to recur repeatedly.

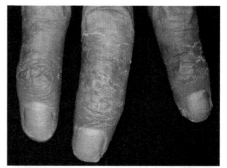

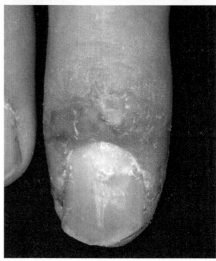

Fig. 25.14 *Candida* **paronychia.**

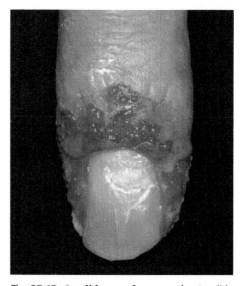

Fig. 25.15 *Candida* **onychomycosis.** *Candida* has infected the entire nail, causing deformity.

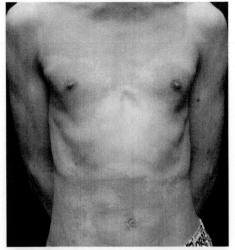

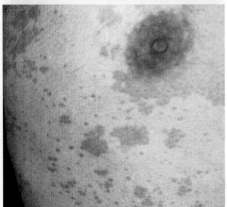

Fig. 25.16 Pityriasis versicolor, tinea versicolor.

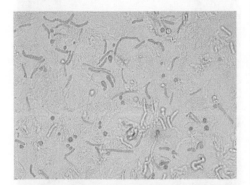

Fig. 25.17 *Malassezia furfur.* Long, thin hyphae and spherical spores are observed in the scales of pityriasis versicolor by direct microscopy with KOH solution to which Parker ink is added.

Malassezia infections

Pityriasis versicolor, tinea versicolor

- This is a superficial infection caused by fungal yeasts of the genus *Malassezia, Malassezia globosa* in particular.
- Light brown patches or hypopigmented macules 1–3 cm in diameter appear on the upper trunk of young men and women, sometimes coalescing into larger macules.
- Scales exfoliate in large amounts from the eruptions when scraped.
- For diagnosis, microscopic examination with sodium hydroxide solution or Wood's lamp (yellow-orange fluorescence) is important.

Clinical features

Pityriasis versicolor begins as light brown patches or hypopigmented macules of 5–20 mm diameter, most frequently on the trunk but sometimes on the upper arms and neck (Fig. 25.16). They gradually enlarge and coalesce. Pityriasis versicolor in which brown patches are produced is called pityriasis versicolor nigra; pityriasis versicolor in which hypopigmented macules occur is called pityriasis versicolor alba. The flat lesions resemble a disorder of skin color but large amounts of pityroid scales detach when scraped. The patches tend to be asymptomatic, although there may be mild reddening or itching.

Epidemiology and causes

Fungi of the genus *Malassezia* are resident in the seborrheic areas and are biphasic, existing as spherical spores or short hyphae. Pityriasis versicolor tends to occur in spring and summer, when perspiration increases. It is found most frequently in young men and women around the age of 20. The cause of pigmentation abnormality in this disorder is unknown but it is thought that substances produced by *Malassezia* cause abnormalities of melanin synthesis.

Laboratory findings and diagnosis

Short dermatophytes and spherical spores are observed microscopically with potassium hydroxide solution in a specimen taken from a scale. This is called "spaghetti and meatballs" appearance (Fig. 25.17). The extent of spread can be observed as a fluorescent yellowish-orange area under Wood's light.

Differential diagnosis

Potassium hydroxide direct microscopy of the scales is necessary for differential diagnosis. Differential diagnosis must consider the clinical features, including erythemas and an abundance of pityriatic scaling from scraping, and the course of progression. Pityriasis versicolor is differentiated from vitiligo, pityriasis simplex, pityriasis rosea (Gibert), and leukoderma pseudosyphiliticum.

Treatment

Pityriasis versicolor heals relatively easily in about 2 weeks with topical imidazole antifungal agents. It often recurs in summer. The abnormality in skin color may remain for many years after treatment.

Malassezia folliculitis

This is folliculitis caused by fungi of the genus *Malassezia*. A red follicular papule 2–3 mm in diameter occurs (Fig. 25.18), sometimes accompanied by a small pustule. Itching and sharp pain are present. It accompanies pityriasis versicolor or seborrheic dermatitis in some cases. It often occurs on the upper back of adolescent men and women. Some cases need differentiation from acne vulgaris, folliculitis, and pustular drug eruption. Diagnosis is done by potassium hydroxide microscopy. Pityrosporum folliculitis responds well to topical antifungal agents.

Subcutaneous mycoses

Sporotrichosis

- *Sporothrix schenckii* in the soil enters the human body through a minor injury. Farmers and infants are most commonly affected.
- A red papule or pustule first occurs, forming a firm subcutaneous nodule or ulcer.
- A granuloma containing asteroid bodies is found histopathologically. Sporotrichin test is positive.
- Oral antifungal drugs such as itraconazole and potassium iodide, and thermotherapy are effective.

Clinical features

After a latency of 8–30 days, a red papule or pustule occurs at the site of fungal invasion (Fig. 25.19). The eruption gradually enlarges to an infiltrative subcutaneous nodule up to 4 cm in diameter. The nodule

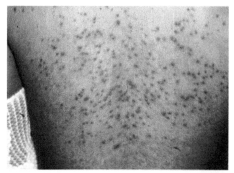
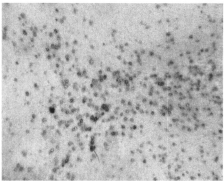

Fig. 25.18 *Malassezia* folliculitis.

MEMO 25–9 Skin disorders caused by fungi of the genus *Malassezia*

Malassezia fungi cause pityriasis versicolor and *Malassezia* folliculitis, as described in this chapter. These bacteria are thought to be a factor in the genesis or aggravation of seborrheic dermatitis and atopic dermatitis (see Chapter 7).

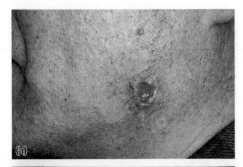

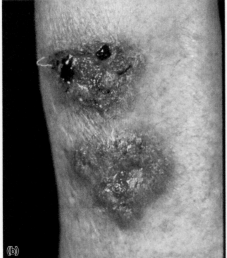

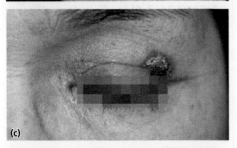

Fig. 25.19 Sporotrichosis. It most frequently occurs in the temperate regions. a: On the face. b: On the lower leg. c: On the eyelid.

easily ruptures, and an intractable ulcer forms. Mild pain may accompany the ulceration; sporotrichosis is otherwise asymptomatic. Many cases are the lymphocutaneous form, in which lesions spread progressively along the lymph vessels. Other subtypes are the fixed form, in which a localized lesion enlarges to form a large ulcerative plaque, and the disseminated form, in which subcutaneous nodules occur systemically by dissemination of fungi. The lymphocutaneous form often occurs on the area between the dorsal hands and forearms of adults; the fixed form frequently occurs on the face and upper arms of children.

Pathogenesis and epidemiology

Sporotrichosis is caused by *Sporothrix schenckii*, a fungus that lives in soil. It occurs most commonly in tropical to temperate regions, in those who often are exposed to the soil, such as farmers, gardeners, and children who play outdoors. *Sporothrix schenckii* invades the dermis through a minor injury, such as a cut, scratch or splinter.

Pathology

A non-specific granulomatous lesion is observed in the layers between the dermis and subcutaneous tissue. Eosin-chromophilic asteroid bodies may be found in the lesion. (See Chapter 18 for asteroid bodies.) In rare cases, spherical spores may be found in giant cells with PAS staining.

Laboratory findings, diagnosis, and differential diagnosis

If a reddish-brown granulomatous lesion or ulcer that does not respond to antibiotics is found, sporotrichosis should be suspected. Crust or exudative fluid is cultured in Sabouraud glucose agar. *Sporothrix schenckii* forms gray to blackish-brown villiform-like colonies at 25°C in 1 week. To confirm the diagnosis, slide culture is used to identify the characteristic dermatophytes with petaloid spores. Exudative fluid or pus is investigated by smear microscopy. Spores are often seen by using PAS or Grocott stain. Sporotrichin intradermal test is a specific test for sporotrichosis.

Non-tuberculous mycobacterial infections, chromoblastomycosis, and pyoderma gangrenosum are differentiated from sporotrichosis.

Treatment

Sporotrichosis tends not to heal spontaneously, and may progress for several years. It heals in 1–3 months with oral itraconazole or potassium iodide, which are extremely effective. Oral terbinafine, thermotherapy, and surgical removal are also useful.

Chromoblastomycosis (synonym: chromomycosis)

- Chromoblastomycosis is a chronic fungal infection of the skin and subcutaneous tissue by pigmented fungi.
- Reddish papules and verrucous plaques form, most frequently on exposed areas such as the legs.
- The lesions develop slowly and form exophytic plaques.

Clinical features

Chromoblastomycosis most commonly affects middle-aged men and women, typically on exposed areas, such as the extremities, legs, and face. A red papule appears and enlarges to form a dark-red elevated plaque with scaling. The lesion tends to heal centrifugally, and it may present a ring or horseshoe appearance (Fig. 25.20). Since abscess or ulcer formation and rupture rarely occur, the lesion tends to be dry. The surface of the lesion may become verrucous. It is called dermatitis verrucosa in some cases. It may form a marked tumor-like mass that has a cauliflower-like appearance. Chromoblastomycosis is nearly asymptomatic. It generally occurs as a solitary lesion that does not heal spontaneously and progresses slowly. There have been some cases that spread lymphogenously or resulted in fatal generalized chromoblastomycosis.

Pathogenesis

Dematiaceous fungi invade the skin through trauma, such as a puncture from a splinter, and form a granulomatous lesion. Most cases are caused by *Fonsecaea pedrosoi*, followed in frequency by *Phialophora verrucosa* and *Cladophialophora carrionii* (*Cladosporium carrionii*). These fungi are resident in soil, plants, and rotting wood. The incubation period is thought to be several years.

Pathology and diagnosis

Large round or polygonal brown cells called sclerotic cells are observed in scales from the lesion by potassium hydroxide direct microscopy. Histopathologically, a

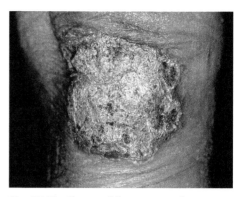

Fig. 25.20 Chromoblastomycosis. The surface of the lesion may appear verrucous.

MEMO 25–10
Dematiaceous fungal infection

"Dematiaceous fungi" is a generic term for fungi that have melanin in their cell walls and form blackish colonies when cultured. Infections caused by these fungi include (1) chromoblastomycosis, in which sclerotic cells are found, (2) pheohyphomycosis, in which sclerotic cells are not found but brown hyphae with septa are found, and (3) tinea nigra, a superficial fungal infection caused by *Hortaea werneckii*, in which black macules appear on the palm.

granulomatous lesion forms in the layers from the dermis to the subcutaneous tissue. The spores are found by H&E staining. Scale culture in Sabouraud glucose agar and PCR is also carried out.

Treatment
When the lesion is small, it is excised with a margin of 5–10 mm of normal skin. Oral itraconazole, flucytosine, terbinafine hydrochloride, and thermotherapy are useful but chromoblastomycosis is often intractable.

Mycetoma
Mycetoma is a chronic granulomatous lesion with subcutaneous induration and multiple fistulae that discharge grains. Mycetoma is classified by the causative microorganism as actinomycetoma (caused by *Nocardia brasiliensis* and similar microorganisms; see Chapter 24) or eumycetoma (caused by *Pseudallescheria boydii*). These microorganisms are resident in the soil. Mycetoma often occurs on the lower extremities of outdoor workers, on the feet in particular. Lesions resembling folliculitis or chronic pyoderma occur and gradually enlarge. Granules are masses of bacteria with diameters of 1–10 mm. The condition progresses slowly over the course of many years, and it may result in joint and bone lesions.

Cutaneous aspergillosis
Cutaneous aspergillosis is caused by fungi of the genus *Aspergillus* (*Aspergillus fumigatus*) that are widely resident in soil. Most cases are lesions in the lung or external auditory canal from opportunistic infection; skin lesions rarely occur. When *Aspergillus* travels hematogenously from a pulmonary lesion to the skin, granulomatous lesions occur (secondary cutaneous aspergillosis) on the whole body. Prolonged bedrest or cast immobilization may induce direct parasitism on the skin resembling tinea corporis or folliculitis (primary cutaneous aspergillosis).

Cutaneous cryptococcosis
The face, neck, and scalp are most commonly involved. Cutaneous cryptococcosis begins with asymptomatic papules and acne-like eruptions that gradually enlarge to form abscesses. The various skin lesions include ulcers, firm subcutaneous nodules, and cellulitis. It is an infection in the layers from the dermis to the subcutaneous tissue caused by *Cryptococcus neoformans*, a fungus that exists in pigeon droppings and soil. The

main subtypes are primary and secondary cutaneous cryptococcosis. The former is caused by direct invasion by the fungi into an external injury. The latter is caused by hematogenous dissemination from pulmonary granulomas. It may be found as an opportunistic infection in people who are on immunosuppressants for long periods or in AIDS patients.

Cutaneous cryptococcosis is diagnosed when microscopic observation shows characteristically thick, capsulated spores in the pus. Histopathological tests, fungal culture, and measurement of *Cryptococcus neoformans* antigen or antibody in the serum are useful for diagnosis.

Paracoccidioidomycosis (synonym: South American blastomycosis)

Paracoccidioidomycosis is a disease of Latin America. However, it may be found elsewhere as an imported fungal infection. A pulmonary lesion first forms as the result of inhalation, and the infection then spreads hematogenously to the skin and mucosa. Papules and ulcers form on the whole body (Fig. 25.21). It tends to be accompanied by swelling of the lymph nodes. Histopathologically, the spores resemble the wheel of a ship (Fig. 25.22). It is a chronic granulomatous fungal infection by *Paracoccidioides brasiliensis*.

Coccidioidomycosis

This disease is endemic to desert areas of the southwestern United States and Latin America. *Coccidioides immitis* aspirated into the lungs induces a pulmonary lesion, and the infection disseminates hematogenously to the skin, causing papules, most commonly on the medial area of the face, such as the nasal region or nasolabial groove, and on the extremities. The papules gradually enlarge to form nodules and plaques.

North American blastomycosis

This occurs on the North American continent and in parts of Africa. A pulmonary lesion occurs and readily spreads to the skin and bones. Verrucous papules, nodules, and ulcers form on the face and in the oral mucosa. The causative fungus is *Blastomyces dermatitidis*.

Histoplasmosis

This is an infection by *Histoplasma capsulatum* var. *capsulatum*. It occurs in tropical, subtropical, and temperate areas of the world, particularly in the Mississippi Valley

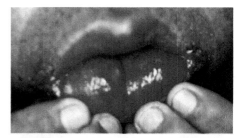
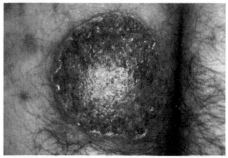
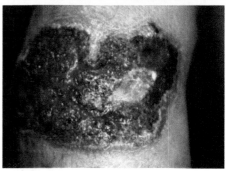

Fig. 25.21-1 Paracoccidioidomycosis.

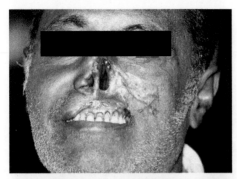

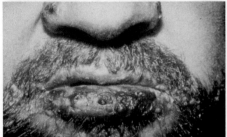

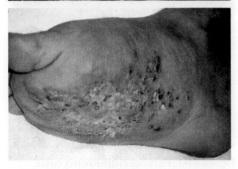

Fig. 25.21-2 Paracoccidioidomycosis.

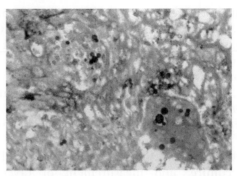

Fig. 25.22 Histopathology of paracoccidioidomycosis (Grocott stain). Dark-stained spores are present in the dermis.

and Africa. The fungus is thought to inhabit bat-infested caves. It may infect humans by aspiration. The infection spreads hematogenously from the lungs and forms skin lesions.

Cutaneous mucormycosis

This is also called zygomycosis. It is usually caused by fungi of the order Mucorales. These fungi are widely present in the environment. Patients with immunodeficiency or severe diabetes are prone to this infection. The cutaneous symptoms include subcutaneous nodules and gangrene.

Cutaneous protothecosis

Caused by algae such as *Prototheca wickerhamii*, this occurs as an opportunistic infection in immunodeficient patients. Verrucous plaques and nodules form on the extremities.

CHAPTER 26

Mycobacterial infections

Mycobacterial infections are caused by bacteria of the genus *Mycobacterium*. These bacteria stain well with Ziehl–Neelsen staining and do not decolorize even when decolorizing agents such as hydrochloric acid alcohol are added; hence, they are called acid-fast bacteria. Of the species in this genus, three are the main pathogens for human skin: *Mycobacterium tuberculosis*, non-tuberculous (atypical) *Mycobacterium marinum*, and *Mycobacterium leprae* (MEMO). Diseases caused by these mycobacteria are introduced in this chapter.

Mycobacterium tuberculosis infections

Epidemiology and classification

Tuberculosis is an infection caused by *Mycobacterium tuberculosis*, or by *Mycobacterium bovis* in rare cases. *Mycobacterium tuberculosis* is an aerobic bacillus of 2–4 mm by 0.3–0.6 mm. It often causes airborne infection (MEMO, see Chapter 23). Generally, mycobacterial infections do not develop into tuberculosis. The

---

MEMO 26–1 Classification of mycobacterial infections

Mycobacteria include tuberculosis bacteria (*Mycobacterium tuberculosis*), non-tuberculosis (atypical) bacteria, and leprosy bacteria (*Mycobacterium leprae*). These are the pathogens of the diseases listed below.

Causative *Mycobacterium*	Diagnostic name	Examination	Treatment
Mycobacterium tuberculosis	Tuberculosis of the skin	Tuberculin reaction (+)	Short-term chemotherapy
	Tuberculid	Tuberculin reaction (++)	Short-term chemotherapy
Non-tuberculosis *Mycobacteria*	Non-tuberculous mycobacterial infection	Tuberculin reaction may be positive in some cases.	Tetracycline New quinolone Thermotherapy and other
Mycobacterium leprae	Leprosy	Smear test of the skin (− to +)	Multidrug therapy, new quinolone

---

Shimizu's Dermatology, Second Edition. Hiroshi Shimizu.

infection is often asymptomatic or latent; however, prior infection may develop into tuberculosis in immunodeficient patients (e.g., elderly people and patients with HIV infection). The lifetime risk of tuberculosis in people with latent infection is estimated as 10%. Skin lesions occur in about 0.1% of patients with tuberculosis. The main type is tuberculosis of the skin (true cutaneous tuberculosis, accounting for 15% of tuberculosis cases with skin lesions), in which *Mycobacterium tuberculosis* causes lesions directly in the skin. Tuberculid is an allergic skin reaction to *Mycobacterium tuberculosis*, accounting for 85% of cases of tuberculosis infection. Tuberculosis of the skin is subclassified by clinical features and mechanisms (Table 26.1).

Treatment
The treatments are generally the same as those for pulmonary tuberculosis. Short-term chemotherapy is carried out. Multidrug therapy using the three drugs isoniazid (INH), rifampicin (RFP), and pyrazinamide (PZA), plus either ethambutol hydrochloride (EB) or streptomycin (SM), is carried out for 2 months; then INH plus either RFP or EB is continued for 4 months. Long-term treatment may cause side effects: peripheral neuropathy for INH and optic nerve inflammation for EB. Tuberculid may be temporarily aggravated by treatments.

(True) Cutaneous tuberculosis

Scrofuloderma
- This is the most common true cutaneous tuberculosis. It most frequently occurs in the neck region.
- It begins as painless subcutaneous nodules. It is characterized by fistula formation and pus discharge from cold abscesses.
- Scrofuloderma occurs when a focus of tuberculosis in extracutaneous organs, such as in the neck lymph nodes, affects the skin.

Clinical features and pathogenesis
This type of true cutaneous tuberculosis occurs when lesions in the lungs, lymph nodes, bones, muscles, and tendons directly spread and affect the skin. It frequently occurs in the lymph nodes of the neck region. A painless, light-pink subcutaneous nodule appears

Table 26.1 Classification of tuberculosis.

Disease	Mechanism of skin infection	Frequent site	Lesions in other organs (e.g., lungs)	Caseous necrosis in pathological tissue	Tubercle bacillus in cutaneous tissue	Remarks
Tuberculosis of the skin						
1 Scrofuloderma	Endogenous spread	Neck	+	+++	++	Cold abscess
2 Lupus vulgaris	Exogenous infection/ endogenous spread	Face	+/–	+	+	Differentiate from DLE and sarcoidosis
3 Warty TB	Exogenous infection	Extremities	+/–	++	+	Affects those who have a history of tuberculosis
Tuberculid						
1 Erythema induratum	Endogenous spread	Lower legs	+/–	+++	+/–	See Chapter 18
2 Papulonecrotic tuberculid	Endogenous spread	Extensor surfaces of the extremities	+/–	+	–	Multiple, contralateral eruptions. Vasculitis-like papules and ulcers are present.
3 Lichen scrofulosorum	Endogenous spread	Trunk	+	-	–	Most frequently occurs after BCG vaccination
4 Tuberculid of the penis	Endogenous spread	Shaft and glans of penis	+	+	–	Painful ulceration is present.

BCG, bacille Calmette–Guérin; DLE, discoid lupus erythematosus.

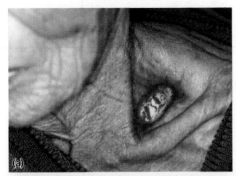

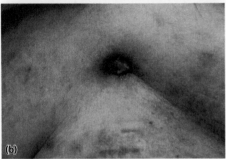

Fig. 26.1 Scrofuloderma. Cold abscess without redness or flushing is present. a: On the neck. b: On the chest.

**MEMO 26–2
QuantiFERON-TB2G (QFT)**

QuantiFERON-TB2G is a new blood test for tuberculosis infection. The results are unaffected by the bacillus Calmette–Guérin vaccination. It is characterized by a higher specificity than that of the tuberculin reaction. *Mycobacterium tuberculosis*-specific protein and lymphocytes in peripheral blood are mixed and cultured, then the level of IFN-γ, a marker for cellular immunity, is measured. If the IFN-γ, level is elevated, cellular immunity against *Mycobacterium tuberculosis* is activated.

first. It softens over the course of several months to form a fistula in the skin, from which pus is discharged (Fig. 26.1). The lesion is not accompanied by reddening or heat sensation; it is called a cold abscess. At a previously formed scrofuloderma, ulceration and characteristic cord-like scarring occur. It is largely asymptomatic.

Diagnosis and treatment

Abundant *Mycobacterium tuberculosis* is found in the pus and tissue. Diagnosis is made by isolating the bacteria from tissue or pus, or by PCR analysis. The original focus of tuberculosis below the skin lesion should be thoroughly treated.

Lupus vulgaris

- Reddish-brown papules appear on the face and neck, coalescing into elevated, infiltrative plaques.
- This condition is caused when *Mycobacterium tuberculosis* disseminates hematogenously or lymphogenously from a focus of extracutaneous tuberculosis.
- It is rarely seen today.
- It progresses extremely slowly. It progresses to squamous cell carcinoma in rare cases.

Clinical features

A single or several unilateral, reddish-brown papules first appear on the face, neck or arms, coalescing into erythematous plaques. The surface of the papule exfoliates, and the center scars. Papules recur on the scarred areas, gradually and repeatedly enlarging and coalescing. This leads to the formation of large, firm, elastic, infiltrative plaques (Fig. 26.2 and Fig. 26.3). It is usually asymptomatic. At the periphery there are small reddish-yellow or brown nodules. Yellowish-brown papules resembling apple jelly are observed by diascopy. Lupus vulgaris progresses extremely slowly, over the course of many years. In addition to preexisting lesions, ulceration and atrophy occur, sometimes leading to squamous cell carcinoma.

Pathogenesis

Mycobacterium tuberculosis is thought to disseminate hematogenously or lymphogenously from a focus of tuberculosis in extracutaneous organs, such as the lungs and the lymph nodes. This dissemination causes a tubercle to form in the skin.

Pathology

An epithelioid cell granuloma containing Langhans giant cells forms in the dermis. Generally, caseous necrosis is found at the center of the lesion. Caseous necrosis is not found in many cases, and mycobacteria are not found in the stain in many cases.

Diagnosis

Lupus vulgaris is diagnosed by the clinical features, the pathology, and the strong positivity in the tuberculin skin test. *Mycobacterium tuberculosis* is often negative in cultures of tissue and in smears. Cultures of pus tend to be positive. PCR is useful, but false positives are possible.

Differential diagnosis

Discoid lupus erythematosus, sarcoidosis, syphilis, and sporotrichosis should be differentiated from lupus vulgaris.

Treatment and prognosis

Lupus vulgaris responds well to antituberculosis drugs. Although the prognosis is good, it leaves distinct scarring. Treatment may induce acute necrosis or circulatory failure, which may lead to the formation of large ulcers.

Warty tuberculosis, tuberculosis verrucosa cutis
Clinical features and pathology

Warty tuberculosis occurs most frequently at the ends of the extremities and in the buttocks, which are prone to injury (Fig. 26.4).

Several small nodules coalesce and enlarge, forming erythematous plaques with a verrucous periphery. The lesions enlarge centrifugally and tend to heal at the center or to scar. There is inflammation with histopathological atypism. Tumors consisting of Langhans giant cells are found in the upper layer of the dermis. *Mycobacteria* are not found in the stain in many cases.

Pathogenesis

Warty tuberculosis is a true cutaneous tuberculosis caused by *Mycobacterium tuberculosis*. It occurs from inoculation of organisms into the skin of a previously infected patient, who usually has a moderate or high degree of immunity.

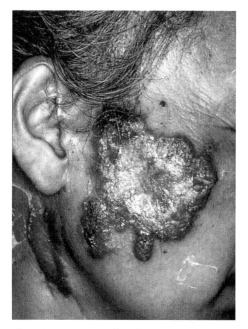

Fig. 26.2 Lupus vulgaris. A large, firm, infiltrative, and elevated plaque on the cheek.

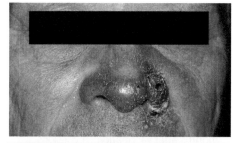

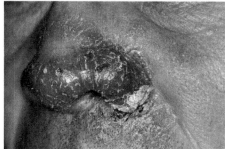

Fig. 26.3 Lupus vulgaris. An infiltrative plaque on the nose.

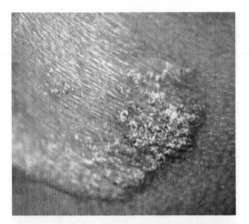

Fig. 26.4 Warty tuberculosis, tuberculosis verrucosa cutis. A keratotic erythematous plaque with a verrucous periphery enlarges centrifugally. The center of the lesion shows a tendency to heal.

MEMO 26–3 Lupus

Lupus is a general term for diseases in which erosive, erythematous ulceration occurs on the face. The name is Latin for "wolf" and it comes from the facial appearance that was thought to resemble the bites of a wolf. Until the 19th century, lupus was most commonly caused by cutaneous tuberculosis. Cutaneous tuberculosis has been called lupus vulgaris. In recent years, the prevalence of lupus vulgaris has drastically decreased. The term "lupus" now almost always refers to lupus erythematosus, an autoimmune disease (see Chapter 12).

Diagnosis and differential diagnosis

Identification of *Mycobacterium tuberculosis* is made by tuberculin skin test and pathological findings in the skin. Diagnosis is done by isolating bacteria from the tissue or pus or by PCR analysis. Differentiation from verruca vulgaris, chromoblastomycosis, lupus vulgaris, and tinea cruris is important. Warty tuberculosis responds well to antituberculosis drugs.

Tuberculid

Eruptions that are thought to be caused by immunological reaction against *Mycobacterium tuberculosis* are called tuberculid. Patients with tuberculid often have a focus of extracutaneous tuberculosis, such as in the lungs. It is thought to be an immunological reaction of the skin to hematogenous dissemination of *Mycobacterium tuberculosis* or to antigens related to *Mycobacterium tuberculosis* in the initially infected lesion. Tuberculid occurs in individuals who have strong cellular immunity against *Mycobacterium tuberculosis*. A remarkably strong reaction is observed in the tuberculin skin tests of such individuals. *Mycobacterium tuberculosis* is not detected in the tuberculid lesions but PCR may be positive. A good response to antituberculosis drugs is characteristic of tuberculid.

Erythema induratum (EI)
Refer to Chapter 18.

Papulonecrotic tuberculid
This is thought to be vasculitis caused by allergic reaction to *Mycobacterium tuberculosis*. It occurs in young people, most frequently on the extensor surfaces of the

---

MEMO 26–4 Bacillus Calmette–Guérin (BCG) granuloma

Infection of *Mycobacterium bovis* occurs in rare cases after BCG vaccination. Subcutaneous nodules appear or enlargement of the lymph nodes occurs in the axillary fossae 1–6 months after vaccination. The lesions spontaneously disappear in several months in many cases, but ulceration may form.

extremities, particularly on the elbows and popliteal fossae. Multiple contralateral dark red papules with a diameter of 1 cm or less appear and necrotize, forming pustules and ulcerations. These heal with scarring. The eruptions occur in succession and progress slowly, with new eruptions presenting together with old ones. It is necessary to differentiate papulonecrotic tuberculid from cutaneous small vessel vasculitis (see Chapter 11) and pityriasis lichenoides (see Chapter 15). Antituberculosis drugs are useful.

Lichen scrofulosorum

Scattered or aggregated flat and elevated papules of one to several millimeters in diameter and of normal skin color to red appear on the trunk and extremities. The papules coalesce to form plaques. Some cases are follicle associated. Lichen scrofulosorum is nearly asymptomatic. Histopathologically, epithelial cells and Langhans giant cells are found at the peripheries of the follicles and sweat glands. Caseous necrosis is not present, nor is *Mycobacterium tuberculosis* detected in tissue culture. Antituberculosis drugs are useful. Most cases heal in 1–2 months.

Tuberculid of the penis, penile tuberculid

Tuberculid of the penis is papulonecrotic tuberculid (described earlier) localized on the penis. It tends to occur in patients with nephrotuberculosis and bladder tuberculosis. A painful ulcer forms on the glans and shaft of the penis. It is necessary to differentiate tuberculid of the penis clinically from penile cancer.

Non-tuberculous mycobacterial infections

Non-tuberculous mycobacteriosis (NTM) is a general term for infections caused by non-tuberculous *Mycobacteria* other than *Mycobacterium tuberculosis* and *Mycobacterium leprae* (Fig. 26.5). There are about 30 non-tuberculous *Mycobacteria* that are pathogenic to humans. Identification of the bacterial type is done by PCR DDH (DNA-DNA hybridization) after mycobacterial culture.

Mycobacterium marinum infection (synonyms: fish tank granuloma, swimming pool granuloma)

Aquarium staff and tropical fish breeders are most commonly affected.

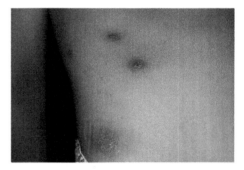

Fig. 26.5-1 Non-tuberculous mycobacterial infection.

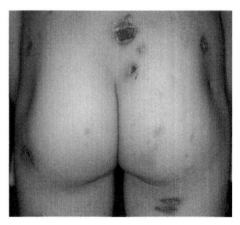

Fig. 26.5-2 Non-tuberculous mycobacterial infection.

- Contaminated water from a swimming pool or a tropical fish tank enters a minor injury, causing infection. Nodules, exfoliation, and ulceration occur.
- Tetracyclines and new quinolone antibiotics are effective treatments.

Clinical features

Mycobacterium marinum infection is the most frequently found non-tuberculous mycobacterial infection that affects the skin. Because *Mycobacterium marinum* favors freshwater environments and its optimal temperature for growth is 30–33°C, most cases of infection are from water from swimming pools or tropical fish tanks. Aquarium staff and tropical fish breeders are commonly infected. The onset is after a 2-week incubation period of infection in an external injury. Areas that are subjected to external friction, such as the dorsum of the fingers and joints, are most commonly involved. Red plaques accompanied by central pustules and crusting occur (Fig. 26.6-1). Scaling and verrucous plaques occur later on. The eruptions are solitary in most cases. However, *Mycobacterium marinum* may be disseminated by lymph flow or spread systemically in some cases.

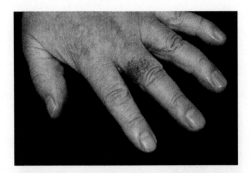

Fig. 26.6-1 *Mycobacterium marinum* infection.

Pathology

Non-specific inflammation mixed with epithelioid cell granulomas is found. Histopathological detection of *Mycobacteria* is difficult.

Diagnosis and differential diagnosis

Mycobacterium marinum infection is suspected when skin lesions in patients whose occupation involves fish are examined. *Mycobacteria* are detected from pus, skin tissue or cultured fish tank water.

Sporotrichosis and other deep mycoses, various forms of cutaneous tuberculosis, and foreign body granuloma should be differentiated from *Mycobacterium marinum* infection.

Treatment

The infection heals in 2–3 months with the administration of tetracycline or new quinolone antibiotics. It is necessary to continue treatments for a period of several months or longer than a year in some cases. Surgical removal and local thermotherapy (42°C for 1–2 h per day) are helpful.

Mycobacterium avium-intracellulare complex infection

Nodules, ulcers, and subcutaneous induration occur on areas subjected to pressure. The extremities and buttocks are most commonly involved. Antituberculosis drugs are used in combination with either macrolide or new quinolone antibiotics for most cases. Surgical removal may be helpful for localized skin lesions.

Mycobacterium fortuitum infection, *Mycobacterium chelonae* infection

A cold abscess, fistula, ulcer or nodule occurs (Fig. 26.6-2). Antituberculosis drugs are used in combination with either macrolide or new quinolone antibiotics; however, these infections are often refractory. Incision, drainage of pus, debridement, and excision are also carried out.

Mycobacterium leprae infection (synonyms: leprosy, Hansen's disease)

- This is a chronic infection caused by *Mycobacterium leprae*. The skin and peripheral nerves are mainly involved. It is characterized by plaques accompanied by decreased sensation.

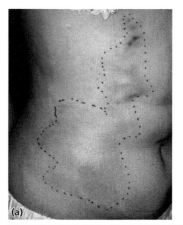

(a)

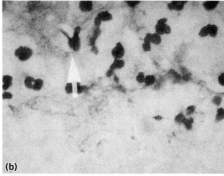

(b)

Fig. 26.6-2 *Mycobacterium fortuitum* **infection in a woman in her 20s.** a: Pulsating nodules and abscesses occur over a large area of the trunk. Pus is discharged in large amounts by puncture. b: *Mycobacteria fortuitum* appear red in Ziehl–Neelsen staining (arrow).

MEMO 26–5 WHO classification of Hansen's disease (leprosy)

To facilitate diagnosis and decision making about treatment, a classification specified by the WHO is often used. When six or more lesions are found or *Mycobacteria* are identified in a skin smear test, the case is classified as multibacillary type (MB). When five or fewer lesions are found and *Mycobacteria* are not identified, the case is classified as paucibacillary type (PB). Among paucibacillary cases, those with only one lesion are called single-lesion paucibacillary type (SLPB). See Figure for a comparison between the WHO classification and the Ridley & Jopling classification.

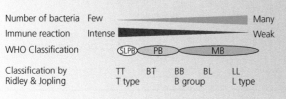

Number of bacteria	Few		Many
Immune reaction	Intense		Weak
WHO Classification	SLPB PB		MB
Classification by Ridley & Jopling	TT BT T type	BB BL B group	LL L type

- It is classified into tuberculoid leprosy (T type) and lepromatous leprosy (L type). In L type, which is more severe than T type, *Mycobacterium leprae* proliferates throughout the entire body to form nodules.
- Multidrug therapy including DDS (dapsone) is the main treatment.

Pathogenesis

Leprosy is an infection caused by *Mycobacterium leprae*. It is thought that infection occurs via the invasion of bacteria in the skin through a minor external injury, or through the mucosa of an infant. Infection often occurs via close contact between parents and children.

Clinical features and classification

Leprosy is subclassified by the strength of the host's cellular immunity against *Mycobacterium leprae* (Table 26.2 and Fig. 26.7). Ring-shaped erythema, leukoderma, and plaques form, accompanied by decreased sensation (Fig. 26.8).

Table 26.2 Classification of leprosy.

Classification by number of bacteria	Paucibacillary (PB)	Multibacillary (MB)
Immunological classification (Ridley–Jopling)	I TT	BT BB BL LL (B)
Cellular immunity	Good	Low/none
Localized immunity	Th1, IL-2, IFN-γ, IL-12	Th2, CD8 T cell, IL-4, IL-5, IL-10
Smear test of the skin	Negative	Positive
Mycobacterium leprae	Few/hard to find	Many
Number of eruptions	Few	Many
Distribution of eruptions	Asymmetrical	Symmetrical
Nature of eruptions	Macules (annular), sharply demarcated	Erythema (annular), papules, nodules
Surface of eruptions	Dry, glabrous	Glossy, smooth
Sensory abnormality of the lesion	Severe (sensations of touch, pain, and temperature)	Mild or none
Pathological findings	Epithelioid cell granuloma, giant cells, inflammatory cell infiltration in the nerve	Histiocytic granuloma, foamy change of histiocytes
Pathological finding of *Mycobacterium leprae*	Negative	Positive
Main basis for diagnosis	Sensory abnormality of the lesion	Finding of *Mycobacterium leprae* in smear test
Infectiousness	None	Contagious

Adapted from the website of the Infectious Disease Surveillance Center, National Institute of Infectious Diseases at http://idsc.nih.go.jp/disease/leprosy/page03.html

There are some cases in which treatments or psychological stress induce an inflammatory reaction and the symptoms rapidly aggravate (leprae reaction). Multiple nodular erythema-like eruptions (see Chapter 18) accompanied by perspiration and arthralgia may occur on the whole body during the leprosy reaction (erythema nodosum leprosum).

Pathology

An epithelioid cell granuloma consisting mainly of Langhans giant cells and macrophages forms in either of the subtypes. In T type (paucibacillary), as the result of cellular immunity, multiple sites of lymphatic infiltration are seen at the periphery of granulomas. In L type (multibacillary), which lacks inflammatory cells, the proliferation of *Mycobacterium leprae* is observed in macrophages.

Laboratory findings and diagnosis

Leprosy is diagnosed by skin lesions such as leukoderma that are accompanied by reduced sensation, hypertrophy of the peripheral nerves (the great auricular and

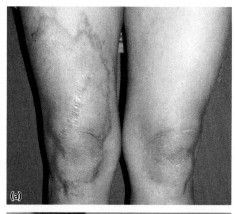
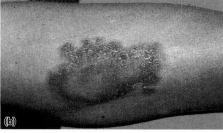

Fig. 26.8 Leprosy, Hansen's disease.
a: T leprosy(paucibacillary type). Annular erythema on the right thigh. b: L leprosy (multibacillary type). A flat, elevated purple plaque on the right upper arm.

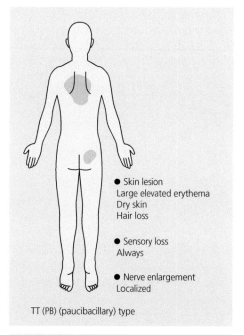

- Skin lesion
  Large elevated erythema
  Dry skin
  Hair loss

- Sensory loss
  Always

- Nerve enlargement
  Localized

TT (PB) (paucibacillary) type

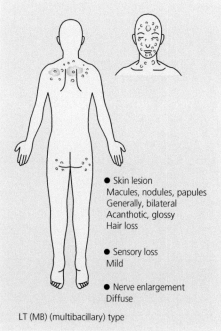

- Skin lesion
  Macules, nodules, papules
  Generally, bilateral
  Acanthotic, glossy
  Hair loss

- Sensory loss
  Mild

- Nerve enlargement
  Diffuse

LT (MB) (multibacillary) type

Fig. 26.7 Comparison between tuberculoid leprosy and lepromatous leprosy.

ulnar nerves), neurological disorder, and histopathological findings. Skin smear, PCR, and measurement of antibody levels against PGL-1 are useful in the diagnosis and classification of leprosy subtypes.

Differential diagnosis

Leprosy should be differentiated from cutaneous tuberculosis, syphilis, cutaneous mycoses, diseases that are accompanied by peripheral nerve impairment, including diabetes and syringomyelia, and mycosis fungoides.

Treatment

Multidrug therapy for each subtype is recommended by the WHO. Non-steroidal antiinflammatory drugs or oral steroids are administered when the leprosy reaction causes sharp pain.

CHAPTER 27
Sexually transmitted infections

Infections whose main transmission route is sexual intercourse or sexual activity are generally called sexually transmitted infections (STI). The rapidly increasing number of STI cases has become a serious social issue. This chapter introduces the STIs that are not discussed in other chapters, such as syphilis, chancroid, and lymphogranuloma venereum (chlamydia).

Syphilis

- The causative bacterium is the spirochete *Treponema pallidum*.
- The various mucocutaneous symptoms include ulceration of the genitals and eruptions over the whole body.
- In primary syphilis, the lesions are localized. Genital lesions, hard ulcerative chancres, and regional lymph node enlargement occur.
- In secondary syphilis, the lesions are caused by systemic spread of the bacteria. Syphilitic roseola, papular syphilide, condylomata lata, and syphilitic alopecia occur. In some HIV-positive cases, secondary syphilis progresses to neurosyphilis.
- Tertiary syphilis: syphilis today rarely progresses to this stage.
- In latent syphilis, the serological reaction is positive for syphilis, with no other symptoms. In many cases, no symptoms occur for the rest of life.
- In congenital syphilis (transplacental infection), the clinical features of primary syphilis are absent.
- Diagnosis is made by the characteristic clinical features, serological test, and detection of the pathogenic microbe. Penicillin antibiotics are administered.

Classification and pathogenesis

Syphilis is caused by the spirochete *Treponema pallidum* via contact infection (acquired syphilis) or intrauterine infection (congenital syphilis). Acquired syphilis is

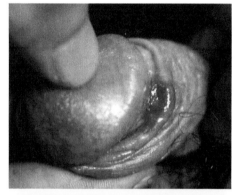

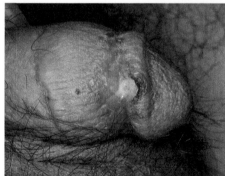

Fig. 27.1 Initial sclerosis. A firm, asymptomatic papule with a diameter of 1–2 cm occurs on the border of the glans penis and foreskin.

Shimizu's Dermatology, Second Edition. Hiroshi Shimizu.
© 2017 John Wiley & Sons, Ltd. Published 2017 by John Wiley & Sons, Ltd.

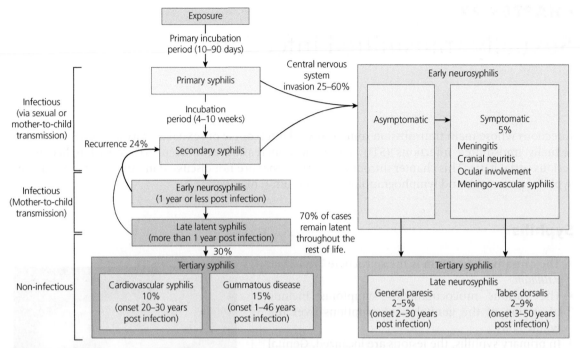

Fig. 27.2 Clinical course of syphilis. Adapted from Golden MR, et al. Update on syphilis: resurgence of an old problem. *JAMA* 2003; 290: 1510.

caused by sexual activity in most cases; however, it may be transmitted non-sexually by healthcare workers. In rare cases, syphilis may be transmitted by transfusion or by mother-to-child transmission from the birth canal or breast feeding.

Clinical features
Syphilis progresses in a characteristic recurring course of lesions appearing on the skin and mucosa followed by an asymptomatic period (Fig. 27.1). Congenital syphilis has a specific course.

Primary syphilis
After the average initial incubation period of 3 weeks (10–90 days), a firm papule occurs at the site invaded by *Treponema pallidum*, gradually ulcerating into a hard chancre (early chancre) (Fig. 27.2). Numerous *Treponema pallidum* bacteria are present on the surface of the hard chancre. The lesion at this stage is highly contagious. Soon after ulceration, the regional lymph node enlarges. The lesion and the lymph node enlargement are asymptomatic, spontaneously disappearing without being noticed in about 3 weeks in

many cases. After this period, an asymptomatic period of about 4–10 weeks continues until the occurrence of secondary syphilis. Infiltration in the central nerves is observed in some cases.

Secondary syphilis

The *Treponema pallidum* bacteria disseminate to the whole body, leading to the various eruptions described below. The antibody titer peaks at this stage. The eruptions spontaneously disappear in several weeks to several months, progressing to latent syphilis. The *Treponema pallidum* bacteria infiltrate the central nervous system and may cause symptomatic neurosyphilis in some cases that accompany HIV infection.

Macular syphilide, roseolar rash

Multiple asymptomatic light pink erythemas 5–20 mm in diameter occur on the whole body surface, markedly on the palms and soles (Fig. 27.3). These are accompanied by slight fever and systemic fatigue. The skin lesions disappear in several days.

Papular syphilide

Two to 3 weeks after the onset of macular syphilide, multiple vivid red papules 5–10 mm in diameter appear, most frequently on the trunk (Fig. 27.4) and most severely on the palms and soles. It is asymptomatic. The lesions on the palms and soles are small scaling plaques resembling the lesions of psoriasis. Figure 27.5 shows the symptoms of syphilitic psoriasis.

Condylomata lata

Highly infectious, moist, flatly elevated papules appear on the intertriginous areas of the anus, genitals, axillary fossae, and inframammary region (Fig. 27.6). *Treponema pallidum* bacteria are observed in high concentrations in the lesions.

Pustular (ulcerative) syphilide

Multiple pustules occur. Papular syphilide may progress to pustular syphilis in some cases. Immunocompromised patients are most likely to be affected.

Syphilitic paronychia

This paronychia is associated with syphilis. There are no clinically characteristic findings in syphilitic paronychia.

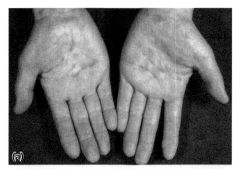

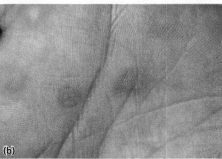

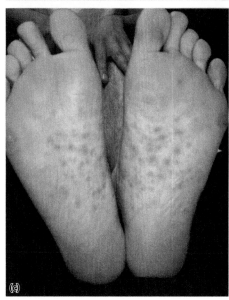

Fig. 27.3 Macular syphilide, roseolar rash. a: Erythema up to 1 cm in diameter that is slightly infiltrative at the edge, on the palms. b: Close-up of a lesion in another case. The erythema is partially infiltrative. c: Lesions on the soles. All cases are asymptomatic.

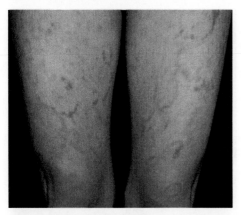

Fig. 27.4 Papular syphilide.

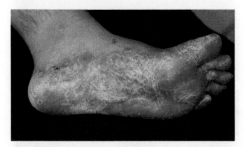

Fig. 27.5 Psoriatic syphilide.

Syphilitic alopecia

Six months after infection, multiple patches of hair loss of 5–20 mm diameter appear and spread gradually over the entire scalp. It should be differentiated from alopecia areata.

Syphilitic mucous eruptions

Grayish-white mucosal lesions form in the oral cavity and on the tongue and tonsils (Fig. 27.7). They are highly contagious.

Latent syphilis

After spontaneous healing of the symptoms of secondary syphilis, serological reaction is positive for syphilis, with no other symptoms. Patients at this stage are often found via health examinations by chance. The symptoms of secondary syphilis recur in about one-quarter of cases of latent syphilis within 1 year after onset of the disease, which is called early latent syphilis. Latent syphilis that occurs after that period is called late latent syphilis. About 30% of latent syphilis cases progress to tertiary syphilis; some of that 30% return to latent syphilis. About 70% of latent syphilis cases remain latent throughout the rest of life. Late latent syphilis is not very contagious but there remains a risk of congenital syphilis through mother-to-child transmission.

Tertiary syphilis

Plaques resembling those of psoriasis and ulcerating granulomatous subcutaneous nodules (gumma) occur. Granulomatous lesions form in multiple organs, including the liver. Cardiovascular syphilis symptoms, such as myocarditis and aortic aneurysm, also occur. In recent years, these symptoms of tertiary syphilis have been declining because treatments using antibiotics have progressed.

Neurosyphilis

Treponema pallidum infiltrates the central nervous system in some cases at the stages of primary and secondary syphilis, and asymptomatic or symptomatic neurosyphilis develops. In early neurosyphilis, meningitis and eye symptoms occur. If untreated, some cases of early neurosyphilis progress to general paresis and myelophthistic anemia (late neurosyphilis).

Congenital syphilis

Treponema pallidum passed through the placenta from the mother infects the child. Intrauterine infection in early pregnancy may result in stillbirth or miscarriage. Therefore, congenital syphilis is usually caused by infection after the first trimester, when the placenta is completely formed. The infection is systemic and hematogenous; congenital syphilis begins with secondary syphilis, without primary syphilis.

Within 6 months after birth, symptoms of secondary syphilis appear (early congenital syphilis). Symptoms of tertiary syphilis appear after late childhood (late congenital syphilis). In early congenital syphilis, premature facial aging, radial scarring around the mouth called Parrot's lines, syphilitic nephritis, and pseudo-paralysis from the sharp pain of osteochondritis (Parrot's pseudo-paralysis) are present. In late congenital syphilis, Hutchinson's triad (barrel-shaped incisors [Hutchinson's tooth], ocular interstitial keratitis, and impairment of the vestibulocochlear nerve) becomes pronounced.

Pathology

Swelling and proliferation of the vascular endothelium and perivascular infiltration of plasma cells and lymphocytes are determined by skin biopsy of a syphilitic eruption. Epithelioid cell granuloma is observed in patients with tertiary syphilis.

Laboratory findings and diagnosis

Treponema pallidum is investigated by serological test and microscopy. Because this bacterium cannot be cultured, specimens are collected and directly investigated by microscopy from moist lesions, such as early chancre, condylomata lata, enanthema in the oral cavity, blisters or pustules. *Treponema pallidum* stains bluish-black in Parker ink and shines in dark-field examination.

Serological tests are useful for finding, screening, and determining the progression of syphilis. Nevertheless, the tests are negative in the fourth to sixth weeks after infection. The main examinations are serological test for syphilis (STS) using lipid antigen (cardiolipin), treponemal hemagglutination (TPHA) assay, *Treponema pallidum* latex agglutination (TPLA) test, and fluorescent treponemal antibody absorption test (FTA-ABS).

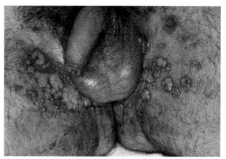
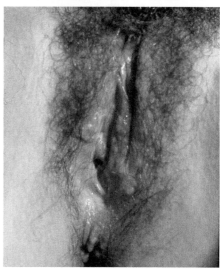

Fig. 27.6 Condylomata lata. Multiple, flatly elevated infiltrative eruptions. These coalesce in some areas.

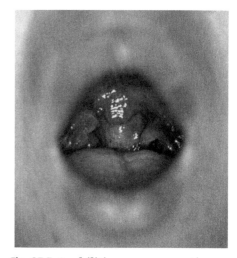

Fig. 27.7 Syphilitic mucous eruptions. Severe edema in the pharyngeal tonsils.

Table 27.1 Interpretation of STS and TPHA results, and courses of action.

STS	TPHA	Interpretation	Course of action
−	−	**Not syphilis**	
		Immediately after exposure to *Treponema***	Re-examination in several weeks, if necessary
−	+	**Syphilis after treatment**	
		Syphilis, many years after onset*	Confirm the results by FTA-ABS.
		Non-specific inflammatory reaction (e.g., alveolar pyorrhea)*	
		Zone phenomenon (STS was false negative from high concentration of antigen.)*	Dilute the serum and make reexamination.
+	−	**Early-stage syphilis infection**	Make reexamination after a certain period of time; confirm by FTA-ABS.
		BFP caused by other disease	Investigate for diseases other than syphilis, such as autoimmune diseases.
+	+	**Syphilis**	Initiate treatment.
		BFP and non-specific reaction*	Confirm by FTA-ABS.

* Very rare.
BFP, biological false positive; STS, serological test for syphilis; TPHA, treponemal hemagglutination.
Adapted from Sugahara T, et al. *Treponema pallidum. Nippon Rinsho* 1990; S48: 408–412.

The STS results show positive in the early stages of infection, and the elevation of antibody titer closely relates to disease progression. STS is effective for screening and is used as an index of therapeutic performance. Wassermann reaction, glass plate test, and rapid plasma reagin card test are used.

Because of their high specificity, TPHA, TPLA, and FTA-ABS are used to confirm the diagnosis. Table 27.1 compares the STS and TPHA tests. The incidence and progression of syphilis are determined by the combination of STS and TPHA.

Treatment

Oral penicillin antibiotics are the first-line treatment. Penicillin-resistant strains have not been found so far. Macrolide or tetracycline drugs are given to patients with penicillin hypersensitivity. Although the administration of antibiotics at the early stage kills *Treponema pallidum* quickly and effectively, the residue of dead *Treponema pallidum* may cause a toxic reaction; within several hours after drug intake, a fever of about 40°C occurs and the syphilis eruptions aggravate (Jarisch–Herxheimer reaction). This condition spontaneously disappears in 1–2 days in many cases.

MEMO 27-1 HIV and syphilis

Sexually transmitted superinfection of HIV and syphilis has been increasing. Syphilis patients who are immunocompromised from HIV infection are prone to severe symptoms of secondary syphilis. Those cases are often difficult to cure by the usual syphilis treatments. The spread of neurosyphilis in HIV-positive patients has become a serious problem. HIV-positive patients may have atypical clinical findings of syphilis, serological findings, and responses to treatments.

Generally, antibiotics are administered for 4 weeks for primary and secondary syphilis, and for 8 weeks for tertiary syphilis. The patient is regarded as cured when the STS quantitative value has fallen to one-quarter of the initial value. HIV carriers may not respond well to treatment, so a long period of treatment may be necessary. Reinfection of *Treponema pallidum* through new sexual activity is not rare.

Chancroid

Pathogenesis and epidemiology
Chancroid is a sexually transmitted infection caused by the *Haemophilus ducreyi* bacterium. This Gram-negative bacillus stains well in Unna–Pappenheim stain. Chancroid is most common in tropical and subtropical countries.

Clinical features
Three to 7 days after infection, a red papule occurs on the coronal sulcus, foreskin, labium or vaginal opening and becomes pustular, leading to ulceration. The ulcer is accompanied by severe pain and a pustular coat at the center. The ulcer is soft to the touch, without induration at the periphery. It begins as a single lesion but rapidly spreads to form multiple lesions via autoinoculation. Painful unilateral swellings called buboes occur in the inguinal lymph node in 25–60% of all patients with chancroid.

Laboratory findings and diagnosis
Chancroid is often diagnosed by the clinical features. It can be differentiated from syphilitic chancres, which are generally painless, hard and indurated, and accompanied by painless lymph node swelling.

Treatment
Azithromycin, ceftriaxone, and erythromycin are the first-line drugs.

Lymphogranuloma venereum (synonyms: lymphogranulomatosis inguinale, chlamydia)

- This is an infection by bacteria of the genus *Chlamydia*.

- It is transmitted by sexual activity. One to 2 weeks after infection, a small papule or vesicle appears on the genitalia. One to 2 weeks after the onset of the skin lesion, fever and swelling occur in lymph nodes of the groin and thighs.
- Lymphogranuloma venereum occurs most frequently in the tropics.

Definition and symptoms

Lymphogranuloma venereum is caused by *Chlamydia trachomatis* L1, L2 or L3. Several days after infection, a small herpes simplex-like papule 1 mm in diameter occurs singly on the genitalia or anus. The skin lesion is asymptomatic and heals unnoticed (primary stage). One to 4 weeks later, systemic symptoms such as fever and splenohepatomegaly occur. The regional lymph node becomes firm and swollen, and the ruptures, discharging pus. The inguinal lymph node of men and the anorectal lymph node of women are often involved (secondary stage). In women, there may be vulvar lymphatic edema, elephantiasis-like change or urethral or rectal stenosis (esthiomène) (third stage: several years after onset and later).

Laboratory findings, diagnosis, and treatment

Culture test using pus, antibody detection from serum, an antigen test from the lesion and PCR test are carried. The Frei test, an intradermal test using fluid taken from the patient's lymph node, is no longer conducted. Tetracycline and macrolide antibiotics are administered orally.

CHAPTER 28

Skin diseases caused by arthropods (insects, spiders, crustaceans) and other noxious animals

Various cutaneous symptoms are caused by arthropods. Contact dermatitis, allergic reactions, and secondary infections occur from arthropod bites or stings, or from contact with the scales. Cutaneous symptoms may occur when arthropods or their body parts or toxins enter the human body or remain in the skin. Pathogens transmitted by arthropods may cause systemic symptoms. Cutaneous diseases related to arthropods are discussed in this chapter.

Diseases caused by insects and other noxious animals

Insect bites

Insect bite is a general term for the dermatitis caused by the bite or sting of a mosquito, gnat, horsefly, bee or other insect. Bites are thought to be allergic reactions to substances that originate from insects and are injected into the human body while the insects are sucking blood, or to the histamines contained in the insect venom. The severity of the clinical symptoms depends largely on the age of the patient and the severity of the allergic reaction. Immediately after an insect bite, an itchy wheal or erythema appears. There are two major clinical types of insect bites: those of immediate hypersensitivity, in which symptoms subside in 1–2 h, and those of delayed hypersensitivity, in which erythema or blistering may occur 1–2 days after the bite (Fig. 28.1). Treatments are topical steroids for eruptions and oral antihistamines for itching lesions. Bee stings require careful systemic observation, because they may cause anaphylactic reactions.

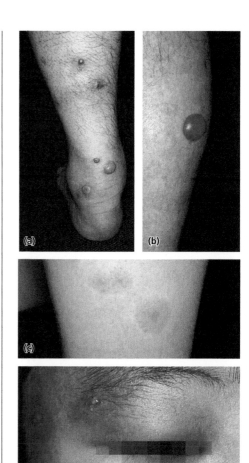

Fig. 28.1-1 Insect bite. a,b: Tense blisters on the lower leg. c: Itching erythema on the lower leg. d: Insect bite on the eyebrow. Severe edema occurred around the lesion.

Shimizu's Dermatology, Second Edition. Hiroshi Shimizu.
© 2017 John Wiley & Sons, Ltd. Published 2017 by John Wiley & Sons, Ltd.

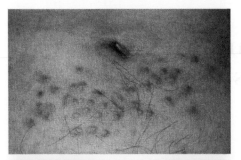

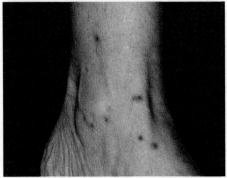

Fig. 28.1-2 Insect bite. Multiple small, itching papules of about 5 mm in diameter on the abdomen and ankle.

MEMO 28–1 Bee stings

A bee sting is usually not life threatening; however, it is necessary to take special care for persons with a history of bee stings or with high levels of IgE antibody to bee venom. An epinephrine autoinjector is used as an emergency treatment for anaphylaxis caused by bee stings.

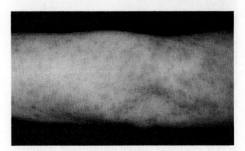

Fig. 28.2 Caterpillar dermatitis. Punctate itching erythema occurs, accompanied by pruritus and blistering in some areas of the lesion.

Hypersensitivity to mosquito bites

After a mosquito bite, an allergic reaction occurs to the saliva of the mosquito, sometimes leading to systemic symptoms such as high fever, liver dysfunction, and lymph node enlargement. Localized symptoms such as blisters and bloody blisters form, and swelling, induration, necrosis, and ulceration occur later. During the course of hypersensitivity to mosquito bites, the histopathological symptoms may resemble those of hydroa vacciniforme (see Chapter 13). Hypersensitivity to mosquito bites may occur as a symptom of chronic active Epstein–Barr virus infection. In such cases, hemophagocytic syndrome and NK/T cell lymphoma may occur later and result in a poor prognosis.

Caterpillar dermatitis

This is also called lepidopteran dermatitis. About 2% of caterpillars are toxic. The urticating hairs of larval moths (caterpillars), including those of the tussock moth, tea tussock moth, and yellowtail moth, cause caterpillar dermatitis. Urticating hairs remaining on the adult moth may also cause caterpillar dermatitis. The hairs may be suspended in the air. Patients are often those who have been working outdoors without knowing that there were caterpillars nearby. Some species (e.g., *Monema flavescens*) have venomous spines that cause symptoms similar to those of caterpillar dermatitis. The affected site has tingling pain. Punctate, itchy erythema is followed by vesicles and papules (Fig. 28.2). Aggregated or linear lesions may be found. The affected site should not be rubbed with the hand. The urticating hairs are removed by washing with water or using adhesive tape, and topical steroids are applied.

Dermatitis linearis

The hemolymph of the *Paederus fuscipes Curtis* beetle comes into contact with the skin, causing dermatitis linearis. This beetle is about 7 mm in length and is found in fields and grasslands. Two to 3 hours after contact, characteristic linear erythematous skin lesions with burning sensation occur (Fig. 28.3). Vesicles, swelling, erosion, and ulceration also occur. The causative substance is thought to be pederin. The lesions heal with pigmentation in about 2 weeks.

Scabies

- This is an infestation of the mite *Sarcoptes scabiei hominis*. Multiple papules occur. Intense itching is present, worsening at night.
- The genitals, trunk, and interdigital areas are most frequently involved. "Tunnels" (burrows) are formed in the interdigital area.
- It may be transmitted by bedclothes or skin-to-skin contact. It often occurs as a sexually transmitted infection or in-hospital epidemic.
- Oral ivermectin, benzyl benzoate, and topical γ-benzenehexachloride (BHC) are the main treatments.

Clinical features

Small multiple light pink papules of 2–5 mm in diameter occur on the trunk, genitals, thighs, inner arms, and interdigital areas (Fig. 28.4). Small nodules may form in the genitals and axillary fossae. Both the papules and the nodules are accompanied by intense itching that worsens when the skin is warmed, such as at bedtime. Patients with scabies often complain of difficulty sleeping because of the itching. Scratching of the skin lesions may lead to the formation of non-specific eczematous plaques. When the interdigital areas and palms are involved, there may be slightly elevated, grayish-white linear lesions (mite burrows) several millimeters in length, in which the female insects lay eggs. Blistering occurs in some cases (Fig. 28.4-2). The infection may occur in the nails, in which case

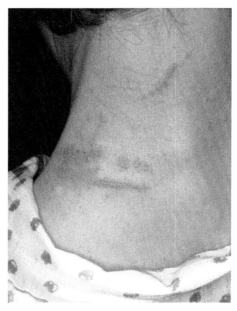

Fig. 28.3 **Dermatitis linearis.**

MEMO 28–2 Myiasis

Flies lay eggs in necrotic tissue. Eggs and maggots are present at the site. It is necessary to remove the maggots by incising the affected site.

MEMO 28–3 Maggot therapy

Specially prepared medical maggots are used to remove necrotic tissue. This therapy may be used for treating diabetic gangrene.

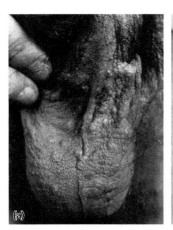
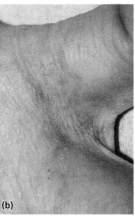

(a)   (b)

Fig. 28.4-1 **Scabies.** a: Small multiple nodules on the scrotum, which characterizes scabies. b: Erythema and papules in the interdigital area. It is accompanied by "tunnels" (burrows).

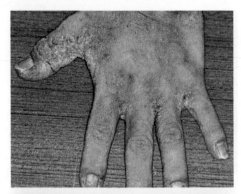

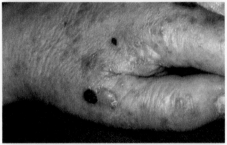

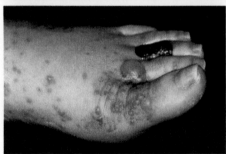

Fig. 28.4-2 Scabies on the hand and foot of an elderly person. Distinct blistering is present.

MEMO 28–4 Bedbugs, *Cimex lectularius*

An adult bedbug is about 8 mm long. Bedbugs inhabit bedding and mattresses and suck human blood. The clinical features and treatments are the same as for insect bites.

---

thickening of the nail plate, resembling tinea unguium, is observed.

When people with immunosuppression or poor hygiene are infected, the mites proliferate in large numbers and cause generalized hyperkeratosis. This condition, which is called hyperkeratotic scabies or Norwegian scabies, is highly contagious.

Pathogenesis

Scabies is an infestation in the stratum corneum. The mite is ovoid and has body dimensions of 0.4 × 0.3 mm for males and 0.2 × 0.15 mm for females, with four pairs of legs at the adult stage (Fig. 28.5). A mated female forms a mite burrow in the stratum corneum and lays 2–4 eggs daily there, dying in 4–6 weeks. Eggs incubate for 3–5 days. The mites inhabit creases in the skin or the hair follicles and grow to adult stage in 10–14 days.

Scabies infestation is caused by direct skin-to-skin contact or indirect contact through bedclothes or clothing. The incubation period is about 1 month. Scabies often occurs within a family and at hospitals and elderly care homes. It is included in sexually transmitted infections.

Diagnosis

When small, disseminated papules accompanied by intense itching are found on the trunk, mite burrows should be carefully sought in the interdigital areas. Multiple papules on the genitals, particularly on the scrotum or labia majora, should be carefully examined. To confirm the diagnosis, a specimen that includes the stratum corneum is removed from the skin by pinching with tweezers or scraping with a scalpel; direct identification of the mite body or eggs is carried out by light microscopy and using potassium hydroxide solution. The likelihood of detecting the mite or its eggs is low for a single site. It is necessary to collect specimens from multiple sites. The mite body is sometimes found on the skin directly by dermoscopy (see Chapter 3). It is helpful to inquire about symptoms of scabies among the patient's family members and sexual partners, and to conduct history taking on sexual activity.

Differential diagnosis

Insect bites, eczema, dermatitis, and urticaria are differentiated from scabies. Mite burrows and nodules on the genitals are useful for differentiation; however, differentiation is often difficult.

Treatment

Oral ivermectin is the first-line treatment. It is effective against adult mites but not eggs. Reexamination is done 1 week after administration, and if scabies is found, the ivermectin is readministered. Ivermectin may cause liver dysfunction as a side effect. Topical application of sulfur and camphor lotion, crotamiton cream, benzyl benzoate, and γ-BHC is helpful. It is important to apply the ointment to the entire body skin below the neck. Antihistamines may be used, if necessary. Ordinary infection countermeasures are sufficient for scabies. Isolation of the patient is unnecessary. In many cases, itchiness and nodules persist after the mites have been killed off. It is necessary to discontinue the administration of ivermectin.

Pediculosis

Definition and classification

An allergic reaction is induced by a louse that parasitizes human skin to suck blood, causing intense itching. The three main lice causing pediculosis are *Pediculus capitis* (head lice, 2–4 mm long, inhabiting head hair), *Pediculus humanus* (clothing or body lice, 2–4 mm long, inhabiting clothing), and *Phthirus pubis* (pubic or crab lice, 1 mm long, inhabiting pubic hair; Fig. 28.6). It is impossible to distinguish between *Pediculus capitis* and *P. humanus* by appearance.

Clinical features

A louse parasitizes a hair shaft and lays eggs on the hair. The eggs incubate for about 1 week. The lice mature in about 3 weeks and lay 3–5 eggs per day. Itching is the result of an allergic reaction caused by bloodsucking lice. Intense itching occurs 1–2 months after the first contact with lice. Eruptions do not usually occur.

Pathogenesis

Pediculus capitis infestation may become epidemic among schoolchildren during group activities at schools or daycare centers. *Phthirus pubis* infestation is caused most frequently by sexual intercourse. The eyebrows are involved in rare cases. *Pediculus humanus* infestation can become epidemic in environments with poor hygiene.

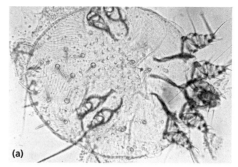

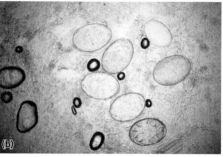

Fig. 28.5 *Sarcoptes scabiei* var. *hominis*. a: *Sarcoptes scabiei* var. *hominis* has four pairs of legs. b: Eggs of *Sarcoptes scabiei* var. *hominis*.

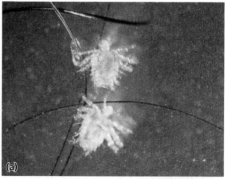

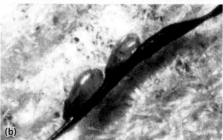

Fig. 28.6 *Phthirus pubis*. a: Adult *Phthirus pubis*. b: Eggs of *Phthirus pubis* on pubic hair.

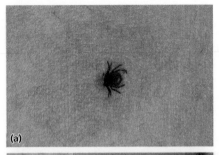

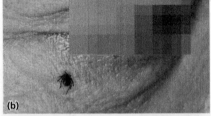

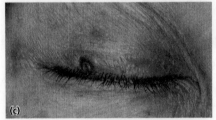

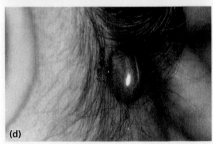

Fig. 28.7 A tick bite. a: The shoulder 2 h after the bite. The legs of the ticks are still moving. b: A tick bite on the lower eyelid. c: A tick bite on the eyelid. The patient thought it was a wart. d: A tick on the neck after sucking blood.

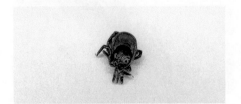

Fig. 28.8 An ixodid tick removed from human skin. They are generally 2–8 mm long.

Diagnosis and treatment

When pediculosis is suspected, itching on the head or genitals is the patient's main complaint. It is important to search for lice and eggs attached to the hair. Phenothrin shampoos and powders are helpful but are ineffective against the eggs. In recent years, species that are resistant to phenothrin have been found. Family members and sexual partners are also treated to avoid "ping-pong infestation," in which the disease repeatedly rebounds from untreated to treated people. Combs that can eliminate the eggs and lice may be used. The affected hair is shaved in some cases. *Pediculus humanus* can be eliminated by bathing, changing clothing, and washing clothes daily.

Tick bites
Clinical features

Tick bites are caused by ixodid (hard) ticks. Because ticks of the family Ixodidae tend not to be felt when they crawl on human skin, they are able to attach insidiously to the face, arms or even the trunk or genitals of humans (Fig. 28.7). The bite tends to be painless. The main symptoms are inflammation around the bite, erythema, edematous swelling, bleeding, and blistering. The mouthpart is firmly fixed in the skin while sucking blood; a tick is often found when the complaint has been a wart or skin tumor. A tick that has sucked its fill of blood falls naturally from the skin. *Borrelia* spirochetes may be transmitted by a tick bite, leading to Lyme disease (described later in this chapter).

Pathogenesis

Ixodidae are 2–8 mm long (Fig. 28.8) and tend to inhabit grasslands and woods. They burrow into the skin of humans and animals to suck blood. *Orientia tsutsugamushi* is classified with the Ixodidae.

Treatment

If a tick is forcefully pulled while sucking blood, it may tear, leaving the mouthpart in the skin. This can lead to foreign body granuloma. The whole tick, including the mouthpart, should be removed by either inserting scissors into the bite spot or excising or punching the site out with the tick attached.

Oral administration of tetracycline or penicillin antibiotics for 1–2 weeks after removal is advised as a prophylactic against Lyme disease.

Skin diseases transmitted by insects and other animals

Lyme disease, Lyme borreliosis

- This infection is caused by the spirochete bacterium *Borrelia burgdorferi sensu lato*, transmitted by ticks of the family Ixodidae.
- It occurs most frequently in the USA, Scandinavia, and central Europe, in spring and summer.
- It begins as erythema chronicum migrans (first stage) and progresses to arthritis and cerebral meningitis (second stage) and then to dysfunction of the joints and central nervous system (third stage).
- Tetracycline antibiotics are the first-line treatment.

Clinical features

Lyme disease occurs from *Borrelia burgdorferi* infection transmitted by the bite of an ixodid tick. The course follows repeated remissions and recurrences. It is divided into three stages (Table 28.1).

First stage (erythema period)

After an incubation of 1–36 days, an erythema or papule occurs at the bite in about 80% of all cases. The skin lesion centrifugally enlarges within several days, forming a characteristic ring-shaped lesion (erythema chronicum migrans) (Fig. 28.9 and Fig. 28.10). The periphery is vivid red and sometimes elevated. There is discoloration at the center. It is asymptomatic and may become as large as 40 cm in diameter. Influenza-like symptoms such as fever, headache, and general malaise are often present. These subside in several weeks.

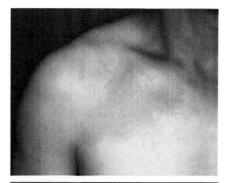
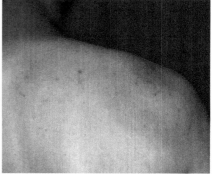
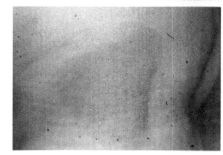

Fig. 28.9 Erythema chronicum migrans at the first stage of Lyme disease. Ring-shaped eruptions characterized by a bright red periphery appear after a tick bite.

Table 28.1 Stages and symptoms of Lyme disease.

Stage	Course of disease	Clinical findings
First stage (Erythema period)	Up to 1 month	Erythema chronicum migrans, influenza-like symptoms (fever, headache, generalized malaise, arthralgia)
Second stage (Dissemination period)	Several weeks to several months	Multiple erythema chronicum migrans, lymphocytoma cutis, migratory arthritis, neurological symptoms (incl. cerebral meningitis), heart block
Third stage (Chronic period)	Several months to several years	Acrodermatitis chronica atrophicans, chronic arthritis, chronic encephalomeningitis

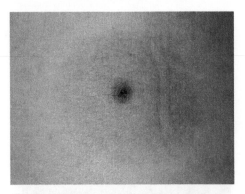

Fig. 28.10 Erythema chronicum migrans.

MEMO 28–5 *Borrelia* infection and skin diseases

Serum anti-*Borrelia* antibody and tissue PCR tests may be positive in patients with lichen sclerosus (see Chapter 18), localized scleroderma (see Chapter 12), and eosinophilic fasciitis (see Chapter 12). These disorders may accompany Lyme disease.

Second stage (dissemination period)

Within a few days to a few weeks after infection, *Borrelia burgdorferi* spread hematogenously to the whole body and cause various organ symptoms. Migratory arthritis, muscle pain, neurological symptoms (facial palsy, cerebral meningitis, and painful radiculoneuritis), and heart block may occur. Multiple small erythema chronicum migrans occur on the whole body in about 20% of all cases. When the bite is on the ear, it may cause lymphocytoma cutis (see Chapter 21).

Third stage (chronic period)

Several months to several years after onset, chronic neurological symptoms (polyneuropathy, mood disorder, and schizophrenia) and knee joint inflammation occur. Acrodermatitis chronica atrophicans occurs 1 year after onset or later. The third-stage symptoms are most commonly seen in the elderly in Europe. Asymptomatic infiltrative edematous erythema first occurs on the dorsa of the hands and feet, and the lesions gradually enlarge and atrophy. The skin becomes so thin that subcutaneous vessels can be seen.

Epidemiology

Lyme disease was first recorded in 1975 from a study of epidemic infections whose main symptoms were erythema and arthritis, done in Lyme, Connecticut (USA). Lyme disease is seen mainly in the USA, Scandinavia, and Central Europe.

Pathogenesis

Lyme disease is caused by *Borellia burgdorferi*, a spirochete bacterium that is most frequently transmitted by the ixodid tick *Ixodae ovatus*. *Borrelia burgdorferi* inhabits the midgut of the tick and tends to invade the human body when the tick burrows into the skin for 24–48 h or longer.

Laboratory findings

- **Detection of specific antibody:** for cases in which infection is thought to occur in the USA, the anti-*Borrelia burgdorferi* antibody test is done.
- **Detection of bacteria:** the bacteria are isolated from the skin lesion for culturing. *Borrelia* proteins (e.g., OspC) can be detected by Western blot, and *Borrelia* DNA can be identified by nested PCR.

Diagnosis and differential diagnosis

Diagnosis can be made by finding the tick bite and by erythema chronicum migrans. To confirm the diagnosis, antibody tests or bacterial culture are carried out.

Treatment

Doxycycline (tetracycline antibiotics) or penicillin is administered orally. Ceftriaxone is used at the second and third stages of the disease, because it is transported to the nerves in sufficient concentrations. The symptoms often improve after administration of these drugs for 3–4 weeks.

Scrub typhus, tsutsugamushi disease

- This rickettsial infection is caused by the obligate intracellular bacterium *Orientia tsutsugamushi*, which is transmitted by the *Leptotrombidium akamushi* mite.
- The three main symptomatic features are high fever, presence of the tick bite, and light pink eruptions on the trunk.
- Tetracycline antibiotics and chloramphenicol are effective treatments.

Clinical features

Five to 14 days after a bite by the *Leptotrombidium akamushi* mite, a fever of about 40°C occurs, accompanied by sudden chills and headache (Fig. 28.11). Careful observation may reveal the bite of that mite, generally on the trunk, genitals or axillary fossae. The bite presents infiltrative erythema of 1–2 cm in diameter with black crusts at the center. Two to 7 days after onset, light pink eruptions of 2–5 mm in diameter appear on the trunk and extremities, disappearing in 7–10 days. There is systemic painful swelling of the lymph nodes, conjunctival congestion, pharyngeal reddening, splenohepatomegaly, liver dysfunction, and disseminated intravascular coagulation (DIC).

Pathogenesis and epidemiology

Scrub typhus disease is a rickettsial infection caused by the obligate intracellular bacterium *Orientia tsutsugamushi* and transmitted by the *Leptotrombidium akamushi*, *pallidum*, and *scutellare* mites. When these feed on humans and the duration of blood sucking exceeds 6 h, rickettsia invades the human body and causes scrub typhus. Fewer than 1% of all *Leptotrombidium akamushi*

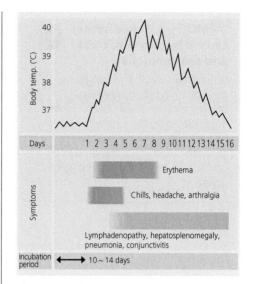

Fig. 28.11 Clinical course of scrub typhus, i.e., tsutsugamushi disease.

MEMO 28–6 Skin diseases caused by jellyfish, coral, and sea anemones

An eruption may be caused by the sting of a jellyfish, coral or sea anemone in the ocean. Some marine organisms sting humans with the nematocysts on their tentacles, or they otherwise injure human skin by contact. Systemic symptoms may be severe.

---

are thought to carry *Orientia tsutsugamushi*. Scrub typhus is not transmitted from human to human.

Diagnosis and differential diagnosis

If the bite and eruptions go unnoticed, the diagnosis will be delayed or misdiagnosed as another febrile disease, such as influenza. Diagnosis is done by identification of elevated antirickettsial IgM antibodies, elevated IgG in the pair serum test or detection of rickettsial DNA by nested PCR test of peripheral blood. Other rickettsial diseases, such as *Rickettsia japonica* infection and Rocky Mountain spotted fever, should be carefully differentiated from scrub typhus (Table 28.2).

Treatment

Chloramphenicol or tetracycline antibiotics are administered in the early stages.

Leishmaniasis
Definition

Leishmaniasis is a parasitic infection caused by protozoa of the genus *Leishmania* in the family Trypanosoma. There are several types of pathogenic *Leishmania*. *Leishmania* protozoa are transmitted to humans by bloodsucking sand flies. Infection may occur through the sharing of needles by drug-addicted people. Leishmaniasis is classified into three subtypes by *Leishmania* species. The distribution and clinical features differ for each type.

Clinical features and classification
(Old World) Cutaneous leishmaniasis

The causative protozoan of cutaneous leishmaniasis is *Leishmania tropica*, which is predominantly distributed in Africa. The hosts are dogs and rodents. A painless papule appears at the bite and progresses to an ulcer accompanied by induration and enlargement. The skin lesion heals with scarring in about 1 year.

Mucocutaneous leishmaniasis

The causative protozoan of mucocutaneous leishmaniasis is *Leishmania braziliensis*. Tumors and odorous ulcers form, mainly on the face. For decades after an infection, secondary ulcerations occur involving the skin and mucosa, and bone destruction occurs in the ears, nasal cavity, oral cavity, and pharynx.

Table 28.2 Comparisons between tsutsugamushi disease and diseases that resemble it.

	Tsutsugamushi disease	Japanese spotted fever	Rocky Mountain spotted fever
Rickettsia pathogen	*Orientia tsutsugamushi*	*Rickettsia japonica*	*Rickettsia rickettsii*
Incubation period	10–14 days	2–8 days	3–12 days
Season of common infection	Autumn, winter, spring (new type); summer (classical type)	April to October	Early summer
Erythema	Most commonly on the trunk, little subcutaneous bleeding	Extremities tend to be involved.	Most of the body, large ecchymosis
	Palms and soles are not involved.	Palms and soles are also involved.	Necrosis in the ends of fingers and toes, tip of the nose, and ears
Bite	Large (about 10 mm in diameter)	Small (about 5 mm in diameter)	Not found
Swelling in lymph nodes	Systemic	Localized	(−)
Treatment		Tetracycline, chloramphenicol	

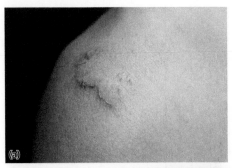

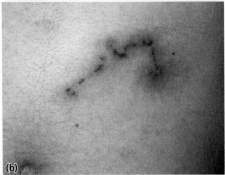

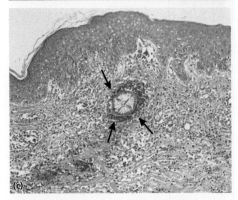

Fig. 28.12 Creeping eruption. a,b: Cutaneous gnathostomiasis caused by linear movement of a parasitic larva in human skin. c: Histopathology of creeping eruption (arrows show the parasitic larva in the skin).

Visceral leishmaniasis

This is also called kala-azar. The causative protozoan of visceral leishmaniasis is *Leishmania donovani*. The main symptoms are fever, fatigue, splenohepatomegaly, and swelling of the lymph nodes. Multiple hard papules may occur on the face 1 year after onset (post kala-azar dermal leishmaniasis).

Diagnosis and treatment

A history of sandfly bites or travel to an endemic area is important for diagnosis. The causative protozoan of leishmaniasis is detected from skin lesions, blood or bone marrow. Miltefosine and sodium stibogluconate are administered.

Diseases caused by parasitic worms

Creeping eruptions (synonym: cutaneous larva migrans)

A cutaneous parasitic larva causes a linear eruption called a "creeping eruption" when it moves in the skin (Fig. 28.12). Two frequent types of creeping eruption are described here: cutaneous larva migrans and cutaneous gnathostomiasis.

Cutaneous larva migrans

This is the most common cause of creeping eruptions worldwide. Hookworm larvae from dogs, cats, and other mammals are the most common cause of creeping eruptions, which tend to occur in tropical and subtropical areas. A few days after skin contact with contaminated sand or soil, characteristically pruritic linear or serpiginous erythema occurs. The feet, buttocks, and genitals are frequently involved.

Cutaneous gnathostomiasis

This results from the ingestion of the third-stage larvae of the *Gnathostoma spinigerum* nematode, which is transmitted by eating raw snake, freshwater fish or frog. Several weeks to several months after a contaminated animal is eaten, localized edema and induration occur. The larva continues to move, causing linear eruptions in the trunk and thighs. Common endemic areas are Southeast Asia (especially Thailand and Japan) and Latin America (mainly Mexico and Ecuador). Other species may cause creeping eruptions, such as the larva of *Spinometra mansoni* (found in amphibian and poultry meat) and nematodes of the superfamily Spiruroidea (found in soft-shelled tortoises and squid). Treatment is removal of the parasite. Oral albendazole and ivermectin are effective.

Lymphatic filariasis

The causative filarial worms of lymphatic filariasis, *Wuchereria bancrofti* and *Brugia malayi*, are carried by mosquitoes. The filarial worms are widely distributed in tropical and subtropical areas. These parasitic nematodes, which invade the human body and inhabit the lymph system, mature in several months. They cause fever, inflammation in lymph nodes and lymph vessels, and epididymitis, leading to lymphatic edema or testicular hydrocele that progresses to elephantiasis (see Chapter 11). Diethylcarbamazine and ivermectin are administered.

APPENDIX
Main genodermatoses and their causative genes and proteins

Disease	Type	Chapter to refer	OMIM number	Inheritance pattern	Causal protein/gene
Epidermolysis bullosa (EB)					
EB simplex (EBS)	Localized	Chapter 14	131800	AD	Keratin (K) 5, K14
	DowlingMeara type	Chapter 14	131760	AD	K5, K14
	Other generalized types	Chapter 14	131900	AD	K5, K14
	EBS associated with muscular dystrophy	Chapter 14	226670	AR	Plectin
	JEB associated with pyloric atresia	Chapter 14	612138	AR	Plectin
Junctional EB (JEB)	Herlitz JEB	Chapter 14	226700	AR	Laminin 332 (LAMA3, LAMB3, LAMC2)
	Non-Herlitz JEB	Chapter 14	226650	AR	Laminin 332, type VII collagen
	JEB associated with pyloric atresia	Chapter 14	226730	AR	Integrin α6 β4
Dystrophic EB (DEB)	Autosomal dominant dystrophic type	Chapter 14	131750	AD	Type VII collagen
	Recessive, severe generalized type	Chapter 14	226600	AR	Type VII collagen
	Recessive, "other, generalized" type	Chapter 14	32200	AR	Type VII collagen
Other genetic blistering diseases	Hailey–Hailey disease	Chapter 14	169600	AD	ATP2C1
	Skin fragility syndrome	Chapter 14	604536	AR	PKP1
Keratotic disorders					
Ichthyosis	Ichthyosis vulgaris	Chapter 15	146700	SD	Filaggrin
	X-linked ichthyosis	Chapter 15	308100	XR	Steroid sulfatase
	Lamellar ichthyosis	Chapter 15	242100	AR	Transglutaminase I
	Epidermolytic ichthyosis	Chapter 15	113800	AD	K1, K10
	Epidermolytic ichthyosis	Chapter 15	113800	AD	K2
	Harlequin ichthyosis	Chapter 15	242500	AR	ABCA12

Shimizu's Dermatology, Second Edition. Hiroshi Shimizu.
© 2017 John Wiley & Sons, Ltd. Published 2017 by John Wiley & Sons, Ltd.

Disease	Type	Chapter to refer	OMIM number	Inheritance pattern	Causal protein/gene
	Netherton syndrome	Chapter 15	256500	AD	SPINK5
	KID syndrome	Chapter 15	242150	AD	Connexin26
	Sjögren–Larsson syndrome	Chapter 15	270200	AR	ALDH3A2
	Dorfman–Chanarin syndrome	Chapter 15	275630	AR	ABHD5 (CGI58)
	Loricrin keratoderma	Chapter 15		AD	LOR
	Ichthyosis with confetti	Chapter 15	609165	AD	KRT10 (KRT1)
	Congenital ichthyosiform erythroderma	Chapter 15		AR	ABCA12, TGM1, ALOXE3, CYP4F22, PNPLA1, LIPN, CERS3, NIPAL4, ALOX12B, ST14
Palmoplantar keratoderma	Vörner syndrome	Chapter 15	144200	AD	K9
	Mal de Meleda	Chapter 15	248300	AR	SLURP1
	Vohwinkel syndrome (classical type)	Chapter 15	124500	AD	Connexin2
	Keratosis palmoplantaris linearis	Chapter 15	148700	AD	K1, Desmoplakin, Desmoglein I
	Pachyonychia congenita type I	Chapter 15	167200	AD	K6A, K16
	Pachyonychia congenita type II	Chapter 15	167200	AD	K6B, K17
	Papillon–Lefèvre syndrome	Chapter 15	245000	AR	Cathepsin C
	Punctate palmoplantar keratoderma type 1	Chapter 15	148600	AD	AAGAB
	Nagashima-type palmoplantar keratosis	Chapter 15	615598	AR	SERPINB7
Keratosis pilaris	Darier's disease	Chapter 15	124200	AD	SERCA2
Erythrokeratodermias	Erythrokeratoderma variabilis	Chapter 15	133200	AD	GJB3, GJB4
	Progressive symmetrical erythrokeratodermia	Chapter 15	602036	AD	Loricrin
Disorders of skin color	Oculocutaneous albinism type IA	Chapter 16	203100	AR	Tyrosinase
	Type IB	Chapter 16	606952	AR	Tyrosinase
	Type II	Chapter 16	203200	AR	P Protein
	Type III	Chapter 16	203290	AR	TYRP1
	Type IV	Chapter 16	606574	AR	MATP
	Chédiak–Higashi syndrome	Chapter 16	214500	AR	LYST
	Hermansky–Pudlak syndrome	Chapter 16	203300	AR	HPS1, AP3B1, HPS3, HPS4
	Piebaldism	Chapter 16	172800	AD	KIT

Continued

Disease	Type	Chapter to refer	OMIM number	Inheritance pattern	Causal protein/gene
	Dyschromatosis symmetrica hereditaria (Toyama)	Chapter 16	127400	AD	ADAR1
	Waardenburg–Klein syndrome type I	Chapter 16	193500	AD	PAX3
	Acropigmentatio reticularis	Chapter 16	615537	AD	ADAM10
	Dyschromatosis universalis hereditaria	Chapter 16	127500	AD	ABCB6
Neurocutaneous syndromes	Neurofibromatosis type I	Chapter 20	162200	AD	NF1
	Neurofibromatosis type II	Chapter 20	101000	AD	NF2
	Tuberous sclerosis	Chapter 20	191100	AD	TSC1, TSC2
	Peutz–Jeghers syndrome	Chapter 20	175200	AD	STK11/LKB1
	Gardner syndrome	Chapter 20	175100	AD	APC
	Cowden syndrome	Chapter 20	158350	AD	PTEN
	Incontinentia pigmenti	Chapter 20	308310	XD	NEMO
	LEOPARD syndrome	Chapter 20	151100	AD	PTPN11
	Basal cell nevus syndrome	Chapter 20	109400	AD	PTCH
	Dyskeratosis congenita (X-linked recessive)	Chapter 20	305000	XR	DKC1
	Dyskeratosis congenita (dominant)	Chapter 20	127500	AD	TERC
	Dyskeratosis congenita (recessive)	Chapter 20	224230	AR	NOLA3, NOLA2
	Hereditary hemorrhagic telangiectasia type I	Chapter 20	187300	AD	ENG
	Type II	Chapter 20	600376	AD	ACVRL
Genodermatoses associated with connective tissue	Hypermobility type	Chapter 18	130010	AD, AR	Type III collagen, Tenascin-X
	Vascular type	Chapter 18	130050	AD	Type III collagen
	Kyphoscoliosis type	Chapter 18	225400	AR	Lysine hydroxylase
	Arthrochalasia type	Chapter 18	130060	AD	Type I collagen
	Dermatosparaxis type	Chapter 18	225410	AR	ADAMTS2
	Marfan syndrome	Chapter 18	154700	AD	Fibrillin-1
	Pseudoxanthoma elasticum	Chapter 18	264800	AR	ABCC6
	Congenital generalized lipodystrophy type 1	Chapter 18	608594	AR	AGPAT2
Metabolic disorders	Acrodermatitis enteropathica	Chapter 17	201100	AR	SLC39A4
	Menkes' kinky hair disease	Chapter 17	309400	XR	ATP7A
	Congenital erythropoietic porphyria	Chapter 17	263700	AR	UROS

Disease	Type	Chapter to refer	OMIM number	Inheritance pattern	Causal protein/ gene
	Erythropoietic protoporphyria	Chapter 17	177000	AD	FECH
	Acute intermittent porphyria	Chapter 17	176000	AD	HMBS
	Variegate porphyria	Chapter 17	176200	AD	PPOX
	Porphyria cutanea tarda	Chapter 17	176100	AD	UROD
	Fabry's disease	Chapter 17	301500	XR	α-galactosidase A
	Kanzaki's disease	Chapter 17	104170	AR	NAGA
	Lipoid proteinosis	Chapter 17	247100	AR	ECM1
	Familial primary localized cutaneous amyloidosis	Chapter 17	105250	AD	OSMR
Other	Werner syndrome	Chapter 18	277700	AR	WRN (RECQL2)
	Bloom syndrome	Chapter 18	210900	AR	BLM (RECQL3)
	Rothmund–Thomson syndrome	Chapter 18	268400	AR	RTS (RECQL4)
	Progeria	Chapter 18	176670	AR	LMNA
	Xeroderma pigmentosum group A	Chapter 13	278700	AR	XPA
	Group B	Chapter 13	133510	AR	XPB/ERCC3
	Group C	Chapter 13	278720	AR	XPC
	Group D	Chapter 13	278730	AR	XPD/ERCC2
	Group E	Chapter 13	278740	AR	DDB2
	Group F	Chapter 13	278760	AR	ERCC4
	Group G	Chapter 13	278780	AR	ERCC5
	Variant	Chapter 13	278750	AR	POLH
	Cockayne syndrome type A	Chapter 18	216400	AR	CSA
	Type B	Chapter 18	133540	AR	CSB
	Ataxia telangiectasia	Chapter 11	208900	AR	ATM
	Wiskott–Aldrich syndrome	Chapter 7	301000	XR	WAS
	Hyper immunoglobulin E syndrome	Chapter 7	147060	AD	STAT3
	(Hereditary) angioedema	Chapter 8	106100	AD	C1NH
	Familial hidradenitis suppurativa	Chapter 8	142690	AD	NCSTN, PSEN1, PSENEN
	Acral peeling skin syndrome	Chapter 8	609796	AR	TGM5
	Autosomal recessive hypotrichosis/wooly hair	Chapter 8	604379, 278150	AR	LIPH, P2RY5
	Olmsted syndrome	Chapter 8	614594	AD	TRPV3
	SAM syndrome	Chapter 8		AR	DSG1

AD, autosomal dominant, AR, autosomal recessive; SD, autosomal semi-dominant; XD: X-linked dominant, XR: X-linked recessive.

Index

Shimizu's Dermatology, Second Edition. Hiroshi Shimizu.
© 2017 John Wiley & Sons, Ltd. Published 2017 by John Wiley & Sons, Ltd.

Printed and bound by CPI Group (UK) Ltd, Croydon, CR0 4YY

16/04/2025

14658511-0001